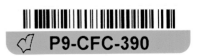

OBESITY

Mechanisms and Clinical Management

OBESITY

Mechanisms and Clinical Management

Editor

Robert H. Eckel, M.D.

Professor of Medicine
Division of Endocrinology, Metabolism and Diabetes
Division of Cardiology
Charles A. Boettcher II Endowed Chair in Atherosclerosis
Professor of Physiology and Biophysics
Program Director, Adult General Clinical Research Center
University of Colorado Health Sciences Center and University
  of Colorado Hospital
Denver, Colorado

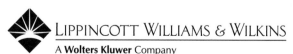
LIPPINCOTT WILLIAMS & WILKINS
A **Wolters Kluwer** Company
Philadelphia • Baltimore • New York • London
Buenos Aires • Hong Kong • Sydney • Tokyo

Acquisitions Editor: Brian Brown
Developmental Editor: Joanne Bersin
Production Editor: Christiana Sahl
Manufacturing Manager: Colin Warnock
Cover Designer: David Levy
Compositor: Lippincott Williams & Wilkins Desktop Division
Printer: Maple Press

© **2003 by LIPPINCOTT WILLIAMS & WILKINS**
530 Walnut Street
Philadelphia, PA 19106 USA
LWW.com

Printed in the USA

Library of Congress Cataloging-in-Publication Data

Eckel, Robert H.
    Obesity : mechanisms and clinical management / Robert H. Eckel.
      p. cm.
    Includes bibliographical references and index.
    ISBN 0-7817-2844-4
    1. Obesity. I. Title.

  RC628 .E355 2003
  616.3'98—dc21

                                  200234136

10 9 8 7 6 5 4 3 2 1

To my wonderful wives,
the late Sharon Cress Eckel and Margaret Scarborough Eckel

Their support and encouragement have meant so much to me
throughout my years in the science of medicine.

Contents

Contributing Authors   *ix*

Preface   *xiii*

Acknowledgments   *xv*

I.   Etiology, Pathophysiology, and Assessment

1. Obesity: A Disease or a Physiologic Adaptation for Survival?   3
    Robert H. Eckel

2. Genetic Influences on Obesity   31
    *David B. Allison, Angelo Pietrobelli, Myles S. Faith, Kevin R. Fontaine,
    Eva Gropp, and José R. Fernández*

3. Environmental Influences on Obesity   75
    James O. Hill and William T. Donahoo

4. Pediatric Obesity   91
    William H. Dietz

5. Human Body Composition   103
    *Daniel J. Hoffman, Rebecca K. Huber-Miller, David B. Allison,
    ZiMian Wang, Wei Shen, and Steven B. Heymsfield*

6. Neuroendocrine Control of Energy Balance   128
    Nicholas A. Tritos and Eleftheria Maratos-Flier

7. Endocrine Control of Fuel Partitioning   147
    Samyah Shadid and Michael D. Jensen

II.   Comorbidities

8. Heart Disease   181
    Paul Poirier and Martin A. Alpert

9. Sleep-Disordered Breathing   202
    Tracey D. Robinson and Ronald R. Grunstein

10. Obesity and Type II Diabetes Mellitus   229
    Robert R. Henry and Sunder Mudaliar

11. Obesity, Hypertension, and Renal Disease   273
    *John E. Hall, Daniel W. Jones, Jeffrey Henegar, Terry M. Dwyer,
    and Jay J. Kuo*

12. Hepatobiliary Complications of Obesity   301
Gregory T. Everson and Marcelo Kugelmas

13. Cancer   327
David Heber

14. Endocrine Disorders and Obesity   345
Margaret E. Wierman

15. Psychosocial Complications of Obesity and Dieting   358
Suzanne Phelan and Thomas A. Wadden

16. Dyslipidemia of the Metabolic Syndrome   378
John D. Brunzell

17. Orthopedic Complications   399
David T. Felson and Susan L. Edmond

III. Therapeutics

18. Behavioral Treatment of Obesity: Strategies to Improve Outcome
and Predictors of Success   415
Rena R. Wing and Suzanne Phelan

19. Nutrition and Obesity   436
Adam Drewnowski and Victoria A. Warren-Mears

20. Treatment of Obesity with Drugs in the New Millennium   449
George A. Bray

21. Exercise   476
William J. Wilkinson and Steven N. Blair

22. Surgical Treatment of Obesity   503
Rifat Latifi and Harvey J. Sugerman

23. The Economic Impact of Overweight, Obesity, and Weight Loss   523
Anne M. Wolf, JoAnn E. Manson, and Graham A. Colditz

24. Treatment of Childhood Obesity   550
Sarah E. Barlow

Appendix A.   Body Mass Index   567

Subject Index   569

Contributing Authors

David B. Allison, Ph.D. *Professor and Head of Statistical Genetics, Department of Biostatistics, University of Alabama at Birmingham, Birmingham, Alabama*

Martin A. Alpert, M.D. *Clinical Professor, Department of Internal Medicine, University of Missouri-Columbia School of Medicine, Columbia; Chairman of the Department of Medicine, Department of Internal Medicine, St. John's Mercy Medical Center, St. Louis, Missouri*

Sarah E. Barlow, M.D., M.P.H. *Assistant Professor, Department of Pediatrics, St. Louis University School of Medicine; Division of Gastroenterology and Hepatology, Department of Pediatrics, Cardinal Glennon Children's Hospital, St. Louis, Missouri*

Steven N. Blair, P.E.D. *Director of Research, The Cooper Institute, Dallas, Texas*

George A. Bray, M.D. *Boyd Professor, Department of Medicine, Pennington Biomedical Research Center, Louisiana State University, Baton Rouge, Louisiana*

John D. Brunzell, M.D. *Professor, Department of Medicine, University of Washington School of Medicine; Program Director, General Clinical Research Center, University of Washington Medical Center, Seattle, Washington*

Graham A. Colditz, M.D., D.P.H. *Professor of Epidemiology, Harvard School of Public Health; Head, Chronic Disease Epidemiology Group, Channing Laboratory; Department of Medicine, Harvard Medical School and Brigham and Women's Hospital, Boston, Massachusetts*

William H. Dietz, M.D., Ph.D. *Director, Division of Nutrition and Physical Activity, Centers for Disease Control and Prevention, Atlanta, Georgia*

William T. Donahoo, M.D. *Assistant Professor, Department of Medicine, University of Colorado Health Sciences Center, Denver, Colorado*

Adam Drewnowski, Ph.D. *Professor, Departments of Epidemiology and Medicine; Director, Center for Public Health Nutrition, University of Washington, Seattle, Washington*

Terry M. Dwyer, M.D., Ph.D. *Professor, Departments of Physiology and Biophysics, University of Mississippi Medical Center, Jackson, Mississippi*

Robert H. Eckel, M.D. *Professor of Medicine, Division of Endocrinology, Metabolism and Diabetes, Division of Cardiology; Charles A. Boettcher II Endowed Chair in Atherosclerosis; Professor of Physiology and Biophysics; Program Director, Adult General Clinical Research Center; University of Colorado Health Sciences Center and University of Colorado Hospital, Denver, Colorado*

Susan L. Edmond, D.Sc. *Associate Professor, Department of Developmental and Rehabilitative Services, University of Medicine and Dentistry New Jersey, Newark, New Jersey*

Gregory T. Everson, M.D., F.A.C.E.P. *Professor of Medicine, Department of Hepatology, University of Colorado Health Sciences Center; Director of Hepatology, University of Colorado Hospital, Denver, Colorado*

Myles S. Faith, M.D. *Assistant Professor, Department of Psychiatry, Weight and Eating Disorders Program, University of Pennsylvania, Philadelphia, Pennsylvania*

David T. Felson, M.D., M.P.H. *Professor of Medicine and Public Health, Clinical Epidemiology Research and Training Unit, Boston University School of Medicine, Boston, Massachusetts*

José R. Fernández, M.D. *Assistant Professor, Department of Nutrition Sciences, University of Alabama at Birmingham, Birmingham, Alabama*

Kevin R. Fontaine, M.D. *Assistant Professor, Department of Rheumatology, Johns Hopkins University, Baltimore, Maryland*

Eva Gropp, M.D. *Obesity Research Center, St. Luke's-Roosevelt Hospital; Institute of Human Nutrition, Columbia University College of Physicians & Surgeons, New York, New York*

Ronald R. Grunstein, B.S., Ph.D., M.D., F.R.A.C.P. *Associate Professor, Department of Medicine, University of Sydney; Head, Centre for Respiratory Failure and Sleep Disorders, Royal Prince Alfred Hospital, Sydney, Australia*

John E. Hall, Ph.D. *Guyton Professor and Chair, Department of Physiology and Biophysics; Director, Center for Excellence in Cardiovascular-Renal Research, University of Mississippi Medical Center, Jackson, Mississippi*

David Heber, M.D., Ph.D., F.A.C.P., F.A.C.N. *Professor, Department of Medicine; Director, Center for Human Nutrition, David Geffen School of Medicine at the University of California, Los Angeles, Los Angeles, California*

Jeffrey Henegar, Ph.D. *Assistant Professor, Department of Pathology; Director of Electron Microscopy, Department of Pathology, University of Mississippi Medical Center, Jackson, Mississippi*

Robert R. Henry, M.D. *Professor in Residence, Department of Medicine, University of California at San Diego; Chief of Diabetes, Endocrinology, and Metabolism, Department of Medicine, VA San Diego Healthcare System, San Diego, California*

Steven B. Heymsfield, M.D. *Professor, Department of Medicine, Obesity Research Center, Columbia University; Attending Physician, St. Luke's-Roosevelt Hospital, New York, New York*

James O. Hill, Ph.D. *Professor, Department of Pediatrics, University of Colorado Health Sciences Center, Denver, Colorado*

Daniel J. Hoffman, M.D. *Assistant Professor, Department of Nutritional Science, Rutgers, The State University of New Jersey, New Brunswick, New Jersey*

Rebecca K. Huber-Miller, M.S., R.D. *Doctoral student, Department of Nutrition, Columbia University Institute of Human Nutrition, New York, New York*

Michael D. Jensen, M.D. *Consultant, Department of Internal Medicine, Division of Endocrinology, Mayo Clinic, Rochester, Minnesota*

Daniel W. Jones, M.D. *Executive Associate Dean; Herbert G. Langford Professor of Medicine; Associate Vice Chancellor for Health Affairs, University of Mississippi Medical Center, Jackson, Mississippi*

Marcelo Kugelmas, M.D. *Assistant Professor, Department of Medicine, University of Colorado Health Sciences Center, Denver, Colorado*

Jay J. Kuo, Ph.D. *Instructor, Department of Physiology and Biophysics, University of Mississippi Medical Center, Jackson, Mississippi*

Rifat Latifi, M.D. *Department of Surgery, University of Arizona, Tucson, Arizona*

Eleftheria Maratos-Flier, M.D. *Associate Professor, Department of Medicine, Harvard Medical School; Head, Section on Obesity, Research Division, Joslin Diabetes Center, Boston, Massachusetts*

JoAnn E. Manson, M.D., D.P.H. *Professor of Medicine, Harvard Medical School; Chief, Division of Preventive Medicine, Brigham and Women's Hospital, Boston, Massachusetts*

Sunder Mudaliar, M.D., M.R.C.P., F.A.C.E. *Assistant Clinical Professor, Division of Endocrinology, Department of Medicine, University of California at San Diego; Staff Physician, Diabetes Metabolism Section, VA San Diego Healthcare System, San Diego, California*

Suzanne Phelan, Ph.D. *Postdoctoral Fellow, Department of Psychiatry, Brown Medical School, Providence, Rhode Island*

Angelo Pietrobelli, M.D. *Staff Physician, Pediatric Clinic, Verona University Medical School; Pediatric Unit, Policlinic G.B. Rossi, Verona, Italy*

Paul Poirier, M.D., F.R.C.P.C., F.A.C.C. *Cardiac Rehabilitation Program Director, Department of Cardiology, Quebec Heart and Lung Institute, Sainte-Foy, Quebec, Canada*

Tracey D. Robinson, M.B.B.S., F.R.A.C.P. *Postgraduate student, Department of Medicine, University of Sydney; Staff Specialist, Department of Respiratory Medicine, Westmead Hospital, Sydney, Australia*

Samyah Shadid, M.D. *Research Fellow, Endocrine Research Unit, Mayo Clinic, Rochester, Minnesota*

Wei Shen, M.D. *Research Scientist, Columbia University Institute of Human Nutrition; Research Scientist, Obesity Research Center, St. Luke's-Roosevelt Hospital, Columbia University College of Physicians and Surgeons, New York, New York*

Harvey J. Sugerman, M.S., M.D. *David M. Hume Professor, Department of Surgery, Virginia Commonwealth University; Chief, Department of General Medicine, Division of Trauma Surgery, Medical College of Virginia Hospitals, Richmond, Virginia*

Nicholas A. Tritos, M.D., D.Sc. *Instructor in Medicine, Department of Medicine, Harvard Medical School; Joslin Diabetes Center; Staff Physician, Department of Medicine, Beth Israel Deaconess Medical Center, Boston, Massachusetts*

Thomas A. Wadden, Ph.D. *Professor of Psychology, Department of Psychiatry, University of Pennsylvania School of Medicine, Philadelphia, Pennsylvania*

ZiMian Wang, Ph.D.   *Associate Research Scientist, Institute of Human Nutrition, Columbia University; Research Associate, Obesity Research Center, St. Luke's-Roosevelt Hospital, New York, New York*

Victoria A. Warren-Mears, Ph.D., R.D.   *Assistant Professor and Clinical Coordinator, Dietetic Internship Program, Oregon Health & Science University, Portland, Oregon*

Margaret E. Wierman, M.D.   *Professor, Department of Medicine, Physiology and Biophysics, University of Colorado; Chief, Department of Medicine, Division of Endocrinology, Veterans Affairs Medical Center, Denver, Colorado*

William J. Wilkinson, M.D., M.S.   *Director, Center for Weight Management Research, Division of Integrated Health Research, The Cooper Institute, Dallas, Texas*

Rena R. Wing, Ph.D.   *Professor, Department of Psychiatry and Human Behavior, Brown Medical School; Director, Weight Control and Diabetes Research Center, The Miriam Hospital, Providence, Rhode Island*

Anne M. Wolf, M.S., R.D.   *Instructor of Research, Department of Health Evaluation Sciences, University of Virginia School of Medicine, Charlottesville, Virginia*

Preface

We live in an age in which overweight (body mass index [BMI] of 25.0 to 29.9 kilograms per meter [kg/m^2]) and obesity (BMI greater than 30.0 kg/m^2) have become epidemic, with the increase in the prevalence of obesity expected to reach nearly 50% by the year 2025 for developed countries. These are not the result of a virus or another contagion but rather a manifestation of the ancient principle of "survival of the fittest" that is now misplaced in time. Overweight and obesity are no longer advantages for a world that, despite socioeconomic deprivation, has more than sufficient food for most, and little need to expend energy to obtain it. Furthermore, the human lifespan is no longer only a few decades, in which the devastating effects of excess body fat are less prominent; instead, it often reaches eight to nine decades, so that the comorbid effects of excess adipose tissue accumulate, often becoming life-threatening.

Increasingly, physicians and related health care professionals of every subspecialty are facing the sequelae of the overweight and obesity epidemic in their clinics and hospitals. Yet, few medical problems are as frustrating to treat. The failure of physicians and health care specialists to deal systematically and effectively with this increasing problem of the late twentieth and early twenty-first centuries has provided an incentive for patients to turn to the many programs advertised with alluring distortions that claim to have "quick and lasting cures for this terrible *cosmetic* problem" of our time. The allegation that the media is filled with mixed messages about the treatment of overweight and obesity is a gross understatement; in fact, many appealing claims are actually fraudulent, lacking even a hint of scientific support, and the public becomes more rather than less independent in their therapeutic approaches. Now is the time for the medical profession to step forward and to become informed about weight regulation, the mechanisms of development of overweight and obesity, and the many associated comorbidities that impact almost every subspecialty of medicine. Only with this knowledge can a comprehensive approach to therapeutics be effectively implemented.

A text for clinicians on the mechanisms for the development of overweight and obesity and the related clinical management is more than timely. The purpose of this text is to provide the interested reader with a strong scientific background on why overweight and obesity have become epidemic in adults and children; this includes a discussion of the importance of the impacts of both genetics and the environment. The community studying obesity has focused on BMI as its working term for defining obesity, and the validity of this classification system is extensively addressed. Of necessity, chapters are devoted to both sides of the energy balance equation to determine the relative roles of energy intake and energy expenditure in the etiology of overweight and obesity. Once the stage is set, the many comorbidities of excess body fat are covered in detail, with particular emphasis on clinical assessment and related therapeutics.

The comorbidities of overweight and obesity receive special attention because aggressive treatment in these areas may help one to prevent the potentially fatal complications of excess adipose tissue. As overweight and obesity increase, so does the incidence of diabetes and hypertension, in particular. Coronary heart disease, stroke, and congestive heart failure are fully expected to follow this pattern as well. Contributing to these relationships are the prevalent lipid and lipoprotein abnormalities and the obstructive sleep apnea that are seen in the overweight and obese. Effective therapies for all of these co-morbidities are currently available, and their use should be strongly encouraged, even in the absence of effective and sustained weight reduction. Clinicians who assess large numbers of overweight and obese patients in their practices list the area of orthopedics as the one with the most common and most burdensome complaints. The risk for certain malignancies, hepatocellular and biliary diseases, endocrine abnormalities and psychosocial disorders in overweight and obese patients is also addressed.

Finally, of equal importance is the series of sound, evidence-based discussions of therapy. These include approaches to the lifestyle (e.g., behavior, nutrition, physical activity), pharmacotherapeutic, and surgical forms of treatment. Of course, rarely does any of these stand alone, so the most efficacious therapy depends on the establishment of effective communication among therapists who are working together to accomplish the treatment goals. Realistically, weight reduction of only 10% may be enough to have a substantial benefit on the patient's health. Also important to note are the high rates of recidivism for reduced-overweight or reduced-obese patients. The expectation of weight regain is essential in the effective long-term management of the overweight and obese conditions. The book concludes with a discussion of the tremendous economic burden that the overweight and obesity epidemic has created. This burden will only escalate in the coming years.

We hope that *Obesity: Mechanisms and Clinical Management* provides clinicians with the necessary firm foundation of the etiology of overweight and obesity, including the principles of body weight regulation. The absence of this knowledge makes the implementation of therapeutic strategies even more difficult. We also expect that this knowledge will lead to an improved clinical approach to, and more aggressive treatment of, the comorbidities of overweight and obesity. Finally, although the successful treatment of obesity can be accomplished in many patients, the text supports the adage that "an ounce of prevention is worth a pound of cure."

Robert H. Eckel

Acknowledgments

I acknowledge my two former mentors, Edwin L. Bierman, M.D., and John D. Brunzell, M.D., as well as my M.D. and Ph.D. postdoctoral fellows with whom I have worked. I would also like to thank the National Institute of Diabetes, Digestive and Kidney Diseases and the National Center for Research Resources (General Clinical Research Center) for their ongoing support of my research in obesity.

PART I

Etiology, Pathophysiology, and Assessment

1

Obesity: A Disease or a Physiologic Adaptation for Survival?

Robert H. Eckel

A disease is a condition of a living plant, animal, or human that impairs normal functioning and implies a condition of ill health. If obesity is a disease—a position that is supported by many, including a number of organizations (1), consensus conferences (2), and experts in the field (3)—it has now reached epidemic proportions. Using the definition of overweight as 25.0 to 29.9 kilograms per meter squared (kg/m^2) and obesity as equal to or more than 30.0 kg/m^2 in adults (4,5), Flegal and Troiano (6) estimate that 26% of the population of the United States is obese and that 61% is overweight. Moreover, the problem of relative adiposity is increasing throughout the world (4). According to Kopelman (4), if the current trend in body mass index (BMI) continues, 40% of the United States population will be labeled obese by 2025.

Adolescents in the 85th and 95th percentiles have been represented as "at risk" and "overweight," respectively (7). However, because the 85th percentile in both children and adolescents approximates a BMI of 25 kg/m^2 and the 95th percentile approximates a BMI of 30 kg/m^2, the most recent recommendation is to use a similar range of BMIs in children as in adults (8). For both adults and children, BMIs of 25 and 30 kg/m^2 are below the mean for many segments of the population, including Hispanics, Native Americans, and African Americans (9,10). If this "disease" were virally induced as was suggested by Dhurandhar et al. (11), by now Congress would have funded research for developing antiviral drugs, analogous to the funds which it provided for human immunodeficiency virus and the related acquired immune deficiency syndrome in the last decade. However, despite the increasing attention to obesity as a "disease" of increasing prevalence, the solutions seem even further away.

OBESITY AS A DISEASE?

Definition of the Disease

Adipose tissue is the body's largest energy reservoir. The triglyceride storage pool in the average normal-weight man and woman with 15% and 25% adipose tissue, respectively, amounts to 10 and 15 kg, respectively. In the average normal-weight man and woman, total body fat stores amount to approximately 88,000 and 132,000 kcal (about 370 and 555 MJ), respectively. This is about three to six times the amount stored as protein (roughly 24,000 kcal or 100 MJ). These fuel depots are used to meet the needs of tissues during exercise, stress, and periods of food deprivation lasting from 60 to 90 days (12,13).

To classify a condition as a disease, typically a pathologic basis is needed. However, unlike pulmonary thromboembolism, rheumatoid arthritis, or hepatitis C, conditions for which criteria for diagnosis are reasonably well established, the definition of obesity is limited to the BMI and to increases in adipocyte cell size (hypertrophy) and/or cell number (hyperplasia) (3). If an increase in adipocyte volume alone would be considered diagnostic, corresponding criteria have not yet been established. Moreover, even if criteria with an acceptable level of sensitivity were established, increases in adipocyte volume might be present in some regions of adipose tissue even though the individual's BMI is less than 25 kg/m^2. The use of adipocyte number for diagnostic assessment is even more difficult because hyperplasia is typically preceded by hypertrophy (14), a generalization that is open to question. Examples to the contrary from transgenic rodents include mice with adipose tissue–specific overexpression of the insulin-mediated glucose transporter GLUT-4 (15) or the α_2-adrenergic receptor (16). In summary, the pathologic criteria that are needed to label obesity as a disease have not yet been established.

Single Gene Defects

Substantial evidence indicates that obesity rarely results from single gene mutations; it is instead polygenic. However, in this genetic age, an increasing number of single gene defects responsible for the obese phenotype have been identified in humans. As Chapter 2 outlines in more detail, most of the known single gene defects are associated with other phenotypes including mental retardation, endocrine (reproductive) disorders, and/or malformations (see Table 2.4 in Chapter 2). Today, the most common single gene mutation associated with obesity in the absence of mental retardation is that of the melanocortin-4 receptor (MC4R) (17). A number of other mutations have also been identified, and the related hyperphagic obesity can present with either dominant or recessive patterns of inheritance (18). The consequences of mutations in MC4R do not appear to be accompanied by other pathophysiologic defects. Because of the high prevalence of this genetic modification (i.e., represents about 4% of patients with severe obesity [17]) and in the absence of accompanying morphologic and/or functional abnormalities, this mutation could perhaps be viewed as "beneficial" for survival rather than as harmful. Of course, this advantage is appreciated only in environments in which adequate sources of energy intake are not available.

Comorbidities as Diseases

When lifespan continues into the eighth and ninth decade, the consequences of excess body fat are anything but advantageous. As other chapters in this text relate, obesity is either directly or indirectly associated with an increased incidence and prevalence of heart disease and stroke (Chapter 8), obstructive sleep apnea (Chapter 9), type II diabetes mellitus (Chapter 10), dyslipidemia (Chapter 16), hypertension (Chapter 11), hepatobiliary disease (Chapter 12), cancer (Chapter 13), endocrine disorders (Chapter 14), psychosocial disturbances (Chapter 15), and orthopedic complications (Chapter 17). Clearly, these outcomes are measurable not only clinically but also pathologically in both gross and microscopic examinations.

Using relative hazards associated with elevated BMI in six United States studies (Alameda Community Health Study, Framingham Heart Study, Tecumseh Community Health Study, American Cancer Society Cancer Protection Study 1, National Health and Nutrition Survey 1 Epidemiological Follow-Up Study 1, and Nurses Health Study), the national distribution of adult BMI, and the estimates of population size and total deaths from the same period, Allison et al. (19) calculated that the annual number of deaths attributable to obesity was 280,000. When hazard ratios were calculated from data for nonsmokers or never-smokers only, this figure was increased by 16% and by 34% in

TABLE 1.1. *Estimates of obesity-attributable mortality in United States adults*

Rank	Cause of death	Number	Role of obesity
1	Diseases of the heart	725,192	+++
2	Malignant neoplasms	549,838	++
3	Cerebrovascular diseases	167,366	++
4	Chronic lower respiratory diseases	124,181	+
5	Accidents	97,860	+
6	Diabetes mellitus	68,399	+++
7	Influenza and pneumonia	63,730	+
8	Alzheimer disease	44,536	0
9	Nephritis, nephrotic syndrome, and nephrosis	35,525	+
10	Septicemia	30,680	+
11	Intentional self-harm (suicide)	29,199	+
12	Chronic liver disease and cirrhosis	26,259	+
13	Essential (primary) hypertension and hypertensive renal disease	16,968	++
14	Assault (homocide)	16,889	0
15	Aortic aneurysm and dissection	15,807	++
16	Other	378,970	+
	TOTAL	**2,391,399**	

The approximate role of obesity, from 0 to ++++, in the pathophysiology for each of the causes of death is simply an estimate.

Data are for the 15 most common causes of death + "Other" in 1999 and the estimated contribution of obesity based on the prevalence of obesity in each of the categories of disease.

Data from Hoyert DL, Arias E, Smith BL, et al. Deaths: final data for 1999. *National Vital Statistics Reports* 2001;49:1–113, with permission.

"ostensibly healthy weight-stable nonsmokers or never smokers." Although these deaths were variably attributable to underlying diseases, such as coronary heart disease, stroke, and diabetes in Framingham (20), obesity was rarely listed as the cause of death; it was more likely to be noted as the associated comorbidity.

When the prevalence of obesity-related comorbidities is examined, age-based and gender-based distributions must be considered. In addition, the criteria used to stipulate the specific comorbidity must be specified. Nevertheless, when estimates of the contributory role of obesity are made for the causes of death in 1999 (Table 1.1), the importance of obesity in contributing to mortality through a number of different pathophysiologic mechanisms may be identified. Recently, criteria for the metabolic syndrome were developed by the National Cholesterol Education Program Adult Treatment Panel III (21). For diagnosis, three or more of the following five components must be present: (a) a waist circumference greater than 102 cm for men and more than 88 cm for women; (b) a fasting triglyceride level higher than 150 mg per dL; (c) a high-density lipoprotein (HDL) cholesterol level less than 40 mg per dL for men and less than 50 mg per dL for women; (d) blood pressure higher than 130/85; and (e) a fasting serum glucose concentration greater than 110 mg per dL. Based on these criteria, the age-adjusted prevalence of the metabolic syndrome in adults 20 years or older is 23.7% (22). Based on data from the 2000 census, 47 million United States citizens are thus afflicted. All of the criteria for the metabolic syndrome point to obesity as an underlying disorder.

Basis for the Definition of Obesity as a Disease

The National Institutes of Health held a Consensus Development Conference on the Health Implications of Obesity in 1985. After presentations by 19 experts in relevant areas of obesity science, a panel of 15 impartial senior-level professionals came to the conclusion that obesity is a disease (2). Although the panelists agreed that the amount of body fat is a continuum within populations, the conclusion that was reached was that an increase in body weight of 20% or more above the desirable body weight is associated with a plethora of comorbidities in addition to excess mortality and that it thus constitutes a health hazard. The panel did note that the precise determination of body fat requires technically sophisticated methodologies that are not readily available to most clinicians and that BMI as an assessment of body fat has limitations. Despite this limitation, because significant health risks (e.g., diabetes, hypertension, heart disease, and others) can occur in some individuals at lower percentages of increased body fat, clinical concern about excess adiposity was extended to this population. (Even though this manuscript is frequently cited in support of approaching obesity as a disease, the term disease is never mentioned in the manuscript.)

The value of this decision by a group of "unbiased" professionals centers in the current thrust of the "obesity as a disease" argument regarding health care reimbursement for a disorder that was estimated in 1998 to amount to 5.5% to 7.8% of total health care expenditures (23). If obesity were considered a disease, early therapeutic and preventive strategies to diminish this epidemic would be implemented and reimbursed. Presently, reimbursement almost always relates to the comorbidities of obesity, such as hypertension, obstructive sleep apnea, and dyslipidemia. Recently, the metabolic syndrome has been given an *International Classification of Diseases* code (in the ninth revision), providing yet another disease category under which reimbursements for some obese patients may be filed. Moreover, even though the Internal Revenue Service now considers the expenses for obesity evaluation and treatment to be medically related tax deductions (24), the high level of expenditures that is necessary for health claims to receive deductions is unlikely to provide the financial incentive that is necessary for most obese individuals to seek additional attention.

In the United States, the importance of obesity as a health problem was highlighted in *Healthy People 2010,* a comprehensive nationwide health-promotion and disease-prevention program orchestrated by the United States Department of Health and Human Services (25). In late 2001, the Surgeon General's call to action notably highlights the need to prevent an increase in overweight individuals and obesity in late 2001 (26). Clearly, the lobbying effort of both professional organizations and lay groups is directed towards future reimbursement for obesity as a disease. The bigger concern is whether the health care system can absorb these costs.

Presently the health care budget in the United States is about $190 billion (27). Using these figures and an average estimate that 6.7% of this budget is obesity related, obesity-related expenses could result in a cost of $12.7 billion. Of course, some of these expenses are presently covered under obesity-related comorbidities, but many are not. These would then be added to the economic burden indicated by the following figures. Each year, about $33 billion is spent in the United States on weight-loss programs, including dietary, exercise, and behavior modifications (28). In fact, a recent bill to prevent obesity that was proposed by Senators Frist, Bingaman, and Dodd ("Improved nutrition and physical activity act" or "Impact," available in May 2002) estimated the annual cost of obesity in the United States as $117 billion. Although the source for this amount is not stated in the bill, incorporating even a small proportion of such costs into health care reimbursement is unthinkable.

If obesity is not a disease but rather a metabolic adaptation for survival in settings of food deprivation, would this fact affect the view of health care economists? The answer may be yes; however, if a preventive strategy is accompanied by sufficient evidenced-based documentation that obesity prevention or treatment modifies hard outcomes (e.g., death, myocardial infarction, stroke, and type II diabetes), the result may be not only clinically effective but also cost saving. Ultimately, this may translate into the same type of "quality-adjusted life-year saved" assessments that have been applied in other areas of medicine. Recent examples include $10,983 per life-year saved for repeated colonoscopy for colorectal carcinoma screening beginning at 50 years of age (29) and $22,256 per life-year saved for hepatitis A vaccines administered to patients with chronic hepatitis C at 30 years of age (30). To reach an "acceptable" median level of cost of $42,000 per life-year saved (31) for obesity using the assumption of the present 26% prevalence of obesity, the cost would be about $14,000 for each life-year saved if only 10% of the obese population were benefitted. The debate about whether obesity is a disease may then be irrelevant when this approach to obesity outcome–related expenditures is used.

OBESITY AS A SURVIVAL ADVANTAGE

Despite the magnitude of the health problem of obesity and its comorbidities today, substantial evidence from history illustrates that the consequences of obesity are far from unfavorable. Adipose tissue remains the predominant storage depot of energy as triacylglycerol. As was noted above, if typical fat depots of 10 and 15 kg for the average adult man and woman, respectively, are assumed, the energy stored therein is sufficient for 60 to 90 days of starvation at a level of energy expenditure of 6 MJ a day (12,13). Energy is also available from protein, but the amount of stored protein can provide only approximately one-half of the stored quantity of protein before life-threatening loss of lean tissue ensues (32). However, expanded adipose tissue mass preserves protein mass (33) (Fig. 1.1).

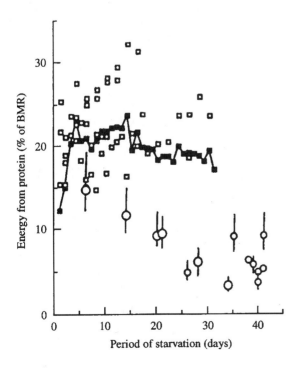

FIG. 1.1. The effect of starvation in lean subjects (*solid squares*) from the Benedict study (179) and from other studies (*open squares*) versus obese subjects (*open circles* from groups of subjects and *small squares* from individual subjects) in the studies of Elia (32) and Elia, Stubbs, and Henry (128). (From Elia M. Hunger disease. *Clin Nutr* 2000; 19:379–386, with permission.)

Adipose Tissue Functions

Adipose tissue has other important functions that are both related to and independent of energy storage (34) (Table 1.2). These include the synthesis and secretion of various proteins that regulate adipose tissue fuel flux, insulin sensitivity, vasomotor tone, cell turnover, inflammation, coagulation, and conversion of androgens to estrogens. Many of these proteins (i.e., those that regulate insulin action, cell proliferation, thrombosis, vascular reactivity, and the inflammatory response) may be related to the survival advantage of obesity.

In addition to periods of food deprivation, other important periods of energy provision include pregnancy and lactation. Low maternal weight before pregnancy and poor weight gain during pregnancy increase the prevalence of low–birth-weight infants (35,36). Although lactation does occur in the absence of abundant adipose tissue stores, energy intakes must increase with a body composition of this type in order to maintain breast milk quantity and quality (37).

In addition, adipose tissue acts as insulation and protects against the adverse effects of cold air or water (38). It also has an important role in fertility. The age at which menarche occurs is at least partially attributable to adipose tissue content (39,40), and, as fat mass decreases with exercise or eating disorders, oligomenorrhea and amenorrhea may result (41). Although the mechanisms for the reproductive function of adipose tissue remain controversial, leptin appears to be important. Not only is leptin able to induce reproductive maturation in female rodents (42), but the decrease in leptin that occurs with weight reduction and loss of adipose tissue mass appears to be partially responsible for the altered function of the hypothalamic–pituitary–ovarian (testicular) axis (43). Bone

---

TABLE 1.2. *Roles of proteins secreted from human adipose tissue*

Regulation of adipose tissue fuel flux	
Adenosine	Kather et al. (182)
Leptin	Friedman and Halaas (150)
Acylation-stimulating protein	Sniderman et al. (183)
Regulation of insulin action	
Adiponectin	Weyer et al. (184)
TNF-α + soluble receptor	Moller (185)
Regulation of vasomotor tone	
Angiotensinogen	Van Harmelen et al. (186)
Angiotensin-converting enzyme	Gorzelniak et al. (187)
PGI$_2$	Fink et al. (188)
Regulation of cell turnover	
PGI$_2$	Negrel et al. (189)
TGF-β	Alessi et al. (190)
IGF-I	Wabitsch et al. (191)
Regulation of coagulation	
Plasminogen activator inhibitor-1	Crandall et al. (192)
PGI$_2$	McCarty (193)
Regulation of inflammation	
TNF-α + soluble receptor	McDermott (194)
Interleukin-6	Hirano et al. (195)
Adipsin	Esterbauer et al. (196)
Steroid conversion, reproduction, bone mass	
Cytochrome P450–dependent aromatase	Bulun et al. (197)
17β-hydroxysteroid oxidoreductase	Crobould et al. (198)
Other	
Agouti signal protein	Voisey et al. (199)

Abbreviations: IGF, insulin-like growth factor; PGI, prostaglandin I; TGF, transforming growth factor; TNF, tumor necrosis factor.

mass and adipose mass are also highly related (44), and obesity protects against the development of osteoporosis (45). When osteoporosis occurs in obese patients, a workup for Cushing syndrome is mandatory.

Environmental Influences on Adipose Tissue Mass

The present environment of food availability and decreased physical activity favors an increase in adipose tissue mass. Although evidence from adoption and twin studies support a genetic basis for body fatness (46–48), the gene pool has changed little, so this does not explain the epidemic of overweight individuals and obesity that has been encountered in the last two decades. Even if genetics could explain a large percentage of the overweight and obesity epidemic, the literature is mixed regarding which component of energy balance is etiologic. Moreover, variable data on the contributions of alterations in energy expenditure to changes in fat mass over time do not clarify the mechanism of the genetic impact (49). Thus, the environment must be examined as the cause.

Influences of the environment on body fatness could work through increases in energy intake and/or decreases in energy expenditure. As Chapter 3 reviews, data on food intake are contradictory, with some studies showing no change in caloric consumption (50,51) and others demonstrating increases (52,53). Evidence supporting a higher consumption of dietary fat as etiologic is equally as unconvincing as that which demonstrates no relationship between dietary fat and weight change (54,55). Some believe that the overconsumption of dietary carbohydrates resulting from the "fat is bad" mentality of the late twentieth century is etiologic (56,57). However, when examining intakes for populations, caution must be used in making conclusions about cause and effect; for example, using such an approach, the increase in overweight and obese individuals can be attributed to the consumption of diet beverages. Reductions in physical activity also contribute to the positive energy balance that, in turn, results in increases in weight and adipose tissue over time (58). Activity data, which have been collected only in the United States since 1985, reveal that 60% of the United States population has no regular pattern of physical activity and that 25% reports no physical activity (59). Many people in the United States and in the rest of the civilized world are increasingly "desk bound" in their occupations, and this lifestyle is supported by the many advances of the modern world.

Substantial evidence from migratory patterns of populations indicates not only that food is more available and more energy dense but also that the physical activity profiles of past generations have been exchanged for a more sedentary lifestyle. Examples from these include the Samoans within the Samoan archipelago and Hawaii (60), the Pima Indians of Mexico and Arizona (61), the Japanese-American immigrants (62), and the West African Diaspora and its migrations out of Africa to the United Kingdom and the United States (63). In these instances, fatness results when the stresses of life in a more deprived setting are replaced by the conveniences of the modern world. One conclusion that seems tenable is that the body creates an excess adipose tissue reservoir in preparation for less favorable environmental conditions.

Another relatively recent example of the impact of the environment on body weight regulation and obesity prevalence was the experience of the Dutch population during the famine of World War II (1944 to 1945). During this 6-month period of food rationing in the Netherlands, infant size was substantially decreased and infant mortality was significantly increased (64). A similar experience was seen in Leningrad and Odessa at the same time (65). Moreover, when food deprivation in the Netherlands was greatest during the third trimester, the incidence of obesity in the offspring was decreased, whereas food deprivation in the first trimester produced a much higher rate of obesity in the offspring (66). The authors concluded that the early deprivation likely caused damage to the hypothalamic centers, which regulate food intake and growth; when deprivation occurs later in gestation, a defect in adipogenesis may be responsible. This experience suggests that the regulation of adipose tissue mass at least partially relates to the intrauterine environment and that it may differ during the course of the prenatal period.

Overfeeding and Obesity

The response to forced overfeeding, which is somewhat unrealistic, remains one way to determine the genetic predisposition to overweight and/or obesity. In general, overfeeding rodents results in weight gain and adipose tissue accumulation; however, this response is typically dependent on the rodent strain (67) and likely on the thermogenic response of the rodent to overfeeding (68). In female baboons that are overfed during infancy, hypertrophic obesity develops after puberty (69). However, variable amounts of intragastric overfeeding in adult male rhesus monkeys resulted in weight gain, but this was also accompanied by reductions in *ad libitum* food intake (70). When the intragastric overfeeding period was discontinued in these monkeys, normal energy intake stabilized over a period of several months and their body weights dropped rapidly. Some monkeys returned to their initial body weight, whereas some net weight gain occurred in others.

A number of overfeeding experiments have been performed in humans. Bouchard et al. (71) performed one of the the longest and best studies for determining the genetic basis of the metabolic and anatomic response to excess calories. In his study, 12 pairs of identical twins were overfed by 84,000 kcal over 100 days. The average weight gain was 8.1 kg, but a range of 4.3 kg to 13.3 kg was observed. Although 63% of the excess calories were stored, predicting an increased cost of weight maintenance at an expanded body weight (72), about one-third of the excess calories were not stored, thus implying that thermogenic mechanisms in response to overfeeding also occurred. Twin pairs were similar in their response, with three times more variance in weight gain and in the increase in adipose tissue among pairs than within pairs. An even greater similarity within twin pairs was noted in the changes in regional adipose tissue mass. Moreover, within 4 months of overfeeding, 82%, 74%, and 100% of the overfeeding gain in body weight, fat mass, and fat-free mass, respectively, were lost (72).

The classic overfeeding studies of Sims et al. (73) also demonstrated that massive caloric overfeeding, which, in this experiment, was accompanied by substantial increases in physical activity, resulted in variable weight gain; an increased thermogenic response; and, for most participants, resumption of their initial body weight after overfeeding was discontinued. More recently, research subjects at the Mayo Clinic who were overfed 1,000 kcal per day for 8 weeks experienced increases in fat from 58 g to 687 g and in fat-free mass from 17 g to 78 g (74). Although energy expenditure increased in most subjects, this ranged from −100 kcal to +360 kcal. The greatest predictor of the change in weight and fat mass during this relatively brief period of overfeeding was the individual's increase in non–exercise-associated thermogenesis (NEAT), or fidgeting. Presently the genetic basis of NEAT remains undefined, but NEAT may be extremely important in determining the response to the environmental factors that lead to obesity regardless of whether it results from the expression of one or many genes.

Reduced Obesity Predicts Resumption of the Obese State

Achieving weight reduction is difficult for obese patients, and it may be more difficult to sustain (75–77). The term reduced obesity defines the behavioral and metabolic status of an obese person or animal after weight reduction and isocaloric weight maintenance. Similar responses may also occur in weight-reduced normal-weight organisms. Although these variables and intervals are probably influenced by the amount of weight reduction and the duration of the weight-reduced state among other factors, they are poorly defined and thus they require additional elucidation.

In general, the adaptations of the reduced obese state appear to work in a manner that predicts resumption of the obese weight (Table 1.3). After successful weight reduction and months of maintenance of the reduced obese state, increases in appetite (78,79) and a preference for energy-dense foods (i.e., those containing fat and sugar) (80) are observed. This increase in appetite may be partially related to decreases in leptin, which in at least one study (81) predicted the increase in body weight after weight reduction; other studies (82,83) have not reported the same effect. In a recent report, Cummings et al. (84) suggest that changes in the gastrointestinal hormone ghrelin may also contribute to weight regain after successful diet-induced weight reduction. Normally, levels of ghrelin increase before the meal and fall after the meal; however, Cummings et al. (84) found that during maintenance of the reduced obese state, 24-hour areas under the curve for ghrelin were actually increased, rather than decreased, compared to the baseline.

Regain of weight is also favored by changes in energy expenditure. With weight reduction, the basal metabolic rate falls in proportion to the loss of lean body mass (85). In many subjects, the energy expended in the form of physical activity does not increase (86–88). Klem et al. (89) gathered a nonrandom sample of "successful" reduced obese subjects into the National Weight Loss Registry. In more than 90% of these subjects, a combination of a diet restricted in fat and exercise of more than 500 kcal daily was necessary to maintain a BMI of 25 kg/m^2 (90,91).

Finally, isocaloric maintenance of the reduced obese state modifies the physiologic processes that promote fat storage. This includes increases in insulin sensitivity (92,93), decreases in fat oxidation (94,95), and tissue-specific changes in lipoprotein-lipase (LPL) activity. Although increases in insulin sensitivity after weight reduction and the maintenance of the reduced obese state have been shown to predict weight regain (96), conflicting reports have been made (5,97).

TABLE 1.3. *The reduced obese state: possible predictors of weight regain*

Increased appetite	Doucet et al. (78)
Decreased leptin	Mavri et al. (81)
Increased ghrelin	Cummings et al. (84)
Preference for energy-dense foods	Drewnowski and Holden-Wiltse (80)
Reductions in energy expenditure	
Basal metabolic rate	Astrup et al. (85)
Physical activity	Weigle (87)
Increased insulin sensitivity	Yost et al. (96)
Increased respiratory quotient	Froidevaux et al. (94)
Changes in LPL	
Increased adipose tissue LPL	Schwartz and Brunzell (100)
Decreased skeletal muscle LPL	Eckel et al. (101)

Abbreviation: LPL, lipoprotein lipase.

Lean

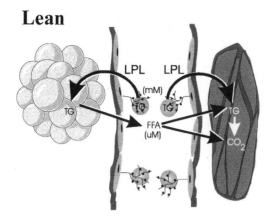

Reduced-Obese

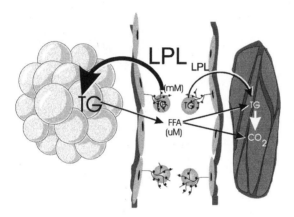

FIG. 1.2. Tissue-specific changes in lipoprotein lipase (LPL) in the reduced obese state. LPL, which is shown bound to the glycocalyx of capillary endothelial cells, hydrolyzes the triglyceride (TG) core of circulating TG-rich lipoproteins, very low density lipoproteins, and chylomicrons, resulting in the production of free fatty acids (FFA) and monoacylglycerol, which are then taken up by adipose tissue and muscle. There the FFAs are either stored (adipose tissue) or stored and/or oxidized (muscle).

LPL hydrolyzes the triglyceride core of circulating triglyceride-rich lipoproteins to provide fatty acid fuels for the LPL-producing tissues of the body, including adipose tissue and muscle. After 3 months of sustained weight reduction, the activity of the fasting enzyme in adipose tissue either remains unchanged or increased (98–100), and the response of LPL to insulin and meals is increased (98). In skeletal muscle, LPL levels are reduced in comparison to the levels that were present before weight reduction (99). These changes in macronutrient partitioning and presumably in storage (Fig. 1.2) do not occur in a vacuum; instead, they are permitted by a setting in which energy intake is greater than energy expenditure.

Overall, these changes in behavior and metabolism are probably important for explaining the relatively low success rate of sustained weight reduction, and they point to the potential role of obesity in defending the organism during food deprivation.

Evidence that Obesity Promotes Survival

Death from starvation is almost always accompanied by marked, if not complete, loss of adipose tissue (102). This is illustrated by adult necropsies performed during the Irish famine of 1847 (103), World War I (104), and World War II (105), as well as in children who were victims of starvation in Kharkov (106). In general, the loss of subcutaneous adipose tissue precedes the loss of fat located elsewhere or of muscle mass (105) (Fig. 1.3). During prolonged periods of food deprivation, the amount of weight reduction varied from 15% over 5 months (107) to nearly 25% over 3 years (108) in World War I, from 22% to 26% during the Russian famine of 1920 to 1922 (109), and from 9.3% to 13.6% among Parisian civilians during World War II (110). More recent studies have ascertained that, for men, a reduction in body fat to less than 4% and in fat mass to less than 2.5 kg reaches a level that is inconsistent with good health (111). Generally, this results in a BMI of about 13 kg/m^2, a level of estimated fatness that separates survivors from nonsurvivors in men. In women, a much greater variability in BMI is seen in survivors versus nonsurvivors (13) (Fig. 1.4). However, more recent data provided by the famine in Somalia suggest that a BMI of less than 10 kg/m^2 can support life as long as the individual receives specialized care (12). However, in Somalia, starving male patients had more severe edema and a poorer prognosis than females at any given level of severity of starvation.

As the previous statement suggests, *women* appear to withstand semistarvation and starvation better than *men*. In addition to the experience in Somalia, other examples include the 1941 to 1942 famine in the Greek cities of Athens and Piraeus (112) (Fig. 1.5), the German siege of Leningrad from 1941 to 1942 (113), and the Dutch famine in 1945 (114) (Fig. 1.6). Although the data accrued from these unfortunate incidents of history are far from satisfactory, the percentage increase in starvation-related mortality in Greece was lower in women than in men. In Leningrad, the peak incidence of and the rise in death mortality were delayed by 2 to 5 months in women versus men. In the Netherlands, the mortality for men increased by 169% while that for women was only

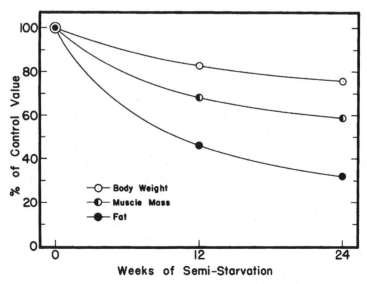

FIG. 1.3. Percentage changes in body weight, muscle mass, and fat during semistarvation in the Minnesota experiment. In this experiment, 32 men weighing 69.3 kg with a body composition of 13.9% fat at baseline voluntarily ingested an average of 1,570 kcal per day for 24 weeks. Body fat was estimated by specific gravity. (From Keys A, Brozek J, Henschel A, et al. *Body fat in biology of human starvation.* Vol. 1. Minneapolis: University of Minnesota Press, 1950:161–183, with permission.)

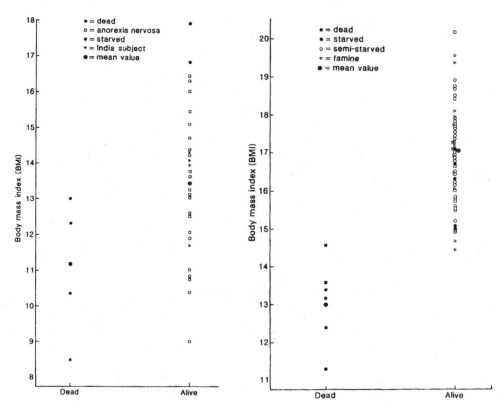

FIG. 1.4. Body mass index (BMI) and limits of survival in men and women. Comparisons of BMIs of male and female survivors versus those of nonsurvivors are portrayed. (Data from Henry CJK. Body mass index and the limits of human survival. *Eur J Clin Nutr* 1990;44: 329–335, with permission.)

72%. One of the factors that most likely contributes to the relative survival advantage of women versus men is the increased fat stores in women. Moreover, the smaller fat cells and reduced metabolic activity of pelvic versus abdominal fat provide a survival advantage in periods of starvation, and they could protect against the pathologic seque-lae of central adipose tissue deposition that is more typical in men during periods of caloric excess.

In the "Minnesota Experiment," or semistarvation experiment, of Keys et al. (102), the adipose tissue dramatically responded to refeeding, predicting the following return of body weight (Fig. 1.7). In more recent experiments, the pattern of lean and fat tissue deposition during the refeeding period appears to be due to individual differences in energy partitioning; in other words, the disproportionate gain in fat versus lean tissue is a consequence of a relative greater reduction in thermogenesis that enhances energy effi-ciency (115). This metabolic efficiency may actually occur in response to low energy intakes (116), although this view is controversial (117,118).

Until the late eighteenth century, individual life expectancy was only 25 to 35 years (119). Even at the beginning of the twentieth century, the average lifespan in the United States was less than 50 years (120). By the early 1900s, survival increased to 55 years (121), and for those born in the G7 countries today (i.e., Canada, France, Germany, Italy, Japan, United Kingdom, United States), the progressive decline in mortality predicts a longevity of nearly 80 years (122). In fact, in a recent and provocative report by Oeppen

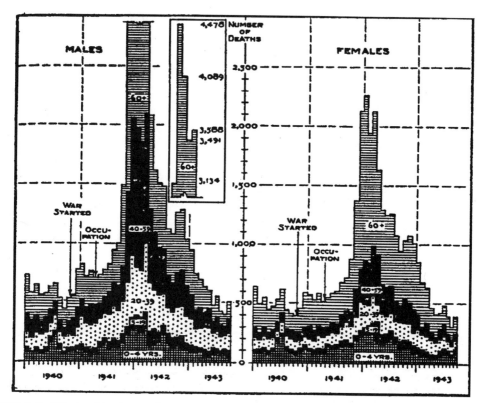

FIG. 1.5. Effects of famine on the population of Greece. Shown is the number of deaths by age for men and women in Athens and Piraeus during the period of World War II, 1940–1943. (From Valaoras VG. Some effects of famine on the population of Greece. *Milbank Memorial Fund Quarterly* 1946;24:215–234, with permission.)

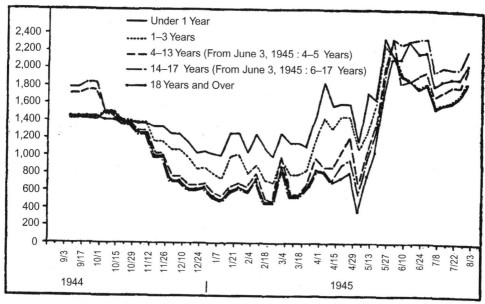

FIG. 1.6. Average calories per day for various age groups. The data portrayed represent the average calories per day by weekly periods for food rations distributed daily to various age groups in the Western Netherlands from September 3, 1944 to August 5, 1945. (From Dols MJL, van Arcken DJAM. Food supply and nutrition in the Netherlands during and after World War II. *Milbank Memorial Fund Quarterly* 1946;24:319–355, with permission.)

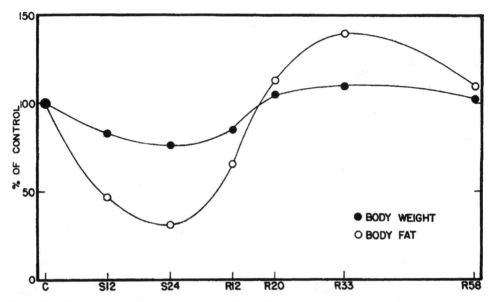

FIG. 1.7. The recovery of body weight and body fat, expressed as a percentage of control, after 24 weeks of semistarvation (1,570 kcal per day) in 32 men in the Minnesota Experiment. During the first 12 weeks of rehabilitation (R1–R12), subjects were divided into four groups consisting of four different caloric levels ranging from 2,378 to 3,392 kcal per day (average 2,896 kcal per day) with or without protein and vitamin supplementation. (From Keys A, Brozek J, Henschel A, et al. *Body fat in biology of human starvation.* Vol. 1. Minneapolis: University of Minnesota Press, 1950:161–183, with permission.)

and Vaupel (123), they indicate that, if the current trends in survival continue, by 2070 the average lifespan could be extended by 12 to 15 years. Although the increasing incidence and prevalence of obesity may ultimately modify this trend, the data available today for obese individuals older than 65 years of age may not indicate an earlier demise (124). However, because a maximum lifespan exists for all mammals (Fig. 1.8), death rarely occurs without it being attributed to one or more "natural or degenerative causes." Although senescence is accepted as the biology of aging, death is still attributed to the failure of one or more organs, and the increased survivorship of these times is largely a function of medical intervention (120).

Evidence indicates that obesity prolongs survival in periods of food deprivation (102,125). In the Irish hunger strikes, the lifespan ranged from 45 to 73 days (32), in which longevity could be predicted by a normal amount of fat mass before starvation. However, prolonged fasts of up to 400 days have been accomplished by obese subjects who fasted for therapeutic reasons (126,127). A number of metabolic factors explain these results (Table 1.4). As has already been noted and portrayed (Fig. 1.1), obese individuals have more body protein (fat-free mass) than lean individuals, but during starvation they excrete less nitrogen than their lean counterparts (128). In addition, within weeks of the onset of starvation, the energy contribution from protein remains the same in lean subjects, but it progressively decreases in obese individuals (33). Other metabolic differences observed in the obese versus the lean include a decreased rate of protein oxidation (128), a decreased rate in the rise of circulating ketone bodies and of the indices of the mitochondrial redox state (129), a greater production of glucose from gluconeo-

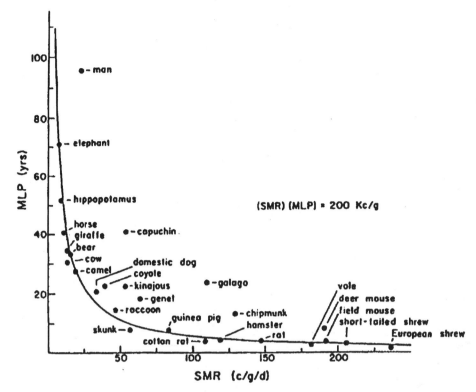

FIG. 1.8. Relationship between maximum lifespan potential *(MLP)* and specific metabolic rate *(SMR)* expressed as calories consumed per gram of body weight per day in a variety of mammalian species (180). (From Weiss KM. Are the known chronic diseases related to the human lifespan and its evolution? *Am J Hum Biol* 1989;1:307–319, with permission.)

genesis by the kidney (130), and a lower deterioration in glucose tolerance (131). The reduced rise in ketogenesis and in the indices of the mitochondrial redox state indicate the relative preservation of glucose as the dominant energy source for the brain in the obese individual. The experiments of Elia et al. (128) portray this nicely (Fig. 1.9). Overall, these differences in the metabolic response to starvation in obese versus lean individuals are not trivial, and they most likely contribute to the prolonged survival that is seen in those with expanded adipose tissue mass.

TABLE 1.4. *Metabolic differences between lean and obese individuals during starvation*

Rate of rise of ketone bodies over 3–4 days	Lean > obese
Ketone body concentration at 3–4 days	Lean > obese
Rate of rise of 3-hydroxybutyrate/acetoacetate ratio	Lean > obese
Concentration of 3-hydroxybutyrate/acetoacetate ratio	Lean > obese
Deterioration of glucose tolerance	Lean > obese
Protein oxidation at 60 h	Lean > obese
Nitrogen excretion	Lean > obese
Renal gluconeogenesis	Lean < obese

From Elia M. Hunger disease. *Clin Nutr* 2000;19:379–386, with permission.

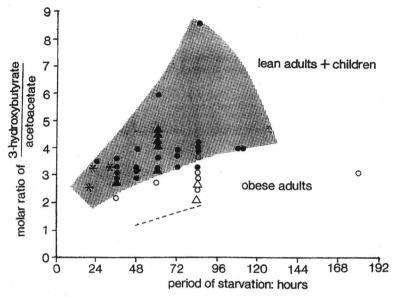

FIG. 1.9. The effect of total starvation on the plasma molar ratio of 3-hydroxybutyrate to ace-toacetate in children (*) and lean (*solid symbols*) and obese (*open symbols*) adults. (From Elia M, Stubbs R, Henry CJK. Differences in fat, carbohydrate, and protein metabolism between lean and obese subjects undergoing total starvation. *Obes Res* 1999;7:597–604, with permission.)

The Thrifty Genotype

As Bray (132,133) has repeatedly pointed out in historical reviews, obesity has been exemplified since the Paleolithic period, approximately 23,000 to 25,000 years ago (134). As Fig. 1.10 demonstrates, Venus figurines portraying female obesity have been located in many sites throughout Europe and the Middle East. The most famous of these is the "Venus of Willendorf" made of limestone, which is the only one that has been discovered in Austria. These figurines have been viewed as representing primordial deities reflecting the bounty of the earth. These artistic records of history may also represent the longevity associated with obesity at a time when the lifespan was only two decades (125).

The concept of the "thrifty genotype" was initially proposed by Neel (135) in 1962 and was revisited in 1982 (136) and 1998 (137). Although his initial interpretation of genes beneficial to survival in a "hunter–gatherer" type of environment related more to diabetes than to obesity, the most recent view focuses more on obesity and it also includes hypertension (137). The putative genes would operate such that carriers are predisposed to extract scarce resources more efficiently from the environment. In the modern world in which the "hunter–gatherer" concept is fading and the lifespan extends far past the reproductive age, these genes are no longer beneficial and they can, in fact, be detrimental. Now called *pleiotropic,* these genes may also predispose their carriers to physiologic degeneration or loss of function during their middle or later years of life (138). This model thus provides a theoretical basis for explaining aging and the many degenerative diseases that accompany the extended lifespan.

As Gerber and Crews (121) outline, the "thrifty and/or pleiotropic" model of degenerative diseases with aging can be applied at two levels. First, specific risk factors associated with

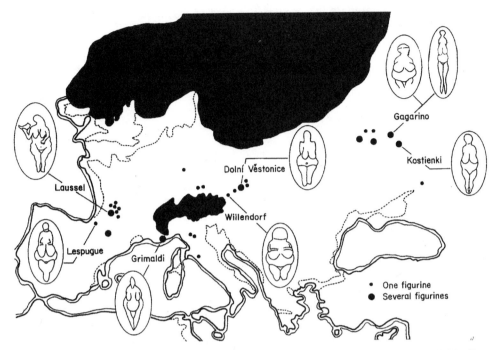

FIG. 1.10. Approximate location of Paleolithic "Venus" figurines in Europe and the Middle East about 22,000 BC. (From Bray G. Historical framework for the development of ideas about obesity. In: Bray GA, Bouchard C, James WPT, eds. *Handbook of obesity.* New York: Marcel Dekker Inc, 1998:1–29, with permission.)

degenerative diseases follow either the accumulation (thrifty) or the scarcity or loss (nonthrifty) of specific nutrients, metabolites, stores, or deposits. Second, some degenerative diseases result from the antagonistic effects of thrifty genotypes that have high selective value during development. These effects then predispose their carriers to the risk factors associated with degenerative diseases. The transition from obesity to type II diabetes and then to the additional risk factors for cardiovascular disease, such as dyslipidemia, the prothrombotic state, and hypertension, is a well-documented example of the proposed model.

Biologic Considerations of the Thrifty or Pleiotropic Genotype

A gene or genes that favorably modify energy storage during periods of food deprivation and that could ultimately result in degenerative diseases during midlife and late life generally are genes that at least have some influence on energy balance. Ideally, candidate genes would operate to enhance energy intake and metabolic efficiency in a way that partitions fuels for storage rather than for oxidative metabolism. Because of the limited capacity for carbohydrate storage, these genes would need to influence lipid uptake and storage mechanisms. The plethora of metabolic effects of insulin satisfy these criteria, so a gene or genes that enhance insulin sensitivity in the periphery is worthy of serious consideration.

In an insulin-sensitive environment, anabolism is the rule. This is related to the multiple effects of insulin that promote fuel uptake and storage in peripheral tissues (Table 1.5). In protein metabolism, insulin increases amino acid uptake and protein synthesis

TABLE 1.5. *Insulin action in insulin-sensitive tissues*

Protein metabolism	
Increases amino acid uptake	Lerner (200)
Inhibits proteolysis	Miers et al. (201)
Increases protein synthesis	Kimball et al. (202)
Glucose metabolism	
Increases glucose transport (adipose tissue, muscle)	Ryder et al. (203)
Increases glycogen synthesis	Srivastava and Pandey (204)
Inhibits hepatic and renal glucose production	Cherrington et al. (205)
Lipid metabolism	
Inhibits lipolysis	Bergman (206)
Increases fatty acid and triglyceride synthesis (liver)	Sparks and Sparks (207)
Increases adipose tissue lipoprotein lipase	Sadur and Eckel (208)
Inhibits skeletal muscle lipoprotein lipase	Farese et al. (209)
Inhibits very low density lipoprotein secretion	Lewis and Steiner (210)

and inhibits proteolysis. Insulin modifies carbohydrate metabolism by increasing glucose uptake and glycogen synthesis in muscle and adipose tissue and by increasing glycogen synthesis and inhibiting glucose production in the liver and kidney. Finally, in lipid metabolism, insulin inhibits adipose tissue lipolysis of stored triacylglycerol (the most sensitive parameter of insulin action); increases lipoprotein-derived fatty acid uptake by its effect on adipose tissue LPL; inhibits the secretion of very low density lipoprotein from the liver; and inhibits skeletal muscle LPL modestly, thus decreasing the availability of circulating lipoprotein-derived fatty acids to muscle. All of these effects of insulin work to enhance energy storage and thus to protect the organism against periods of nutrient deprivation. However, insulin is also known to inhibit food intake when it is infused into the third ventricle in baboons and rodents (139,140). How this parameter of insulin action relates to energy balance in the periphery remains unclear.

A substantial amount of evidence provides support for the concept that insulin sensitivity promotes weight gain and insulin resistance protects against weight gain (141–144). Some epidemiologic studies (145,146) indicate that fasting hyperinsulinemia—a marker of insulin resistance—or more likely insulin resistance itself predicts weight maintenance; however, not all studies (147,148) support this. Nevertheless, several recent studies have demonstrated that increased insulin sensitivity is a predictor of weight (fat) gain or of the rebound of obesity after successful weight reduction (96). In these cases as well, alternative data do exist (97).

Graphical depictions (Fig. 1.11) indicate that, when the thrifty gene effects of insulin sensitivity are manifested, increases in adipocyte number and/or size and insulin resis-

FIG. 1.11. The progression of insulin sensitivity in leanness **(A)** to obesity **(B)**, which represents the intermediate metabolic paradigm, to the insulin resistance of type II diabetes mellitus **(C)**. In the setting of insulin sensitivity, insulin-mediated glucose uptake and glycogen deposition in skeletal muscle is enhanced with relative sparing of fatty acid oxidation and the uptake of lipids with storage in adipose tissue. The liver remains responsive to insulin-mediated suppression of hepatic glucose production. In obesity, defects in all aspects of insulin action ultimately result; however, insulin secretion increases, resulting in hyperinsulinemia but preservation of glucose tolerance. With persistence of insulin resistance and islet failure, insulin secretion fails. In this metabolic setting, insulin resistance increases, including resistance to insulin suppression of hepatic glucose production, and further defects in insulin-mediated glucose disposal and hyperglycemia result. Because of persistent and worsening insulin action in adipose tissue, fat mass fails to increase further.

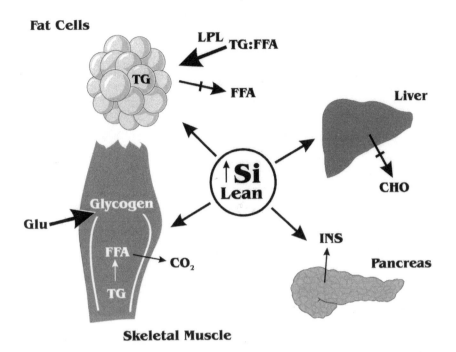

A

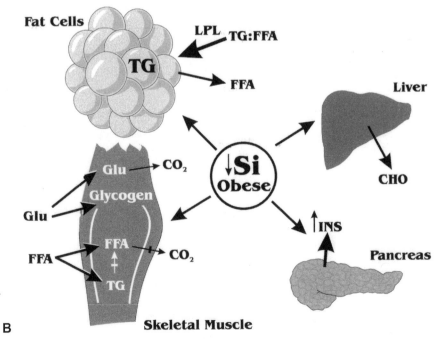

B

(continued on next page)

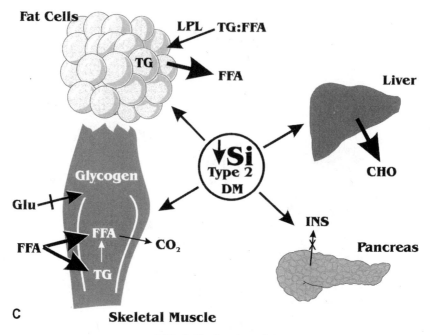

FIG. 1.11. *Continued.*

tance, as manifested by hyperinsulinemia, ultimately result. In adipose tissue, insulin resistance to the antilipolytic effects of insulin and the insulin stimulatory effects on LPL become apparent. Moreover, with the development of obesity, insulin resistance in tissues also results in defects in insulin-mediated glucose transport and glycogen synthesis, with increases in triacylglycerol accumulation and fatty acid oxidation in muscle and lack of suppression of glucose production by the liver and kidney. Over years, the continued stress of the insulin-resistant environment on the pancreas produces an inability to maintain insulin secretion, and type II diabetes results. Of interest is recent evidence from insulin receptor knockout mice suggesting that the islet defect may also be a consequence of insulin resistance (149). Whether the propensity to develop diabetes relates to the function of the same gene, thus demonstrating its pleiotropic qualities, or to a separate gene must still be elucidated.

Several genes have been entertained as candidates for the thrifty or pleiotropic gene hypothesis or at least for the "thrifty" component. Leptin is a cytokine secreted by adipocytes that regulates energy balance at the levels of intake and expenditure (150). Moreover, although leptin appears to be the long-explored factor that communicates between the periphery (adipose tissue) and the hypothalamus regarding fat mass (adipostat), "favorable" mutations of leptin result not only in obesity but also in reproductive incompetence and infertility (151).

MC4R is expressed in hypothalamic nuclei and is involved in the regulation of energy balance (152,153). Indirect evidence for this was provided when the agouti obesity syndrome in mice was found to be a consequence of chronic inhibition of MC4R signaling (152). Furthermore, mice with a deletion of the MC4R gene have a phenotype indistinguishable from the agouti, and mice with heterozygous knockouts of MC4R have an intermediate phenotype (154). A recent discovery indicates that up to 4% of obesity in some populations may be related to mutations in MC4R (17). Moreover, those with heterozygous mutations of MC4R are predisposed to obesity, likely as a result of haploinsufficiency (155,156). The variable penetrance of obesity in heterozygotes indicates that other genes and/or environmental influences are important in the development of the obese phenotype.

Presently, the gene that best meets the qualifications for the thrifty or pleiotropic gene is the nuclear receptor peroxisome proliferator-activated receptor γ (PPARγ). This gene product is activated by fatty acids or fatty acid derivatives and forms heterodimers with other nuclear receptors, such as the retinoid X receptor (RXR), to modify the gene transcription of numerous target genes with specific PPAR response elements (157). The PPARγ gene product is particularly relevant because one of the ligands for its activation is the class of drugs called thiazolidinediones, which are currently used to improve insulin sensitivity in the treatment of type II diabetes and other insulin-resistant states (158). Studies in cultured adipocytes show that thiazolidinediones enhance adipocyte differentiation (159) and that *in vivo* they produce weight gain in both animals and humans (160–162). Although some of the weight gain can be attributed to fluid retention (161), the predominant explanation is an increase in adipose tissue.

PPARγ action is not only reflected by increasing adipocyte differentiation and insulin action but also by a number of other effects (Table 1.6). These include its influence on insulin secretion, cell cycle control, immunomodulation, inflammation, atherosclerosis, myocardial function, and carcinogenesis (157). Of added relevance is the fact that naturally occurring mutations in PPARγ and induced haploinsufficiency in mice heterozygous for PPARγ produce interesting modifications in receptor biology. For example, the Pro12Ala PPARγ mutation in humans has variably been associated with obesity (163); diabetes (164); protection from diabetes (163,165); reductions in glucose and arginine-mediated insulin secretion (166); and diverse effects on atherosclerotic risk, including a lipid and lipoprotein phenotype consistent with familial combined hyperlipidemia (167), reductions in total and non–high-density lipoprotein cholesterol (168) and postheparin LPL (169), and reductions in coronary heart disease (170). Alternatively, this mutation has had no metabolic effect in some populations (171,172). However, other mutations in PPARγ have also been linked to human obesity, either directly (173) or via their influence on other obesity-related proteins, such as leptin (174).

Serendipitously, mice heterozygous for PPARγ (PPARγ +/–) or normal mice treated with PPARγ or RXR antagonists are spared adipocyte hypertrophy, they are more insulin sensitive, they are relatively hyperleptinemic with reductions in muscle and liver triacylglycerol levels and increases in fatty acid oxidation, and they have enhanced immune (T-cell and B-cell) function (175–178). When PPARγ +/– mice are treated with a PPARγ or a RXR antagonist, a dramatic metabolic effect characterized by marked reductions in white adipose tissue, leptin, and energy expenditure; increases in triacylglycerol accu-

TABLE 1.6. *Paroxisome proliferator-activated receptor γ actions*

Increased adipocyte differentiation	Fajas et al. (211)
Increased insulin sensitivity	Sood et al. (212)
Increased insulin secretion	Kawai et al. (213)
Cell cycle regulation	Altiok et al. (214)
Immunomodulation	Clark et al. (215)
Reduced atherosclerosis	Molavi et al. (216)
Enhanced myocardial function	Khandoudi et al. (217)
Carcinogenesis	Fajas et al. (211)

mulation in muscle and liver; and decreases in insulin sensitivity is observed (178). A role for RXR in this response is supported by the relative leanness and the increased energy expenditure found in mice with a knockout of RXRγ (90).

Together these data suggest that PPARγ has a pivotal role in adipose tissue biology and insulin action that is modified by the number of PPARγ alleles. The critical role of this gene is also exemplified by embryonic lethality in its absence (175). With a lifespan that extends past the "beneficial" effects of PPARγ gene expression on survival, the pleiotropic downside may be metabolic disorders, atherosclerosis, or malignancy. Much about this fascinating candidate for the thrifty or pleiotropic gene remains to be learned. Moreover, the hope is that, with the human genome sequence now in hand, many more genes that act alone or in concert to produce obesity will likely be uncovered.

CONCLUSIONS

Is obesity a disease or an adaptation for survival? Does this even make a difference? The answer is yes. The impact of the environment is the same with either view; however, the atmosphere in which health care professionals and their patients operate may be profoundly and differentially influenced by the opinion of science, government, health care reimbursement organizations, and the marketplace, which includes pharmaceutical companies, weight loss programs, and over-the-counter products. Although referring to obesity as a disease is politically correct, the criteria for obesity to be called a disease are insufficiently delineated; moreover, abundant evidence indicates that, when famine or semistarvation occur, obesity could be a participant's best friend. Without question, the complications of obesity are diseases. However, an acknowledgment of the importance of obesity over the history of humankind helps the health care professional and the patient to develop an understanding about the facts of excess body fat. This newfound knowledge can modify the behavior of both so that guilt is removed and both can now approach the difficulties of treatment with a greater appreciation of the barriers. With some degree of ambivalence, what was once "thrifty" and beneficial must now be accepted as "pleiotropic" and potentially harmful.

REFERENCES

1. World Health Organization. *Obesity: preventing and managing the global epidemic.* Albany, NY: World Health Organization, 2000.
2. National Institutes of Health Consensus Development Panel on the Health Implications of Obesity. Health implications of obesity. *Ann Intern Med* 1985;103:147–151.
3. Bray GA. Etiology and pathogenesis of obesity. *Clin Cornerstone* 1999;2:1–15.
4. Kopelman PG. Obesity as a medical problem. *Nature* 2000;404:635–643.
5. National Institutes of Health. Clinical guidelines on the identification, evaluation, and treatment of overweight and obesity in adults—the evidence report. *Obes Res* 1998;6:51S–209S.
6. Flegal KM, Troiano RP. Changes in the distribution of body mass index of adults and children in the US population. *Int J Obes Relat Metab Disord* 2000;24:807–818.
7. Himes JH, Dietz WH. Guidelines for overweight in adolescent preventive services: recommendations from an expert committee. *Am J Clin Nutr* 1994;59:307–316.
8. Flegal KM, Ogden CL, Wei R, et al. Prevalence of overweight in US children: comparison of US growth charts from the Centers for Disease Control and Prevention with other reference values for body mass index. *Am J Clin Nutr* 2001;73:1086–1093.
9. Bolen JC, Rhodes L, Powell-Griner EE, et al. State-specific prevalence of selected health behaviors, by race and ethnicity—Behavioral Risk Factor Surveillance System, 1997. *MMWR Morb Mortal Wkly Rep* 2000;49:1–60.
10. Strauss RS, Pollack HA. Epidemic increase in childhood overweight, 1986–1998. *JAMA* 2001;286:2845–2848.
11. Dhurandhar NV, Kulkarni PR, Ajinkya SM, et al. Association of adenovirus infection with human obesity. *Obes Res* 1997;5:464–469.
12. Collins S. The limit of human adaptation to starvation. *Nat Med* 1995;1:810–814.
13. Henry CJK. Body mass index and the limits of human survival. *Eur J Clin Nutr* 1990;44:329–335.
14. Hirsch J, Batchelor B. Adipose tissue cellularity in human obesity. *Clin Endocrinol Metab* 1976;5:299–311.

15. Shepherd PR, Gnudi L, Tozzo E, et al. Adipose cell hyperplasia and enhanced glucose disposal in transgenic mice overexpressing GLUT4 selectively in adipose tissue. *J Biol Chem* 1993;268:22243–22246.
16. Valet P, Grujic D, Wade J, et al. Expression of human alpha 2-adrenergic receptors in adipose tissue of beta 3-adrenergic receptor–deficient mice promotes diet-induced obesity. *J Biol Chem* 2000;275:34797–34802.
17. Vaisse C. Melanocortin-4 receptor mutations are a frequent and heterogenous cause of morbid obesity. *J Clin Invest* 2000;106:253–262.
18. Farooqi IS, Yeo GS, Keogh JM, et al. Dominant and recessive inheritance of morbid obesity associated with melanocortin 4 receptor deficiency. *J Clin Invest* 2000;106:271–279.
19. Allison DB, Fontaine KR, Manson JE, et al. Annual deaths attributable to obesity in the United States. *JAMA* 1999;282:1530–1538.
20. Dawber TR, Moore FE. Epidemiological approaches to heart disease: the Framingham Study. *Am J Public Health* 1951;41:279–286.
21. National Cholesterol Education Program. Executive summary of the third report of the National Cholesterol Education Program (NCEP) Expert Panel on Detection, Evaluation, and Treatment of High Blood Cholesterol in Adults (Adult Treatment Panel III). *JAMA* 2001;285:2486–2497.
22. Ford ES, Giles WH, Dietz WH. Prevalence of the metabolic syndrome among US adults: findings from the third National Health and Nutrition Examination Survey. *JAMA* 2002;287:356–359.
23. Kortt MA, Langley PC, Cox ER. A review of cost-of-illness studies on obesity. *Clin Ther* 1998;20:772–779.
24. Internal Revenue Service, Department of Treasury. *Medical and dental expenses for use in preparing 2001 returns.* Washington, D.C.: United States Government Printing Office, 2002.
25. United States Department of Health and Human Services. *Healthy people 2010,* 2nd ed. Washington, D.C.: United States Government Printing Office, 2000.
26. Deitel M. The Surgeon-General's call to action to prevent an increase in overweight and obesity: released Dec. 13, 2001. *Obes Surg* 2002;12:3–4.
27. Lovern E, Gardner J. Too little or just right? Bush lays his healthcare budget on the table, but Democrats—and some Republicans—say $190 billion falls short. *Modern Health Care* 2002;32:6–7.
28. Espinoza G, Scott S. The real skinny: forgoing fad diets, seven once-obese people go from hefty to healthy by cutting calories and gaining resolve. *Time* 2002 Feb 11:88.
29. Sonnenberg A, Delco F. Cost-effectiveness of a single colonoscopy in screening for colorectal cancer. *Arch Intern Med* 2002;162:163–168.
30. Jacobs RJ, Koff RS, Meyerhoff AS. The cost-effectiveness of vaccinating chronic hepatitis C patients against hepatitis A. *Am J Gastroenterol* 2002;97:427–434.
31. Tengs TO, Adams ME, Pliskin JS, et al. Five-hundred life-saving interventions and their cost-effectiveness. *Risk Analysis* 1995;15:369–390.
32. Elia M. Effect of starvation and very low calorie diets on protein–energy interrelationships in lean and obese subjects. In: Scrimshaw NS, Schurch B, eds. *Protein–energy interactions.* Lausanne, Switzerland: Nestlé Foundation. 1992:249.
33. Elia M. Hunger disease. *Clin Nutr* 2000;19:379–386.
34. Fruhbeck G, Gomez-Ambrosi J, Muruzabal FJ, et al. The adipocyte: a model for integration of endocrine and metabolic signaling in energy metabolism regulation. *Am J Physiol Endocrinol Metab* 2001;280:E827–E847.
35. Lechtig A, Yarborough C, Delgado H, et al. Influence of maternal nutrition on birth weight. *Am J Clin Nutr* 1975;28:1223–1233.
36. van der Spuy ZM, Steer PJ, McCusker M, et al. Outcome of pregnancy in underweight women after spontaneous and induced ovulation. *BMJ* 1988;296:962–965.
37. Prentice AM, Goldberg GR, Prentice A. Body mass index and lactation performance. *Eur J Clin Nutr* 1994;48: S78–S79.
38. Rennie DW, Covino BG, Howell BJ, et al. Physical insulation of Korean diving women. *J Appl Physiol* 1962; 17:961–966.
39. Frisch RE, McArthur JW. Menstrual cycles: fatness as a determinant of minimum weight for height necessary for their maintenance or onset. *Science* 1974;185:949–951.
40. Wattigney WA, Srinivasan SR, Chen W, et al. Secular trend of earlier onset of menarche with increasing obesity in black and white girls: the Bogalusa Heart Study. *Ethn Dis* 1999;9:181–189.
41. Solomon CG, Hu FB, Dunaif A, et al. Long or highly irregular menstrual cycles as a marker for risk of type 2 diabetes mellitus. *JAMA* 2001;286:2421–2426.
42. Chehab FF, Mounzih K, Lu R, et al. Early onset of reproductive function in normal female mice treated with leptin. *Science* 1997;275:88–90.
43. Kopp W, Blum WF, von Prittwitz S, et al. Low leptin levels predict amenorrhea in underweight and eating disordered females. *Mol Psychiatry* 1997;2:335–340.
44. Fogelholm GM, Sievanen HT, Kukkonen-Harjula TK, et al. Bone mineral density during reduction, maintenance and regain of body weight in premenopausal, obese women. *Osteoporos Int* 2001;12:199–206.
45. Albala C, Yanez M, Devoto E, et al. Obesity as a protective factor for postmenopausal osteoporosis. *Int J Obes Relat Metab Disord* 1996;20:1027–1032.
46. Nelson TL, Vogler GP, Pedersen NL, et al. Genetic and environmental influences on body fat distribution, fasting insulin levels and CVD: are the influences shared? *Twin Res* 2000;3:43–50.
47. Price RA, Gottesman II. Body fat in identical twins reared apart: roles for genes and environment. *Behav Genet* 1991;21:1–7.

48. Stunkard AJ, Sorensen TI, Hanis C, et al. An adoption study of human obesity. *N Engl J Med* 1986;314: 193–198.
49. Goran MI. Energy metabolism and obesity. *Med Clin North Am* 2000;84:347–362.
50. Posner BM, Franz MM, Quatromoni PA, et al. Secular trends in diet and risk factors for cardiovascular disease: the Framingham Study. *J Am Diet Assoc* 1995;95:171–179.
51. Stephen AM, Wald NJ. Trends in individual consumption of dietary fat in the United States, 1920–1984. *Am J Clin Nutr* 1990;71:775–788.
52. Binkley JK, Eales J, Jekanowski M. The relation between dietary change and rising US obesity. *Int J Obes Relat Metab Disord* 2000;24:1032–1039.
53. Briefel RR, McDowell MA, Alaimo K, et al. Total energy intake of the US population: the third National Health and Nutrition Examination Survey, 1988–1991. *Am J Clin Nutr* 1995;62:1072S–1080S.
54. Bray GA, Popkin BM. Dietary fat intake does affect obesity! *Am J Clin Nutr* 1998;68:1157–1173.
55. Willett WC. Dietary fat and obesity: an unconvincing relation. *Am J Clin Nutr* 1998;68:1149–1150.
56. Ludwig DS. Dietary glycemic index and obesity. *J Nutr* 2000;130:280S–283S.
57. Stubbs RJ, Mazlan N, Whybrow S. Carbohydrates, appetite and feeding behavior in humans. *J Nutr* 2001;131: 2775S–2781S.
58. Weinsier RL, Hunter GR, Heini AF, et al. The etiology of obesity: relative contribution of metabolic factors, diet, and physical activity. *Am J Med* 1998;105:145–150.
59. United States Department of Health and Human Services. *Physical activity and health.* Washington, D.C.: United States Government Printing Office, 1996.
60. McGarvey ST. Obesity in Samoans and a perspective on its etiology in Polynesians. *Am J Clin Nutr* 1991;53: 1586S–1594S.
61. Ravussin E, Valencia ME, Esparza J, et al. Effects of a traditional lifestyle on obesity in Pima Indians. *Diabetes Care* 1994;17:1067–1074.
62. Hara H, Egusa G, Yamakido M. Incidence of non–insulin-dependent diabetes mellitus and its risk factors in Japanese-Americans living in Hawaii and Los Angeles. *Diabetes Med* 1996;13:S133–S142.
63. Osei K. Metabolic consequences of the West African Diaspora: lessons from the thrifty gene. *J Lab Clin Med* 1999;133:98–111.
64. Smith CA. Effects of maternal undernutrition upon the newborn infants in Holland. *J Pediatr* 1947;30: 229–243.
65. Antonov AN. Children born during the siege of Leningrad in 1942. *J Pediatr* 1942;30:250–259.
66. Ravelli GP, Stein ZA, Susser MW. Obesity in young men after famine exposure in utero and early infancy. *N Engl J Med* 1976;295:349–353.
67. West DB, Boozer CN, Moody DL, et al. Dietary obesity in nine inbred mouse strains. *Am J Physiol* 1992;262: R1025–R1032.
68. Gong TW, Stern JS, Horwitz BH. High fat feeding increases brown fat GDP binding in lean but not obese Zucker rats. *J Nutr* 1990;120:786–792.
69. Lewis DS, Jackson EM, Mott GE. Effect of energy intake on postprandial plasma hormones and triglyceride concentrations in infant female baboons (Papio species). *J Clin Endocrinol Metab* 1992;74:920–926.
70. Jen KL, Hansen BC. Feeding behavior during experimentally induced obesity in monkeys. *Physiol Behav* 1984; 33:863–869.
71. Bouchard C, Tremblay A, Despres JP, et al. The response to long-term overfeeding in identical twins. *N Engl J Med* 1990;322:1477–1482.
72. Tremblay A, Despres JP, Theriault G, et al. Overfeeding and energy expenditure in humans. *Am J Clin Nutr* 1992;56:857–862.
73. Sims EA, Danforth E Jr, Horton ES, et al. Endocrine and metabolic effects of experimental obesity in man. *Recent Prog Horm Res* 1973;29:457–496.
74. Levine JA, Eberhardt NL, Jensen MD. Role of nonexercise activity thermogenesis in resistance to fat gain in humans. *Science* 1999;283:212–214.
75. Bartlett SJ, Faith MS, Fontaine KR, et al. Is the prevalence of successful weight loss and maintenance higher in the general community than the research clinic? *Obes Res* 1999;7:407–413.
76. Dyer RG. Traditional treatment of obesity: does it work? *Baillieres Clin Endocrinol Metab* 1994;8:661–688.
77. Wing RR, Hill JO. Successful weight loss maintenance. *Annu Rev Nutr* 2001;21:323–341.
78. Doucet E, Imbeault P, St Pierre S, et al. Appetite after weight loss by energy restriction and a low-fat diet-exercise follow-up. *Int J Obes Relat Metab Disord* 2000;24:906–914.
79. McGuire MT, Wing RR, Klem ML, et al. What predicts weight regain in a group of successful weight losers? *J Consult Clin Psychol* 1999;67:177–185.
80. Drewnowski A, Holden-Wiltse J. Taste responses and food preferences in obese women: effects of weight cycling. *Int J Obes Relat Metab Disord* 1992;16:639–648.
81. Mavri A, Stegnar M, Sabovic M. Do baseline serum leptin levels predict weight regain after dieting in obese women? *Diabetes Obes Metab* 2001;3:293–296.
82. Nagy TR, Davies SL, Hunter GR, et al. Serum leptin concentrations and weight gain in postobese, postmenopausal women. *Obes Res* 1998;6:257–261.
83. Wing RR, Sinha MK, Considine RV, et al. Relationship between weight loss maintenance and changes in serum leptin levels. *Horm Metab Res* 1996;28:698–703.

84. Cummings D, Weigle DS, Frayo R, et al. Plasma ghrelin levels after diet-induced weight loss or gastric bypass surgery. *N Engl J Med* 2002;346:1623.
85. Astrup A, Gotzsche PC, van de Werken K, et al. Meta-analysis of resting metabolic rate in formerly obese subjects. *Am J Clin Nutr* 1999;69:1117–1122.
86. van Gemert WG, Westerterp KR, van Acker BA, et al. Energy, substrate and protein metabolism in morbid obesity before, during and after massive weight loss. *Int J Obes Relat Metab Disord* 2000;24:711–718.
87. Weigle DS. Contribution of decreased body mass to diminished thermic effect of exercise in reduced-obese men. *Int J Obes* 1988;12:567–578.
88. Weinsier RL, Hunter GR, Zuckerman PA, et al. Energy expenditure and free-living physical activity in black and white women: comparison before and after weight loss. *Am J Clin Nutr* 2000;71:1138–1146.
89. Klem ML, Wing RR, McGuire MT, et al. A descriptive study of individuals successful at long-term maintenance of substantial weight loss. *Am J Clin Nutr* 1997;66:239–246.
90. McGuire MT, Wing RR, Klem ML, Hill JO. Behavioral strategies of individuals who have maintained long-term weight losses. *Obes Res* 1999;7:334–341
91. McGuire MT, Wing RR, Klem ML, et al. Long-term maintenance of weight loss: do people who lose weight through various weight loss methods use different behaviors to maintain their weight? *Int J Obes Relat Metab Disord* 1998;22:572–577.
92. Friedman JE, Dohm GL, Leggett-Frazier N, et al. Restoration of insulin responsiveness in skeletal muscle of morbidly obese patients after weight loss. Effect on muscle glucose transport and glucose transporter GLUT4. *J Clin Invest* 1992;89:701–705.
93. Henry RR, Wiest-Kent TA, Scheaffer L, et al. Metabolic consequences of very-low-calorie diet therapy in obese non–insulin-dependent diabetic and nondiabetic subjects. *Diabetes* 1986;35:155–164.
94. Froidevaux F, Schutz Y, Christin L, Jequier E. Energy expenditure in obese women before and during weight loss, after refeeding, and in the weight-relapse period. *Am J Clin Nutr* 1993;57:35–42.
95. Kelley DE, Goodpaster B, Wing RR, et al. Skeletal muscle fatty acid metabolism in association with insulin resistance, obesity, and weight loss. *Am J Physiol* 1999;277:E1130–E1141.
96. Yost TJ, Jensen DR, Eckel RH. Weight regain following sustained weight reduction is predicted by relative insulin sensitivity. *Obes Res* 1995;3:583–587.
97. Wing RR. Insulin sensitivity as a predictor of weight regain. *Obes Res* 1997;5:24–29.
98. Eckel RH, Yost TJ. Weight reduction increases adipose-tissue lipoprotein-lipase responsiveness in obese women. *J Clin Invest* 1987;80:992–997.
99. Kern PA, Ong JM, Saffari B, et al. The effects of weight loss on the activity and expression of adipose-tissue lipoprotein lipase in very obese humans. *N Engl J Med* 1990;322:1053–1059.
100. Schwartz RS, Brunzell JD. Increased adipose-tissue lipoprotein-lipase activity in moderately obese men after weight reduction. *Lancet* 1978;1:1230–1231.
101. Eckel RH, Yost TJ, Jensen DR. Sustained weight reduction in moderately obese women results in decreased activity of skeletal muscle lipoprotein lipase. *Eur J Clin Invest* 1995;25:396–402.
102. Keys A, Brozek J, Henschel A, et al. *Body fat in biology of human starvation.* Vol. 1. Minneapolis: University of Minnesota Press, 1950:161–183.
103. Donovan D. Observations sure les maladies particulieres produites par la famine de l'annee 1847, et sur les effects morbides causes par une nourriture insuffisante. *J Med Chir Pharm* 1848;7:305–314.
104. Schittenhelm A, Schlect H. Uber Odemkrankheit mit hypertonischer Brady-kardie. *Berl Klin Ws* 1918;55:1138–1142.
105. Leyton GB. Effects of slow starvation. *Lancet* 1946;2:73–79.
106. Nicolaeff L. Influence de l'inanition sur la morphologie des organes infantiles. *Presse Med* 1923;2:1007–1009.
107. Hehir P. Effects of chronic starvation during the siege of Kut. *BMJ* 1922;1:865–868.
108. Rubner M. Der Gesundheitszustand in Allgemeinen. In: Bumm, ed. 1928:65–86.
109. Ivanovsky A. Physical modifications of the population of Russia under famine. *Am J Phys Anthropol* 1923;6:331–353.
110. Tremolieres J. Enseignements de la guerre dans le domeaine de l'alimentation en France. In: Bigwood, ed. 1947:205–231.
111. Friedl K, Moore RJ, Martinez-Lopez L, et al. Lower limit of body fat in healthy active men. *J Appl Physiol* 1994;77:933–940.
112. Valaoras VG. Some effects of famine on the population of Greece. *Milbank Memorial Fund Quarterly* 1946;24:215–234.
113. Brozek J, Wells S, Keys A. Medical aspects of semistarvation in Leningrad (siege 1941–1942). *Am Rev Soviet Med* 1946;4:70–86.
114. Dols MJL, van Arcken DJAM. Food supply and nutrition in the Netherlands during and after World War II. *Milbank Memorial Fund Quarterly* 1946;24:319–355.
115. Dulloo AG, Jacquet J, Girardier L. Autoregulation of body composition during weight recovery in human: the Minnesota Experiment revisited. *Int J Obes Relat Metab Disord* 1996;20:393–405.
116. Shetty P. Adaptive changes in basal metabolic rate and lean body mass in chronic undernutrition. *Hum Nutr Clin Nutr* 1984;38C:443–451.
117. Ferro-Luzzi A, Petracchi C, Kuriyan R, et al. Basal metabolism of weight-stable chronically undernourished men and women: lack of metabolic adaption and ethnic differences. *Am J Clin Nutr* 1997;66:1086–1093.

118. Shetty P. Adaptation to low energy intakes: the responses and limits to low intake in infants, children and adults. *Eur J Clin Nutr* 1999;53:S14–S33.
119. Roberts JM. *A history of Europe.* New York: Allen Lane, 1997.
120. Weiss KM. Are the known chronic diseases related to the human lifespan and its evolution? *Am J Hum Biol* 1989;1:307–319.
121. Gerber L, Crews D. Evolutionary perspectives on chronic degenerative diseases. *Evolutionary Medicine* 1994: 443–469.
122. Tuljapurkar S, Li N, Boe C. A universal pattern of mortality decline in the G7 countries. *Nature* 2000;405: 789–792.
123. Oeppen J, Vaupel JW. Demography. Broken limits to life expectancy. *Science* 2002;296:1029–1031.
124. Heiat A, Vaccarino V, Krumholz HM. An evidence-based assessment of federal guidelines for overweight and obesity as they apply to elderly persons. *Arch Intern Med* 2001;161:1194–1203.
125. Lev-Ran A. Human obesity: an evolutionary approach to understanding our bulging waistline. *Diabetes Metab Res Rev* 2001;17:347–362.
126. Stewart W, Fleming L. Features of a successful therapeutic fast of 382 days' duration. *Postgrad Med J* 1973;49: 203–209.
127. Thomson T, Glasg M, Runcie J, et al. Treatment of obesity by total fasting for up to 249 days. *Lancet* 1966;ii:992–999.
128. Elia M, Stubbs R, Henry C. Differences in fat, carbohydrate, and protein metabolism between lean and obese subjects undergoing total starvation. *Obes Res* 1999;7:597–604.
129. Elia M. The inter-organ flux of substrates in fed and fasted man, as indicated by arteriovenous balance studies. *Nutr Res Rev* 1991;4:3–31.
130. Owen O, Smalley KJ, D'Alessio A, et al. Protein, fat, and carbohydrate requirements during starvation: anaplerosis and cataplerosis. *Am J Clin Nutr* 1998;68:12–34.
131. Goschke H. Mechanism of glucose intolerance during fasting: differences between lean and obese subjects. *Metabolism* 1977;26:1147–1153.
132. Bray GA. Obesity: historical development of scientific and cultural ideas. *Int J Obes* 1990;14:909–926.
133. Bray G. Historical framework for the development of ideas about obesity. In: Bray GA, Bouchard C, James WPT, eds. *Handbook of obesity.* New York: Marcel Dekker Inc, 1998:1–29.
134. Gamble C. *The Paleolithic settlement of Europe.* Cambridge: Cambridge University Press, 1986.
135. Neel J. Diabetes mellitus: A "thrifty" genotype rendered detrimental by "progress?" *Am J Hum Genet* 1962;14: 353–362.
136. Neel J. The thrifty genotype revisited. In: Kobberling J, Tattersall R, eds. *The genetics of diabetes mellitus.* Amsterdam: Academic Press, 1982:S2–S9.
137. Neel J. The "thrifty genotype" in 1998. *Nutr Rev* 1999;57:S2–S9.
138. Williams GC. Pleiotropy, natural selection, and the evolution of senescence. *Evolution* 1957;11:398–411.
139. Ikeda H, West DB, Pustek JJ, et al. Intraventricular insulin reduces food intake and body weight of lean but not obese Zucker rats. *Appetite* 1986;7:381–386.
140. Woods SC, Lotter EC, McKay LD, et al. Chronic intracerebroventricular infusion of insulin reduces food intake and body weight of baboons. *Nature* 1979;282:503–505.
141. Assali AR, Beigel Y, Schreibman R, et al. Weight gain and insulin resistance during nicotine replacement therapy. *Clin Cardiol* 1999;22:357–360.
142. Eckel RH. Insulin resistance: an adaptation for weight maintenance. *Lancet* 1992;340:1452–1453.
143. Swinburn BA, Nyomba BL, Saad MF, et al. Insulin resistance associated with lower rates of weight gain in Pima Indians. *J Clin Invest* 1991;88:168–173.
144. Travers SH, Jeffers B, Eckel RH. Insulin resistance during puberty and future fat accumulation. *J Clin Endocrinol Metab* 2002;87:3814–3818.
145. Hodge AM, Dowse GK, Alberti KG, et al. Relationship of insulin resistance to weight gain in nondiabetic Asian Indian, Creole, and Chinese Mauritians. Mauritius Non-communicable Disease Study Group. *Metabolism* 1996;45:627–633.
146. Valdez R, Mitchell BD, Haffner SM, et al. Predictors of weight change in a bi-ethnic population. The San Antonio Heart Study. *Int J Obes Relat Metab Disord* 1994;18:85–91.
147. Odeleye OE, de Courten M, Pettitt DJ, Ravussin E. Fasting hyperinsulinemia is a predictor of increased body weight gain and obesity in Pima Indian children. *Diabetes* 1997;46:1341–1345.
148. Schwartz MW, Boyko EJ, Kahn SE, et al. Reduced insulin secretion: an independent predictor of body weight gain. *J Clin Endocrinol Metab* 1995;80:1571–1576.
149. Kulkarni RN, Bruning JC, Winnay JN, et al. Tissue-specific knockout of the insulin receptor in pancreatic beta cells creates an insulin secretory defect similar to that in type 2 diabetes. *Cell* 1999;96:329–339.
150. Friedman JM, Halaas JL. Leptin and the regulation of body weight in mammals. *Nature* 1998;395:763–770.
151. Chehab F, Lim M, Lu R. Correction of the sterility defect in homozygous obese female mice by treatment with the human recombinant leptin. *Nat Genet* 1996;12:318–320.
152. Fan W, Boston B, Kesterson R, et al. Role of melanocortinergic neurons in feeding and the agouti obesity syndrome. *Nature* 1997;385:165–168.
153. Mountjoy KG, Mortrud MT, Low MJ, et al. Localization of the melanocortin-4 receptor (MC4-R) in neuroendocrine and autonomic control circuits in the brain. *Mol Endocrinol* 1994;8:1298–1308.

154. Huszar D. Targeted disruptions of the melanocortin-4 receptor results in obesity in mice. *Cell* 1997;88:131–141.
155. Cody J. Haplosufficiency of the melanocortin-4 receptor gene in individuals with deletions of 18q. *Hum Genet* 1999;105:424–427.
156. Cone R. Haploinsufficiency of the melanocortin-4 receptor: part of a thrifty genotype. *J Clin Invest* 2000;106:185–187.
157. Auwerx J. PPARγ: the ultimate thrifty gene. *Diabetologia* 1999;42:1033–1049.
158. Lenhard JM. PPAR gamma/RXR as a molecular target for diabetes. *Receptors Channels* 2001;7:249–258.
159. Spiegelman BM. PPAR-gamma: adipogenic regulator and thiazolidinedione receptor. *Diabetes* 1998;47:507–514.
160. Bar-Tana J. Peroxisome proliferator-activated receptor gamma (PPARgamma) activation and its consequences in humans. *Toxicol Lett* 2001;120:9–19.
161. Chilcott J, Tappenden P, Jones ML, et al. A systematic review of the clinical effectiveness of pioglitazone in the treatment of type 2 diabetes mellitus. *Clin Ther* 2001;23:1792–1823.
162. Kubota N, Terauchi Y, Miki H, et al. PPAR gamma mediates high-fat diet-induced adipocyte hypertrophy and insulin resistance. *Mol Cell* 1999;4:597–609.
163. Li WD, Lee JH, Price RA. The peroxisome proliferator-activated receptor gamma 2 Pro12Ala mutation is associated with early onset extreme obesity and reduced fasting glucose. *Mol Genet Metab* 2000;70:159–161.
164. Evans D, de Heer J, Hagemann C, et al. Association between the P12A and c1431t polymorphisms in the peroxisome proliferator activated receptor gamma (PPAR gamma) gene and type 2 diabetes. *Exp Clin Endocrinol Diabetes* 2001;109:151–154.
165. Mori H, Ikegami H, Kawaguchi Y, et al. The Pro12→Ala substitution in PPAR-gamma is associated with resistance to development of diabetes in the general population: possible involvement in impairment of insulin secretion in individuals with type 2 diabetes. *Diabetes* 2001;50:891–894.
166. Stefan N, Fritsche A, Haring H, et al. Effect of experimental elevation of free fatty acids on insulin secretion and insulin sensitivity in healthy carriers of the Pro12Ala polymorphism of the peroxisome proliferator-activated receptor-gamma2 gene. *Diabetes* 2001;50:1143–1148.
167. Swarbrick MM, Chapman CM, McQuillan BM, et al. A Pro12Ala polymorphism in the human peroxisome proliferator-activated receptor-gamma 2 is associated with combined hyperlipidaemia in obesity. *Eur J Endocrinol* 2001;144:277–282.
168. Iwata E, Matsuda H, Fukuda T, et al. Mutations of the peroxisome proliferator-activated receptor gamma (PPAR gamma) gene in a Japanese population: the Pro12Ala mutation in PPAR gamma 2 is associated with lower concentrations of serum total and non-HDL cholesterol. *Diabetologia* 2001;44:1354–1355.
169. Schneider J, Kreuzer J, Hamann A, et al. The proline 12 alanine substitution in the peroxisome proliferator-activated receptor-gamma2 gene is associated with lower lipoprotein lipase activity in vivo. *Diabetes* 2002;51:867–870.
170. Wang XL, Oosterhof J, Duarte N. Peroxisome proliferator-activated receptor gamma C161→T polymorphism and coronary artery disease. *Cardiovasc Res* 1999;44:588–594.
171. Clement K, Hercberg S, Passinge B, et al. The Pro115Gln and Pro12Ala PPAR gamma gene mutations in obesity and type 2 diabetes. *Int J Obes Relat Metab Disord* 2000;24:391–393.
172. Mori Y, Kim-Motoyama H, Katakura T, et al. Effect of the Pro12Ala variant of the human peroxisome proliferator-activated receptor gamma 2 gene on adiposity, fat distribution, and insulin sensitivity in Japanese men. *Biochem Biophys Res Commun* 1998;251:195–198.
173. Ristow M, Muller-Wieland D, Pfeiffer A, et al. Obesity associated with a mutation in a genetic regulator of adipocyte differentiation. *N Engl J Med* 1998;339:953–959.
174. Meirhaeghe A, Fajas L, Helbecque N, et al. A genetic polymorphism of the peroxisome proliferator-activated receptor gamma gene influences plasma leptin levels in obese humans. *Hum Mol Genet* 1998;7:435–440.
175. Miles PD, Barak Y, He W, et al. Improved insulin-sensitivity in mice heterozygous for PPAR-gamma deficiency. *J Clin Invest* 2000;105:287–292.
176. Setoguchi K, Misaki Y, Terauchi Y, et al. Peroxisome proliferator-activated receptor-gamma haploinsufficiency enhances B cell proliferative responses and exacerbates experimentally induced arthritis. *J Clin Invest* 2001;108:1667–1675.
177. Yamauchi T, Kamon J, Waki H, et al. The mechanisms by which both heterozygous peroxisome proliferator-activated receptor gamma (PPARgamma) deficiency and PPARgamma agonist improve insulin resistance. *J Biol Chem* 2001;276:41245–41254.
178. Yamauchi T, Waki H, Kamon J, et al. Inhibition of RXR and PPARgamma ameliorates diet-induced obesity and type 2 diabetes. *J Clin Invest* 2001;108:1001–1013.
178a. Brown NS, Smart A, Sharma V, et al. Thyroid hormone resistance and increased metabolic rate in the RXR-gamma–deficient mouse. *J Clin Invest* 2000;106:73–79.
179. Benedict FG. *A study of prolonged fasting.* Publication no. 201. Washington, D.C.: Carnegie Institution, 1915: 1–416.
180. Cutler RG. Evolutionary biology of senescence. In: Behnke J, Finch C, Moment G, eds. *The biology of aging.* New York: Plenum Publishing, 1978:311–360.
181. Hoyert DL, Arias E, Smith BL, et al. Deaths: final data for 1999. *National Vital Statistics Reports* 2001;49:1–113.
182. Kather H, Wieland E, Scheurer A, et al. Influences of variation in total energy intake and dietary composition on regulation of fat cell lipolysis in ideal-weight subjects. *J Clin Invest* 1987;80:566–572.
183. Sniderman AD, Maslowska M, Cianflone K. Of mice and men (and women) and the acylation-stimulating protein pathway. *Curr Opin Lipidol* 2000;11:291–296.

184. Weyer C, Funahashi T, Tanaka S, et al. Hypoadiponectinemia in obesity and type 2 diabetes: close association with insulin resistance and hyperinsulinemia. *J Clin Endocrinol Metab* 2001;86:1930–1935.
185. Moller DE. Potential role of TNF-alpha in the pathogenesis of insulin resistance and type 2 diabetes. *Trends Endocrinol Metab* 2000;11:212–217.
186. van Harmelen V, Ariapart P, Hoffstedt J, et al. Increased adipose angiotensinogen gene expression in human obesity. *Obes Res* 2000;8:337–341.
187. Gorzelniak K, Engeli S, Janke J, et al. Hormonal regulation of the human adipose-tissue renin–angiotensin system: relationship to obesity and hypertension. *J Hypertens* 2002;20:965–973.
188. Fink AN, Frishman WH, Azizad M, et al. Use of prostacyclin and its analogues in the treatment of cardiovascular disease. *Heart Dis* 1999;1:29–40.
189. Negrel R, Gaillard D, Ailhaud G. Prostacyclin as a potent effector of adipose-cell differentiation. *Biochem J* 1989;257:399–405.
190. Alessi MC, Bastelica D, Morange P, et al. Plasminogen activator inhibitor 1, transforming growth factor-beta1, and BMI are closely associated in human adipose tissue during morbid obesity. *Diabetes* 2000;49:1374–1380.
191. Wabitsch M, Hauner H, Heinze E, et al. The role of growth hormone/insulin-like growth factors in adipocyte differentiation. *Metabolism* 1995;44:45–49.
192. Crandall DL, Quinet EM, Morgan GA, et al. Synthesis and secretion of plasminogen activator inhibitor-1 by human preadipocytes. *J Clin Endocrinol Metab* 1999;84:3222–3227.
193. McCarty MF. Hemostatic concomitants of syndrome X. *Med Hypotheses* 1995;44:179–193.
194. McDermott MF. TNF and TNFR biology in health and disease. *Cell Mol Biol* 2001;47:619–635.
195. Hirano T, Ishihara K, Hibi M. Roles of STAT3 in mediating the cell growth, differentiation and survival signals relayed through the IL-6 family of cytokine receptors. *Oncogene* 2000;19:2548–2556.
196. Esterbauer H, Krempler F, Oberkofler H, et al. The complement system: a pathway linking host defense and adipocyte biology. *Eur J Clin Invest* 1999;29:653–656.
197. Bulun SE, Mahendroo MS, Simpson ER. Aromatase gene expression in adipose tissue: relationship to breast cancer. *J Steroid Biochem Mol Biol* 1994;49:319–326.
198. Corbould AM, Judd SJ, Rodgers RJ. Expression of types 1, 2, and 3 17 beta-hydroxysteroid dehydrogenase in subcutaneous abdominal and intra-abdominal adipose tissue of women. *J Clin Endocrinol Metab* 1998;83:187–194.
199. Voisey J, van Daal A. Agouti: from mouse to man, from skin to fat. *Pigment Cell Res* 2002;15:10–18.
200. Lerner J. Effectors of amino acid transport processes in animal cell membranes. *Comp Biochem Physiol A* 1985; 81:713–739.
201. Miers WR, Barrett EJ. The role of insulin and other hormones in the regulation of amino acid and protein metabolism in humans. *J Basic Clin Physiol Pharmacol* 1998;9:235–253.
202. Kimball SR, Vary TC, Jefferson LS. Regulation of protein synthesis by insulin. *Annu Rev Physiol* 1994;56:321–348.
203. Ryder JW, Chibalin AV, Zierath JR. Intracellular mechanisms underlying increases in glucose uptake in response to insulin or exercise in skeletal muscle. *Acta Physiol Scand* 2001;171:249–257.
204. Srivastava AK, Pandey SK. Potential mechanism(s) involved in the regulation of glycogen synthesis by insulin. *Mol Cell Biochem* 1998;182:135–141.
205. Cherrington AD, Edgerton D, Sindelar DK. The direct and indirect effects of insulin on hepatic glucose production in vivo. *Diabetologia* 1998;41:987–996.
206. Bergman RN. Non-esterified fatty acids and the liver: why is insulin secreted into the portal vein? *Diabetologia* 2000;43:946–952.
207. Sparks JD, Sparks CE. Insulin regulation of triacylglycerol-rich lipoprotein synthesis and secretion. *Biochim Biophys Acta* 1994;1215:9–32.
208. Sadur CN, Eckel RH. Insulin stimulation of adipose tissue lipoprotein lipase. Use of the euglycemic clamp technique. *J Clin Invest* 1982;69:1119–1125.
209. Farese RV Jr, Yost TJ, Eckel RH. Tissue-specific regulation of lipoprotein lipase activity by insulin/glucose in normal-weight humans. *Metabolism* 1991;40:214–216.
210. Lewis GF, Steiner G. Acute effects of insulin in the control of VLDL production in humans. Implications for the insulin-resistant state. *Diabetes Care* 1996;19:390–393.
211. Fajas L, Debril MB, Auwerx J. Peroxisome proliferator-activated receptor-gamma: from adipogenesis to carcinogenesis. *J Mol Endocrinol* 2001;27:1–9.
212. Sood V, Colleran K, Burge MR. Thiazolidinediones: a comparative review of approved uses. *Diabetes Technol Ther* 2000;2:429–440.
213. Kawai T, Hirose H, Seto Y, et al. Troglitazone ameliorates lipotoxicity in the beta cell line INS-1 expressing PPAR gamma. *Diabetes Res Clin Pract* 2002;56:83–92.
214. Altiok S, Xu M, Spiegelman BM. PPARgamma induces cell cycle withdrawal: inhibition of E2F/DP DNA-binding activity via down-regulation of PP2A. *Genes Dev* 1997;11:1987–1998.
215. Clark RB, Bishop-Bailey D, Estrada-Hernandez T, et al. The nuclear receptor PPAR gamma and immunoregulation: PPAR gamma mediates inhibition of helper T cell responses. *J Immunol* 2000;164:1364–1371.
216. Molavi B, Rasouli N, Mehta JL. Peroxisome proliferator-activated receptor ligands as antiatherogenic agents: panacea or another Pandora's box? *J Cardiovasc Pharmacol Ther* 2002;7:1–8.
217. Khandoudi N, Delerive P, Berrebi-Bertrand I, et al. Rosiglitazone, a peroxisome proliferator-activated receptor-gamma, inhibits the Jun NH(2)-terminal kinase/activating protein 1 pathway and protects the heart from ischemia/reperfusion injury. *Diabetes* 2002;51:1507–1514.

2

Genetic Influences on Obesity

David B. Allison, Angelo Pietrobelli, Myles S. Faith, Kevin R. Fontaine,
Eva Gropp, and José R. Fernández

This chapter reviews studies regarding the genetic influences on obesity or, more generally, adiposity. This task is challenging because this area has become so active that it is becoming a field unto itself. Moreover, in what has been called the "postgenomics" era (1), the boundaries between genetic research (which more and more is known as "functional genomics") and other areas, such as physiology, are becoming less distinct. The authors consider this a desirable and exciting turn of events. This chapter attempts to capture some of this excitement and to focus a bit more on areas in which new progress is being made (e.g., linkage studies and mutation detection) or on those that hold great promise for progress in the near future (e.g., pharmacogenomics and large-scale expression studies). In doing so, somewhat lesser attention had to be given to other important areas that have been well reviewed elsewhere. Two notable areas that are not discussed at any length are the commingling and segregation analyses that provided the earliest evidence for major genes (2–4) and the results of association tests with candidate genes. Association tests with candidate genes have become so numerous that they almost require a review of their own. Although a number of intriguing association findings have been reported, very few have been convincingly shown to be associated with obesity when the body of data is reviewed. The most notable exception is the melanocortin-4 receptor (MC4R) gene polymorphisms, which have been proven to be associated with obesity. For a thorough, if not exhaustive, review, see Rankinen et al. (5). Alternatively, some topics that have been studied for a long time but that have not been thoroughly reviewed elsewhere in the literature on obesity (e.g., selective breeding studies) are covered.

This chapter begins by reviewing the evidence for the genetic influences on adiposity, including selective breeding studies in nonhuman animals, followed by twin, family, and adoption studies in humans. The potential role of genetic factors is reviewed by explaining differences in obesity rates among populations of different ethnicity. The discussion then shifts to the common fallacy that a genetic influence on adiposity implies that behavior is not involved and to the evidence that genes may influence the development of obesity largely through their effects on food intake and activity behaviors. Subsequently, a review of what genetic studies have revealed about the environmental influences on human obesity is included. This is followed by an examination of the quantitative trait locus (QTL) linkage studies conducted in both nonhumans and humans that have provided more modern evidence for major gene effects. The relatively recent identification of humans with obesity caused by mutations in single genes is described next. Finally, the conclusion discusses the newer areas of pharmacogenomics and large-scale gene-expression studies and how they have and can be used to study obesity.

EVIDENCE FOR GENETIC EFFECTS

Selection Studies

Obesity is probably a highly polygenic and complex disorder (5,6). Because of this, obesity is not inherited in a typical mendelian fashion. Thus, to the casual observer, its genetic component is less immediately obvious, and, for many years, the genetic contribution to obesity was doubted. Many geneticists consider the ability to breed selectively for increased or decreased values of a quantitative trait to be among the strongest evidence possible for a genetic influence on that trait (7,8). By this criterion, exceptionally strong evidence for genetic influences on a number of obesity-related traits has existed for at least decades in laboratory animals (9) and even longer in agricultural livestock (10,11). The number of selection experiments conducted in various species is enormous, and an exhaustive review is beyond the scope of this chapter. Because studies of laboratory animals are slightly better known, they are not commented on in detail here (12). Instead, a selective summary highlights the range of species and phenotypes for which such effects have been demonstrated, focusing mainly on agriculture and aquaculture.

Figure 2.1 illustrates the ironic fact that while technologic alterations of the environment have led to ever fatter humans (13), the use of genetic technology (selective breed-

Changes in Pig Backfat and Human Mean BMI

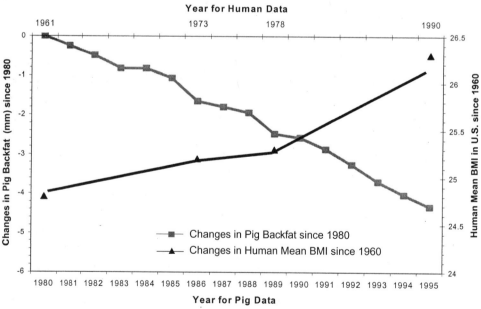

FIG. 2.1. Opposite changes in human body mass indexes (BMIs) among United States adults and back-fat thickness of the Canadian Yorkshire pig over the recent past. Pig data are from the Canadian Swine Breeders Association. Changes in back-fat thickness were measured in millimeters and were adjusted to 100 kg. The study included animals born between 1980 and 1995. Human data were taken from the National Health and Nutrition Examination Surveys, 1960 to 1991 as reported in Kuczmarski RJ, Flegal KM, Campbell SM, et al. Increasing prevalence of overweight among US adults. *JAMA* 1994;272:205–211, with permission. Mean BMI was determined for a United States population of men and women aged 20 through 74 years and was measured during four different 3-year to 5-year periods between 1960 and 1991.

ing) has led to ever leaner swine (14). This figure dramatically shows the powerful effects that manipulations of both the genotype and the environment can have.

Table 2.1 summarizes some selective breeding experiments for obesity-related traits. As the table shows, a large number of obesity-related traits have been successfully manipulated by selective breeding in a wide diversity of species, which demonstrates several important things. First, the large number and diversity of species indicate that genetic influences on adiposity are not some strange anomaly confined to mice but that they exist across species and that no reason exists for believing that humans are an exception. The patterns of results indicate a strong degree of genetic correlation among many of these traits and probably suggest that many genes are involved in these traits. Second, the traits that have been successfully selected include those related to the amount and distribution of adiposity, the metabolic aspects, and the behavioral aspects. This implies that genetic effects probably operate on each of these traits. Moreover, it highlights the fact that numerous animal models exist for studying specific obesity-related traits, and that more can be generated with just a few generations of selection. Some of these models have yet to be well exploited. For example, fish have ample body fat, but most have little to no subcutaneous adipose tissue. Virtually all of their body fat is intramuscular (IM) (70). IM fat has recently generated great interest because of its potential role in human health (71). Thus, the study of these strains of fish selected for more or less body fat either alone or in comparison to mammalian species that have a lot of IM and non-IM body fat (72) may yield important insights into the genetic causes and effects of IM fat.

Twin, Family, and Adoption Studies

Twin studies have been an integral part of research into the genetics of obesity (6). Dating back more than 100 years to Galton (73), twin studies examining the genetics of body composition proliferated in the 1970s through the 1990s and they continue today. Detailed reviews of twin studies are provided elsewhere (74). One of the fundamental goals of twin studies is to decompose interindividual differences in body fat into the following three components: heritability (h^2), shared environment (c^2), and nonshared environment (e^2). *Heritability* is defined as the proportion of within-population variance in a trait (e.g., body fat) that is due to within-population genetic variations. *Shared environment* refers to those aspects of the environment that are perfectly correlated among siblings in the same household (e.g., number of televisions in the home or number of pieces of exercise equipment). Finally, *nonshared environment* refers to those aspects of the home environment that are not correlated among siblings (e.g., differential parenting toward siblings). By examining the pattern of correlations among pairs of individuals who share differing degrees of genetic kinship, the correlations can be mathematically decomposed into proportions of phenotypic variance resulting from genetic and environmental factors. For derivations and details, see Neale and Cardon (75) and Fisher (76).

Reviews of the literature on twins suggest that, on balance, genes account for approximately 50% to 80% of the variation in body mass, with the remaining variance being attributable to nonshared environmental influences (6,74). Heritability estimates appear to be higher in children and adolescents (77,78). A remarkably consistent finding across all ages is the apparent lack of common environmental influences on body fat, an intriguing dilemma that was explored by Hopper (79).

Family designs offer an alternative to the classic twin design for estimating heritability by testing patterns of phenotypic associations among family members (74). Nuclear family designs that examine only sibling–sibling or parent–sibling correlations cannot disentangle the genetic from the environmental influences. However, the combination of

TABLE 2.1. *Some obesity-related traits that have been shown to respond to selective breeding*

Phenotype	Mouse	Rat	Mink	Rabbit	Turkey	Chicken	Ducks	Quail	Pigs	Sheep	Cattle	Salmon	Trout	Guppy fish
Weight	Allen and McCarthy (15); Eisen (16); Falconer (17)	Levin et al. (18)	Lagerkvist et al. (19)	—	Nestor (20)	Vanwambek et al. (21)	Farhat and Chavaz (22)	Marks (23,24)	Newton et al. (25)	Ghoneim et al. (26)	Koch (27)	Refstie and Steine (28)	—	Ryman (29)
Growth rate	Sutherland et al. (30)	Notter et al. (31)	—	—	—	Konarzewski et al. (32)	Maruyama et al. (33)	Marks (24)	Sather and Fredeen (34); Standal (35)	Vesely and Peters (36)	Andersen et al. (37); Perry and Arthur (38)	Gjedrem (39)	Kincaid et al. (40)	—
Fat mass or percent	Allen and McCarthy (15); Beniwal et al. (41); Sharp et al. (42)	Levin et al. (18)	—	Piles and Pla (43)	—	Geraert et al. (44)	Farhat and Chavaz (22)	Marks (45)	Standal (35)	—	Aass and Vangen (46)	Gjedrem (39)	—	—
Fat distribution	Allen and McCarthy (15); Hayes and McCarthy (47)	—	—	—	—	—	Baeza et al. (48); Maruyama et al. (33)	Marks and Washburn (49)	Standal (35)	—	—	Gjedrem (39)	—	—

Trait								
Lean mass and/or muscle mass	Hooper (50); Beniwal et al. (41)	Notter et al. (31)	—	—	Farhat and Chavaz (22)	Marks (51)	Standal (35)	—
Food intake	Meyer and Hill (52); Parker and Bhatti (53)	—	Pym and Nicholls (54); O'Sullivan et al. (55)	Farhat and Chavaz (22)	Marks (56)	Cameron et al. (57); Vangen (58)	—	Aass and Vangen (46)
Feed efficiency	Eisen and Durrant (59); Kownacki et al. (60)	Notter et al. (31)	Pym and Nicholls (54); O'Sullivan et al. (55)	—	Marks (56)	Sather and Fredeen (34); Vangen (58)	Rompala et al. (61)	—
Intramuscular fat	—	—	—	Baeza et al. (48)	—	Serra et al. (63)	—	Hernandez et al. (62)
Activity	Swallow et al. (64,65); Zhan et al. (66)	—	—	—	—	—	—	Aass and Vangen (46)
Resting metabolic rate (RMR) or temperature	Rhodes et al. (67); Kownacki et al. (68)	—	Konarzewski et al. (32)	—	Maeda et al. (69)	—	Rompala et al. (61)	—

parental information and twin data can yield estimates of heritability, as well as estimates for the nonparental shared environment, the nonshared environment, and assortative mating. Using this method, Maes et al. (80) estimated the heritability of the sum of skinfolds to be 0.79 for men and 0.90 for women. Still other investigators have conducted "extended family designs" to estimate heritability from analyses of first-degree and second-degree relationships (81,82).

Adoption studies provide yet another approach for estimating heritability based on the similarity of adopted children's body weight to that of their adoptive and biologic parents, respectively. Sørensen and Stunkard (83) and Maes et al. (84) provide thorough reviews of this literature, including the Danish study (85), the Iowa study (86), the Colorado study (87), the Quebec study (81), and the Take Off Pounds Sensibly (TOPS) study (88). On balance, the studies reliably show that adopted children are more similar to their biologic parents than to their adoptive parents. What is particularly striking is the low correlation between adoptive children and parents, with correlations that are roughly in the range of 0.0 to 0.1. Recent analyses of the Colorado adoption study suggest heritability estimates of approximately 0.35 to 0.65 for children from 2 to 9 years of age (87).

Extensions of the classic twin design have been developed to provide more precise and perhaps more accurate information on genetic contributions to obesity. A recent method using "virtual twins" bypasses an inherent limitation of the classic twin design—its inability to estimate simultaneously variance resulting from the shared environment and genetic dominance (i.e., interactions among different genetic loci). This design uses information on monozygotic (MZ) and dizygotic (DZ) twins in addition to that of so-called virtual twins, which are same-sex, age-matched unrelated siblings reared together since infancy (89). Virtual twin pairs consist of either two adoptees or one biologic offspring and one adopted child. Using data from these pairs, the researcher can simultaneously estimate additive genetic, dominant and/or nonadditive genetic, shared environmental, and nonshared environmental influences on a phenotype. Using this method, Segal and Allison (90) found that the common environment may have a stronger impact than the previous studies suggested. They found that almost all of the genetic influences were due to dominance or to other nonadditive effects (61%), with shared and nonshared environmental influences accounting for 25% and 14% of the variance, respectively.

Another extension of the classic twin design is the study of extended twinships. Maes et al. (74) analyzed data from the Virginia 30,000 sample—a pooled database that combines information on more than 14,500 MZ and DZ twins and their parents, siblings, spouses, and children, when available. The results of their "stealth model" indicate that, for women, body mass index (BMI) variation could be partitioned as follows: 39% additive genetics, 26% dominant genetics, 7% to 8% "special environment" (i.e., shared by siblings but no other family members), and 27% nonshared environment.

Finally, to bypass the potential confounds introduced by twin cohabitation, Allison et al. (91) estimated the heritability of BMI among an international sample of MZ twins reared apart (MZAs). Twins from Finland, Japan, and the United States were investigated. Structural equation modeling indicated heritability estimates of 50% to 70%, confirming the results of the previous classic twin studies, as well as those of prior studies of MZAs.

When looking across the twin, adoption, and family studies, a notable divergence of heritability estimates is seen. Possible reasons for this heterogeneity are reviewed by Maes et al. (84). First, twin studies typically yield higher heritability estimates than other family designs. These heritability estimates may be more accurate because twins are perfectly matched for age and sex (for MZ twins). Moreover, twin designs are better able to detect genetic dominance and other forms of nonadditivity. A second issue concerns the nuances of statistical modeling. For example, the few twin studies that modeled particular "twin environment" parameters as part of the analysis (92) yielded smaller heritability estimates than did the balance of studies that did not model such parameters. Maes et al. (84) note that this approach may underestimate dominance effects. Finally, as Maes et al. (74) demonstrate, inconsistent heritability estimates can result from sample size variability. Progressively larger sample sizes yield more consistent heritability estimates, and hence they provide a clearer picture of the probable magnitude of genetic influence. Despite these issues, the balance of twin, adoption, and family studies provides unequivocal support for the notion of genetic influences on body fat. When one considers all of these factors and looks across all classes of information, heritability estimates higher than 0.50 and somewhere around 0.70 appear most reasonable given the current knowledge.

Ethnic Differences and Admixture Studies

One arena that may be underexplored as a source of important information about the genetic influences on obesity is that of ethnic differences. The ethnic diversity of the United States has permitted the identification of differences in obesity-related phenotypes among European Americans and other ethnic groups, such as African Americans (93), Asian Americans (94), Pima Indians (95,96), and Puerto Ricans (97).

The observation of ethnic differences in obesity levels opens the question of what relative contributions among-group differences in genetic and environmental factors make to these among-group phenotypic differences. In addition to the influence of genes, phenotypic differences among populations might also result from the effect of environmental factors. One such factor, or marker, thereof that has frequently been conjectured as potentially accounting for observed ethnic differences in obesity is socioeconomic status (SES). Therefore, one may ask whether the observed among-group phenotypic differences remain after controlling for SES. Harrell and Gore (98) observed that, after controlling for income and education—two indicators of SES—African-American women remained more than twice as likely as to be obese than European-American women. Furthermore, as Allison et al. (99) discuss, several studies indicate that the differences in obesity-related traits between African-American and European-American women remain, even after removing the effect of SES.

When considering genetic influences on differences among ethnic groups in adiposity, the reader must remember (as was pointed out in the previous section) that twin, family, and adoption studies, which estimate the heritability of adiposity measures, are estimating the fraction of the *within-population* variation in adiposity that is due to *within-population* genotypic variations. Heritability estimates from traditional twin, family, and adoption studies say nothing about the source of among-population differences in adiposity. Estimating the sources of among-population variations requires alternative study designs.

One such design is built on the recognition that, within any self-defined ethnic group, substantial genotypic variations usually exist among members. Some of these within-group genotypic variations are the result of differential degrees of genetic admixture from two or more ancestral populations. So, for example, among people who define themselves as African Americans, the proportion of their genome that is descended from Africans, Europeans, and/or Native Americans varies substantially from person to person. If the hypothesis is that the genetic aspects of African ancestry predispose individuals to greater adiposity, then, even within a group of individuals who all define themselves as *African American,* those with a greater degree of African ancestry will demonstrate greater degrees of adiposity. Therefore, if the degree of admixture from ancestral populations that individuals have within a current admixed ethnic group is estimated, then those individual admixture estimates can be correlated with individual adiposity measurements. Significant nonzero correlations in the predicted direction would suggest that some nonzero proportion of the observed differences *among* ethnic groups is genetic in origin. Methods have been established for estimating the degree of individual admixture based on DNA markers (100).

Williams et al. (101) present an application of the use of individual genetic admixture in obesity-related phenotypes. These authors used an admixed sample from European-American and Pima Indian parental populations to obtain individual estimates of European-American admixture for every subject. Regression analysis of quantitative predictors of type II diabetes mellitus and BMI shows significant inverse relations with individual admixture (IA) when it is controlled for sex and age. More recently, Fernandez et al. (102) showed significant positive correlations between individual African ancestry estimates and BMI among African Americans. Collectively, these two studies suggest that some of the factors that cause Pima Indians and African Americans to have, on average, higher BMIs than European Americans are genetic. Finally, although research designs using populations of admixed ethnic background have yet to be used extensively, they may also result in the identification of specific genetic variants influencing disease-related phenotypes (103). The mapping of disease-related phenotypes in admixed populations is known as *mapping through admixture linkage disequilibrium* (104,105).

GENETIC INFLUENCES ON BEHAVIORAL PHENOTYPES

In the authors' experience, many people mistakenly assume that the statement that genetic factors influence a trait is tantamount to stating that behaviors, such as eating and activity, are not involved. This is a patently incorrect inference. Genetic influences and behavioral influences are not mutually exclusive categories. That genes can influence behavioral traits is well documented (106). Therefore, part of the way in which genes influence the level of adiposity that one achieves may be through their effects on behaviors. This section reviews the evidence concerning this possibility that has been obtained in both humans and nonhuman animals.

Human Studies

An important, yet surprisingly understudied, issue in the human literature concerns genetic influences on behavioral phenotypes. Ironically, "behavioral" genetic studies of human obesity have historically paid greater attention to body composition and metabolic phenotypes than to behavior *per se* (107). Recognizing the potential contributions of eating and physical activity to obesity onset (108), researchers have begun to bridge behavioral measurements with genetic designs. One of the first systematic twin investigations of human eating behavior collected 7-day food and beverage records from the "free-living environment" (109–113). These studies found that genes accounted for approximately 65% of the variance in total caloric intake and 70% to 80% of the variance in beverage intake (109,110). Other twin studies using self-report methods appear to confirm genetic influences on food intake, attitudes, and preferences (114–121).

Of course, reporting inaccuracies are a major concern when energy intake is estimated by self-report methods (122). Therefore, Faith et al. (123) recently conducted the first twin study to estimate the heritability of *ad libitum* caloric intake that used *behaviorally measured* food intake from a buffet meal eaten in the laboratory. Genes accounted for 24% to 33% of the variance in total caloric intake, and they influenced macronutrient-specific intake.

Even less research has been conducted on the genetics of physical activity in humans (124–126). Analysis of the Quebec family study revealed that approximately 30% of the variance in the level of habitual physical activity, which was estimated from activity records, was due to genetic factors. One noteworthy study of more than 4,000 twin pairs from the Finnish twin registry reported a heritability estimate of 62% for reported physical activity. Using a co-twin control design, Samaras et al. (127) recently illustrated how the interaction of genetics and physical activity levels can have an impact on obesity. Among identical twins who were discordant for participation in moderate-intensity physical activity, corresponding differences with respect to total body fat were found. Specifically, a 2-hour-per-week difference in physical activity among twins was associated with a 1.4-kg difference in total body fat on average. The interaction of physical activity regimens with genetic variations remains a ripe area for research (126).

Animal Studies

Intake

Several lines of evidence indicate that genetic influences on food intake exist in animals. First, a number of mutations have been identified that result in extreme pathologic alterations in food intake. Nelson and Young (128) summarized these well.

> Inactivation of the tyrosine hydroxylase (TH) gene results in dopamine-deficient mice that are adipsic and aphagic. Neurotrophin three receptor (NT-3) –/– mice fail to ingest food and die within 24 h[ours] of birth...as do the Brn-3a–/– mice that lack suckling behavior and perish without evidence of milk ingestion. Hexa–/– and Hexb–/– mice stop feeding behavior at approximately three months of age. Reduced spontaneous "behavior" accompanies impaired drinking responses to water deprivation in angiotensin II type receptor (AT2)-deficient mice. The inability to synthesize noradrenaline and adrenaline due to targeted deletion of the gene for β-hydroxylase (dbh) results in increased food intake corresponding to a higher metabolic rate. (pg. 457)

Moreover, numerous genes that, when mutated in particular ways, confer marked obesity in rodents have been identified (Table 2.2). Although these animal models are clearly *genetically obese,* their obesity is often, but by no means always, largely due to hyperphagia (184). This is true for many of the animals listed in Table 2.2. This is quite dramatically illustrated in the case of the *ob/ob* mouse (185). When fed *ad libitum*, this mouse tends to be about two to three times as heavy as normal controls. In contrast, when these animals have their food intake restricted to the same levels as the normal controls, although they are still heavier than controls, they are far less so (186,187). This is a clear example of genes influencing the development of obesity largely, although not exclusively, through their influence on behavior.

Second, clear evidence indicates that selective breeding can produce large changes in food intake in animals such as pigs (57,58), salmon (39,188), mice (52), chickens (54,189), and ducks (22). This provides support that for the idea of genetic effects on food intake even in cases in which a markedly disturbed "syndromic" obesity is not present.

Third, at least one QTL mapping study has detected a significant QTL for food intake in chickens (190), and at least two studies have detected QTLs for food intake–related variables in mice (191,192). These suggest that some of the genes involved may be of sufficient magnitude to be individually detectable.

Finally, the complexity of the ways in which genes may influence food intake are illustrated by targeted disruption of the thy-1 gene (193). Under ordinary circumstances, mice adjust their ingestive behavior to be more similar to that of other mice in the environment. Thus, social facilitation or inhibition of specific feeding behaviors in the mouse is observed. However, among *thy-1* knockout mice, this social facilitation response is elim-

TABLE 2.2. *Knockout mutants and transgenic models with effects on body composition*

Gene	Major effect on food intake?	Other phenotypic characteristics	Reference
Obesity predisposing mutations (p-locus fat-associated) ATPase	—	Highly increased body fat content	West et al. (129)
5-HT$_{1b}$	—	Increased aggression and impulsivity, reduced or absent locomotor stimulation to some serotonergic drugs, increased vulnerability to drugs of abuse	Scearce-Levie et al. (130)
5-HT$_{2c}$	Yes	Obesity, seizures, nonresponsive to fenfluramines, hyperphagic, insulin resistant	Tecott et al. (131)
Agouti	Yes	Increased diabetes, obesity, tumor susceptibility, and embryonic lethality	Siracusa et al. (132)
β$_1$/β$_2$-Adrenoceptor	—	Increased epididymal and perirenal fat, predisposition to the development of obesity	Din et al. (133)
β$_3$-Adrenoreceptor	Yes	Increased food intake, increased total body fat, decreased lean body mass, predisposition to the development of obesity	Revelli et al. (134)
Bombesin receptor subtype 3	Yes	Mild obesity association with hypertension and impairment of glucose metabolism, reduced metabolic rate, increased feeding efficiency and subsequent hyperphagia	Ohki-Hamazaki et al. (135)
CART	Yes	Increased weight and fat mass	Asnicar et al. (136)
CCK-A receptor	Yes	OLETF rats are diabetic, hyperphagic, and obese; slow patterns of ingestion consistent with a satiety deficit secondary to CCK insensitivity	Schwartz et al. (137)
COX-2 (heterozygous knockouts)	—	Elevated serum leptin	Fain et al. (138)
CYP19 (aromatase)	No	Cannot synthesize endogenous estrogens; progressively accumulate excess intraabdominal adipose tissue; increased adipocyte volume at gonadal and infrarenal sites; reduced spontaneous physical activity levels, reduced glucose oxidation, reduced lean body mass	Jones et al. (139)
ER-α	No	Increased epididymal, perirenal, and inguinal adipose tissue with advancing age; increased epididymal and perirenal adipocyte size and number; insulin resistance and impaired glucose tolerance; reduced energy expenditure	Heine et al. (140)
Fabpi (in males)	—	Increased adiposity; high plasma triglyceride levels	Vassileva et al. (141)
Fat	No	Increased obesity, but lack of hyperphagia and hypercorticism; mild, male-biased diabetes syndrome	Leiter et al. (142)
Follicle-stimulating hormone receptor	—	Obesity and skeletal abnormalities	Danilovich et al. (143)
G-protein alpha subunit (maternal allele)	No	Hypometabolic, normal sensitivity to sympathetic stimulation but decreased activity of the sympathetic nervous system, decreased physical activity and resting energy expenditure	Yu et al. (144)
ICAM-1	—	Increased obesity, hyperinsulinemia, hyperlipemia; males develop hyperglycemia, glucosuria, polyuria, and nephropathy	Matsui et al. (145)
LEP	Yes	Profound obesity, Type II diabetes, hyperphagia	Zhang et al. (146)
LEP-R	Yes	Early-onset morbid obesity, hyperphagia, reduced energy expenditure, hypercortisolemia, alterations in glucose homeostasis, dyslipidemia, infertility due to hypogonadotropic hypogonadism	Clement et al. (147)

MC3R	No	Increased adiposity, reduced lean mass, increased feed efficiency, hypophagic	Chen et al. (148)
MC4R	Yes	Hyperphagia, tendency toward tall stature, hyperinsulinemia, preserved reproductive function	Farooqi et al. (149)
Nhlh2	—	Adult-onset obesity with impaired gonadal growth associated with puberty	Good et al. (150)
Orexin	Yes	Rapid eye movement sleep dysregulation, reduced levels of physical activity	Chemelli et al. (151); Hara et al. (152)
PAI-1	—	Faster weight gain under high-fat diet with no effect on stroma cells; obese animals show elevated plasma triglyceride and decreased plasma glucose levels; nonobese animals display 62% higher plasma insulin levels than the wild-type litter mates	Morange et al. (153)
POMC	—	Increased obesity, defective adrenal development, and altered pigmentation	Yaswen et al. (154)
PPARα	No	Lack of hepatic peroxisomal proliferation, increased obesity, hypercholesterolemia, normal triglycerides and stable caloric intake, sexual dimorphism, steatosis	Costet et al. (155)
PPARγ	—	Protection from insulin resistance under a high-fat diet, overexpression and hypersecretion of leptin, smaller adipocytes, decreased fat mass	Kubota et al. (156)
Preadipocyte factor-1 (PREF-1/DLK-1)	—	Growth retardation; imprinted mode of inheritance in heterozygous form	Moon et al. (157)
Steroidogenic factor-1 (SF-1)	No	Decreased activity level	Majdic et al. (158)
TUB	—	Slow weight gain, retinal and cochlear degeneration, impaired fertility	Stubdal et al. (159)
Obesity resistance mutations			
DAT	—	Resistant to diet-induced obesity, markedly hyperactive; females show inability to lactate and impaired capability to care for their offspring	Gainetdinov et al. (160)
DGAT	—	Lean, resistant to diet-induced obesity, increased energy expenditure and increased activity, altered triglyceride metabolism	Smith et al. (161)
Fabpi (in females)	—	Decreased adiposity, reduced plasma cholesterol level	Vassileva et al. (141)
G-protein alpha subunit (paternal allele)	No	Hypermetabolic, normal sensitivity to sympathetic stimulation but increased activity of the sympathetic nervous system, increased physical activity and resting energy expenditure	Yu et al. (144)
HMG1C	No	Deficiency in fat tissue, resistant to diet-induced obesity, reduction in the obesity induced by leptin deficiency	Anand and Chada (162)
IKKβ (heterozygote knockouts)	—	Reduced glucose, insulin, and free fatty acid concentrations	Yuan et al. (163)
Klotho gene	No	Barely detectable amount of white adipose tissue, brown adipose tissue preserved, increased glucose tolerance and insulin sensitivity, lower body temperature, no difference in food intake	Mori et al. (164)
Mahogany	Yes	Decreased obesity and hyperinsulinemia, increased linear growth, hyperphagia, increased RMR	Dinulescu et al. (165)
MCH	Yes	Hypophagia, increased RMR	Shimada et al. (166)
Perilipin	Yes	Hyperphagia but reduced body fat mass and increased protein content; smaller adipocytes, lower plasma leptin levels, and elevated basal rate of lipolysis; resistant to diet-induced obesity	Martinez-Botas et al. (167)
Protein kinase A	—	Lean, resistant to diet-induced obesity, increased basal rate of lipolysis	Planas et al. (168)
PTP-1B	Yes	Enhanced insulin sensitivity, obesity resistant in response to high fat diet but phenotypically similar to normal on chow, increased RMR, increased food intake relative to body mass, increased core temperature	Elchebly et al. (169); Kennedy (170); Klaman et al. (171)

(continued)

41

TABLE 2.2. *Continued.*

Gene	Major effect on food intake?	Other phenotypic characteristics	Reference
Obesity resistance mutations (contd.)			
TNF-α	—	Reduced body weight but no prevention from weight gain, lower plasma glucose and plasma insulin levels, improved glucose tolerance and insulin sensitivity	Ventre et al. (172); Uysal et al. (173)
TNF-α receptor (p75)	—	Only in male animals: lower body weight and lower plasma insulin levels, improvement in chronic insulin sensitivity, decreased weight gain under a high fat diet	Schreyer et al. (174)
UCP-1	—	Cold sensitive, lean, normal resting metabolic rate, normal feed efficiency, high respiration rate	Monemdjou et al. (175)
UCP-3 (overexpression in skeletal muscle)[a]	Yes	Hyperphagia, reduced weight and adiposity, lower fasting glucose and insulin, normal activity, increased muscle temperature but normal core temperature	Clapham et al. (176)
VGF	—	Increased RMR, increased activity	Hahm et al. (177)
Myostatin	—	Massive muscling; marked leanness	McPherron et al. (178); McPherron and Lee (179)
FOXC2 (transgenic overexpressors)	—	Reduced fat, serum glucose, and serum insulin; white adipose tissue takes on appearance of brown adipose tissue	Cederberg et al. (180)
VLDL receptor	—	Leanness despite high fat diet; increased postprandial plasma triglycerides	Goudriaan et al. (181)

Abbreviations: ATPase, adenosine triphosphatase; CART, cocaine- and amphetamine-regulated transcript; CCK-A, cholecystokinin-A; COX-2, cyclooxygenase-2; CYP, cytochrome P450 enzyme; DAT, dopamine transporter; DGAT, diacylglycerol acyltransferase; ER, estrogen receptor; HMG, human menopausal gonadotropin; HMG1C, high motility group 1c; 5-HT, 5-hydroxytryptamine; ICAM-1, intracellular adhesion molecule-1; IKK, IKappa B kinase; MC3R, melanocortin-3 receptor; MCH, mean corpuscular hemoglobin; OLETF, Otsuka Long-Evans Tokushima Fatty; PAI-1, plasminogen activator inhibitor; POMC, proopiomelanocortin; PPARα, peroxisome proliferator-activated receptor α; PTP-1B, protein tyrosine phosphatase-1B; RMR, resting metabolic rate; TNF, tumor necrosis factor; UCP, uncoupling protein; VLDL, very low density lipoprotein.

[a]Targeted disruption of the UCP-3 gene does not alter any obesity-related phenotype obviously (182). Discrepancies between these types of experimental manipulations have been previously reported (183), and they may indicate functional redundancy between the targeted gene and other known or unknown genes.

inated. Social facilitation effects on feeding in humans have also been shown to exist, and they are fairly large (113). This suggests the possibility that some of the genetic influences on food intake and body weight may involve responsiveness to social stimuli that affect food intake.

Activity

Several selection experiments have shown that mice can be selected for activity levels (194). In some cases, the types of activity measures used may be highly influenced by anxiety levels and the genes for anxiety (195). However, total activity has been estimated to have a heritability of more than 54% among male albino mice from the ICR strain (196). Interestingly, Dunnington et al. (196) found a negative correlation between total activity and body weight, suggesting that the genetic effects on body weight in these male mice may work in part through their effects on activity–energy expenditure.

Recently, Swallow et al. (64,65) and Zhan et al. (66) published data on the effects of at least 14 generations of selection for increased spontaneous activity, such as wheel running. Several interesting findings emerged. First, clear increases in wheel running were seen among both male and female mice, indicating the clear genetic influence on this aspect of spontaneous activity. Second, the response to selection was quite specific. In other words, although total activity via wheel running increased dramatically, this occurred solely through an increase in revolutions per minute rather than through an increase in the number of minutes the mice chose to run. This indicates that genes may, in ways that are far from understood, influence the tendency to engage in highly specific forms of activity. It further suggests that, in human studies of the genetics of activity, extremely broad measures of activity may not be optimal. Finally, as the study by Dunnington et al. (196) predicted, male mice selected for high activity were lighter. However, female mice showed no such effect on weight. This sex difference in the effects of activity on body weight has been observed in several other studies in rodents (65). This may also have public health and clinical applications, because the result suggests that interventions producing modest changes in spontaneous activity may not affect body weight in women.

WHAT GENETIC STUDIES INDICATE ABOUT THE ENVIRONMENT

Some of the most important contributions of genetically informative studies include their ability to provide information about the environment as well (106). An example of a genetic study that tells about an interesting gene by environmental interaction in mice is depicted in Fig. 2.2. Genetic studies of obesity in humans have given enlightenment about the types of environmental influences that seem important and about how enduring these influences are, and they have pointed toward specific environmental influences.

Common or Shared Versus Unique or Environmental Influences

As was previously discussed, twin, adoption, and family studies reveal a substantial genetic influence on relative body weight across the age span. However, an equally important finding from this literature concerns the nature of environmental influences on obesity. Specifically, genetic studies reveal with rare exception that environmental influences on obesity are *not* those shared by siblings living in the same household (i.e., the common environment). Rather, the unique environment or life experiences that are uncorrelated among siblings appear to promote differences in body weight. Thus, factors, such as differential treatment by parents or peers and/or unique experiences outside of the

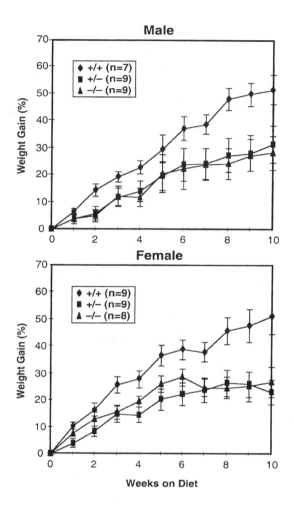

FIG. 2.2. Protein tyrosine phosphatase-1B (PTP-1B): An obesity-resistance gene and an illustration of a gene by environment interaction. (From Elchebly M, Payette P, Michaliszyn E, et al. Increased insulin sensitivity and obesity resistance in mice lacking the protein tyrosine phosphatase-1B gene. *Science* 1999;283:1544–1548, with permission.)

home, may be more important than the ways in which siblings are treated similarly by their parents. This counterintuitive finding casts the understanding of the environment's role in obesity onset into an entirely new light. To the extent that unique environmental influences on adolescent obesity exist, they may be gender and ethnicity specific (197).

Methodologically, certain behavior–genetic designs have limited power to detect common environmental effects. This is true of the classic twin design. Moreover, in the classic twin design, nonadditive genetic effects and common environmental effects are perfectly confounded; thus, they cannot be simultaneously estimated. Therefore, a large nonadditive effect could obscure a smaller common environmental effect (90), and substantial data from both human and nonhuman animals indicate that many significant sources of nonadditive genetic variation for adiposity exist (198,199). The use of the virtual twin methodology, which was previously mentioned, may offer a potential solution to this methodologic challenge. In the first application of this method to weight and BMI, Segal and Allison (90) found that the common environment accounted for 25% of the variance in BMI ($p = 0.0113$). By contrast, the unique environment accounted for only 14% of the variance. These results raise the intriguing possibility that previous studies may have underestimated the magnitude of common environmental influences on BMI. Further research is needed to confirm and extend this initial finding.

Transience

Lay theories of obesity often claim that obesity originates from some early environmental experiences that maintain obesity over a lifetime. Statements such as, "It is in the early formative years that the eating and exercise behaviors we will take with us throughout life are established," are often heard. By contrast, behavioral–genetic studies paint a different picture of the environmental influences on obesity. Environmental influences on obesity appear transient, promoting obesity at a specific point but not necessarily beyond the given moment. Thus, with time, different environmental variables may operate to maintain the obese condition. Evidence from both twin and adoption studies support this finding. In an analysis of the Colorado Adoption Study, Cardon (87) tested the genetic–environmental underpinnings of BMI from the ages of 0 to 9 years. The results indicated that the consistency in BMI across these years was primarily due to genetic factors. By contrast, environmental influences were age specific (i.e., the life experiences promoting obesity at the age of 3 years differed from those at the age of 4 years, which differed from those at the age of 5, and so on). Similar results emerged from the analysis by Fabsitz et al. (200) of middle-aged men in the National Academy of Sciences–National Research Council (NAS–NRC) twin registry, thus indicating that environmental influences are largely age specific and that they do not explain the consistency in BMI over time. Finally, the longitudinal analysis of twin birth weights and adult BMIs by Allison et al. (201) yielded similar conclusions about the intrauterine environment. The implications of these results for obesity are that treatment via "one-shot" environmental inoculations is unlikely to have a sustaining clinical impact for weight loss. Environmental changes that become sustained and consistent facets of everyday living will be more likely to have greater effects.

Specific Environmental Influences

Finally, genetic designs can also provide new insights regarding specific environmental variables. The analysis by Price et al. (86) of the Iowa adoption study found that the BMIs of adopted children were more strongly associated with their biologic mothers' BMIs rather than those of their adoptive mothers. However, they also found evidence for a direct causal effect of the following two environmental factors on children's BMIs: (a) a rural rather than an urban upbringing and (b) the presence of disturbance in the adoptive home environment. The exact mechanisms through which these effects operate are unknown, but they clearly warrant further investigation. This study illustrates the potential advantages of infusing precise environmental measures into genetic studies.

QUANTITATIVE TRAIT LOCUS MAPPING STUDIES

QTL mapping studies have been conducted in many livestock, laboratory, and free-living species ranging from swine and cattle to mice and rats to deer and humans (202–205). This section provides a brief and selective overview of this work.

Mice

Because of the advantages of using mouse models, the vast majority of nonhuman work has been conducted on this species, and this area of research is described in greater detail. Geneticists have capitalized on the advantages of inbreeding and mating crosses in animal models to understand genetic influences in complex traits. Figure 2.3 depicts the different mating populations obtained from the cross of two parental inbred strains

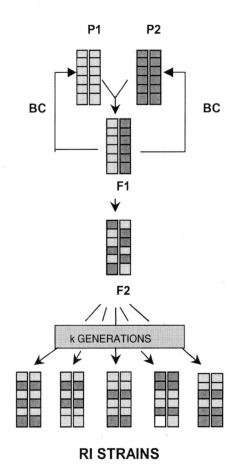

RI STRAINS

FIG. 2.3. Mouse model used for quantitative trait locus mapping.

that differ on a phenotype. Many of the initial findings leading the identification of DNA sequences influencing obesity were based on the identification of QTLs across the mouse genome that are associated with obesity traits.

QTL discovery is considered the first step in the identification of genes influencing complex traits (206). This approach, however, is limited by low resolution and low precision of the DNA region (207). In other words, even when regions of the genome can be identified as harboring QTL, the region that plausibly contains the QTL is often quite

TABLE 2.3. *Quantitative trait loci identification for body weight measures on crosses with strain C57BL/6J in one parental line*

Parental strain mated with C57BL/6J	Chromosome												Reference
	1	4	5	6	7	9	11	13	14	15	17	X	
CASTT/Ei	—	—	—	—	—	—	—	—	—	X	—	—	Mehrabian et al. (208)
A/JXM. spretus	—	—	—	—	—	—	—	—	—	—	—	X	Dragani et al. (209)
KK/H1Lt	—	—	—	—	X	—	—	—	—	—	—	—	Taylor et al. (210)
KK-A(y)	—	X	—	X	—	—	—	—	—	—	—	—	Suto et al. (211)
DBA/2J	X	X	X	X	X	X	X	X	X	—	X	—	Keightley et al. (212)
DBA/2J (males only)	—	X	—	X	—	—	—	—	—	—	—	—	Fernandez et al. (213)

large. This makes moving from an identified region that harbors a QTL to identifying the gene itself difficult. Table 2.3 summarizes findings reported in the literature for QTLs for body weight for those crosses with the strain C57/BL6 as one of the parents. As Table 2.3 illustrates, despite the use of a mouse model, different studies report different findings in different chromosomes, thus reflecting a lack of clear replication.

The following paragraphs describe some examples of mating crosses and their contributions to QTL determination for different obesity-related traits. A comprehensive summary of QTL findings in animal models for obesity can found in Perusse et al. (204) or online at *http://obesite.chaire.ulaval.ca/qtl.html* (Accessed May 28, 2002).

Recombinant Inbred Strains

Although recombinant inbred (RI) strains have been a powerful tool for studying the genetics of other phenotypes, such as alcohol consumption, they have not been greatly used in the field of obesity. Hyman et al. (214) and Paigen (215) independently reported QTLs for sensitivity to dietary (fat) atherosclerosis using RI populations. A combined RI-F_2 approach was used by Fernandez et al. (213) to suggest QTL influencing body weight in females but not in males using the BXD RI series.

Intercrosses

The frequent use of intercrossed populations in QTL studies is a response to the influence of genetic recombination and independent segregation acting to produce genetically unique individuals. Besides the various reports for QTL influencing weight (5,205), findings have also been reported in different mouse strains and in other phenotypes, such as adiposity (210), lipoproteins (216), and energy balance (217).

Backcrosses

The use of backcrosses on experimental designs has provided information about QTL influencing fat, weight, and cholesterol levels (205,218,219) across the mouse genome. Recently, Reifsnyder et al. (220) used this approach in nominating QTL for diabetes predisposition and adiposity, and they suggested that the maternal environment interacts with a genotype to establish diabetes-related phenotypes.

Selected Lines

Mouse lines selected for extreme phenotypes are valuable when identifying QTL. Selected lines were used by Keightley et al. (212) to explore the genetic basis of body weight, identifying 11 QTLs across the mouse genome. Selected lines are also useful as parental populations for intercross studies, such as the one presented by Horvat et al. (221) using an F_2 obesity model that resulted from long-term selected lines for high or low body fat. The genome-wide QTL analysis of this study nominated QTL for body fat in chromosomes 2, 12, 15, and X.

Outbred Populations

These populations are created from the intermating of various inbred strains, thus creating a genetically heterogeneous stock. These stocks are extremely useful as a method to increase the resolution of QTL mapping (222). This approach, although it has not yet been used in obesity research, has been applied to other disease-related phenotypes such as psychologic traits in mice (223).

Congenic Strains

Once a QTL has been localized to a region of the genome, the region must be narrowed down to a smaller region. This can be accomplished in several ways. One way is through the use of congenic strains. The development of congenic strains involves the iterative use of a selective breeding strategy to create pairs of complementary strains of mice so that both strains are homozygous at all loci and both strains are identical at all loci except for those loci at a very small portion of the genome that lies within the previously identified QTL. This effectively increases the power by taking a quantitative trait that is inherently polygenic and making it functionally monogenic (or at least oligogenic). The development of congenic strains can be achieved by testing an average of only 20 markers by the third generation of selective breeding via a genotyping strategy that is described elsewhere (224). By successfully slicing up the QTL-containing interval, the congenic strains can theoretically be used to localize the causative gene precisely.

Agriculture

Studies involving a variety of agricultural and aquacultural species, such as cows, sheep, and pigs, are relatively advanced (202,225). The reason for this is obvious. Significant economic incentives exist for manipulating the obesity levels and/or body composition of livestock to increase efficiency, reduce dependence on dwindling resources, and improve the quality and flavor of the animal products that humans consume. Because many of the animals studied (e.g., cattle) are no less genetically similar to humans than are mice (226), they provide viable models and potentially useful information to the studies of the genetics of human obesity and body composition. Likewise, because the sequence of the human genome is now reasonably well established (227), humans can serve as good "models" for livestock genetics (228).

In many ways, livestock genetics represents a middle ground between the mouse and human. This is true both from the perspective of generation time and in the ability to conduct controlled breeding. The substantial progress made in the mouse is a result of the ability to completely control breeding and of the short generation time, which allows the creation of extremely powerful studies. In contrast, human studies are difficult, partially because of the inability to control breeding. Livestock lie somewhere in between. Like humans, they tend to be outbred, but to a lesser extent. Moreover, breeding can be controlled, but the generation time is generally too long and the cost of animals too high for inbred lines to be established.

Significant progress has been made in locating QTLs for obesity-related traits in livestock. The callipyge mutation, a mutation resulting in marked leanness and muscular hypertrophy in selected anatomic regions has been mapped to a relatively narrow interval on the distal end of chromosome 18 in the ovine genome (229). The myostatin gene, originally localized by QTL mapping methods (230), has now been cloned (231). This gene confers marked leanness and massive muscling, and it has been found to produce parallel effects in mice and cattle. Significant QTLs have also been detected for growth and body composition in chickens (232), cattle (233–237), pigs (238–248), trout (249), and other species. Some of these findings may be of great value to medical researchers given the traits studied. For example, because these studies often include terminal carcass studies, which obviously cannot be done in human QTL mapping, they have identified QTLs for traits such as *marbling,* which is the livestock nomenclature for IM adipose tissue, that is now believed to be of great potential importance in the development of human insulin resistance and diabetes (250). Clearly, studies of agricultural and aquacultural genetics have much to contribute to the understanding of obesity.

Humans

Currently, at least 30 different mapping studies for human obesity are underway (204,251). The inherent difficulties are several-fold. First, statistical power tends to be quite low. Second, the areas of the genome identified as containing likely obesity QTLs tend to be very large (typically 20 to 40 centimorgans), making identification of the genes themselves difficult with positional cloning techniques. One solution that is currently being explored is the possibility of pooling data from multiple studies to increase power and precision. Moreover, a massive amount of multiple testing is conducted over multiple genetic markers, multiple phenotypes, multiple subgroups, and multiple statistical techniques. All of this multiplicity greatly increases the likelihood of type 1 errors, creating further interpretive difficulty. Thus, this field may well be replete with false-positive findings. Because of this, findings derived from mapping studies should be interpreted with caution until they have been replicated, ideally by different investigators. Three areas (on chromosomes 2, 10, and 20) have been replicated to the point where most investigators in the area now believe the evidence that these areas harbor true QTL is compelling. Investigations are now underway in several laboratories to locate the specific genes involved (5).

SINGLE-GENE MUTATIONS AND RARE SYNDROMES

Most cases of "garden-variety" obesity may result from the combined effects of multiple genes and multiple environmental factors, not one of which necessarily has an overwhelming effect. However, an increasing number of cases in which obesity may stem from the overwhelming influence of variation at a single genetic locus have been recognized. This section first reviews identified single-gene obesities, followed by a description of various syndromes involving mental retardation or lipodystrophy where the exact genes involved may not have been identified. The discussion continues with a more methodologically oriented discussion regarding the identification of such unusual individuals. Finally, the clinical implications of this developing research are considered.

Identified Single-Gene Mutations

Significant progress has been made in the characterization of specific genes involved in the syndromes related to obesity (5,204). In this section, a selection of single-gene mutations related to cases of human obesity are briefly described in a review that is more illustrative than it is exhaustive. For a more detailed approach, see Perusse et al. (204). The first identification of individuals with single-gene obesities was published in the 1990s.

The gene whose mutations contributing to obesity may be the most prevalent is the melanocortin-4 receptor (MC4R) gene. Hinney et al. (252) described six female obese subjects with mutations in the MC4R gene, two with the CTCT deletion at codon 211, and four others with a novel mutation at position 35, leading to a premature stop codon that generated a truncated protein product. Hinney et al. (252) also described seven other extremely obese subjects with missense mutations in MC4R of unknown significance. Gu et al. (253) identified a woman with a BMI of 57 who was heterozygous for an Ile137Thr polymorphism in the MC4R gene. However, no clear association between this polymorphism and obesity was found in her pedigree. More cases of obesity that have apparently resulted from polymorphisms in the MC4R gene have been identified (149,254). MC4R mutations have been suggested as the most frequent single-gene cause of obesity, but the insufficient availability of information precludes making confident statements about the prevalence of or attributable risk associated with this or any other putative obesity gene.

Krude et al. (255) identified two children with marked obesity who had mutations in the proopiomelanocortin (POMC) gene. This gene is involved in some of the same physiologic pathways as some of the melanocortin and agouti genes, which seem to be involved in both feeding and pigmentation. Interestingly, like the POMC knockout mouse that both is obese and develops an orange coat, these children both were obese and both had vivid red hair.

Nothen et al. (256) found an obese man (BMI of 37) who was homozygous for a 13 base-pair deletion in exon 1 of the dopamine receptor D$_4$ (DRD4) gene. This caused a premature stop codon that, in all likelihood, produced a nonfunctional protein. In contrast, an individual who was homozygous for a Val194Gly mutation in the DRD4 gene was identified and was reported to have a pattern of low weight overall.

Ristow et al. (257) identified a number of individuals who had mutations in the peroxisome proliferator-activated receptor γ2 (PPARγ2) gene. The identified mutation was a Pro115Gln mutation that apparently promotes adipocyte proliferation.

Perhaps the best-known single-gene mutation involves the recently isolated hormone leptin, the product of the obesity gene leptin (LEP) (258). Leptin, which is produced by fat cells, is thought to be critical in the regulation of body fat and body weight. Leptin's effects are mediated through a specific receptor, LEPR, which has been cloned and characterized (259). To date, the authors suspect that many thousands of people have been screened for LEP and LEPR mutations. Thus far, however, very few individuals have been found to have mutations that appear to confer obesity (5). Strobel et al. (260) and Ozata et al. (261) described a family of Turkish origin with three obese members who carried a homozygous missense mutation in LEP that is associated with a low serum level of leptin. Farooqi et al. (262) recently reported a significant clinical response to recombinant human leptin in a 9-year-old severely obese girl with a congenital leptin deficiency. Over 12 months, the girl lost 16.4 kg of weight, 15.6 kg of which was fat mass. Individuals with mutations in the LEPR gene have also been identified (5), but common polymorphisms in this gene do not appear to be major contributors to BMI variation in the general population (263).

Lipodystrophies

Lipodystrophies can be defined as marked abnormalities of body fat distribution. One form of lipodystrophy occurs in the lower half of the female body, where it is characterized by swollen deposition of subcutaneous fat (264). Ketterings (264) and others (265–267) have suggested that lipodystrophy, typically a rare autosomal recessive genetic disorder, can cause psychologic problems in early age and, in later life, heavy, painful legs; edema; and varicose veins.

Congenital generalized lipodystrophy, also called also Berardinelli–Seip syndrome, is a rare autosomal recessive genetic disorder characterized by a near-complete absence of adipose tissue and marked insulin resistance from birth. A locus has been identified for this disease on chromosome 9q34 (268–270). A subtype of general lipodystrophy is familial partial lipodystrophy or Dunnigan variety, a highly penetrant autosomal dominant disorder characterized by a dramatic loss of subcutaneous adipose tissue from the extremities and trunk and excess fat deposition in the head and neck (271,272). Speckman et al. (272) have localized a gene for this disease to chromosome 1q21-q23.

Dercum disease (*adiposis dolorosa*) is a rare autosomal dominant condition that is characterized by painful fatty deposits. The cause is unknown, and no specific treatment is available (266,267). Steroids, lidocaine, or analgesics may relieve pain. Surgical treatment consists of liposuction of the adipose masses (266). Fagher et al. (265) analyzed the activity of fat cells in 13 patients and concluded that no known metabolic pathogenic factor can explain this uncommon disease.

A new form of lipodystrophy is a syndrome of peripheral lipodystrophy, central adiposity, dyslipidemia, and insulin resistance that has emerged since the introduction of human immunodeficiency virus type 1 (HIV-1) protease inhibitors, which are a component of the antiretroviral drug combination regimen. In this case, the adipose tissue deposits are not associated with physical pain (273,274). Discussion about possible treatment options for these body shape changes and metabolic disturbance is ongoing, but, thus far, no options exist for changing drug treatment in patients with HIV (274). This area seems ripe for pharmacogenetic research, as is discussed later in this chapter.

Finally, multiple symmetric lipomatosis, also known as Launois–Bensaude syndrome or Madelung disease, is a rare disorder that is predominantly seen in middle-aged male patients (275). The mode of inheritance is not yet known. This disorder is characterized by large subcutaneous fat masses that are distributed around the neck, shoulders, and trunk and that are often associated with nervous system abnormalities. Kratz et al. (275) reported characteristic clinical findings of this disease in two 9-year-old children with associated mild mental retardation. Multiple symmetric lipomatosis appears to be a new neurometabolic disorder with heterogeneous clinical expression, the pathogenesis of which is still unknown.

Syndromes Associated with Mental Retardation

This section briefly reviews the syndromes associated with both mental retardation and obesity (276–278) (Table 2.4).

Prader–Willi Syndrome

In Prader–Willi syndrome (PWS), most patients have three to four megabase deletions in the paternally derived chromosome at 15q11.2, while other patients display uniparental disomy (e.g., two maternally derived chromosomal regions at 15q11). A small number of other cases have microdeletions in the imprinting center at 15q11-q13 (5). The syndrome is characterized by severe obesity, mild to moderate mental retardation, hypogonadism, hypotonia, short stature, and small hands and feet (279). PWS has an incidence of 1 per 10,000 to 15,000 livebirths (280). Massive obesity usually develops within the first year of life (281).

Bardet–Biedl Syndrome

The genetic heterogeneity of Bardet–Biedl syndrome, a rare autosomal disease, has been confirmed by the identification of five different chromosomal regions (chromosome 11q13, 16q21, 3p13-p12, 15q22.3-23, and 2q31) (282–285). Main features of this syndrome include generalized obesity with ubiquitous fat deposition, mental retardation, retinal dystrophy, polydactyly, hypogonadism, and congenital heart defects (286).

TABLE 2.4. *Rare, presumably genetic syndromes involving both obesity and mental retardation*

Syndrome	Obesity	Mental retardation	Chromosome locus	Candidate gene
Rare				
Prader–Willi	Severe	Mild to moderate	15q11–q13	SNRPN
Bardet–Biedl	Generalized	Mild	11q13	—
			16q21	—
			3p13–p12	—
			15q22.3–23	MY09A
			2q31	—
Cohen	Truncal	Mild	8q22–q23	—
Carpenter	Truncal gluteal	Mild	Autosomal recessive trait	—
Börjeson	Truncal	Mild	Xq26.3	FGF13
Down	Generalized	Mild to severe	Trisomy 21	—
Very rare				
Achondroplasia	Generalized	Mild	4p16.3	FGFR3
Albright	Generalized	Moderate	15q	—
Angelman with obesity	Generalized	Mild	15q11–q13	—
Carbohydrate-deficient glycoprotein syndrome type IA	Truncal gluteal	Severe	16p13	PMM2
Choroideremia	Truncal	Moderate	Xq21.1–21.2	—
Mental retardation, epileptic seizures, hypogonadism, macrocephaly, and obesity	Generalized	Mild to moderate	Xp22.13–21.1	—
Pseudohypoparathyroidism	Generalized	Mild	20q13.3	GNAS1
Wilson–Turner	Generalized	Mild	Xp21.1–q22	—

Cohen Syndrome

Cohen syndrome is determined by an anomaly on the long arm of chromosome 8 (8q22-q23). This autosomal recessive syndrome presents with facial, oral, ocular, and spinal abnormalities; generalized muscular hypotonia; mental retardation; and truncal obesity (287).

Carpenter Syndrome

Carpenter syndrome is transmitted in an autosomal recessive manner (288). The Carpenter syndrome is characterized by short hands, polydactyly (syndactyly), coxa vara, mental retardation, hypogonadism, hernia, congenital heart disease, craniofacial abnormalities, and obesity (289).

Börjeson–Forssman–Lehmann Syndrome

Börjeson–Forssman–Lehmann syndrome is an X-linked syndrome with the chromosomal region of the disorder in the long arm of the X chromosome (q26-q27) (290). The main features consist of mental retardation, epilepsy, a high level of abdominal fat, a short neck, muscular hypotonia, and hypogonadism (291).

Down Syndrome

Trisomy 21 is a genetic disorder with either a portion of or a complete extra chromosome at chromosome 21. The prevalence is 1 in 600 to 800 livebirths. Signs at birth include a flat facial profile, the absence of the Moro reflex, muscular hypotonia, a dysplastic ear, oblique palpebral fissures, and dysplastic middle phalanx of the fifth finger. Congenital heart disease is frequent, and skeletal abnormalities and visual problems are present. Immune function is generally depressed, and mental retardation is extremely common among patients with Down syndrome who are overweight and obese (292). The obesity predisposition among individuals with Down syndrome appears to be partially due to a reduced metabolic rate (277,293).

Other Syndromes

Some other very rare syndromes associated with both obesity and mental retardation include MOMO (macrosomia, obesity, macrocephaly, and ocular abnormalities) syndrome (294,295); achondroplasia (296); Albright hereditary osteodystrophy and other pseudohypoparathyroidisms (297–299); a new form of Angelman syndrome with obesity (300); carbohydrate-deficient glycoprotein syndrome type IA (CDGS1A) (301); choroideremia with deafness (302); MEHMO (mental retardation, epileptic seizures, hypogonadism, microcephaly, and obesity) syndrome (303); and Wilson–Turner syndrome (290). Engelen et al. (304) described a patient with psychomotor retardation, mild obesity, pes equinovarus, strabismus, and facial anomalies. They found *de novo* translocations between the long arms of chromosomes 14 and 18 (304). The authors reported a single-gene variant proceeding obesity in humans. Recently, a young girl was identified who phenotypically was quite unusual, as she was extremely obese and had a voracious appetite. Cytogenetic analysis revealed a fusion of the short arm of chromosome 1 to the long arm of chromosome 6. Further study revealed a disruption of the SIM1 gene (305). SIM1 knockout mouse models were subsequently generated and were shown to be fatter than normal controls, thus confirming the role of SIM1 in the regulation of adiposity (306). Finally, a new syndrome form of X-linked inheritance of mental retardation associated with obesity, MRXS7, has been localized to chromosome Xp11.3-q23 in a large Pakistani family. The ten affected men show clinical manifestations that include mental retardation, mild obesity, and hypogonadism (278).

Searching for the Phenotypically "Odd" Cases in Mutation Detection

Four centuries ago, in *Novum organum*, Francis Bacon wrote, "Errors of Nature, Sports and Monsters correct the understanding in regard to ordinary things and reveal general forms. For whoever knows the ways of Nature will more easily notice her deviations; and on the other hand, whoever knows her deviations will more accurately describe her ways." "Sport" is an archaic term used by farmers to describe a phenotypically unusual animal that occasionally arises in livestock.

Nowhere has Bacon's enjoinder (307) met with better success than in the study of the genetics of obesity. Coleman (reviewed in Johnson et al. [308]) first observed the mutants *ob, db, tub,* and *fat* when they spontaneously appeared in laboratory mice. These mutant models, along with the agouti mouse (309) were the "original" five obesity mutations studied (310), all of which have now been cloned, thus greatly vitalizing the field. Indeed, the most influential single finding in the obesity field in several decades is surely the discovery of leptin (146), which stemmed directly from Coleman's astute detection of a *sport* in the Jackson Laboratory's colony. More recently, significant advances in understanding the genetics and physiology of obesity have arisen with other investigators, who have observed the unexpected *sport* in studies of knockout animals. For example, the intracellular adhesion molecule (ICAM) gene came under careful study because of its suspected physiologic effects (311). However, it was unexpectedly found to be an important gene for body composition. This discovery illustrates the importance of being open to the unexpected finding.

Examples

Among humans, attentiveness to the unusual obesity phenotype has also provided important insights. For example, among the small number of obese humans currently identified as having obesity resulting from mutations in single genes, most show a unique pattern or cluster of phenotypes. For example, individuals with leptin mutations not only are massively obese, but they also, not surprisingly, have essentially no circulating serum leptin (187). In contrast, individuals with leptin receptor mutations have enormously high levels of circulating leptin, and, like the *db/db* mouse that also suffers from a homozygous mutation in the leptin receptor gene, they do not reach full sexual maturity despite achieving chronological adulthood (187). Individuals with the POMC mutation, like the agouti mouse, have reddish-orange hair (255). Individuals with certain PPARγ mutations are not only obese, but, given their obesity, they also show unusually low levels of insulin. These phenotypic patterns or clusters are easier to identify after the individual with the mutation has been identified. However, the thoughtful investigator could perhaps identify some of these in advance and could then use this knowledge to guide mutation detection in human research. Tables 2.2 and 2.5 list several animal models that exhibit not only obesity or marked obesity resistance (i.e., the tendency to stay thin or lean despite the opportunity to become obese, a phenotype that may be of as much interest for obesity gene mapping studies as obesity itself is [318,319]), but also some other characteristic phenotypic patterns. A prospective collection of DNA samples from humans with such pheno-

TABLE 2.5. *Some potential "sports"*

Animal model	Syndrome	Human equivalent?
5-HT$_{2c}$ receptor knockout (131)	Obesity, seizures; nonresponsive to fenfluramines; hyperphagic; insulin resistant	". . . case of Hernandez syndrome . . . 16-year-old Brazilian girl . . . psychomotor retardation, epilepsy, a bulbous nose and obesity" (312)
Tubby (307)	Obesity, retinal degeneration, cochlear degeneration	". . . case of identical female twins . . . presented with retinal degeneration, obesity, and mental retardation . . ." (287)
DGAT (161)	Obesity resistance, failure to lactate	". . . survey of women . . . risk factors for delayed onset of lactation included ... heavy/obese body build . . ." (313)
Orexin/hypocretin-deficient mice (316,317)	Narcolepsy, reduced food intake, possibly reduced metabolic rate	"Obesity appeared as an unexpected association in this case series, with 11 of the 16 narcoleptic patients found to be overweight at the time of diagnosis" (314)
An example of human syndrome in search of a gene	Adiposis dolorosa with obesity and painful lipomas	"Dercum disease consists of multiple, painful lipomata and occurs in obese, postmenopausal women" (315)
ICAM-1—deficient mice (311)	Late-onset obesity without overeating, accompanied by inflammatory and immune defects	Unknown
Nhlh2 knockout mice (150)	Adult-onset obesity with impaired gonadal growth associated with puberty	Unknown

Abbreviations: 5-HT, 5-hydroxytryptamine; ICAM-1, intracellular adhesion molecule-1.

typic characteristics, with examination for potential mutations in the human homologues of these murine model obesity or obesity-resistance genes, might be useful. This represents another potentially fruitful area for future research.

Methodology

The idea of advance identification of potential *sports* based on knowledge from murine obesity or obesity-resistance models is a sound one. However, it may not lead to all the interesting phenotypic clusters that are available for detection among humans. Considering other approaches that begin with humans may be useful. For example, Allison et al. (320,321) published two papers in which they used cluster analytic methodology to identify distinct subtypes of obesity. This was done among unrelated individuals. Some of these subtypes possibly are strongly heritable, perhaps even in a mendelian fashion. One way of examining this would be an attempt to derive clusters of specific obesity subtypes simultaneously within a context of genetically informative design. An example of this in the context of eating disorders was reported by Bulik et al. (322), who used a sample of female twins. A program of research in which highly specific unique patterns of obesity derived from cluster analytic methods (323) are applied to family data so that clusters, which are highly heritable, perhaps in a mendelian fashion, are identified, may be envisioned. Subsequently, these could be validated in separate samples of family data, and, finally, to the extent that they hold up, a search could then be conducted for specific genes causing these unique subtypes of obesity using QTL mapping technology and mutation-detection approaches. Such approaches may not be a study of garden-variety obesity *per se*, which most people believe is enormously heterogeneous, but they might narrow the phenotype to a distinct subtype of obesity with a much more homogeneous origin. The researcher may then be in a better position to detect specific genetic effects.

Responding to Phenotypically or Genotypically Unusual Obese Persons in the Clinic

The identification of individuals with obesity that results from single-gene mutations and the possibility of more such identification in the future raise a new series of questions regarding how clinicians respond to extremely obese or obese people with unusual clinical presentations (324). When such individuals do present, a reasonable consideration is to obtain a DNA sample and to send it to a laboratory that will screen it for potential obesity-promoting mutations in a number of genes. Such screening, if successful, might lead to an interesting scientific discovery, may offer the patient an explanation for the obesity, and may possibly even guide treatment.

However, although a greater understanding of the role that genetic factors play in the development and expression of obesity is rapidly developing, the medical community at this time is not in a strong position to offer obese individuals highly sophisticated genetic counseling. Indeed, even if DNA collection from severely obese individuals was conducted, establishing the genetic causes of a given individual's obesity, given the current level of understanding, is unlikely. Moreover, even with identification of genes that are responsible for an individual's obesity, with rare exceptions (e.g., leptin mutation), a specific treatment would not be available to address this cause. Thus, the clinician must be honest with obese patients and study subjects, indicating to them in no uncertain terms that a direct and immediate benefit is unlikely (although it is possible) to result from the collection of their DNA. However, through their willingness to participate in treatment studies, they do help with continued development and refinement of the understanding of the genetics of obesity. Nonetheless, even if they do not benefit from the studies, the growing evidence that genetics plays a prominent role in obesity may give these obese individuals "peace of mind," knowing that their obesity is not due to the stereotypic character traits that are thought to be associated with obesity (e.g., laziness, gluttony, and poor self-control) (325). This, in and of itself, may prove therapeutic, at least with regard to their psychosocial functioning and subjective well-being.

Assuming that the ability to identify and understand the role that genes play in obesity continues to increase, the medical community must begin to anticipate and address, at least in a preliminary way, the practical and ethical issues that are likely to emerge. Among them are (a) the development of shared common protocols for the collection of DNA, (b) a consensus on issues pertaining to confidentiality, (c) the development of comprehensive consent forms that anticipate and address potential future "human subject" issues, (d) the most effective ways to obtain and analyze DNA, and (e) the translation of advances in the screening and identification of obesity genes to clinical practice. The interested reader is referred to other resources (326,327) for detailed information on the specific procedures involved in the collection and analysis of DNA and the potential clinical implications of advances in the understanding of the genetics of obesity.

MICROARRAY GENE-EXPRESSION STUDIES

What Are Microarrays?

One important aspect of modern genetics is "functional genomics." Here, the function of genes is examined with multiple methods. The examination of the pattern of gene expression of many genes in one or more tissues, experimental conditions, or genetic backgrounds is one useful approach.

A powerful instrument for understanding the function of known or unknown DNA sequences is high-density arrays of oligonucleotides or complementary DNAs. These *microarrays* work by hybridization of labeled RNA or DNA in solution to DNA molecules attached at precise locations on a surface. Although this technique has been used for decades (328), a recent technical achievement has increased the experimental efficiency and information content—arrays of thousands of genes per square centimeter can now be produced (329), thus allowing the quantification of gene expression on a genome-wide level for a large set of genes in any particular tissue. The most widespread application of microarray technology is expression profiling, which is the gene-by-gene determination of differences in messenger RNA abundance between two preparations (329,330).

Data Analysis

An area requiring careful attention when using microarrays is data analysis. Although detailed descriptions of data analysis are beyond the scope of this chapter, a few central themes can be highlighted. Microarray experiments are typically characterized by an extraordinarily large number of variables (genes) being studied on a very small number of objects (e.g., a small number of mice). This creates the need to consider multiple testing issues, to use statistical procedures that are adaptable to small samples, and to find ways in which the large number of variables may somehow be used to augment the information provided by a very small number of objects. One means of doing this is by treating the unit of observation as the gene, rather than as the object (e.g., mouse, tumor, and human). Generally, this is what is done in the common clustering procedures that are applied. In these procedures, the data matrix is effectively transposed from its usual form of an n rows by p columns matrix, in which n is the number of objects and p is the number of variables, to a *p* rows by *n* columns matrix. Cluster analysis is then performed on this matrix to obtain families of genes that appear to be coexpressed. If a gene with a previously unidentified function is found to cluster with a variety of other genes of known and similar function, this novel gene may have a similar function. Other methods for determining whether differences across groups or conditions are statistically significant are being developed, and if significant, they seek to estimate what the magnitude of this difference is (331,332). Finally, a number of important statistical measurement issues accompanying the use of microarrays have yet to be dealt with fully. Important developments, which are likely to come in the next few years, are needed in this area. Researchers using microarrays are advised to consider data analysis issues carefully and not to rely solely on loosely articulated conventions for a determination of how to analyze their data appropriately.

Examples

The characterization of gene expression in adipose tissue has been a topic of investigation for many years (333,334). Recent studies employing microarray technology take advantage of the large number of genes that can be examined simultaneously. An analysis of gene expression in human adipose tissue by Gabrielsson et al. (335) resulted in the identification of numerous genes that had not previously reported to be expressed in adipocytes. Soukas et al. (336) found a number of genes associated with adipocyte differentiation that were dysregulated in the adipose tissue of *ob/ob* mice. Nadler et al. (337) showed that a decrease in the expression of genes normally involved in adipogenesis is associated with obesity in mice. Lee et al. (338) presented a gene-expression profile of the aging brain in mice and reported that retardation of the aging process occurs as a result of caloric restriction. Ferrante et al. (339) used microarrays to examine the effects of leptin on hepatic gene expression.

Although the use of microarrays extends to a wide range of analytic methods, well-established techniques, such as differential polymerase chain reaction and Northern blot analysis, are still applied. Oishi et al. (340) characterized the difference in gene expression in bovine adipose tissue due to fattening using reverse transcriptase polymerase chain reaction. They discovered three unknown genes that are expressed in adipocytes after fattening, but not before. Two recent publications (341,342) focused on the tissue-specific gene expression of humans and rats in visceral adipose tissue. Genes that are specifically expressed in visceral adipose tissue were identified by Northern blot analysis in both species. The Northern blot technique is also commonly used to confirm microarray data or to establish thresholds for reliable fold changes (336).

Other Possible Uses of Microarrays

Microarrays can highly flexible uses. For example, if a researcher is interested in pharmacogenetics and in exploring the genetic mediators of drug response, he or she might look for changes in gene-expression levels that occur with exposure to a drug that tends to produce weight gain and then might evaluate whether the amount of weight gain produced is correlated with gene-expression level. To rule out the possibility that the overexpressed or underexpressed genes among high weight gainers are simply genes that are associated with weight gain *per se*, rather than with weight gain induced by the drug under study, he or she might then replicate the study using animals that gain weight via forced feeding, instead of via ingestion of a drug. Obviously, an infinite number of different designs can use multiple microarray conditions to narrow down and tease out the genes involved in a particular response.

PHARMACOGENOMICS

Defining Pharmacogenomics

The terms *pharmacogenetics* and *pharmacogenomics* are often used interchangeably, and they will appear so here. However, some people use *pharmacogenetics* to connote studies of one or a few genes and *pharmacogenomics* to refer to the study of many genes or whole genomes. *Pharmacogenomics* has been defined as "the study of the genetic basis for the differences between individuals in responses to drugs" (343, pg. 440). By this definition, pharmacogenetics may therefore be viewed as a special case in the study of gene–environment interactions. Emilien et al. (344) more broadly defines *pharmaco-genomics* as "the application of genomic technologies such as gene sequencing, statistical genetics, and gene-expression analysis to drugs in clinical development and on the market" (pg. 391). Pharmacogenetics may be the most applied subfield in the genetics of human obesity as one of its chief goals is to provide information that allows the clinician "to tailor drug prescriptions to individual genotype" (343, pg. 440). The most obvious example of this is the discovery of leptin-deficient people who are uniquely susceptible to the beneficial effects of exogenous leptin (262). However, pharmacogenomics can also serve the cause of more basic discovery by helping to point out previously unknown or unconfirmed pathways through which certain drugs work. One reason to think that pharmacogenomics may offer a unique window of opportunity in this regard is the nature of the phenotype being studied. In pharmacogenomics, the phenotype is some response to a known stimulus, which is the drug under study. Often this stimulus can be given in a greatly controlled manner. Thus, in pharmacogenomic studies of weight gain in response to a drug, the study does not simply examine a large number of people who all happen to have gained weight, but it instead looks at subjects who are likely to have done so at very different times, in different ways, and for different reasons, as is the case in most genetic studies of obesity. Therefore, the heterogeneity that plagues studies of complex traits in general and in obesity particularly (6,345) is most likely markedly reduced. Moreover, because the researcher often has some knowledge about how drugs that influence body weight work, the candidate genes can be selected with much greater sagacity.

A large number of drugs cause weight loss (346) or weight gain (347). Table 2.6 lists classes of drugs with effects on body weight. Obviously, within any class, substantial variability exists in terms of effect on weight. To what extent does genetic variability mediate or moderate individual responsivity to various pharmacologic agents in terms of weight change? Gross et al. (358) offered an example of this supposition when they attempted to study the influence of the sparteine and/or debrisoquine genetic polymorphism on the disposition of dexfenfluramine (the antiobesity agent removed from the market in 1997). They found that the metabolism of dexfenfluramine was impaired in poor metabolizers of debrisoquine, and they therefore concluded that the cytochrome P450 CYP2D6, the isoenzyme deficient in poor metabolizers of debrisoquine, must also be involved in the metabolism of dexfenfluramine. Beyond this, to the authors' knowledge, little work has been published on the pharmacogenetics of weight change beyond the area of antipsychotic agents as of the writing of this chapter; even the work that is available has been minimal.

The ability of antipsychotic agents or neuroleptics to induce weight gain is well known. This is especially true for the newer so-called atypical agents, with the exception

TABLE 2.6. *Drugs or classes of drugs with effects on body weight*

Drug or class of drugs	Reference	Comments	Example of candidate genes
Weight gain			
Antipsychotics	Allison et al. (348)	Marked variability among drugs in this class with some (e.g., clozapine) producing substantial weight gain and others (e.g., ziprasidone) producing none	Dopamine, serotonin, histamine, adrenergic receptors
Tricyclic antidepressants	Bernstein (349)	—	Glucocorticoid receptor
Monoamine oxidase inhibitors	Bernstein (349)	—	Dopa decarboxylase gene
Protease inhibitors (and possibly other antivirals)	Kotler (350), Lenhard et al. (351)	Accompanied by unusual metabolic and anatomic changes	PPARγ, DGAT, HMG1C
Valproic acid	Sachs and Guille (352)	—	PPARδ
Lithium	Bernstein (349)	—	Thyroid hormone receptor
Oral contraceptives	Kaunitz (353)	—	Estrogen receptors
Weight loss			
Selective serotonin reuptake inhibitor antidepressants	Edwards and Anderson (354)	Some reports of weight gain also found for these drugs	Serotonin receptors, serotonin transporter gene
Nicotine	Perkins (355)	Effect can be studied by examining weight gain after withdrawal	Nicotinic receptors
Topiramate	Perucca (356)		GABA receptors, glutamate (AMPA) receptors
Agents intended to produce weight loss	Bray and Greenway (346)	Many prescription drugs, such as phentermine, orlistat, and sibutramine, as well as compounds in development, such as leptin and axokine	Cathecholamine receptors
Methylphenidate	Schertz et al. (357)		Dopamine receptor D_4 gene

Abbreviations: AMPA, α-amino-3-hydroxy-5-methyl-4-isoxazolepropionic acid; DGAT, diacyglycerol acyltransferase; GABA, γ-aminobutyric acid; HMG1C, high motility group 1c; PPAR, peroxisome proliferator-activated receptor.

of ziprasidone (348). These drugs are often antagonists of the same catecholamine receptors that antiobesity agents stimulate. Thus, these receptors are excellent candidate genes. One example is the 5-hydroxytryptamine 2C (5-HT_{2C}) receptor (359). Many antipsychotics that cause marked weight gain are potent antagonists of the 5-HT_{2C} receptor. Moreover, 5-HT_{2C} agonists, such as sibutramine, are effective weight loss agents (360), and mice made null for the 5-HT_{2C} receptor by knockout techniques become obese (131). At least two studies have examined polymorphisms of the 5-HT_{2C} receptor, and neither found a significant association with the degree of weight gain after taking clozapine (361–363). In addition, Rietschel et al. (364) found no connection between polymorphisms in the D_4 receptor gene and weight gain among 149 patients with schizophrenia taking clozapine. However, most recently, Reynolds et al. (365) found a compelling association between a polymorphism in the promoter region of the 5-HT_{2C} gene and weight gain among individuals taking antipsychotic medication.

Methodologic Issues

A number of methodologic issues are raised by the use of pharmacogenomics (366,367), and this section addresses one that is frequently unappreciated. More specifically, after receiving some treatment (e.g., a drug), different individuals vary with respect to their subsequent change in a certain variable, such as body weight. This variability is often assumed to be variability in *response* to treatment and the search then begins for the causes of this variability. However, if individuals exposed to treatment who then vary in their change in weight are the only ones observed, the investigator is not necessarily observing a variation in *response* to treatment; he or she is simply observing variation in *change*. To draw firm conclusions about the influence of a genetic polymorphism on a response to treatment, a randomized design in which some subjects are assigned to a control condition must be applied. The crucial test is not whether a polymorphism is associated with change scores within a single group but instead is whether a polymorphism exhibits a significant interaction with group assignment when the change score is the dependent variable. In this manner, variation that is variation in response to treatment is separated from variation that is simply variation in change. In fact, from a strict inferential point of view, the conclusion that variation in response to treatment occurs cannot be drawn simply by observing that a variation in change is seen in a variable after receiving treatment. This is true even if a strict (i.e., rigorous) randomized clinical trial is available. This point was recently clarified by Gadbury and Iyer (368). Interestingly, Gadbury and Iyer (368) developed a useful method for determining the possible range for the amount of variability present in a true response to treatment. Investigators might find the use of methods such as that exemplified by Gadbury and Iyer beneficial in determining how great the true variability is in response to treatment before they undertake pharmacogenetic studies. This would then allow them to determine better whether the variability in response to treatment is sufficient enough to warrant the effort for a pharmacogenetics search. Other authors discuss further methodologic issues in pharmacogenetics (369–371).

SUGGESTIONS FOR FUTURE RESEARCH

This review identified several key issues that need to be addressed to move the field forward and to set the stage for reaping clinical benefit from the advances in the understanding of the genetics of obesity. The following is a brief overview of these issues, as well as some recommendations for future research.

Increased Emphasis on the Genetics of Obesity-Promoting Behaviors

Most of the work conducted thus far has focused on genetic determinants of BMI and intermediary phenotypes, such as resting metabolic rate and insulin sensitivity. Although this work promises to elucidate important physiologic pathways, it does not address whether genetic effects exist for every relevant trait of obesity. That is, can the substantial variability in "obesity-promoting" behaviors, such as food intake, eating behavior, and physical activity, be explained genetically? Work in this area has began (107,372), but far more is needed.

A major difficulty with this type of research, however, concerns measurement imprecision. Although measurement technologies have improved greatly (e.g., doubly labeled water to measure food intake and accelerometers to measure physical activity), they tend to be prohibitively expensive and thus they are not available to all investigators. Thus, technologic advances in measurement must be sought. The difficulty of obtaining accurate data should not deter investigators from the pursuit of the behavioral genetics of obesity, but they should instead motivate the development and incorporation of better behavioral measures into genetic studies.

Use of Ethnically Diverse Samples

Another important issue revolves around increasing the ethnic diversity of samples used in genetic studies. Although the sampling of relatively small isolated populations (e.g., Alaskan Natives, Pima Indians, and Mennonites) is advantageous because such populations are thought to exhibit greater homogeneity and linkage disequilibrium, most research has been conducted with samples that predominantly include white persons of European origin (6). Despite the potential disadvantages of studying diverse ethnic groups (e.g., reduced statistical power and practical and social barriers), expansion of the breadth of populations studied is essential. Groups that are currently underrepresented in genetic studies include Cubans, Puerto Ricans, Asians, Arabs, and Native Africans.

Environmental Genetic Interactions in the Expression of Obesity

Although genetic studies indicate that both childhood and adult BMIs are substantially heritable, environmental factors also clearly wield an important influence on human obesity. Several environmental variables appear to promote obesity (373), and, given that the human genome has not changed substantially in the past two decades, these variables are largely responsible for the dramatic rise in overweight and obesity in the developed world (374). Thus, an important direction for future research is forging a greater understanding of gene–environment interactions. Research suggests that the important genetic causes of the change in BMI from young adulthood to middle age act independently of the genetic influences on individual BMI at young adulthood (372). In other words, important ongoing gene–environment interactions and/or gene–age interactions determine how individuals respond within a given environment. Determining the best manner for incorporating environmental influences into genetic research is an exciting area with promise for informing both basic and clinical research.

Combining Databases

Although the existence of a few genes may have particularly substantial effects on obesity in certain subgroups of the population, a large number of relevant genes may account for only a small portion of the total phenotypic variance. The power to map genes that exert small effects will remain unacceptably low because no single investigator can realistically collect large enough sample sizes. A potential solution is to pool data across many investigators and laboratories. A simple way to do this is with the use of meta-analysis; however, the summary statistics derived from this sort of "indirect" pooling are not without limitations (375). Perhaps, the best method for accomplishing this pooling is the combination of raw data from multiple studies. This would increase statistical power but would also require a form of "data sharing" that, given the competition to identify important obesity genes, may prove challenging.

Single-Gene Syndromes Versus Gene Phenotypes of Obesities

Although the identification of a few cases of single-gene obesity syndromes has been successful, these single-gene obesities clearly are rare syndromes, and they do not adequately explain the majority of human obesities that appear to be the result of multiple and interacting phenotypes. As knowledge of the genetic determinants of obesity develops, genetically distinct "obesities" (i.e., manifestations of obesity that are the product of different and distinct gene phenotypes that perhaps require different approaches to their clinical management) may be identified.

Obesity Genes and Response to Antiobesity Medications

An important goal of studying the genetics of obesity is improving the clinical management of obese individuals. Insights derived from the study of genetic factors in the pathogenesis of obesity will offer new avenues for drug development (pharmacogenetics). The potential "modes of action" for these drugs include molecules that decrease food intake, molecules that modify nutrient partitioning, and molecules that increase energy expenditure (376). As the field advances, pharmacogenetics for obesity will likely take the following two general directions: (a) identification of the specific genes and gene products associated with obesity that might become targets for new medications and (b) identification of genes and allelic variations of genes that might affect responses to current antiobesity medications. The possibility of using the understanding of the role genetic differences in the development and expression of obesity to target particular drugs to particular genetic phenotypes of obesity is not difficult to imagine. In other words, understanding the various genetic determinants of different types of obesities may make the design of drugs that are targeted toward these particular obesities possible, thereby reducing the genetic variability in therapeutic responses. This would eliminate the prescription of ineffective drugs and would decrease the chances of adverse drug reactions in "sensitive" individuals (377).

Ethical Issues

Several ethical issues are likely to emerge as this field matures. As was noted previously, given the rapid pace with which advances occur, the potential ethical dilemmas in genetic research on human subjects must be anticipated and addressed (378). Within the context of obesity research, the crucial concerns appear to be (a) the development of common protocols for the collection of genetic material, (b) proper subject education and consent for the collection of genetic material, (c) the maintenance of confidentiality (which is especially critical in studies involving data pooling), and (d) the provision for genetic counseling as the ability to identify polymorphisms improves. As genetic testing becomes widespread and begins to inform clinical practice more explicitly, other important issues, such as guidelines for DNA collection in clinical practice, access to specialty care as a function of the results of testing, and legal issues regarding the use of obesity-related genetic information by insurance companies, will need to be tackled.

Conclusion

Great strides have been made in understanding the genetic determinants of obesity. Although important practical, methodologic, and statistical issues must still be dealt with, the rate of progress in the last decade has been substantial. As the field moves forward, it is poised to make even greater advances, not only in the identification of obesity genes but also in the development and application of genetically based treatments of human obesity.

ACKNOWLEDGMENTS

This work was supported in part by grants R29DK47256, R01DK51716, P30DK26687, K08MH01530, and R01ES09912 from the National Institutes of Health. The authors are grateful to Streamson Chua for his helpful comments.

REFERENCES

1. Eisenberg D, Marcotte EM, Xanarios I, et al. Protein function in the post-genomic era. *Nature* 2000; 405:823–826.
2. Price RA. The case for single gene effects on human obesity. In: Bouchard C, ed. *The genetics of obesity.* Boca Raton, FL: CRC Press, 1994:93–108.
3. Price RA. Strategies for identifying human obesity genes. In Bouchard C, Bray GA, eds. *Regulation of body weight: biological and behavioral mechanisms.* West Sussex, UK: John Wiley and Sons, 1996:239–250.
4. Schork NJ, Allison DB, Theil B. Mixture distributions in human genetics research. *Stat Methods Med Res* 1996; 5:155–178.
5. Rankinen T, Perusse L, Weisnagel SJ, et al. The human obesity gene map: the 2001 update. *Obes Res* 2002;10: 196–243.
6. Comuzzie AG, Allison DB. The search for human obesity genes. *Science* 1998;280:1374–1377.
7. Green EL. *Genetics and probability in animal breeding experiments.* New York: Macmillan Publishers, 1981.
8. Hill WG. Estimation of realized heritabilities from selection experiments, I: Divergent selection. *Biometrics* 1972;28:747–765.
9. Biondini PE, Sutherland TM, Haverland LH. Body composition of mice selected for growth rate. *J Anim Sci* 1968;27:5–12.
10. Herbert R. Statistics of live stock in the United Kingdom, 1853–1863. *J Stat Soc London* 1864;27:520–525.
11. Warwick EJ. Fifty years of progress in breeding beef cattle. *J Anim Sci* 1958;17:922–943.
12. Eisen E. Selection of components for body composition in mice and rats. A review. *Livestock Production Science* 1989;23:17–32.
13. Kuczmarski RJ, Flegal KM, Campbell SM, et al. Increasing prevalence of overweight among US adults. *JAMA* 1994;272:205–211.
14. Cameron ND. *Selection indices and prediction of genetic merit in animal breeding.* New York: CABI Publishing, 1997.
15. Allen P, Mccarthy JC. The effects of selection for high and low body-weight on the proportion and distribution of fat in mice. *Animal Production* 1980;31:1–11.
16. Eisen EJ. Single-trait and antagonistic index selection for litter size and body-weight in mice. *Genetics* 1978; 88:781–811.
17. Falconer DS. Replicated selection for body-weight in mice. *Genet Res* 1973;22:291–321.
18. Levin B, Dunn-Meynell AA, Balkan B, et al. Selective breeding for diet-induced obesity and resistance in Sprague–Dawley rats. *Am J Physiol* 1997;273:R725–R730.
19. Lagerkvist G, Johansson K, Lundeheim N. Selection for litter size, body weight, and pelt quality in mink (Mystela vison): experimental design and direct response of each trait. *J Anim Sci* 1993;71:3261–3272.
20. Nestor KE. Genetics of growth and reproduction in turkey, V: Selection for increased body-weight alone and in combination with increased egg production. *Poult Sci* 1977;56:337–347.
21. Vanwambeke F, Moermans R, Degroote G. Early body-weight selection of broiler breeder males in relation to reproductive and growth performance of their offspring. *Br Poult Sci* 1979;20:565–570.
22. Farhat A, Chavez ER. Comparative performance, blood chemistry, carcass composition of two lines of Pekin ducks reared mixed or separated by sex. *Poult Sci* 2000;79:460–465.
23. Marks HI. Reverse selection in a Japanese quail line previously selected for 4-week body-weight. *Poult Sci* 1980;59:1149–1154.
24. Marks HI. Long-term selection for 4-week body-weight in Japanese quail under different nutritional environments. *Theor Appl Genet* 1978;52:105–111.
25. Newton JR, Cunningham PJ, Zimmerman DR. Selection for ovulation rate in swine—correlated response in age and weight at puberty, daily gain and probe backfat. *J Anim Sci* 1977;44:30–35.
26. Ghoneim KE, Kazzal NT, Mclaren JB. Selection for increased weight of Awassi sheep in Iraq. *Tropical Agriculture* 1975;52:229–232.
27. Koch RM. Selection in beef cattle, III: Correlated response of carcass traits to selection for weaning weight, yearling weight and muscling score in cattle. *J Anim Sci* 1978;47:142–150.
28. Refstie T, Steine TA. Selection experiments with salmon, III: Genetic and environmental sources of variation in length and weight of atlantic salmon in freshwater phase. *Aquaculture* 1978;14:221–234.
29. Ryman N. Two way selection for body-weight in guppy-fish, lebistes reticulatus. *Hereditas* 1973;74:239–245.
30. Sutherland TM, Biondini PE, Ward GM. Selection for growth rate, feed efficiency and body composition in mice. *Genetics* 1974;78:525–540.

31. Notter DR, Dickerson GE, Deshazer JA. Selection for rate and efficiency of lean gain in rat. *Genetics* 1976;84: 125–144.
32. Konarzewski M, Gavin A, McDevitt R, et al. Metabolic and organ mass responses to selection for high growth rates in the domestic chicken (Gallus domesticus). *Physiol Biochem Zool* 2000;73:237–248.
33. Maruyama K, Akbar MK, Turk CM. Growth pattern and carcase development in male ducks selected for growth rate. *Br Poult Sci* 1999;40:233–239.
34. Sather AP, Fredeen HT. Effect of selection for lean growth-rate upon feed-utilization by market hog. *Can J Anim Sci* 1978;58:285–289.
35. Standal N. Selection for low backfat and high growth-rate and vice versa for 9-generations—effect on quantity and quality of lean meat. *Acta Agriculture Scand* 1979;117–121.
36. Vesely JA, Peters HF. Response to selection for weight-per-day-of-age in rambouillet and romnelet sheep. *Can J Anim Sci* 1975;55:1–8.
37. Andersen BB, Fredeen HT, Weiss GM. Correlated response in birth-weight, growth-rate and carcass merit under single-trait selection for yearling weight in beef shorthorn cattle. *Can J Anim Sci* 1974;54:117–125.
38. Perry D, Arthur PF. Correlated response in body composition and fat partitioning to divergent selection for yearling growth rate in Angus cattle. *Livestock Prod Sci* 2000;62:143–153.
39. Gjedrem T. Genetic improvement of cold-water fish species. *Aquaculture Res* 2000;31:25–33.
40. Kincaid HI, Bridges WR, Vonlimbach B. Three generations of selection for growth-rate in fall spawning rainbow trout. *Trans Am Fisheries Soc* 1977;106:621–628.
41. Beniwal BK, Hastings IM, Thompson R, et al. Estimation of changes in genetics parameters in selected lines of mice using REML with an animal model, II: Body weight, body composition and litter size. *Heredity* 1992; 69:361–371.
42. Sharp GL, Hill WG, Robinson A. Effects of selection on growth, body composition and food intake in mice, I: Responses in selected traits. *Genet Res* 1984;43:75–92.
43. Piles M, Blasco A, Pla M. The effect of selection for growth rate on carcass composition and meat characteristics. *Meat Sci* 2000;54:347–355.
44. Geraert PA, Macleod MG, Leclercq B. Energy metabolism in genetically fat and lean chickens: diet- and cold-induced thermogenesis. *J Nutr* 1988;118:1232–1239.
45. Marks HL. Carcass composition, feed intake, and feed efficiency following long-term selection for four-week body weight in Japanese quail. *Poult Sci* 1993;72:1005–1011.
46. Aass L, Vangen O. Effects of selection for high milk yield and growth on carcass and meat quality traits in dual purpose cattle. *Livestock Prod Sci* 1997;52:75–86.
47. Hayes JF, Mccarthy JC. Effects of selection at different ages for high and low body-weight on pattern of fat deposition in mice. *Genet Res* 1976;27:389–433.
48. Baeza E, Carville H, Salichon MR, et al. Effects of selection, over three and four generations, on meat yield and fatness in Muscovy ducks. *Br Poult Sci* 1997;38:359–365.
49. Marks HL, Washburn KW. Body, abdominal fat, and testes weights, and line by sex interactions in Japanese quail divergently selected for plasma cholesterol response to adrenocorticotropin. *Poult Sci* 1991;70: 2395–2401.
50. Hooper AC. Bone length and muscle weight in mice subjected to genetic selection for relative length of tibia and radius. *Life Sci* 1978;22:283–286.
51. Marks HL. Changes in unselected traits accompanying long-term selection for 4-week body-weight in Japanese quail. *Poult Sci* 1979;58:269–274.
52. Meyer K, Hill WG. Mixed model analysis of a selection experiment for food intake in mice. *Genet Res* 1991; 57:71–81.
53. Parker RJ, Bhatti MA. Selection for feed efficiency in mice under ad libitum and restricted feeding terminated by fixed time or quantity of intake. *Can J Genet Cytol* 1984;24:117–122.
54. Pym RA, Nicholls PJ. Selection for food conversion in broilers—direct and correlated responses to selection for body-weight gain, food-consumption and food conversion ratio. *Br Poult Sci* 1979;20:73–86.
55. O'Sullivan NP, Dunnington EA, Siegel PB. Correlated responses in lines of chickens divergently selected for fifty-six-day body weight, I: Growth, feed intake, and feed utilization. *Poult Sci* 1992;71:590–597.
56. Marks HL. Long-term selection for body weight in Japanese quail under different environments. *Poult Sci* 1996;75:1195–1203.
57. Cameron ND, Penman JC, McCullough E. Serum leptin concentration in pigs selected for high or low daily food intake. *Genet Res* 2000;75:209–213.
58. Vangen O. Studies on a 2-trait selection experiment in pigs, III: Correlated responses in daily feed—intake, feed conversion and carcass traits. *Acta Agriculture Scand* 1980;30:125–141.
59. Eisen EJ, Durrant BS. Effects of maternal environment and selection for litter size and body-weight on biomass and feed efficiency in mice. *J Anim Sci* 1980;50:664–679.
60. Kownacki M, Jezierski T, Guszkiewicz A, et al. Effects of selection on the body composition and feed efficiency in mouse. *Genet Polonica* 1979;20:595–603.
61. Rompala RE, Johnson DE, Rumpler WV, et al. Energy utilization of and organ mass of Targhee sheep selected for rate and efficiency of gain and receiving high and low planes of nutrition. *J Anim Sci* 1991;69:1760–1765.
62. Hernandez P, Pla M, Blasco A. Carcass characteristics and meat quality of rabbit lines selected for different objectives, II: Relationships between meat characteristics. *Livestock Prod Sci* 1998;54:125–131.

63. Serra X, Gil F, Perez-Enciso M, et al. A comparison of carcass, meat quality and histochemical characteristics of Iberian (Guadyerbas line) and Landrace pigs. *Livestock Prod Sci* 1998;56:215–223.
64. Swallow JG, Carter PA, Garland T Jr. Artificial selection for increased wheel-running behavior in house mice. *Behav Genet* 1998;28:227–237.
65. Swallow JG, Koteja P, Carter PA, et al. Artificial selection for increased wheel-running activity in house mice results in decreased body mass at maturity. *J Exp Biol* 1999;202:2513–2520.
66. Zhan WZ, Swallow JG, Garland T Jr, et al. Effects of genetic selection and voluntary activity on the medial gastrocnemius muscle in house mice. *J Appl Physiol* 1999;87:2326–2333.
67. Rhodes JS, Koteja P, Swallow JG, et al. Body temperatures of house mice artificially selected for high voluntary wheel-running behavior: repeatability and effect of genetic selection. *Journal Thermal Biology* 2000;25: 391–400.
68. Kownacki M, Keller J, Gebler E. Selection of mice for high weight gains—effect on basal metabolic rate. *Genet Polonica* 1975;16:359–363.
69. Maeda Y, Fukunaga Y, Okamoto S, et al. The changes in body temperature, oxygen consumption, CO_2 production and muscle protein turnover rate by selection for body size in Japanese quail, Coturnix coturnix japonica. Comparative biochemistry and physiology. *Comp Physiol* 1992;103:767–770.
70. Pond CM. *The fats of life.* Cambridge, UK: Cambridge University Press, 1998.
71. Perseghin G, Scifo P, De Cobelli F, et al. Intramyocellular triglyceride content is a determinant of in vivo insulin resistance in humans: a ^{1}H-^{13}C nuclear magnetic resonance spectroscopy assessment in offspring of type 2 diabetic parents. *Diabetes* 1999;48:1600–1606.
72. Mourot J, Kouba M. Development of intra- and intermuscular adipose tissue in growing large white and Meishan pigs. *Reprod Nutr Dev* 1999;39:125–132.
73. Galton F. *Natural inheritance.* London: Macmillan, 1889.
74. Maes HH, Neale MC, Eaves LJ. Genetic and environmental factors in relative body weight and human adiposity. *Behav Genet* 1997;27:325–351.
75. Neale MC, Cardon LR. *Methodology for genetic studies of twins and families.* Dordrecht, the Netherlands: Kluwer Academic Publishers, 1992.
76. Fisher RA. The correlation between relatives on the supposition of Mendelian inheritance. *Trans R Soc Edinb* 1918;52:399–433.
77. Faith MS, Rha S, Neale MC, et al. Evidence for genetic influence on human energy intake: results from a twin study using measured observations. *Behav Genet* 1999;29:145–154.
78. Bodurtha JN, Mosteller M, Hewitt JK, et al. Genetic analysis of anthropometric measures in 11-year-old twins: the Medical College of Virginia twin study. *Pediatr Res* 1990;28:1–4.
79. Hopper JL. Why "common environmental effects" are so uncommon in the literature. In: Spector TD, Snieder H, MacGregor AJ, eds. *Advances in twin and sib-pair analyses.* London: Greenwich Medical Media, 2000.
80. Maes HH, Neale MC, Eaves LJ. Genetic and environmental factors in relative body weight and human adiposity. *Behav Genet* 1997;27:325–351.
81. Bouchard C, Savard R, Depres JP. Body composition in adopted and biological siblings. *Hum Biol* 1985;57: 61–75.
82. Tambs K, Mourn T, Eaves L, et al. Genetic and environmental contributions to the variance of the body mass index in a Norwegian sample of first- and second-degree relatives. *Am J Hum Biol* 1991;3:257–267.
83. Sorenson TIA, Stunkard AJ. Overview of the adoption studies. In: Bouchard C, ed. *The genetics of obesity.* Boca Raton, FL: CRC Press, 1994:49–61.
84. Maes HH, Beunen GP, Vlietinck RF, et al. Inheritance of physical fitness in 10-year-old twins and their parents. *Med Sci Sports Exerc* 1996;28:1479–1491.
85. Stunkard AJ, Sorenson TI, Hanis C, et al. An adoption study of human obesity. *N Engl J Med* 1986;314:193–198.
86. Price RA, Cadoret RJ, Stunkard AJ, et al. Genetic contributions to human fatness: an adoption study. *Am J Psychiatry* 1987;144:1003–1008.
87. Cardon LR. Genetic influences on body mass index in early childhood. In: Turner JR, Cardon LR, Hewitt JK, eds. *Behavior genetic approaches in behavioral medicine.* New York: Plenum Publishing, 1995:133–143.
88. Hartz A, Giefer E, Rimm AA. Relative importance of the effect of family environment and heredity on obesity. *Ann Hum Genet* 1997;41:185–193.
89. Segal NL. *Entwined lives: twins and what they tell us about human behavior.* New York: Plume, 2000.
90. Segal NL, Allison DB. Twins and virtual twins: Bases of relative body weight revisited. *Int J Obes Relat Metab Disord* 2002;26:437–441.
91. Allison DB, Kaprio J, Korkeila M, et al. The heritability of body mass index among an international sample of monozygotic twins reared apart. *Int J Obes* 1996;20:501–506.
92. Bouchard C, Pérusse L, Leblanc C, et al. Inheritance of the amount and distribution of human body fat. *Int J Obes* 1987;12:205–212.
93. Sanchez AM, Reed DR, Price RA. Reduced mortality associated with body mass index (BMI) in African-Americans relative to Caucasians. *Ethnicity Dis* 2000;10:24–30.
94. Suen S, Tam R, Yang V, et al. Comparison of incidences of overweight and obesity between Asian and non–Asian American middle and high schoolers. *FASEB J* 1997;11:2313.
95. Weyer C, Pratley RE, Snitker S, et al. Ethnic differences in insulinemia and sympathetic tone as links between obesity and blood pressure. *Hypertension* 2000;36:531–537.

96. Krosnick A. The diabetes and obesity epidemic among the Pima Indians. *N J Med* 2000;94:31–37.
97. Wang J, Thornton JC, Burastero S, et al. Comparisons for body mass index and body fat percent among Puerto Ricans, blacks, whites and Asians living in the New York City area. *Obes Res* 1996;4:377–384.
98. Harrell JS, Gore SV. Cardiovascular risk factors and socioeconomic status in African American and Caucasian women. *Res Nurs Health* 1998;21:285–295.
99. Allison D, Edlen-Nezin L, Clay-Williams G. Obesity among African American women: prevalence, consequences, causes, and developing research. *Womens Health Res Gender Behav Policy* 1997;3:243–274.
100. Parra EJ, Marcini A, Akey J, et al. Estimating African-American admixture proportions by use of population-specific alleles. *Am J Hum Genet* 1998;63:1839–1851.
101. Williams RC, Long JC, Hanson RL, et al. Individual estimates of European genetic admixture associated with lower body mass index, plasma glucose, and prevalence of type 2 diabetes in Pima Indians. *Am J Hum Genet* 2000;66:527–539.
102. Fernandez JR, Shriver MD, Rafla-Demetrious N, et al. Is African genetic admixture associated with BMI and resting metabolic rate in African American females? *Obese Res* 2001;Suppl 3:87S.
103. Jenkinson CP, Hanson R, Cray K, et al. Association of dopamine D_2 receptor polymorphism Ser311Cys and TaqIA with obesity or type 2 diabetes mellitus in Pima Indians. *Int J Obes Relat Metab Disord* 2000;24:1233–1238.
104. Chakraborty R, Weiss KM. Admixture as a tool for finding linked genes and detecting that difference from allelic association between loci. *Proc Natl Acad Sci U S A* 1988;85:9119–9123.
105. McKeigue PM. Mapping genes underlying ethnic differences in disease risk by linkage disequilibrium in recently admixed populations. *Am J Hum Genet* 1997;60:188–196.
106. Plomin R. The role of inheritance in behavior. *Science* 1990;248:183–188.
107. Faith MS, Johnson SL, Allison DB. Putting the behavior into behavior genetics of obesity. *Behav Genet* 1997;27:423–437.
108. Weinsier RL, Hunter GR, Heini AF, et al. The etiology of obesity: relative contribution of metabolic factors, diet, and physical activity. *Am J Med* 1998;105:145–150.
109. de Castro JM. Social facilitation of eating: effects of social instruction on food intake. *Physiol Behav* 1992;52:749–754.
110. de Castro JM. Heritability of hunger relationships with food intake in free-living humans. *Physiol Behav* 1999;67:249–258.
111. de Castro JM. Genes and environment have gender-independent influences on the eating and drinking of free-living humans. *Physiol Behav* 1998;63:385–395.
112. de Castro JM. Heritability of hunger relationships with food intake in free-living humans. *Physiol Behav* 1993;67:249–258.
113. de Castro JM. Genetic influences on daily intake and meal patterns of humans. *Physiol Behav* 1993;53:777–782.
114. Fabsitz RR, Garrison RJ, Feineib M, et al. A twin analysis of dietary intake: evidence for a need to control for possible environmental differences in MZ and DZ twins. *Behav Genet* 1978;8:15–25.
115. Falciglia GA, Norton PA. Evidence for a genetic influence on preference for some foods. *J Am Diet Assoc* 1994;94:154–158.
116. Faust J. A twin study of personal preferences. *J Biosoc Sci* 1974;6:75–91.
117. Krondl M, Coleman P, Wade J, et al. A twin study examining the genetic influence on food selection. *Hum Nutr Appl Nutr* 1983;37:189–198.
118. Rutherford J, McGuffin P, Katz R, et al. Genetic influences on eating attitudes in a normal female twin population. *Psychol Med* 1993;23:425–436.
119. Yeo MA, Treloar SA, Marks G, et al. What are the causes of individual differences in food consumption and are they modified by personality? *Personality and Individual Differences* 1997;23:535–542.
120. Wade J, Milner J, Krondl M. Evidence for a physiological regulation of food selection and nutrient intake in twins. *Am J Clin Nutr* 1981;34:143–147.
121. van den Bree MB, Eaves LJ, Dwyer JT. Genetic and environmental influences on eating patterns of twins aged ≥50 y. *Am J Clin Nutr* 1999;70:456–465.
122. Wolper C, Heshka S, Heymsfield SB. Measuring food intake: an overview. In: Allison DB, ed. *Handbook of assessment methods for eating behaviors and weight-related problems*. Thousand Oaks, CA: Sage Publications Inc, 1995.
123. Faith MS, Pietrobelli A, Nunez C, et al. Evidence for independent genetic influences on fat mass and body mass index in a child and adolescent twin sample. *Pediatrics* 1998;104:61–67.
124. Bouchard C, Malina RM, Pérusse L. *Genetics of fitness and physical performance*. Champaign, IL: Human Kinetics, 1994.
125. Goran MI. Genetic influences on human energy expenditure and substrate utilization. *Behav Genet* 1997;27:389–399.
126. Pérusse L, Rice T, Province MA, et al. Familial aggregation of amount of distribution of subcutaneous fat and their responses to exercise training in the HERITAGE family study. *Obes Res* 2000;8:140–150.
127. Samaras K, Kelly PJ, Chiano MN, et al. Genetic and environmental influences on total-body fat and central abdominal fat: the effect of physical activity in female twins. *Ann Intern Med* 1999;130:873–882.
128. Nelson RJ, Young KA. Behavior in mice with targeted disruption of single genes. *Neurosci Biobehav Rev* 1998;22:453–462.

129. West D, Dhar M, Webb L, et al. A heterozygous deletion of a novel ATPase gene on mouse chromosome 7 increases body fat. Presented at the North American Association for the Study of Obesity Conference, 2000 Oral Presentations O184 Long Beach, California, October 29 to November 2, 2000.

130. Scearce-Levie K, Chen JP, Gardner E, et al. Molecular and functional diversity of ion channels and receptors. *Ann N Y Acad Sci* 1999;868:701–715.

131. Tecott LH, Sun LM, Akana SF, et al. Eating disorder and epilepsy in mice lacking 5-HT$_{2c}$ serotonin receptors. *Nature* 1995;374:542–546.

132. Siracusa LD. The agouti gene—turned on to yellow. *Trend Genet* 1994;10:43–428.

133. Din N, Sorensen A, Hamilton BS, et al. Beta1/beta2 adrenergic receptor (AR) double knockout mice exhibit mild obesity. Presented at the North American Association for the Study of Obesity Conference, 2000 Poster Presentation PE10.

134. Revelli JP, Preitner F, Samec S, et al. Targeted gene disruption reveals a leptin-independent role for the mouse beta3-adrenoceptor in the regulation of body composition. *J Clin Invest* 1997;100:1098–1126.

135. Ohki-Hamazaki H, Watase K, Yamamoto K, et al. Mice lacking bombesin receptor subtype-3 develop metabolic defects and obesity. *Nature* 1997;390:165–169.

136. Asnicar MA, Smith DP, Yang DD, et al. Absence of cocaine- and amphetamine-regulated transcript results in obesity in mice fed a high caloric diet. *Endocrinology* 2001;142:4394–4400.

137. Schwartz GJ, Whitney A, Skoglund C, et al. Decreased responsiveness to dietary fat in Otsuka–Lomg–Evans Tokushima fatty rats lacking CCK-A receptors. *Am J Physiol* 1999;277:R1144–R1151.

138. Fain JN, Ballou LR, Bahouth SW. Obesity is induced in mice heterozygous for cyclooxygenase-2. *Prostaglandins Other Lipid Mediat* 2001;65:199–209.

139. Jones ME, Thorburn AW, Britt KL, et al. Aromatase-deficient (ArKO) mice have a phenotype of increased adiposity. *Proc Natl Acad Sci U S A* 2000;97:12735–12740.

140. Heine PA, Taylor JA, Iwamoto GA, et al. Increased adipose tissue in male and female estrogen receptor knockout mice. *Proc Natl Acad Sci U S A* 2000;97:12729–12734.

141. Vassileva G, Huwyler L, Poirier K, et al. The intestinal fatty acid binding protein is not essential for dietary fat absorption in mice. *FASEB J* 2000;14:2040–2046.

142. Leiter EH, Kintner J, Flurkey K, et al. Physiologic and endocrinologic characterization of the male sex-biased diabetes in C57BLKS/J mice congenic for the fat mutation at the carboxypeptidase E locus. *Endocrine* 1999; 10:57–66.

143. Danilovich N, Babu PS, Xing WR, et al. Estrogen deficiency, obesity, and skeletal abnormalities in follicle-stimulating hormone receptor knockout (FORKO) female mice. *Endocrinology* 2000;141:4295–4308.

144. Yu S, Gavrilova O, Chen H, et al. Paternal versus maternal transmission of a stimulatory G-protein alpha subunit knockout produces opposite effects on energy metabolism. *J Clin Invest* 2000;105:615–623.

145. Matsui H, Suzuki M, Tsukuda R, et al. Expression of ICAM-1 on glomeruli is associated with progression of diabetic nephropathy in a genetically obese diabetic rat, Wistar fatty. *Diabetes Res Clin Pract* 1996;32:1–9.

146. Zhang Y, Proenca R, Maffei M, et al. Positional cloning of the mouse obese gene and its human homologue. *Nature* 1994;372:425–432.

147. Clement K, Vaisse C, Lahlou N, et al. A mutation in the human leptin receptor gene causes obesity and pituitary dysfunction. *Nature* 1998;392:398–401.

148. Chen AS, Marsh DJ, Trumbauer ME, et al. Inactivation of the mouse melanocortin-3 receptor results in increased fat mass and reduced lean body mass. *Nat Genet* 2000;26:97–102.

149. Farooqi IS, Yeo GS, Keogh JM, et al. Dominant and recessive inheritance of morbid obesity associated with melanocortin 4 receptor deficiency. *J Clin Invest* 2000;106:271–279.

150. Good DJ, Porter FD, Mahon KA, et al. Hypogonadism and obesity in mice with a targeted deletion of the Nhlh2 gene. *Nat Genet* 1997;15:397–401.

151. Chemelli RM, Willie JT, Sinton CM, et al. Narcolepsy in orexin knockout mice: molecular genetics of sleep regulation. *Cell* 1999;98:437–451.

152. Hara J, Beuckmann CT, Nambu T, et al. Genetic ablation of orexin neurons in mice results in narcolepsy, hypophagia, and obesity. *Neuron* 2001;30:345–354.

153. Morange PE, Lijnen HR, Alessi MC, et al. Influence of PAI-1 on adipose tissue growth and metabolic parameters in a murine model of induced obesity. *Physiol Genomics* 2000;4:93–100.

154. Yaswen L, Diehl N, Brennan MB, et al. Obesity in the mouse model of pro-opiomelanocortin deficiency responds to peripheral melanocortin. *Nat Med* 1999;5:1066–1070.

155. Costet P, Legendre C, More J, et al. Peroxisome proliferator-activated receptor alpha-isoform deficiency leads to progressive dyslipidemia with sexually dimorphic obesity and steatosis. *J Biol Chem* 1998;273:29577–29585.

156. Kubota N, Terauchi Y, Miki H, et al. PPAR gamma mediates high-fat diet–induced adipocyte hypertrophy and insulin resistance. *Mol Cell* 1999;4:597–609.

157. Moon YS, Smas CM, Lee K, et al. Mice lacking paternally expressed pref-1/dlk1 display growth retardation and accelerated adiposity. *Mol Cell Biol* 2002;22:5585–5592.

158. Majdic G, Young M, Gomez-Sanchez E, et al. Knockout mice lacking steroidogenic factor 1 are a novel genetic model of hypothalamic obesity. *Endocrinology* 2002;143:607–614.

159. Stubdal H, Lynch CA, Moriarty A, et al. Targeted deletion of the *tub* mouse obesity gene reveals that *tubby* is a loss-of-function mutation. *Mol Cell Biol* 2000;20:878–882.

160. Gainetdinov RR, Jones SR, Caron MG. Functional hyperdopaminergia in dopamine transporter knockout mice. *Biol Psychiatry* 1999;46:303–311.

161. Katz EB, Stenbit AE, Hatton K, et al. Cardiac and adipose tissue abnormalities but not diabetes in mice deficient in GLUT4. *Nature* 1995;377:151–155.
162. Anand A, Chada K. In vivo modulation of HMGIC reduces obesity. *Nat Genet* 2000;24:377–380.
163. Yuan MS, Konstantopoulos N, Lee JS, et al. Reversal of obesity- and diet-induced insulin resistance with salicylates or targeted disruption of IKK beta. *Science* 2001;293:1673–1677.
164. Mori K, Yahata K, Mukoyama M, et al. Disruption of Klotho gene causes an abnormal energy homeostasis in mice. *Biochem Biophys Res Commun* 2000;278:665–670.
165. Dinulescu DM, Fan W, Boston BA, et al. Mahogany (mg) stimulates feeding and increases basal metabolic rate independent of its suppression of agouti. *Proc Natl Acad Sci U S A* 1998;96:12707–12712.
166. Shimada M, Tritos NA, Lowell BB, et al. Mice lacking melanin-concentrating hormone are hypophagic and lean. *Nature* 1998;396:670–674.
167. Martinez-Botaz J, Andreson JB, Tessler D, et al. Absence of pirilipin results in leanness and reverses obesity in *db/db* mice. *Nat Genet* 2000;26:474–479.
168. Planas JV, Cummings DE, Idzerda RL, et al. Mutation of the RII beta subunit of protein kinase A differentially affects lipolysis but not gene induction in white adipose tissue. *J Biol Chem* 1999;274:36281–36287.
169. Elchebly M, Payette P, Michaliszyn E, et al. Increased insulin sensitivity and obesity resistance in mice lacking the protein tyrosine phosphatase-1B gene. *Science* 1999;283:1544–1548.
170. Kennedy BP. Role of protein tyrosine phosphatase-1B in diabetes and obesity. *Biomed Pharmacother* 1999;53:466–470.
171. Klaman LD, Boss O, Peroni OD, et al. Increased energy expenditure, decreased adiposity, and tissue-specific insulin sensitivity in protein-tyrosine phosphatase 1B–deficient mice. *Mol Cell Biol* 2000;20:5479–5489.
172. Ventre J, Doebber T, Wu M, et al. Targeted disruption of the tumor necrosis factor-alpha gene: metabolic consequences in obese and non-obese mice. *Diabetes* 1997;46:1526–1531.
173. Uysal KT, Wiesbrock SM, Marino MW, et al. Protection from obesity-induced insulin resistance in mice lacking TNF-alpha function. *Nature* 1997;389:610–614.
174. Schreyer SA, Chua SC Jr, LeBoeuf RC. Obesity and diabetes in TNF-alpha receptor deficient mice. *J Clin Invest* 1998;102:402–411.
175. Monemdjou S, Hofmann WE, Kozak LP, et al. Increased mitochondrial proton leak in skeletal muscle of UCP1-deficient mice. *Am J Physiol Endocrinol Metab* 2000;279:E941–E946.
176. Clapham JC, Arch JR, Chapman H, et al. Mice overexpressing human uncoupling protein-3 in skeletal muscle are hyperphagic and lean. *Nature* 2000;406:415–418.
177. Hahm S, Mizuno TM, Wu TJ, et al. Targeted deletion of the Vgf gene indicates that the encoded secretory peptide precursor plays a novel role in the regulation of energy balance. *Neuron* 1999;23:537–548.
178. McPherron AC, Lawler AM, Lee SJ. Regulation of skeletal muscle mass in mice by a new TGF-beta superfamily member. *Nature* 1997;387:83–90.
179. McPherron AC, Lee SJ. Double muscling in cattle due to mutations in the myostatin gene. *Proc Natl Acad Sci U S A* 1997;94:12457–12461.
180. Cederberg A, Gronning LM, Ahren B, et al. FoxC2 is a winged helix gene that counteracts obesity, hypertriglyceridemia, and diet-induced insulin resistance. *Cell* 2001;106:563–573.
181. Goudriaan JR, Tacken PJ, Dahlmans VE, et al. Protection from obesity in mice lacking the VLDL receptor. *Arterioscler Thromb Vasc Biol* 2001;21:1488–1493.
182. Vidal-Puig AJ, Grujic D, Zhang CY, et al. Energy metabolism in uncoupling protein 3 gene knockout mice. *J Biol Chem* 2000;275:16258–16266.
183. Magdaleno SM, Curran T. Gene dosage in mice—BAC to the future. *Nat Genet* 1999;22:319–320.
184. Trayhurn P. The development of obesity in animals: the role of genetic susceptibility. *Clin Endocrinol Metab* 1984;13:451–474.
185. Campfield LA, Smith FJ, Guisez Y, et al. Recombinant mouse OB protein: evidence for a peripheral signal linking adiposity and central neural networks. *Science* 1995;269:546–549.
186. Trayhurn P, Fuller L. The development of obesity in genetically diabetic-obese (*db/db*) mice pair fed with lean siblings. The importance of thermoregulatory thermogenesis. *Diabetologia* 1980;19:148–153.
187. Trayhurn P. Biology of leptin—its implications and consequences for the treatment of obesity. *Int J Obes* 2001;25:S26–S28.
188. Thodesen J, Grisdale-Helland B, Helland SJ, et al. Feed intake, growth and feed utilization of offspring from wild and selected Atlantic salmon (Salmo salar). *Aquaculture* 1999;180:237–246.
189. Proudman JA, Mellen WJ, Anderson DL. Utilization in feed in fast- and slow-growing lines of chickens. *Poult Sci* 1970;49:961–972.
190. van Kaam JB, Groenen MA, Bovenhuis H, et al. Whole genome scan in chickens for quantitative trait loci affecting growth and feed efficiency. *Poult Sci* 1999;78:15–23.
191. Blizard DA, Kotlus B, Frank ME. Quantitative trait loci associated with short-term intake of sucrose, saccharin and quinine solutions in laboratory mice. *Chem Senses* 1999;24:373–385.
192. Belknap JK, Crabbe JC, Plomin R, et al. Single-locus control of saccharin intake in Bxd Ty recombinant inbred (RI) mice—some methodological implications for RI strain analysis. *Behav Genet* 1992;22:81–100.
193. Mayeux-Portas V, File SE, Stewart CL, Morris RJ. Mice lacking the cell adhesion molecule Thy-1 fail to use socially transmitted cues to direct their choice of food. *Curr Biol* 2000;10:68–75.
194. Plomin R, DeFries JC, McClearn GE. *Behavioral genetics,* 2nd ed. New York: WH Freeman and Company, 1989.

195. Flint J, Corley R, DeFries JC, et al. A simple genetic basis for a complex psychological trait in laboratory mice. *Science* 1995;269:1432–1435.

196. Dunnington EA, White JM, Vinson WE. Genetic parameters of serum cholesterol levels, activity and growth in mice. *Genetics* 1997;85:659–668.

197. Jacobson KC, Rowe DC. Genetic and shared environmental influences on adolescent BMI: interactions with race and sex. *Behav Genet* 1998;28:265–278.

198. Kluge R, Giesen K, Bahrenberg G, et al. Quantitative trait loci for obesity and insulin resistance (Nob1,Nib2) and their interaction with the leptin receptor allele (LeprA720T/T1044I) in New Zealand obese mice. *Diabetologia* 2000;43:1565–1572.

199. Brockmann GA, Kratzsch J, Haley CS, et al. Single QTL effects, epistasis, and pleiotropy account for two-thirds of the phenotypic F2 variance of growth and DU6i x DBA/2 mice. *Genome Res* 2000;10:1943–1957.

200. Fabsitz RR, Carmelli D, Hewitt JK. Evidence for independent genetic influences on obesity in middle age. *Int J Obes Relat Metab Disord* 1992;16:657–666.

201. Allison DB, Kaprio J, Korkeila M, et al. The heritability of body mass index among an international sample of monozygotic twins reared apart. *Int J Obes Relat Metab Disord* 1996;20:501–506.

202. Georges M. Recent progress in livestock genomics and potential impact on breeding programs. *Theriogenology* 2001;55:15–21.

203. Goosen GJ, Dodds KG, Tate ML, et al. QTL for live weight traits in Pere David's x red deer interspecies hybrids. *J Hered* 1999;90:643–647.

204. Pérusse L, Chagnon YC, Weisnagel SJ, et al. The human obesity gene map: the 2000 update. *Obes Res* 2000; 9:135–169.

205. Pomp D. Genetic dissection of obesity in polygenic animal models. *Behav Genet* 1997;27:285–306.

206. Nadeau JH, Frankel WN. The roads from phenotypic variation to gene discovery: mutagenesis versus QTLs. *Nat Genet* 2000;25:381–384.

207. Coppieters W, Blott S, Farnir F, et al. From phenotype to genotype: towards positional cloning of QTL in livestock? *Arch Anim Breeding* 1999;42:86–92.

208. Mehrabian M, Wen P, Fisler J, et al. Genetic loci controlling body fat, lipoprotein metabolism, and insulin levels in a multifactorial mouse model. *J Clin Invest* 1998;101:2485–2496.

209. Dragani TA, Zeng ZB, Canzian F, et al. Mapping of body weight loci on mouse chromosome X. *Mamm Genome* 1995;6:778–781.

210. Taylor BA, Tarantino LM, Phillips SJ. Gender-influenced obesity QTLs identified in a cross involving the KKtyor II diabetes-prone mouse strain. *Mamm Genome* 1999;10:963–968.

211. Suto J, Matsuura S, Imamura K, et al. Genetics of obesity in KK mouse and effects of A(y) allele on quantitative regulation. *Mamm Genome* 1998;9:506–510.

212. Keightley PD, Hardge T, May L, et al. A genetic map of quantitative trait loci for body weight in the mouse. *Genetics* 1996;142:227–235.

213. Fernandez JR, Allison DB, Tarantino LM, et al. Sex-exclusive quantitative trait loci (QTL) for body weight in mice. *Obes Res* 1999;7:25S.

214. Hyman RW, Frank S, Warden CH, et al. Quantitative trait locus analysis of susceptibility to diet-induced atherosclerosis in recombinant inbred mice. *Biochem Genet* 1994;32:397–407.

215. Paigen B. Genetics of responsiveness to high-fat and high-cholesterol diets in the mouse. *Am J Clin Nutr* 1995; 62:S458–S462.

216. Purcell-Hunh DA, Weinreb A, Castellani LW, et al. Genetic factors in lipoprotein metabolism—analysis of genetic cross between inbred mouse strains NZB/BINJ and SM/J using a complete linkage map approach. *J Clin Invest* 1995;96:1845–1858.

217. Moody DE, Pomp D, Nielsen MK, et al. Identification of quantitative trait loci influencing traits related to energy balance in selection and inbred lines of mice. *Genetics* 1999;152:699–711.

218. Brockmann G, Buitkamp J, Teuscher F, et al. Multilocus fingerprint bands are associated with the growth performance in selected mouse lines: linkage analysis in reference families. *Arch Anim Breeding* 1996;39:477–487.

219. Warden CH, Fisler JS, Shoemaker SM, et al. Identification of 4 chromosomal loci determining obesity in a multifactoral mouse model. *J Clin Invest* 1995;95:1545–1552.

220. Reifsnyder PC, Churchill G, Leiter EH. Maternal environment and genotype interact to establish diabesity in mice. *Genome Res* 2000;10:1568–1578.

221. Horvat S, Bunger L, Falconer VM, et al. Mapping of obesity QTLs in a cross between mouse lines divergently selected on fat content. *Mamm Genome* 2000;11:2–7.

222. Mott R, Talbot CJ, Turri MG, et al. From the cover: a method for fine mapping quantitative trait loci in outbred animal stocks. *Proc Natl Acad Sci U S A* 2000;97:12649–12654.

223. Talbot CJ, Nicod A, Cherny SS, et al. High resolution mapping of quantitative trait loci in outbred mice. *Nat Genet* 1999;21:305–308.

224. Weil MM, Brown BW, Seachitopol DM. Genotype selection to rapidly breed congenics. *Genetics* 1997;146:1061–1069.

225. Rocha J, Pomp D, van Vleck D. QTL analysis in livestock. In: Camp NJ, Cox A, eds. *Quantitative trait loci: methods and protocols.* Totowa, NJ: Humana Press Inc, 2002.

226. Barendse W, Armitage SM, Kossarek LM, et al. A genetic-linkage map of the bovine genome. *Nat Genet* 1994; 6:227–235.

227. Subramanian G, Adams MD, Venter JC, et al. Implications of the human genome for understanding human biology and medicine. *JAMA* 2001;286:2296–2307.
228. Rexroad C. Ham, eggs, and chips—animal genomics. Presented at the meeting of the EC-US Task Force on Biotechnology Research: Mutual Understanding in Valencia, June 21 to 23, 2001.
229. Cockett NE, Jackson SP, Snowder GD, et al. The callipyge phenomenon: evidence for unusual genetic inheritance. *J Anim Sci* 1999;77:221–227.
230. Charlier C, Coppieters W, Farnir F, et al. The MH gene causing double-muscling in cattle maps to bovine chromosome-2. *Mamm Genome* 1995;6:788–792.
231. Grobet L, Poncelet D, Royo LJ, et al. Molecular definition of an allelic series of mutations disrupting the myostatin function and causing double-muscling in cattle. *Mamm Genome* 1998;9:210–213.
232. van Kaam JB, Van Arendonk JA, Groenen MA, et al. Whole genome scan for quantitative trait loci affecting body weight in chickens using a three generation design. *Livestock Prod Sci* 1998;54:133–150.
233. Casas E, Stone RT, Keele JW, et al. Comprehensive search for quantitative trait loci affecting growth and carcass composition of cattle segregating alternative forms of the myostatin gene. *J Anim Sci* 2001;79:854–860.
234. Casas E, Shackleford SD, Keele JW, et al. Quantitative trait loci affecting growth and carcass composition of cattle segregating alternate forms of myostatin. *J Anim Sci* 2000;78:560–569.
235. Elo KT, Vilkki J, de Koning DJ, et al. A quantitative trait locus for live weight maps to bovine chromosome 23. *Mamm Genome* 1999;10:831–835.
236. Sonstegard TS, Garrett WM, Ashwell MS, et al. Comparative map alignment of BTA27 and HSA4 and 8 to identify conserved segments of genome containing fat deposition QTL. *Mamm Genome* 1999;11:682–688.
237. Stone RT, Keele JW, Shackelford SD, et al. A primary screen of the bovine genome for quantitative trait loci affecting carcass and growth traits. *J Anim Sci* 1999;77:1379–1384.
238. Bidanel JP, Milan D, Iannuccelli N, et al. Detection of quantitative trait loci for growth and fatness in pigs. *Genet Sel Evol* 2001;33:289–309.
239. de Koning DJ, Rattink AP, Harlizius B, et al. Genome-wide scan for body composition in pigs reveals important role of imprinting. *Proc Natl Acad Sci U S A* 2000;97:7947–7950.
240. Grindflek E, Szyda J, Liu ZT, et al. Detection of quantitative trait loci for meat quality in a commercial slaughter pig cross. *Mamm Genome* 2001;12:299–304.
241. Malek M, Dekkers JC, Lee HK, et al. A molecular genome scan analysis to identify chromosomal regions influencing economic traits in the pig, I: Growth and body composition. *Mamm Genome* 2001;12:630–636.
242. Malek M, Dekkers JC, Lee HK, et al. A molecular genome scan analysis to identify chromosomal regions influencing economic traits in the pig, II: Meat and muscle composition. *Mamm Genome* 2001;12:637–645.
243. Perez-Enciso M, Clop A, Noguera JL, et al. A QTL on pig chromosome 4 affects fatty acid metabolism: evidence from an Iberian by Landrace intercross. *J Anim Sci* 2000;78:2525–2531.
244. Rattink AP, De Koning DJ, Faivre M, et al. Fine mapping and imprinting analysis for fatness trait QTLs in pigs. *Mamm Genome* 2000;11:656–661.
245. Rohrer GA. Identification of quantitative trait loci affecting birth characters and accumulation of backfat and weight in a Meishan-white composite resource population. *J Anim Sci* 2000;78:2547–2553.
246. Wada Y, Akita T, Awata T, et al. Quantitative trait loci (QTL) analysis in a Meishan x Gottingen cross population. *Anim Genet* 2001;31:376–384.
247. Walling GA, Visscher PM, Andersson L, et al. Combined analyses of data from quantitative trait loci mapping studies: chromosome 4 effects on porcine growth and fatness. *Genetics* 2000;155:1369–1378.
248. Wu XL, Lee C, Jiang J, et al. Mapping a quantitative trait locus for growth and backfat on porcine chromosome 18. *Asian Aust J Anim Sci* 2001;14:1665–1669.
249. Robison BD, Wheeler PA, Sundin K, et al. Composite interval mapping reveals a major locus influencing embryonic development rate in rainbow trout (Oncorhynchus mykiss). *J Hered* 2001;92:16–22.
250. Goodpaster BH, Theriault R, Watkins SC, et al. Intramuscular lipid content is increased in obesity and decreased by weight loss. *Metab Clin Exp* 2000;49:467–472.
251. National Institute of Diabetes, Digestive and Kidney Diseases. *Adi-map: an obesity gene mapping collaborative project. Meeting report.* Bethesda, MD: National Institutes of Health, 2000.
252. Hinney A, Schmidt A, Nottebom K. Several mutations in the melanocortin-4 receptor gene including a nonsense and frameshift mutation associated with dominantly inherited obesity in humans. *J Clin Endocrinol Metab* 1999;84:1483–1486.
253. Gu W, Tu Z, Kleyn PW. Identification and functional analysis of novel melanocortin-4 receptor variants. *Diabetes* 1999;48:635–639.
254. Hebebrand J, Sommerlad C, Geller F, et al. The genetics of obesity: practical implications. *Int J Obes Relat Metab Disord* 2001;25:S10–S17.
255. Krude H, Biebermann H, Luck W, et al. Severe early-onset obesity, adrenal insufficiency and red hair pigmentation caused by POMC mutations in humans. *Nat Genet* 1998;19:155–157.
256. Nothen MM, Cichon S, Hemmer S. Human dopamine D₄ receptor gene: frequent occurrence of a null allele and observation of homozygosity. *Hum Mole Genet* 1994;3:2207–2212.
257. Ristow M, Muller-Wieland D, Pfeiffer A, et al. Obesity associated with a mutation in a genetic regulator of adipocyte differentiation. *N Engl J Med* 1998;339:953–959.
258. Campfield LA, Smith FJ, Burn P. Strategies and potential targets for obesity treatment. *Science* 1998;280:1383–1387.

259. Tartaglia LA, Dembski M, Weng X, et al. Identification and expression cloning of a leptin receptor, OB-R. *Cell* 1995;83:1263–1271.
260. Strobel A, Issad T, Camoin L, et al. A leptin missense mutation associated with hypogonadism and morbid obesity. *Nat Genet* 1998;18:213–215.
261. Ozata M, Ozdemir IC, Licinio J. Human leptin deficiency caused by a missense mutation: multiple endocrine defects, decreased sympathetic tone, and immune system dysfunction indicate new targets for leptin action, greater central than peripheral resistance to the effects of leptin, and spontaneous correction of leptin-mediated defects. *J Clin Endocrinol Metab* 1999;84:3686–3695.
262. Farooqi IS, Jebb SA, Langmack G, et al. Effects of recombinant leptin therapy in a child with congenital leptin deficiency. *N Engl J Med* 1999;341:879–884.
263. Heo M, Leibel RL, Fontaine KR, et al. A meta-analytic investigation of linkage and association of common leptin receptor (LEPR) polymorphisms with body mass index and waist circumference. *Int J Obes Relat Metab Disord* 2002;26:640–646.
264. Ketterings C. Lipodystrophy and its treatment. *Ann Plast Surg* 1988;21:536–543.
265. Fagher B, Monti M, Nilsson-Ehle P, et al. Fat-cell heat production, adipose tissue fatty acids, lipoprotein lipase activity and plasma lipoproteins in adiposis dolorosa. *Clin Sci* 1991;81:793–798.
266. Brodovsky S, Westreich M, Leibowitz A, et al. Adiposis dolorosa (Dercum's disease): 10-year follow up. *Ann Plast Surg* 1994;33:664–668.
267. Reece PH, Wyatt M, O'Flynn P. Dercum's disease (adiposis dolorosa). *J Laryngol Otol* 1999;113:174–176.
268. Garg A, Wilson R, Barnes R, et al. A gene for congenital generalized lipodystrophy maps to human chromosome 9q34. *J Clin Endocrinol Metab* 1999;84:3390–3394.
269. Garg A, Stray-Gundersen J, Parsons D, et al. Skeletal muscle morphology and exercise response in congenital generalized lipodystrophy. *Diabetes Care* 2000;23:1545–1550.
270. Chen D, Garg A. Monogenic disorders of obesity and body fat distribution. *J Lipid Res* 1999;10:1735–1746.
271. Jackson SN, Pinkney J, Bargiotta A, et al. A defect in the regional deposition of adipose tissue (partial lipodystrophy) is encoded by a gene at chromosome 1q. *Am J Hum Genet* 1998;63:534–540.
272. Speckman RA, Garg A, Du F, et al. Mutational and haplotype analyses of families with familial partial lipodystrophy (Dunnigan variety) reveal recurrent missense mutations in the globular C-terminal domain of lamin A/C. *Am J Hum Genet* 2000;66:1192–1198.
273. Baker R, Kotler D, Carr A, et al. Altered body shape in HIV disease: a side effect of therapy? *Aids Patient Care and STDs* 1999;13:395–402.
274. Behrens GM, Stoll M, Schmidt RE. Lipodystrophy syndrome in HIV infection: what is it, what causes it and how can managed? *Drug Safety* 2000;23:57–76.
275. Kratz C, Lenard HG, Ruzicka T, et al. Multiple symmetric lipomatosis: an unusual cause of childhood obesity and mental retardation. *Eur J Pediatr Neurol* 2000;3:63–67.
276. Bray MS, Allison DB. Obesity syndromes. In: Owen JB, Treasure JL, Collier DA, eds. *Animal models of the disorders of eating and body composition disorders.* Dordrecht, the Netherlands: Kluwer Academic Publishers, 2001.
277. Allison BD, Packer-Munter W, Pietrobelli A, et al. Obesity and developmental disabilities: pathogenesis and treatment. *J Dev Phys Disabil* 1998;10:215–255.
278. National Center for Biotechnology Information. OMIM Online Mendelian Inheritance in Man home page. Available at: http://www.ncbi.nlm.nih.gov/omim/. Accessed April 7, 2002.
279. Prader A, Labhart A, Willi H. Syndrome von Adipositas, Kleinwuchs, Kryptorchidismus und Oligophrenia nach hyatonieartigem Zustand im Neugeborenenalter. *Schweiz Med Wochenschr* 1956;86:1260–1261.
280. Di Mario FJ, Dunham B, Burleson JA, et al. An evaluation of autonomic nervous system function in patients with Prader–Willi syndrome. *Pediatrics* 1994;93:76–81.
281. Butler MG, Meaney FJ. Standards for selected anthropometric measurements in Prader–Willi syndrome. *Pediatrics* 1991;88:853–860.
282. Leppert M, Baird L, Anderson KL, et al. Bardet–Biedl syndrome is linked to DNA markers on chromosome 11q and is genetically heterogeneous. *Nat Genet* 1994;7:108–112.
283. Young TL, Penney L, Woods MO. A fifth locus for Bardet–Biedl syndrome maps to chromosome 2q31. *Am J Hum Genet* 1999;64:900–904.
284. Ghadami M, Tomita HA, Najafi MT, et al. Bardet–Biedl syndrome type 3 in an Iranian family: clinical study and confirmation of disease localization. *Am J Med Genet* 2000;94:433–437.
285. Katsanis N, Beales PL, Woods MO, et al. Mutations in MKKS cause obesity, retinal dystrophy and renal malformations associated with Bardet–Biedl syndrome. *Nat Genet* 2000;26:67–70.
286. Elbedour K, Zucker N, Zalzstein E, et al. Cardiac abnormalities in the Bardet–Biedl syndrome: echocardiograph studies of 22 patients [Review]. *Am J Med Genet* 1994;52:164–169.
287. North KN, Fulton AB, Whiteman DA. Identical twins with Cohen syndrome. *Am J Med Genet* 1995;58:54–58.
288. Richieri-Costa A, Pirolo Junior L, Cohen MM Jr. Carpenter syndrome with normal intelligence Brazilian girl born to consanguineous patients. *Am J Med Genet* 1993;47:281–283.
289. Taravath S, Tonsgard JH. Cerebral malformations in carpenter syndrome. *Pediatr Neurol* 1993;9:230–234.
290. Reed DR, Ding Y, Cather C, et al. Human obesity does not segregate with the chromosomal regions of Prader–Willi, Bardet–Biedl, Cohen, Börjeson or Wilson–Turner syndromes. *Int J Obes Relat Metab Disord* 1995;19:599–603.

291. Gecz J, Baker E, Donnelly A. Fibroblast growth factor homologous factor 2 (FHF2): gene structure, expression and mapping to the Börjeson–Forssman–Lehmann syndrome region in Xq26 delineated by a duplication breakpoint in a BFLS-like patient. *Hum Genet* 1999;104:56–63.
292. Kennedy RL, Jones TH, Cuckle HS. Down's syndrome and the thyroid. *Clin Endocrinol* 1992;37:471–476.
293. Allison DB, Paultre F, Pi-Sunyer FX, et al. Is the intra-uterine period really a critical period for the development of obesity? *Int J Obes Relat Metab Disord* 1995;19:397–402.
294. Moretti-Ferreira D, Koiffmann CP, Listik M, et al. Macrosomia, obesity, macrocephaly and ocular abnormalities (MOMO syndrome) in two unrelated patients: delineation of a newly recognized overgrowth syndrome. *Am J Med Genet* 1993;46:555–558.
295. Zannolli R, Mostardini R, Hadjistilianou T, et al. MOMO syndrome: a new possible third case. *Clin Dysmorphol* 2000;9:281–284.
296. Falik-Zaccai TC, Shachak E, Abeliovitch D, et al. Achondroplasia in diverse Jewish and Arab populations in Israel: clinical and molecular characterization. *Isr Med Assoc J* 2000;2:601–604.
297. Patten JL, Johns DR, Valle D, et al. Mutation in the gene encoding the stimulatory G protein of adenylate cyclase in Albright's hereditary osteodystrophy. *N Engl J Med* 1990;322:1412–1419.
298. Rastogi S, Gupta S, Misra PK, et al. Pseudohypoparathyroidism—Albright hereditary osteodystrophy. *Indian J Pediatr* 1998;65:477–480.
299. Ong KK, Amin R, Dunger DB. Pseudohypoparathyroidism—another monogenic obesity syndrome. *Clin Endocrinol* 2000;52:389–391.
300. Gillessen-Kaessbach G, Demuth S, Thiele H, et al. A previously unrecognised phenotype characterised by obesity, muscular hypotonia, and ability to speak in patients with Angelman syndrome caused by an imprinting defect. *Eur J Hum Genet* 1999;7:638–644.
301. Matthijs G, Schollen E, Pardon E, et al. Mutations in PMM2, a phosphomannomutase gene on chromosome 16p13, in carbohydrate-deficient glycoprotein type I syndrome (Jaeken syndrome). *Nat Genet* 1997;16:88–92.
302. Rosenberg T, Niebhur E, Yang HM, et al. Choroidermia, congenital diseases, and mental retardation in a family with an X-chromosomal deletion. *Opthalmic Paediatr Genet* 1987;8:139–143.
303. Steinmuller R, Steinberger D, Muller U. MEHMO (mental retardation, epileptic seizures, hypogonadism and genitalism, microcephaly, obesity), a novel syndrome: assignment of disease locus to Xp21.1-p22.13. *Eur J Hum Genet* 1998;6:201–206.
304. Engelen JJ, Loots WJ, Albrechts JC, et al. Characterization of a de novo unbalanced translocation t(14q18q) using microdissection and fluorescence in situ hybridization. *Am J Med Genet* 1998;75:409–413.
305. Holder JL, Butte NF, Zinn AR. Profound obesity associated with a balanced translocation that disrupts the SIM1 gene. *Hum Mol Genet* 2000;9:101–108.
306. Zinn AR, Butte NF, Holder JL. SIM1 and obesity. *Obes Res* 2000;8:I24.
307. Bacon F. *The novum organum, with other parts of the great instauration.* Chicago, IL: Open Court, 1994.
308. Johnson PR, Greenwood MR, Horwitz BA, et al. Animal models of obesity. *Ann Rev Nutr* 1991;11:325–353.
309. Moussa NM, Claycombe KJ. The yellow mouse obesity syndrome and mechanisms of agouti-induced obesity. *Obes Res* 1999;7:506–514.
310. Chua SC. Monogenic models of obesity. *Behav Genet* 1997;27:277–284.
311. Dong ZM, Gutierrez-Ramos JC, Coxon A, et al. A new class of obesity genes encodes leucocyte adhesion receptors. *Proc Natl Acad Sci U S A* 1997;94:7526–7530.
312. Melo DG, Acosta AX, de Pina-Neto JM. Syndrome of psychomotor retardation, bulbous nose, and epilepsy (Hernandez syndrome): a Brazilian case. *Clin Dysmorphol* 1999;8:301–303.
313. Chapman DJ, Perez-Escamilla R. Identification of risk factors for delayed onset of lactation. *J Am Diet Assoc* 1999;99:450–454.
314. Dahl RE, Holttum J, Trubnick L. A clinical picture of child and adolescent narcolepsy. *J Am Acad Child Adolesc Psychiatry* 1994;33:834–841.
315. Bonatus TJ, Alexander AH. Dercum's disease (adiposis dolorosa)—a case-report and review of the literature. *Clin Orthop* 1986;205:251–253.
316. Sutcliffe JG, de Lecea L. The hypocretins: excitatory neuromodulatory peptides for multiple homeostatic systems, including sleep and feeding. *J Neurol Res* 2000;62:161–168.
317. Chicurel M. The sandman's secrets. *Nature* 2000;407:554–556.
318. Bjorntorp, P. Thrifty genes and human obesity. Are we chasing ghosts? *Lancet* 2001;358:1006–1008.
319. Bulik CM, Allison DB. Genetic epidemiology of thinness. *Obes Rev* 2001;2:107–115.
320. Allison DB, Heshka S, Neale MC, et al. A genetic analysis of relative weight among 4,020 twin pairs, with an emphasis on sex effects. *Health Psychol* 1994;13:362–365.
321. Allison DB, Heshka S, Neale MC, et al. Race effects in the genetics of adolescents' body mass index. *Int J Obes Relat Metab Disord* 1994;18:363–368.
322. Bulik CM, Sullivan PF, Kendler KS. An empirical study of classification of eating disorders. *Am J Psychiatry* 2000;157:886–895.
323. Thomas JG, Olson JM, Tapscott SJ, et al. An efficient and robust statistical modeling approach to discover differentially expressed genes using genomic expression profiles. *Genome Res* 2001;11:12227–12236.
324. Vague J. *Obesities.* London: John Libbey & Company, 1991.
325. Allison DB, Basile VC, Yuker HE. The measurement of attitudes toward and beliefs about obese persons. *Int J Eat Disord* 1991;10:599–607.
326. Barsh GS, Farooqi IS, O'Rahilly S. Genetics of body weight regulation. *Nature* 2000;404:644–651.

327. Farooqi IS, O'Rahilly S. Recent advances in the genetics of severe childhood obesity. *Arch Dis Child* 2000;83: 31–44.
328. Gillespie D, Spiegelman S. A quantitative assay for DNA-RNA hybrids with DNA immobilized on a membrane. *J Mol Biol* 1965;12:829–842.
329. Lipshutz RJ, Fodor SP, Gingeras TR, Lockhart DJ. High density synthetic oligonucleotide arrays. *Nat Genet* 1999;21:20–24.
330. Eisen MB, Brown PO. DNA arrays for analysis of gene expression. *Method Enzymol* 1999;303:179–205.
331. Allison DB, Coffey CS. Two-stage testing in microarray analysis: what is gained? *J Gerontol Biol Sci* 2002; 57A:B189–B192.
332. Allison DB, Gadbury G, Heo M, et al. A mixture model approach for the analysis of microarray gene expression data. *Comput Stat Data Anal* 2002;39:1–20.
333. Ladu MJ, Kapsas H, Palmer WK. Regulation of lipoprotein-lipase in muscle and adipose tissue during exercise. *J Appl Physiol* 1991;71:404–409.
334. Graves RA, Tontonoz P, Platt KA, et al. Identification of a fat-cell enhancer—analysis of requirements for tissue specific gene expression. *J Cell Biochem* 1992;49:219–224.
335. Gabrielsson BL, Carlsson B, Carlsson LM. Partial genome scale analysis of gene expression in human adipose tissue using DNA array. *Obes Res* 2000;8:374–384.
336. Soukas A, Cohen P, Socci ND, et al. Leptin-specific patterns of gene expression in white adipose tissue. *Genes Dev* 2000;14:963–980.
337. Nadler ST, Stoehr JP, Schueler KL, et al. The expression of adipogenic genes is decreased in obesity and diabetes mellitus. *Proc Natl Acad Sci U S A* 2000;99:11371–11376.
338. Lee C, Weindruch R, Prolla TA. Gene-expression profile of the ageing brain in mice. *Nat Genet* 2000;25: 294–297.
339. Ferrante AW, Thearle M, Liao T, et al. Effects of leptin deficiency and short-term repletion on hepatic gene expression in genetically obese mice. *Diabetes* 2001;50:2268–2278.
340. Oishi M, Taniguchi Y, Nishimura K, et al. Characterization of gene expression in bovine adipose tissue before and after fattening. *Anim Genet* 2000;31:166–170.
341. Dussere E, Moulin P, Vidal H. Differences in mRNA expression of the proteins secreted by the adipocytes in human subcutaneous and visceral adipose tissue. *Biochim Biophys Acta* 2000;1500:88–96.
342. Hida K, Wada J, Zhang H, et al. Identification of genes specifically expressed in the accumulated visceral adipose tissue of OLETF rats. *J Lipid Res* 2000;41:1615–1622.
343. Destenaves B, Thomas F. New advances in pharmacogenomics. *Curr Opin Chem Biol* 2000;4:440–444.
344. Emilien G, Ponchon M, Caldas C, et al. Impact of genomics on drug discovery and clinical medicine. *QJM* 2000;93:391–423.
345. Allison DB, Schork NJ. Selected methodological issues in meiotic mapping of obesity genes in humans: issues of power and efficiency. *Behav Genet* 1997;27:401–421.
346. Bray GA, Greenway FL. Current and potential drugs for treatment of obesity. *Endocr Rev* 1999;20:805–875.
347. Cheskin LC, Bartlett SJ, Zayas R, et al. Weight gain and prescription medications: a review. *South Med J* 1999; 92:898–904.
348. Allison DB, Mentore JM, Heo M, et al. Meta-analysis of the effects of anti-psychotic medication on weight gain. *Am J Psychiatry* 1999;156:1686–1696.
349. Bernstein JG. Induction of obesity by psychotropic drugs. *Ann N Y Acad Sci* 1987;499:203–215.
350. Kotler DP. Body composition studies in HIV-infected individuals. *Ann N Y Acad Sci* 2000;904:546–552.
351. Lenhard JM, Furfine ES, Jain RG, et al. HIV protease inhibitors block adipogenesis and increase lipolysis in vitro. *Antivir Res* 2000;47:121–129.
352. Sachs GS, Guille C. Weight gain associated with use of psychotropic medications. *J Clin Psychiatry* 1999;60: 16–19.
353. Kaunitz AM. Long-acting hormonal contraception: assessing impact on bone density, weight, and mood. *Int J Fertil Womens Med* 1999;44:110–117.
354. Edwards JG, Anderson I. Systematic review and guide to selection of selective serotonin reuptake inhibitors. *Drugs* 1999;57:507–533.
355. Perkins KA. Metabolic effects of cigarette smoking. *J Appl Physiol* 1992;72:401–409.
356. Perucca E. A pharmacological and clinical review on topiramate, a new antiepileptic drug. *Pharmacol Res* 1997;35:241–256.
357. Schertz M, Adesman AR, Alfieri NE, et al. Predictors of weight loss in children with attention deficit hyperactivity disorder treated with stimulant medication. *Pediatrics* 1996;98:763–769.
358. Gross AS, Phillips AC, Rieutord A, et al. The influence of the sparteine/debrisoquine genetic polymorphism on the disposition of dexfenfluramine. *Br J Clin Pharmacol* 1996;41:311–317.
359. Murad I, Kremer I, Dobrusin M, et al. A family-based study of the Cys23Ser 5HT2C serotonin receptor polymorphism in schizophrenia. *Am J Med Genet* 2001;105:236–248.
360. Heal DJ, Cheetham SC, Prow MR, et al. A comparison of the effects on central 5-HT function of sibutramine hydrochloride and other weight-modifying agents. *Br J Pharmacol* 1998;125:301–308.
361. Basile VS, Masellis M, Ozdemir V, et al. Pharmacogenetics of antipsychotic induced weight gain and tardive dyskinesia. *Am J Med Genet* 2000;96:O27.
362. Rietschel M, Naber D, Fimmers R, et al. Efficacy and side-effects of clozapine not associated with variation in the 5-HT2C receptor. *Neuroreport* 1997;8:1999–2003.

363. Rietschel M, Naber D, Oberlander H, et al. Efficacy and side-effects of clozapine: testing for association with allelic variation in the dopamine D-4 receptor gene. *Neuropsychopharmacology* 1996;15:491–496.

364. Rietschel M, Krauss H, Fernandez AY, et al. Weight gain and EEG alterations under treatment with clozapine not associated with 5-HT_{2C} variants. *Am J Med Genet* 1997;74:617–617.

365. Reynolds GP, Zhang ZJ, Zhang XB. Association of antipsychotic drug-induced weight gain with a 5-HT_{2C} receptor gene polymorphism. *Lancet* 2002;359:2086–2087.

366. Katz DA, Schork NJ. Power calculations for pharmacogenetic association studies. *Clin Pharmacol Ther* 1999; 65:III27.

367. Lovell DP. Impact of pharmacogenetics on toxicological studies—statistical implications. *J Exp Anim Sci* 1993; 35:259–281.

368. Gadbury GL, Iyer HK. Unit-treatment interaction and its practical consequences. *Biometrics* 2000;56:882–885.

369. Cardon LR, Idury RM, Harris TJ, et al. Testing drug response in the presence of genetic information: sampling issues for clinical trials. *Pharmacogenetics* 2000;10:503–510.

370. Witte JS, Elston RC, Cardon LR. On the relative sample size required for multiple comparisons. *Stat Med* 2000; 19:369–372.

371. Elston RC, Idury RM, Cardon LR, et al. The study of candidate genes in drug trials: sample size considerations. *Stat Med* 1999;18:741–751.

372. Hewitt JK. The genetics of obesity: what have genetic studies told us about the environment. *Behav Genet* 1997; 27:353–358.

373. Price RA, Cadoret RJ, Stunkard AJ, et al. Genetic contributions to human fatness—an adoption study. *Am J Psychiatry* 1987;144:1003–1008.

374. Hill JO, Peters JC. Environmental contributions to the obesity epidemic. *Science* 1998;280:1371–1374.

375. Steinberg KK, Smith SJ, Stroup DF, et al. Comparison of effect estimates from a meta-analysis of summary data from published studies and from a meta-analysis using individual patient data for ovarian cancer studies. *Am J Epidemiol* 1997;145:917–925.

376. Bray G, Bouchard C. Genetics of obesity: research directions. *FASEB J* 1997;11:937–945.

377. Wolf CR, Smith G, Smith RL. Pharmacogenetics. *BMJ* 2001;320:987–990.

378. Cunningham GC. The genetics revolution: ethical, legal, and insurance concerns. *Postgrad Med* 2000;108: 193–202.

3

Environmental Influences on Obesity

James O. Hill and William T. Donahoo

The obesity epidemic has arisen so quickly that it cannot be due to biology alone (1,2). This chapter examines how nongenetic and nonbiologic factors in the environment contribute to body weight regulation, as well as how the degree of influence of these factors has changed over the past few decades as obesity rates have skyrocketed. The epidemic of obesity may not represent abnormal physiology; instead, it may be a natural response to the modern world.

NATURE OF BODY WEIGHT REGULATION

To begin to assess how the environment can impact the development of obesity, the nature of energy balance regulation must first be examined. Some physiologic regulation of energy balance probably occurs. The strongest evidence for this is the surprising stability of body weight over time in most people. Given the large amount of energy that is processed through the body (1 million calories per year for an average adult), even small errors in balancing intake with expenditure can lead to substantial changes in body weight.

Additional support for energy balance regulation comes from short-term overfeeding and underfeeding studies. In response to food restriction, energy expenditure declines, attenuating the loss of body weight and body energy that results from the negative energy balance (3,4). Similarly, when human subjects are overfed, an increase in energy expenditure occurs that serves to attenuate the increase in body weight and body energy that occurs as a consequence of positive energy balance (3–7). However, the changes in energy expenditure are not sufficient to prevent weight gain during overfeeding and weight loss during underfeeding; after the intervention stops, the body weight returns to baseline levels (3–7). For example, Bouchard et al. (8) reported that weight gain during 100 days of overfeeding tends to be more similar with identical twin pairs than between twin pairs.

Further evidence for some regulation of energy balance is shown by the Bettsville One Year Dietary Intake Study, where, for example, one subject had a range of intake from 950 to 3,100 kcal per day and no significant weight changes (Fig. 3.1) (9). In many people, body weight seems to change little despite an enormous day-to-day variation in energy intake.

This suggests the presence of a regulation of energy balance such that either energy expenditure or energy intake can be, to some extent, altered in response to changes in the other. This regulatory system seems to work well to "buffer" periods of slight positive or negative energy balance of the type that occurs from day to day, with the assumption of some periods of negative energy balance and some periods of positive energy balance. The system would also work to compensate for short periods of more severe underfeed-

ENERGY (KJ)

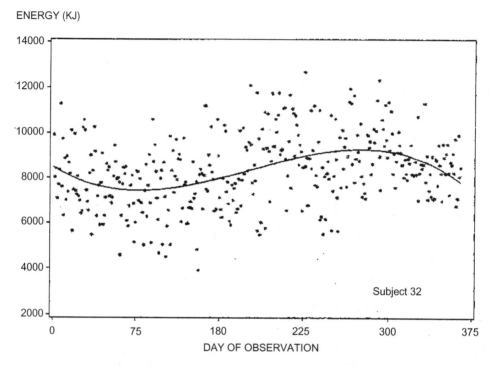

FIG. 3.1. An example of the wide variation in daily energy intake in a single weight-stable person over a year's time. (To convert kilojoules to kilocalories, divide by 4.18.)

ing or overfeeding that might be encountered during a period of food shortage or food surfeit. The system is biased toward a stronger adaptive response to negative energy balance than to positive energy balance, likely because most of humankind's history has been associated with frequent periods of inadequate food availability. Overall, this physiologic regulatory system has served humans well in the past. Is it, however, well suited for the modern world?

In the past, the system has worked sufficiently well that many have argued for the existence of a "set point" for body weight (10). The "set-point" notion dictates that body weight is regulated around some "set point" that is physiologically, and possibly genetically, determined. When body weight rises above the set point, food intake is reduced and energy expenditure is increased until the body weight returns to the set-point level. The opposite pattern occurs when body weight falls below the set point. However, explaining the epidemic of obesity using the set-point theory is difficult. The average United States adult continues to gain weight over the adult years with seemingly little physiologic opposition.

Others have argued against the set point and have instead substituted the term *settling point* (1,11). Those who prefer *settling point* argue that body weight is determined by an interaction of genetics and the environment. Because genetics do not change rapidly, body weight appears constant as long as the environment remains relatively constant. Some "buffering" capacity likely exists within the system so that body weight may remain unchanged as the environment begins to change. However, once the environment affects energy balance to the point that it exceeds the "buffering" capacity of the physiologic energy balance regulatory system, the level at which body weight is regulated would change.

The fact that most adults today are gaining weight suggests either that the regulation of body weight is defective (i.e., the set point is not working) or that factors within the environment are driving up the settling point.

IMPACT OF THE MODERN WORLD ON THE PHYSIOLOGIC REGULATORY SYSTEM

Some of the following important characteristics of the energy balance regulatory system may be problematic in today's environment:

1. The system previously was driven by the high levels of physical activity needed for daily living, and it was aimed at facilitating eating whenever food was available to ensure a sufficient level of food intake, thus avoiding body energy loss.
2. The system is much stronger when responding to a negative energy balance than when facing a positive energy balance.
3. The system is effective at buffering day-to-day variations in energy balance, with the assumption of periods of both positive and negative energy balance.
4. The system can recover quickly after short-term perturbations.

Today's environment requires very little physical activity for most people, and it provides a cheap, easily available, palatable food supply. Thus, the system is no longer driven by physical activity but instead by the availability of food and the physiologic system, which promotes eating. The challenge for the system, opposite of that of previous eras, is increasing the energy expenditure enough to match a high level of energy intake. This is a difficult challenge. The development of human physiology was not for the purpose of allowing the easy restriction of energy intake when food is readily available. One of the major problems with weight management today is that it attempts to regulate weight almost entirely by limiting food intake when human physiology developed for the opposite purpose—to facilitate eating. Put more simply, the modern world encourages humans both to be more sedentary and to eat more. This creates a situation that exceeds the capacity of the physiologic energy balance regulatory system for maintaining body weight at a healthy level.

The environmental influences on energy balance appear to be unidirectional, extremely strong, and sustained. Thus, they exceed the ability of the energy balance regulatory system to act as a "buffer," and they lead to increases in body weight (i.e., obesity) for many. The only way a high level of energy intake can be supported with a low level of physical activity is with the development of obesity. The increased body weight and the increased body fat content allow the body to achieve an energy and macronutrient balance.

ENVIRONMENTAL CHANGES THAT HAVE AN IMPACT ON ENERGY INTAKE

Unfortunately, only primarily correlational data may be used when attempting to identify the environmental factors that affect energy balance. These data must be used with caution because they cannot be used to infer cause and effect. In fact, virtually everything that has occurred as a result of the Industrial Revolution and the more recent Information

Age could be associated with the rise in the incidence of obesity (including the increase in the number of fitness facilities, which has increased from 6,742 in 1987 to 16,983 in 2001) (12). Nonetheless, an examination of how the environment has changed in ways that might be contributing to the obesity epidemic may be worthwhile.

Total Energy Intake

Many environmental factors may be influencing energy intake. Part of the difficulty in addressing this area is in getting accurate information about how energy intake has changed over time. Many studies have assessed total caloric intake in various populations using a variety of methods. Table 3.1 summarizes many such studies. Most studies reveal a decrease in total caloric intake from the 1940s to the 1980s. Only the more recent evaluation of food disappearance data from Italy (13) and the National Health and Nutrition Examination Survey III (NHANES III) (14) suggest that total energy intake might be increasing.

All of these studies are suspect because of limitations in the methodology that is used. For example, studies of food disappearance cannot correct accurately for food that is not consumed or that is consumed by nonhumans. The other studies use a form of dietary recall or dietary records. As the NHANES-III (14) illustrates, energy intake appears to be underreported, particularly in populations such as women and overweight adults. To address this specific question, Heitmann et al. (15) examined trends in reporting dietary energy over time. Using urinary nitrogen to determine protein balance and then applying this to estimate the total energy expenditure, they compared reported energy intake with predicted energy intake in a population studied from 1987 to 1988 and again from 1993 to 1994. They found that the subjects underreported energy intake by 15% in the 1987 sample and by 29% in the 1993 sample, and they found a positive correlation between the degree of underreporting and the degree of excess weight (15). Underreporting of energy that has been ingested appears to be a major issue in these population studies; it has gotten worse over time; it increases with obesity; and therefore it will continue to worsen over time.

Finally, these studies are based on entire populations, so they do not reveal the effect of dietary energy changes on susceptible subgroups. When compilations of multiple studies of dietary intake are made, the variation in energy intake between studies within a given time frame is striking. This is apparent from Table 3.1; in the studies reporting energy intake in the 1980s, a variation between 2,162 and 3,190 kcal per day in men and between 1,530 and 1,880 kcal per day in women can be observed. Although methodologic differences and the differences in study populations explain some of variation, the variation raises the issue of the accuracy of these methods in evaluating the energy intake of susceptible subgroups. The decreases in energy intake seen in many of the studies may be driven by the subgroups of people who are more severely restricting calorie intake in an effort to maintain weight. The more recent data reflecting increases in energy intake despite the concerns for underreporting may be the more accurate reflection of the general population.

One environmental factor that possibly contributes to increased total energy intake and obesity is portion size. One needs to look only as far as the nearest restaurant or convenience store to see that, in the United States, people are served extremely large servings of food. Clearly, portion size has increased dramatically over the past two decades. For example, the present size of a large soda is 32 oz, compared with 8 oz in the 1950s (17). Some research suggests that increased portion size contributes to the increased total

TABLE 3.1. Average daily consumption of energy[a]

Author	Journal	Population	Sex	1940s	1950s	1960s	1970s	1980s	1990s	% for 1960–1980[b]	% for 1980–1990[b]
Posner et al., 1995 (38)	J Am Diet Assoc	Framingham	M	—	—	3,129	2,678	2,273	—	27.36	—
			F	—	—	2,139		1,536	—	28.19	—
Hallfrisch et al., 1990 (37)	J Gerontol	Baltimore LSOA	M	—	—	2,553	2,318	2,162	—	15.32	—
USDA, 1993 (70)		USDA consumption survey	M	—	—	—	—	—	—	6	—
			F	—	—	—	—	—	—	3	—
Heini, 1997 (71)	Am J Med	NHANES and USDA		—	—	—	—	—	—	4	—
Bertheke, 2001 (72)	Br J Nutr	Dutch Longitudinal	M	—	—	—	—	3,190	2,840	—	10.97
Stephen, 1990 (73)	Am J Clin Nutr	United States studies, metaanalysis	M	—	3,030	2,860	2,690	2,480	—	13.29	—
			F	—	1,910	1,860	1,860	1,570	—	15.59	—
Stephen, 1994 (74)	Br J Nutr	United Kingdom studies, metaanalysis	M	3,080	2,920	3,260	2,820	2,710	—	16.87	—
			F	2,200	1,990	2,510	2,140	1,880	—	25.10	—
Zizza, 1997 (13)	Eur J Clin Nutr	Italian food disappearance		—	—	2,838	3,157	3,190	3,300	−12.40	−3.45
Briefel et al., 1995 (14)	Am J Clin Nutr	NHANES	M	—	—	—	—	2,579	2,747	—	−6.51
			F	—	—	—	—	1,573	1,834	—	−16.59
Average				**2,640**	**2,462**	**2,644**	**2,523**	**2,286**	**2,680**	**12.94**	**−3.90**

[a] In kilocalories, based on the decade of the survey.
[b] Represents the change between those decades. A positive percentage change indicates an increase in calories consumed.

Abbreviations: LSOA, Longitudinal Study of Aging; NHANES, National Health and Nutrition Examination Survey; USDA, United States Department of Agriculture.

energy intake (16). Using food disappearance data to corroborate this, between 1970 and 1999, the average United States resident increased consumption of carbonated soda by 109% and consumed 36 more pounds of caloric sweeteners (18).

Dietary Fat

Whether changes in the macronutrient composition of the food supply in the United States contribute to energy intake and obesity is controversial. Dietary fat is one specific macronutrient that has received extensive attention as a major factor contributing to obesity (6). This is due to several factors, including its greater energy density (9 kcal per g versus 4 kcal per g for carbohydrate and protein), its lower dietary-induced thermogenesis, and the lesser increase in fat oxidation versus that of carbohydrates with overfeeding (19). Studies of national energy consumption from fat do show a strong positive relationship with increasing weight (20). Additionally, numerous cross-sectional studies have shown an association between obesity and energy intake as fat (21). Specific food disappearance data from the United States show that the average United States citizen consumed 18 lb more of cheese and 16 lb more of added fats and oils in 1998, compared with the dietary intake in 1970 (18).

The percentage of calories consumed as dietary fat has been decreasing in several study populations (Table 3.2), leading some to conclude that dietary fat may not play an important role in the obesity epidemic. However, in many of these studies, total energy intake is increasing, so that the actual amount of fat that is consumed has not changed. Similarly, even in the studies that show a decrease in the percentage of calories consumed from fat, the decrease is small, and it is still within the range of high-fat diets that reliably produce obesity in animal models (20). Finally, great concern remains about the accuracy of the dietary self-reports used in the studies. Because of the extensive information on the deleterious effects of dietary fat, underreporting of dietary fat likely is even more of a problem than is the underreporting of energy intake described already (13). In a metaanalysis of *ad libitum* feeding studies using low fat versus high fat, Astrup et al. (22) found that low-fat diets resulted in greater weight loss than the control groups (22). Increases in the fat content of the diet may predispose susceptible individuals to obesity, and treatment by decreasing dietary fat is prudent. Vigorous efforts have been made to convince the public that restricting dietary fat is not effective in preventing obesity (22,23), but some have questioned the objectivity of these efforts (24,25).

Energy Density

Diets high in fat are also high in energy density, and some investigators have suggested that the energy density of foods is a more important indicator of total energy intake (26,27). Energy density is defined as the amount of available kilocalories per unit weight of food consumed. Although fat content is a major determinant of energy density, water content is also important, and the combination of fat and water content explains 99% of the variance in energy density (28). Currently, no specific data are available on how the energy density of the food supply has changed over time, but it probably has risen with the increases in the consumption of processed foods and the decreases in the fiber and water content of foods. Similarly, no data correlate energy density with obesity (29). In general, energy-dense foods are highly palatable but not very satiating, so they might be more easily overconsumed (30). Numerous studies show that, with short-term feeding, energy density is a key determinant of intake (26,31). The role of energy density in long-

TABLE 3.2. Average daily percentage of energy consumption as dietary fat based on the decade of the survey

Author	Journal	Population	Sex	1940s	1950s	1960s	1970s	1980s	1990s	% for 1960–1980[a]	% for 1980–1990[a]
Posner, 1995 (38)	J Am Diet Assoc	Framingham	M	—	38.7	39.4	—	38.4	—	2.54	—
			F	—	—	39.7	—	38	—	4.28	—
Hallfrisch, 1990 (37)	J Gerontol	Baltimore LSOA	M	—	—	42	—	34	—	19.05	—
USDA, 1993 (70)	USDA	USDA consumption survey	—	—	—	41	—	37	—	9.76	—
Heini, 1997 (71)	Am J Med	NHANES and USDA	—	—	—	—	—	—	—	11	—
Bertheke, 2001 (72)	Br J Nutr	Dutch Longitudinal	M	—	—	—	—	40	36	—	10.00
			F	—	—	—	—	39	37	—	5.13
Stephen, 1990 (73)	Am J Clin Nutr	United States studies, metaanalysis	—	41.2	37.6	40.5	39.9	37.8	—	6.67	—
Stephen, 1994 (74)	Br J Nutr	United Kingdom studies, metaanalysis	—	33.1	33.2	38.4	40.1	40.3	—	−4.95	—
Zizza, 1997 (13)	Eur J Clin Nutr	Italian food disappearance	—	—	—	25.5	32.8	37.5	38.9	−47.06	−3.73
Popkin, 1996 (75)	N Engl J Med	USDA surveys	—	—	—	38.4	37.5	34.3	—	10.68	—
Average				**37.15**	**36.50**	**38.11**	**37.58**	**37.63**	**37.30**	**1.33**	**3.80**

[a]Represents the change between the decade. A positive percentage change indicates a decrease in the percentage of fat consumption, whereas a negative percentage change indicates an increase.

Abbreviations: LSOA, Longitudinal Study of Aging; NHANES, National Health and Nutrition Examination Survey; USDA, United States Department of Agriculture.

term weight regulation and in populations with an increased risk of obesity, however, needs further delineation.

Dietary Carbohydrate

Dietary carbohydrate (particularly carbohydrate with a high glycemic index) has also been implicated in obesity and related diseases, including cardiovascular disease and diabetes (32–36). As dietary protein intake is fairly constant over time and because the population studies described in Table 3.2 show that the percentage of calories consumed as dietary fat is decreasing, the reported percentage of calories consumed as carbohydrate must be increasing. This is evident in the study conducted by Hallfrisch et al. (37), in which the percentage of calories consumed as carbohydrate increased from 39% in the 1960s to 44% in the 1980s. However, data from the Framingham cohort (38) show no significant change in the percentage of dietary calories from carbohydrate between the 1950s and the 1980s.

Glycemic Index

Rather than the total carbohydrates present, some argue that the glycemic index is the relevant parameter that relates carbohydrate intake to metabolic risk. The glycemic index is defined as the area under the curve of the blood glucose excursion after the ingestion of 50 g of carbohydrate from a given food. This is usually expressed relative to the glycemic curve obtained for glucose or white bread, which is set at 100. The mechanism by which foods with a high glycemic index lead to obesity is based on the idea that these foods lead to a greater increase and then decrease in blood glucose level, thus causing a relative hypoglycemia and overall increases in food intake (34). Obesity would be a consequence of this increased food intake. Indeed, at least one population study (39) using the Nurses Health Study cohort showed an increase in glycemic load (a surrogate for the overall glycemic index in a diet) of 22% between 1980 and 1992. Several studies using this cohort have also shown a relationship between glycemic load and coronary heart disease (34) and diabetes (36). Additionally, numerous studies have shown that energy intake is significantly higher (29% on average) after test meals with a high versus a low glycemic index (34).

Opponents of the glycemic index hypothesis raise several questions about its role in the etiology of obesity. First, some studies are not able to replicate the differences seen in the glycemic index when foods are given as mixed meals, rather than as a single food (40). Second, the glycemic index of many foods has been determined in individuals with type II diabetes (41). Subjects with type II diabetes have insulin resistance and defects in insulin secretion that can vary over time, and this leads to great variation in the response to a test meal and to limited generalization to other populations (40). The glycemic index of a given food also varies with the processing, method of storage, and method of cooking (34). As a practical issue, determining the glycemic index of new foods or foods eaten away from home is difficult (42). Finally, the relationship between hyperinsulinemia caused by a high glycemic index and food intake has not yet been firmly established.

These are only some of the changes in the food supply that may have had an impact on energy intake. Certainly, the use of artificial sweeteners, fat-modified and calorie-modified foods, and diet soft drinks has increased (29). Whether these changes have had an effect on total energy intake is not clear, but the bottom line is that the current environment encourages humans to consume more total calories.

ENVIRONMENTAL CHANGES THAT HAVE AN IMPACT ON ENERGY EXPENDITURE

If the reported data on total energy intake are accurate, then much of the reason for the current obesity epidemic must lie in decreased energy expenditure. As has already been discussed, the energy intake of society in general probably has not decreased substantially in recent years. How has the modern world impacted energy expenditure?

Energy expenditure is usually divided into the following three components: resting metabolic rate (RMR), the thermic effect of food (TEF), and energy expended in physical activity. Figure 3.2 portrays the components of energy expenditure, including the components of energy expended in physical activities. RMR is influenced by body size, particularly by the amount of fat-free mass (FFM) (43). No data that look specifically at RMR over time are available, but, because obesity is associated with an increased FFM (43), one might expect that it has increased. The TEF is the increase in energy expenditure that occurs after the ingestion of food. Some of the TEF is caused by the energy that is needed for digestion, absorption, and storage and oxidation of nutrients, but part of the TEF may be unrelated to these requirements. If dietary fat consumption has increased over time, then the TEF may have decreased over time; however, the contribution of the TEF to total energy expenditure is small, and the significance of such a decrease in the TEF likely is not sufficient enough to explain the increase in obesity. Therefore, the constituent of energy expenditure that probably has been the most altered by the current environment is the energy expended in physical activity.

The energy expended in physical activity can also be divided into several components. Some of these, such as non–exercise-associated thermogenesis (i.e., the energy for posture and other minor activities such as fidgeting), are not likely to vary because of environmental changes (44). However, other components of energy expenditure, including leisure-time energy expenditure, occupational energy expenditure, and the energy expenditure required for daily life, could have been greatly impacted.

Based on data from the Framingham cohort (38), between 1957 and 1960 and 1984 and 1988, overall physical activity as assessed by the questionnaire has increased by 9.5% in men and 9.1% in women. Studies of occupational energy expenditure have shown that

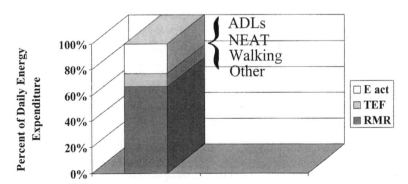

FIG. 3.2. Total daily energy expenditure. The components of energy expenditure and their relative contribution to overall energy expenditure as a percentage of the total daily energy expenditure. The energy of activity is broken down into several of its components, including activities of daily living (ADL) (e.g., personal grooming, cooking, and cleaning), non–exercise-associated thermogenesis (NEAT) (see text for details), daily activities requiring walking, and other components.

energy expenditure related to work type has decreased over the last few decades. More specifically, Wietlisbach et al. (45) in Switzerland found that the percentage of people involved in moderate to high physically intense work activities decreased from 33% in 1984 to 27% in 1992. Furthermore, an inverse relationship between occupational energy expenditure and leisure-time physical activity does not appear to occur; instead, the most sedentary patients at work were also the most sedentary during leisure time (46).

No strong evidence indicates that leisure-time physical activity has recently declined. In the Harvard alumni study (47), 39.4% of men had a physical activity index of more than 2,000 kcal per week in 1962, compared with 43% in 1977. An even more striking finding from this study (47) was that, although 45% of men participated in moderate to vigorous sporting activity in 1962, 80% were participating in such activity in 1977.

One might argue that the use of these studies is not appropriate for determining the effect of the environment on the obesity epidemic because these studies recorded data before the large increase in obesity prevalence. However, studies done by survey or questionnaire on more recent groups have shown results of either no change or of slight increases in physical activity. For example, the Nurses Health Study (39) found no change in physical activity between 1986 and 1994. Additionally, data from the Behavioral Risk Factor Surveillance Survey (48) recently showed that the percentage of adults that reported engaging in recommended levels of physical activity (i.e., moderate intensity activity at least five times per week for more than 30 minutes and/or vigorous activity at least three times per week for more than 20 minutes) has increased from 24.3% in 1990 to 25.4% in 1998.

Based on these studies, the reported percentage of people who have increased their leisure-time activity appears to be increasing. One final study attempted to control for occupational physical activity and then to correlate the change in weight with changes in physical activity (49). This study used military personnel who had a constant and high level of occupational energy expenditure. It then looked at reported leisure-time activity and the prevalence of overweight and obesity (defined as a body mass index [BMI] greater than 25 kilograms per meter squared [kg/m^2]) (49). The authors (49) found that, between 1995 and 1998, the level of activity (greater than 3 days per week at the recommended guidelines of vigorous activity of 3 days or more per week for 20 min) increased in men (65.5% in 1995 to 67.9% in 1998) and women (61.5% in 1995 to 62.8% in 1998). Despite this, a significant increase occurred in the prevalence of obesity in men (54.1% in 1995 versus 58.6% in 1998) and women (21.6% versus 26.1%) (49). Additionally, no independent association was found between increases in weight and changes in physical activity (49). Therefore, data on physical activity is similar to that for the data for energy intake. Based on much of the literature, the population reports eating fewer calories and exercising more, but it is still becoming obese. One may again point out that, in the studies of activity, surveys and questionnaires likely are biased by overreporting similar to the underreporting of the energy-intake side.

Decreases in other aspects of physical activity may be contributing to a decline in total energy expenditure. In particular, advances in technology and information science may have contributed to reducing the amount of physical activity required for daily living and to increasing the time spent in sedentary leisure-time activities. Quantifying the extent to which these environmental changes have contributed to reduced energy expenditure is difficult. However, remote controls, garage door openers, microwave ovens, and numerous other technologic advances probably have made some contributions to reducing total energy expenditure. In today's environment, everything is "drive through." In addition to drive throughs at restaurants, we use drive throughs for banking, dry cleaning, drug purchases, and many other errands. Each drive through represents a reduction in physical activity from the pre–drive-through environment.

Additionally, technologic advances have made sedentary activities more attractive, and people may be spending more of their leisure time in these sedentary pursuits. Television viewing is one such factor. In 1992, adolescents were estimated to watch 22 hours of television per week, while children watched 23 hours per week (50). Additionally, adolescents have been shown to have an energy expenditure that is lower while watching television than it is at rest (extrapolated to 245 kcal per day lower in obese and 109 kcal per day lower in lean) (51). Although these numbers may appear small, these numbers are lower than resting numbers, and the adolescents expend greater amounts of energy sleeping than they would watching television (added to this is the lost energy expenditure and other benefits of increased leisure-time activity). In addition to television viewing, other popular sedentary pursuits include computer and video games and "surfing" the Internet. Thus, physically active leisure-time pursuits have more difficulty competing with sedentary ones today.

Only a relatively small energy imbalance is required to account for the increase in body weight of the United States population over the past two decades. Data from the Coronary Artery Disease in Adults (CARDIA) study (52) show that weight gain over the past 15 years has occurred on the order of 1 to 2 lb per year, with greater weight gain being seen in African Americans than in whites. Theoretically, an energy excess of only 10 to 15 kcal per day will produce 1 lb of weight gain in 1 year. Even if some adaptation of the body to gain weight is allowed, the degree of energy imbalance leading to the obesity epidemic is, on a population basis, probably less than 50 kcal per day. This is equivalent to walking about half a mile less during the day. Believing that technologic advances have reduced walking by at least half a mile per day over the past 15 years is not difficult. Thus, the reduction in physical activity required in daily living and the increase in sedentary leisure-time pursuits may have lowered energy expenditure in a sufficient quantity to account for much of the weight gain seen in the United States population over the past two decades.

CONSEQUENCES OF AN ANCIENT METABOLISM IN A MODERN WORLD

If the physiologic energy balance regulatory system is not sufficient for protecting against the weight gain promoted by the modern environment, obesity may be the natural consequence. One simple explanation for the epidemic of obesity is that, in most people, environmental pressures toward increased food intake and decreased physical activity lead to positive energy balance. This positive energy balance is relatively constant, overcoming the capacity of the physiologic energy balance regulatory system to compensate by increasing energy expenditure. Very little physiologic opposition to weight gain is seen because the drive to increase physical activity in response to positive energy balance appears to be absent. This state of positive energy balance leads to increases in body weight, of which about 20% to 40% is FFM and the remainder is body fat (53). If the behavior (e.g., eating and exercise) remains constant, a new equilibrium of energy balance can be reached metabolically. Because FFM is the primary determinant of resting energy expenditure (REE), REE increases with weight gain (54). Similarly, even without any change in the amount of physical activity performed, the energy expended in physical activity will increase, because of the increased cost of moving a higher mass (i.e., greater body weight). A new equilibrium of energy balance is reached once the body weight has increased to the point that increases in REE and energy expended in physical activity are enough to match energy expenditure to energy intake. Some (54) have even suggested that the increased body fat mass increases fat oxidation to match the high-fat intake seen in Western diets (54). For example, one might assume that the environment leads to increased energy intake of a high-fat diet by 300 kcal per day. Under this condition, weight gain will occur until the total energy expenditure has been increased by 300 kcal per day and until the body fat mass has increased sufficiently so that fat oxidation is equal to fat intake. Then body weight will stabilize and will remain constant unless changes in the usual level of energy intake or energy expenditure occur. The physiologic buffering system seems to act to defend the new higher body weight. Important individual differences in how much weight gain is required to achieve this new equilibrium may be present.

ALTERNATIVES TO BECOMING OBESE IN THE MODERN WORLD

Although most United States adults are overweight or obese, some people avoid weight gain in the current environment. Examination of the strategies used by these individuals to avoid obesity may be useful. The category of nonobese individuals is made up of those who have never been overweight or obese, as well as of those who have been overweight but who are now maintaining a healthy weight. Unfortunately, little is known about the former group; it likely consists of individuals who maintain a healthy weight with little conscious effort and those who expend considerable effort to avoid obesity. The proportion of each subgroup within this group is unknown. Research into the genetics of obesity may eventually identify how the physiologic regulatory system of individuals who maintain weight with no conscious effort differs from that of most the United States population. A better understanding of the cognitive strategies used for body weight maintenance in those who have never been overweight or obese but who must work hard to avoid obesity may also be useful.

The group of individuals who have maintained weight loss for long periods of time, however, has been studied. Individuals in the National Weight Control Registry (NWCR) have maintained an average weight loss of 30 kg for an average of 5.5 years. These individuals appear to devote a considerable effort to maintaining behaviors that facilitate weight maintenance. They report eating a low-fat, high-carbohydrate diet, watching their total energy intake, engaging in high levels of physical activity, and regularly monitoring food intake and body weight (55). They also report that maintaining weight loss is achieved with considerable effort. This effort may be reduced slightly over time (51), but these individuals apparently do not rely on their physiology; rather they rely on their intellect to avoid weight regain.

Apparently, an individual who is not genetically fortunate (i.e., he or she does not have to worry about weight management) can either become obese (the default option), or he or she may exert conscious control over his or her behavior to prevent obesity. Different strategies for resisting the "push" of the environment toward obesity exist. One starting point could be the behaviors that are most commonly reported by subjects in the NWCR. These behaviors include eating a low-fat, high-carbohydrate diet, engaging in high levels of physical activity, and frequent self-monitoring of food intake and body weight, as were mentioned already.

Low-Fat, High-Carbohydrate Diets

Further support for a role for low-fat, high-carbohydrate diets in regulating body weight comes from studies of weight loss maintenance in obese individuals. After weight loss was induced by an energy-restricted diet, weight regain at 2 years was less in subjects who were assigned to an *ad libitum* low-fat diet (5.4 kg) than in those who consumed a fixed energy-intake diet (11.3 kg) (56).

In the Diet and Nutrition Survey of British Adults, for example, the mean BMI was similar in habitual low-fat (less than 35%) and high-fat (greater than 45%) consumers, although the distribution was skewed to the right in the latter group (57).

Physical Activity and Weight Gain

Furthermore, studies in which subjects are followed over time suggest that changes in physical activity are associated with changes in body fatness. This was illustrated in the three studies shown in Table 3.1. In each study, both the self-reported physical activity and the BMI were recorded at baseline and at follow-up 2 to 10 years later. In all studies, the level of physical activity was negatively related to BMI at baseline, and the level of physical activity at follow-up was negatively related to the change in BMI from baseline to follow-up. In two of the three studies, the level of physical activity at baseline was negatively related to the change in BMI from baseline to follow-up. Finally, all of the studies suggested a negative relationship between the change in the level of physical activity and the change in BMI.

Multiple cross-sectional studies in the literature (58–60) have shown a negative correlation between self-reported levels of physical activity and BMI. Moreover, several prospective studies (61–63) have shown that the baseline level of physical activity is negatively associated with weight gain over time and that changes in physical activity are negatively correlated with changes in body weight over time. In addition, studies (64) have shown that high levels of physical activity predict long-term success in weight loss maintenance.

Self-Monitoring and Weight Gain

Data are found for avoiding weight regain. However, do any data exist for primary prevention? Self monitoring has consistently been found to predict success in weight management (64a). Frequent self monitoring may provide an "early warning system" for reduced obese individuals, allowing them to implement predetermined strategies when their weight increases.

IMPLICATIONS FOR PREVENTION AND TREATMENT OF OBESITY

Apparently, the environment is contributing to the obesity epidemic as it encourages overeating and a sedentary lifestyle. Only a minority of the United States population has the ability to resist these pressures and maintain a healthy body weight. In this sense, obesity is a societal problem, and little may be gained from blaming either the patient or genetic factors.

Health care professionals involved in weight management must realize that, for most people, avoiding obesity is an extremely difficult task. Individuals are being asked to oppose their physiologic drives to eat when food is available and to "rest" when physical activity is not required. Achieving a healthy weight in the modern world requires that cognition overcome physiology. Achieving successful weight loss and maintenance of weight loss requires constant vigilance. Overweight and obese patients need help in developing strategies to manage energy intake and energy expenditure in a modern world that facilitates obesity.

HOW CAN THE ENVIRONMENT BE CHANGED?

Interest in changing the environment to one that is more conducive to healthy weights is growing, but no clear strategy for how to do this exists. Some have suggested approaches such as taxing high-fat or "junk" food or soft drinks (65,66). Dr. David

Satcher, the former Surgeon General, suggested several ways of changing the environment in his call to action (67).

Most people think about modifying food intake to achieve changes in body weight or to avoid obesity. This is a bit ironic because high levels of regular physical activity appear to be the best predictor of success in weight loss maintenance (51,61), and they have been shown to be effective in the prevention of weight gain (61–63).

Individuals in the NWCR, for example, report high levels of physical activity. In fact, only 9% of these individuals are able to maintain weight loss with no regular physical activity. Rarely, an individual may be able to achieve long-term weight loss maintenance success without significant amounts of physical activity. This information suggests that a starting point in modifying the environment may be increasing physical activity.

Such a strategy has economic consequences. Until recently, many professions involved substantial amounts of manual labor. Many people were, in essence, paid to be physically active. In the current environment, this is no longer the case, and most people who want to maintain high levels of physical activity have to pay, both with their money (e.g., joining health clubs) and their time. Few people are able to achieve healthy weights with the low levels of physical activity currently seen in the population. Thus, increasing physical activity may be a necessity to combat the obesity epidemic. Because of how human physiology developed and the way in which the current environment encourages eating, food intake may not be able to be restricted sufficiently and consistently enough to avoid obesity.

Finally, Peters et al. (68) note that environmental changes may take some time to bring about; meanwhile, obesity continues to increase. They suggest that body weight regulation should be viewed as a cognitive process and that people should be taught the skills they need to achieve better energy balance within the current environment.

CONCLUSION

That obesity is a serious disease that is associated with an increased risk of many other serious diseases is becoming increasingly clear. A report from the Rand Institute (69) recently documented that obese individuals have more health problems than smokers or drinkers. However, whether the disease of obesity develops from abnormalities in physiology is unclear. The view of obesity put forth in this chapter suggests that, given the genetic and physiologic profile of humans, the development of obesity may be a natural response to the modern-day environment.

If this is the case, modifying human physiology may not be the best strategy for stemming the obesity epidemic. A better strategy may be either changing the environment or understanding how to help people better manage their weight within the environment.

REFERENCES

1. Hill JO, Peters JC. Environmental contributions to the obesity epidemic. *Science* 1998;280:1371–1374.
2. French SA, Story M, Jeffery RW. Environmental influences on eating and physical activity. *Annu Rev Public Health* 2001;22:309–335.
3. Heyman MB, Young VR, Fuss P, et al. Underfeeding and body weight regulation in normal-weight young men. *Am J Physiol* 1992;263:R250–R257.
4. Garby L, Kurzer MS, Lammert O, et al. Effect of 12 weeks' light-moderate underfeeding on 24-hour energy expenditure in normal male and female subjects. *Eur J Clin Nutr* 1988;42:295–300.
5. Roberts SB, Fuss P, Dallal GE, et al. Effects of age on energy expenditure and substrate oxidation during experimental overfeeding in healthy men. *J Gerontol A Biol Sci Med Sci* 1996;51:B148–B157.
6. Hill JO, Melanson EL, Wyatt HT. Dietary fat intake and regulation of energy balance: implications for obesity. *J Nutr* 2000;130:284S–288S.
7. Roberts SB, Young VR, Fuss P, et al. Energy expenditure and subsequent nutrient intakes in overfed young men. *Am J Physiol* 1990;259:R461–R469.

8. Bouchard C, Tremblay A, Despres JP, et al. The response to long-term overfeeding in identical twins. *N Engl J Med* 1990;322:1477–1482.
9. Tarasuk V, Beaton GH. The nature and individuality of within-subject variation in energy intake. *Am J Clin Nutr* 1991;54:464–470.
10. Keesey RE, Corbett SW. Metabolic defense of the body weight set-point. *Association for Research in Nervous and Mental Disease* 1984;62:87–96.
11. Davis JD, Wirtshafter D. Set points or settling points for body weight? A reply to Mrosovsky and Powley. *Behav Biol* 1978;24:405–411.
12. The International Health, Racquet & Sportsclub Association (IHRSA). Industry statistics. 2001. Available at: http//www.ihrsa.org/. Accessed June 20, 2001.
13. Zizza C. The nutrient content of the Italian food supply, 1961–1992. *Eur J Clin Nutr* 1997;51:259–265.
14. Briefel RR, McDowell MA, Alaimo K, et al. Total energy intake of the US population: the third National Health and Nutrition Examination Survey, 1988–1991. *Am J Clin Nutr* 1995;62:1072S–1080S.
15. Heitmann BL, Lissner L, Osler M. Do we eat less fat, or just report so? *Int J Obes Relat Metab Disord* 2000;24:435–442.
16. Edelman B, Engell D, Bronstein P, et al. Environmental effects on the intake of overweight and normal-weight men. *Appetite* 1986;7:71–83.
17. Putnam J. US food supply providing more food and calories. *Food Review*. Washington, D.C.: United States Department of Agriculture, 1999. Available at: http://www.ers.usda.gov/publications/food review/sep1999/frsept99a.pdf. Accessed June 20, 2001.
18. Putnam J, Allshouse J. *Food consumption: food supply and use*. Economic research service. Washington, D.C.: United States Department of Agriculture, 2000. Available at: http://www.ers.usda.gov/briefing/consumption/Supply.htm. Accessed June 20, 2001.
19. Horton TJ, Drougas H, Brachey A, et al. Fat and carbohydrate overfeeding in humans: different effects on energy storage. *Am J Clin Nutr* 1995;62:19–29.
20. Lissner L, Heitmann BL. Dietary fat and obesity: evidence from epidemiology. *Eur J Clin Nutr* 1995;49:79–90.
21. Hill JO, Melanson EL. Overview of the determinants of overweight and obesity: current evidence and research issues. *Med Sci Sports Exerc* 1999;31:S515–S521.
22. Astrup A, Grunwald GK, Melanson EL, et al. The role of low-fat diets in body weight control: a meta-analysis of ad libitum dietary intervention studies. *Int J Obes Relat Metab Disord* 2000;24:1545–1552.
23. Taubes G. Nutrition. What if Americans ate less saturated fat? *Science* 2001;291:2538.
24. Willett WC. Is dietary fat a major determinant of body fat? *Am J Clin Nutr* 1998;67:556S–562S.
25. Astrup A, Hill JO, Saris WH. Dietary fat: at the heart of the matter. *Science* 2001;293:801–804.
26. Rolls BJ, Bell EA. Intake of fat and carbohydrate: role of energy density. *Eur J Clin Nutr* 1999;53:S166–S173.
27. Stubbs RJ, Ritz P, Coward WA, et al. Covert manipulation of the ratio of dietary fat to carbohydrate and energy density: effect on food intake and energy balance in free-living men eating ad libitum. *Am J Clin Nutr* 1995;62:330–337.
28. Grunwald GK, Seagle HM, Peters JC, et al. Quantifying and separating the effects of macronutrient composition and non-energetic food components on energy density. *Br J Nutr* 2001;86:265–276.
29. Drewnowski A. Intense sweeteners and energy density of foods: implications for weight control. *Eur J Clin Nutr* 1999;53:757–763.
30. Drewnowski A. Energy density, palatability, and satiety: implications for weight control. *Nutr Rev* 1998;56:347–353.
31. Rolls BJ, Hammer VA. Fat, carbohydrate, and the regulation of energy intake. *Am J Clin Nutr* 1995;62:1086S–1095S.
32. Ludwig DS. Dietary glycemic index and obesity. *J Nutr* 2000;130:280S–283S.
33. Morris KL, Zemel MB. Glycemic index, cardiovascular disease, and obesity. *Nutr Rev* 1999;57:273–276.
34. Roberts SB. High-glycemic index foods, hunger, and obesity: is there a connection? *Nutr Rev* 2000;58:163–169.
35. Liu S, Willett WC, Stampfer MJ, et al. A prospective study of dietary glycemic load, carbohydrate intake, and risk of coronary heart disease in US women. *Am J Clin Nutr* 2000;71:1455–1461.
36. Salmeron J, Manson JE, Stampfer MJ, et al. Dietary fiber, glycemic load, and risk of non–insulin-dependent diabetes mellitus in women. *JAMA* 1997;277:472–477.
37. Hallfrisch J, Muller D, Drinkwater D, et al. Continuing diet trends in men: the Baltimore Longitudinal Study of Aging (1961–1987). *J Gerontol* 1990;45:M186–M191.
38. Posner BM, Franz MM, Quatromoni PA, et al. Secular trends in diet and risk factors for cardiovascular disease: the Framingham Study. *J Am Diet Assoc* 1995;95:171–179.
39. Hu FB, Stampfer MJ, Manson JE, et al. Trends in the incidence of coronary heart disease and changes in diet and lifestyle in women. *N Engl J Med* 2000;343:530–537.
40. Hollenbeck CB, Coulston AM. The clinical utility of the glycemic index and its application to mixed meals. *Can J Physiol Pharmacol* 1991;69:100–107.
41. Foster-Powell K, Miller JB. International tables of glycemic index [Review]. *Am J Clin Nutr* 1995;62:871S–890S.
42. Saltzman E. The low glycemic index diet: not yet ready for prime time. *Nutr Rev* 1999;57:297.
43. Ravussin E, Lillioja S, Anderson TE, et al. Determinants of 24-hour energy expenditure in man. Methods and results using a respiratory chamber. *J Clin Invest* 1986;78:1568–1578.
44. Levine JA, Eberhardt NL, Jensen MD. Role of nonexercise activity thermogenesis in resistance to fat gain in humans. *Science* 1999;283:212–214.

45. Wietlisbach V, Paccaud F, Rickenbach M, et al. Trends in cardiovascular risk factors (1984–1993) in a Swiss region: results of three population surveys. *Prev Med* 1997;26:523–533.
46. Pomerleau J, McKee M, Robertson A, et al. Physical inactivity in the Baltic countries. *Prev Med* 2000;31: 665–672.
47. Paffenbarger RS, Hyde RT, Wing AL, et al. The association of changes in physical-activity level and other lifestyle characteristics with mortality among men. *N Engl J Med* 1993;328:538–545.
48. Centers for Disease Control and Prevention. Physical activity trends—United States, 1990–1998. *JAMA* 2001; 285:1835.
49. Lindquist CH, Bray RM. Trends in overweight and physical activity among U.S. military personnel, 1995–1998. *Prev Med* 2001;32:57–65.
50. Sweet D, Singh R. *TV viewing and Parental guidance. Consumer guide.* Washington, D.C.: Office of Educational Research and Improvement, United States Department of Education, 1994. Available at: http://www.ed/gov/pubs/OR/ConsumerGuides/tv.html. Accessed June 25, 2001.
51. Klesges RC, Shelton ML, Klesges LM. Effects of television on metabolic rate: potential implications for childhood obesity. *Pediatrics* 1993;91:281–286.
52. Lewis CE, McCreath H, West DE, et al. The obesity epidemic rolls on: 15 years in CARDIA. *Circulation* 2001; 104:II787.
53. National Institutes of Health. Clinical guidelines on the identification, evaluation, and treatment of overweight and obesity in adults—the evidence report. *Obes Res* 1998;6:51S–209S.
54. Flatt JP. Importance of nutrient balance in body weight regulation. *Diabetes Metab Res Rev* 1988;4:571–581.
55. Wing RR, Hill JO. Successful weight loss maintenance. *Annu Rev Nutr* 2001;21:323–341.
56. Toubro S, Astrup A. Randomised comparison of diets for maintaining obese subjects' weight after major weight loss: ad lib, low fat, high carbohydrate diet v fixed energy intake. *BMJ* 1997;314:29–34.
57. Blundell JE, Macdiarmid JI. Passive overconsumption. Fat intake and short-term energy balance. *Ann N Y Acad Sci* 1997;827:392–407.
58. Eck LH, Hackett-Renner C, Klesges LM. Impact of diabetic status, dietary intake, physical activity, and smoking status on body mass index in NHANES II. *Am J Clin Nutr* 1992;56:329–333.
59. Slattery ML, McDonald A, Bild DE, et al. Associations of body fat and its distribution with dietary intake, physical activity, alcohol, and smoking in blacks and whites. *Am J Clin Nutr* 1992;55:943–949.
60. Seidell JC, Cigolini M, Deslypere JP, et al. Body fat distribution in relation to serum lipids and blood pressure in 38-year-old European men: the European fat distribution study. *Atherosclerosis* 1991;86:251–260.
61. Williamson DF, Madans J, Anda RF, et al. Recreational physical activity and ten-year weight change in a US national cohort. *Int J Obes Relat Metab Disord* 1993;17:279–286.
62. French SA, Jeffery RW, Forster JL, et al. Predictors of weight change over two years among a population of working adults: the Healthy Worker Project. *Int J Obes Relat Metab Disord* 1994;18:145–154.
63. Owens JF, Matthews KA, Wing RR, et al. Can physical activity mitigate the effects of aging in middle-aged women? *Circulation* 1992;85:1265–1270.
64. Kayman S, Bruvold W, Stern JS. Maintenance and relapse after weight loss in women: behavioral aspects. *Am J Clin Nutr* 1990;52:800–807.
64a. Baker RC, Kirschenbaum DS. Self-monitoring may be necessary for successful weight control. *Behav Ther* 1993;24:377–394.
65. Brownell, KD. Public policy and the prevention of obesity. In: Fairburn CG, Brownell KD, eds. *Eating disorders and obesity.* New York: Guilford Press, 2001:619–624.
66. Nestle M, Jacobson MF. Halting the obesity epidemic: a public health policy approach. *Public Health Rep* 2000; 115:12–24.
67. Office of the Surgeon General. *The Surgeon General's call to action to prevent and decrease overweight and obesity.* Rockville, MD: United States Department of Health and Human Services, 2000.
68. Peters JC, Wyatt HR, Donahoo WT, et al. From instinct to intellect: the challenge of maintaining healthy weight in the modern world. *Obes Rev* 2002;3:69–74.
69. Sturm R, Wells KB. Does obesity contribute as much to morbidity as poverty or smoking? *Public Health* 2001; 115:229–235.
70. United States Department of Agriculture. *Food consumption and dietary levels of households in the United States.* Report no. 87-H-1. Washington, D.C.: United States Department of Agriculture, 1993.
71. Heini AF, Weinwurm RL. Divergent trends in obesity and fat intake patterns: the American paradox. *Am J Med* 1997;102:259–264.
72. Bertheke PG, de Vente W, Kemper HC, Twisk JW. Longitudinal trends in and tracking of energy and nutrient intake over 20 years in a Dutch cohort of men and women between 13 and 33 years of age: the Amsterdam Growth and Health Longitudinal Study. *Br J Nutr* 2001;85:375–385.
73. Stephen AM, Wald NJ. Trends in individual consumption of dietary fat in the United States. 1920–1984. *Am J Clin Nutr* 1990;52:457–469.
74. Stephen AM, Sieber GM. Trends in individual fat consumption in the UK, 1900–1985. *Br J Nutr* 1994;71: 775–788.
75. Popkin BM, Siega-Riz AM, Haines PS. A comparison of dietary trends among racial and socioeconomic groups in the United States. *N Engl J Med* 1996;335:716–720.

4

Pediatric Obesity

William H. Dietz

ASSESSMENT

In 1994, the Expert Committee on Clinical Guidelines for Overweight in Adolescent Preventive Services was convened by the Maternal and Child Health Bureau (MCHB), the American Academy of Pediatrics, and the American Medical Association with guidance and support from the Centers for Disease Control and Prevention (CDC). The purpose of this committee was to advise the Bright Futures: National Guidelines for Health Supervision of Infants, Children and Adolescents and the Guidelines for Adolescent Preventive Services (GAPS) on the criteria for the identification of adolescent obesity. The expert committee recommended that the body mass index (BMI) be used to identify adolescent obesity, and it developed an algorithm that established who should be treated (1). The committee agreed that all adolescents with a BMI either at or higher than the 95th percentile for their age and gender should be considered overweight and should receive an in-depth assessment. Adolescents with a BMI between the 85th and 95th percentiles should be considered at risk and should be evaluated further. If at-risk adolescents had an additional risk factor, such as a positive family history of cardiovascular disease, parental hypercholesterolemia or obesity, diabetes, elevated blood pressure, elevated total cholesterol level, or an increase of 2 BMI units over the previous year, or if they were concerned about their weight, they should also receive an in-depth assessment. If at-risk individuals lacked an additional risk factor, they should be seen again in 1 year for a second evaluation. In-depth assessments would include the measurement of the pubertal stage, skinfold thicknesses, and lipoprotein fractions. The committee focused only on adolescents, and it made no recommendations regarding the assessment or treatment of younger children.

In 1997, the Childhood Obesity Working Group of the International Obesity Task Force (IOTF) convened an international conference to consider the most appropriate criteria for the assessment of obesity in younger children and preadolescents (2). The workshop attendees agreed that an important goal was making the childhood and adult criteria consistent. The group also agreed that the high reliability and reasonable validity of the BMI as a measure of body fat made it the anthropometric measure best suited to the assessment of obesity. Furthermore, it concluded that the most appropriate process by which to establish the criteria for overweight and obesity was to identify separately the BMI percentiles that corresponded to a BMI of 25 and 30 kilograms per meter squared (kg/m^2) for young adult men and women and to extend the use of percentiles to identify overweight and obesity in younger children. Because a BMI of 25 to 29.9 kg/m^2 in adults identifies overweight, and a BMI of 30 kg/m^2 or more identifies obesity, this approach made the criteria used to identify overweight children and adolescents consistent with the adult criteria.

Two growth charts are now available for use. In the United States, the CDC growth charts have just been revised, and, for the first time, BMI charts for age and gender can be downloaded from the CDC web page (http://www.cdc.gov/growthcharts/. Accessed

August 2002.) (Table 4.1). Because these growth charts are derived from data collected before 1988, they provide a historical reference against which more recent changes in prevalence can be compared. Somewhat fortuitously, a BMI of 30 kg/m² in a young United States adult corresponds to the 95th percentile, and a BMI of 25 kg/m² in a young United States adult corresponds to slightly below the 85th percentile. Therefore, the extension of the adolescent criteria previously identified by the MCHB panel to younger children and adolescents and the use of the CDC growth charts appear warranted.

Because the United States population is not representative of the world's population, an international reference population was recently developed. It used data from six countries to establish the BMI percentiles in young adults that corresponded to a BMI of 25 and 30 kg/m² (3). Use of the international reference population, rather than the United

TABLE 4.1. *Body mass index percentiles by age and gender*

Age (yr)	5th percentile	15th percentile	50th percentile	85th percentile	95th percentile
Males					
2	14.7	15.3	16.6	18.2	19.3
3	14.3	14.9	16.0	17.3	18.2
4	14.0	14.6	15.6	16.9	17.8
5	13.8	14.4	15.4	16.8	17.9
6	13.7	14.3	15.4	17.0	18.4
7	13.7	14.3	15.5	17.4	19.2
8	13.8	14.4	15.8	18.0	20.1
9	14.0	14.6	16.2	18.6	21.1
10	14.2	15.0	16.6	19.4	22.2
11	14.6	15.4	17.2	20.2	23.2
12	15.0	15.8	17.8	21.0	24.2
13	15.5	16.4	18.5	21.9	25.2
14	16.0	17.0	19.2	22.7	26.0
15	16.6	17.6	19.9	23.5	26.8
16	17.1	18.2	20.6	24.2	27.6
17	17.7	18.8	21.2	24.9	28.3
18	18.2	19.4	21.9	25.7	29.0
19	18.7	19.9	22.5	26.4	29.7
20	19.1	20.3	23.0	27.0	30.6
Females					
2	14.4	15.1	16.4	18.0	19.1
3	14.0	14.6	15.7	17.2	18.3
4	13.7	14.2	15.3	16.8	18.0
5	13.5	14.0	15.2	16.8	18.3
6	13.4	14.0	15.2	17.1	18.8
7	13.4	14.1	15.5	17.6	19.7
8	13.5	14.2	15.8	18.3	20.7
9	13.7	14.5	16.3	19.1	21.8
10	14.0	14.9	16.9	20.0	23.0
11	14.4	15.3	17.5	20.9	24.1
12	14.8	15.8	18.1	21.7	25.3
13	15.3	16.3	18.7	22.6	26.3
14	15.8	16.9	19.4	23.3	27.3
15	16.3	17.4	19.9	24.0	28.1
16	16.8	17.9	20.5	24.7	28.9
17	17.2	18.3	20.9	25.2	29.6
18	17.6	18.7	21.3	25.7	30.3
19	17.8	18.9	21.6	26.1	31.0
20	17.8	19.0	21.7	26.5	31.8

Note: A body mass index ≥95th percentile for children of the same age and gender is considered overweight.

States population, to assess overweight in United States children and adolescents increases the prevalence of obesity in United States children and adolescents. In contrast, use of the United States reference population to assess the prevalence of obesity in other populations reduces the prevalence of overweight. Because the United States prevalence estimates were developed from a United States reference population, the United States BMI charts are more suitable for assessing United States children and adolescents.

Based on the CDC criteria, approximately 10% to 15% of children and adolescents are overweight, depending on the age, gender, and ethnic group considered (4). Between the completion of the National Health and Nutrition Examination Survey II (NHANES-II) in 1980 and NHANES-III in 1994, the prevalence of overweight children and adolescents in the United States doubled.

No consensus has yet been achieved with respect to the terminology used to describe the two groups identified by the 85th and 95th percentiles. As was indicated already, the Bright Futures and GAPS expert committee used the terms *at risk of overweight* and *overweight* to describe children and adolescents who fall between the 85th and 95th percentiles and those who fall at or above the 95th percentile of BMI, respectively. In contrast, the terms *overweight* and *obese* are used to describe adults with BMIs of 25.5 to 29.9 kg/m^2 and of 30 kg/m^2 or more, respectively, even though the percentile definitions of *at risk of overweight* and *overweight* for children are based on these adult categories. Although the term *obesity* is sometimes used interchangeably with the term *overweight* to describe children and adolescents, CDC focus group data indicate that many adolescents use the term *obese* to describe massive obesity (5). Therefore, use of the term *overweight* is probably more appropriate when dealing with patients and families.

Because the use of these percentiles to describe children and adolescents was empirically justified by their correspondence to the adult criteria, the IOTF Childhood Obesity Working Group agreed that additional data were needed to confirm that these percentiles accurately identified at-risk children and adolescents. The first confirmation that these criteria were associated with potentially adverse outcomes was a study that demonstrated that approximately 60% of overweight 5-year-old to 10-year-old children identified by a BMI at or above the 95th percentile had at least one additional cardiovascular disease risk factor, such as hyperinsulinemia, elevated blood pressure, or hyperlipidemia (6). Furthermore, 25% of overweight children had two or more additional cardiovascular disease risk factors. However, additional confirmatory studies are still essential.

The measurement and use of visceral fat in the clinical assessment of obesity in children and adolescents remain a subject for further investigation. In adults, visceral adiposity appears to be an important determinant of cardiovascular disease risk factors, such as hypertension, hyperlipidemia, and glucose intolerance (7). In children and adolescents, fewer studies have been conducted. Furthermore, because hypertension, hyperlipidemia, and glucose intolerance occur with a lower prevalence than they do in adults, the predictive value of visceral adiposity for these risk factors necessarily is lower. Nonetheless, visceral fatness in children and adolescents, as measured by magnetic resonance imaging or computed tomography scanning, appears to be directly associated with their blood pressure, insulin levels, and low-density lipoprotein (LDL) cholesterol levels and to be inversely associated with their high-density lipoprotein (HDL) cholesterol levels (8,9). In adults, sufficient data exist to warrant the use of critical values for waist circumference (88 cm in women, 102 cm in men [10]) to evaluate medical risk. However, because the volume of visceral fat is so much lower in children and adolescents, waist circumference is not likely to reflect visceral adiposity. Considerably more research is required to determine whether waist circumference reflects visceral adiposity and whether the addition of waist circumference enhances the sensitivity of BMI as an indicator of the risks of morbidity in overweight children and adolescents.

FACTORS ASSOCIATED WITH THE INCREASED PREVALENCE OF OBESITY

Various environmental changes have accompanied the rapid increases in the prevalence of obesity. These include major changes in food-related behaviors, such as an increased reliance on food consumed outside the home, the increased portion size of foods consumed outside the home, increased soda and juice consumption, and the increased availability of food products in supermarkets (11). The decline of family dinners also appears to affect dietary intake. Children who eat more dinners with other members of their family consume more fruits and vegetables, less fried food at home and away from home, and less soda than children who eat fewer dinners with other family members (12). As of yet, none of these behaviors has been causally related to the development of obesity in children or adolescents.

Preoccupation with weight and restrictive eating behaviors, particularly in preadolescent and adolescent girls, has also occurred coincident with the increase in the prevalence of obesity (13). A new study suggests that such behaviors may have an adverse effect on weight regulation. Girls who are very restrained eaters or who skip meals have more rapid rates of weight gain than do girls who do not exhibit such behaviors (14).

Television viewing consistently appears to be related to the prevalence of obesity in children and adolescents (15,16), and Dietz and Gortmaker (15) have argued that this relationship is causal. The mechanism whereby television viewing may cause obesity may be related either to the inactivity associated with television viewing or to the consumption of the foods advertised on television. The causal linkage between television viewing and obesity has been recently strengthened by a study that demonstrated that an intervention that included reduced television viewing was associated with a reduction in the prevalence of obesity (17) and by a second study that demonstrated that reduced television viewing was associated with a reduced rate of weight gain (18).

PERIODS OF RISK

Approximately one-third of adult obesity begins in childhood (19). Nonetheless, adult obesity that begins in childhood may be associated with more severe obesity in adulthood than that obesity which is of adult onset (20). Three periods of risk may exist in childhood for the development of obesity that persists into adulthood (21). These include the prenatal period, the period of "adiposity" rebound, and adolescence.

High birth weight appears to pose a risk of childhood obesity (22). Infants of diabetic mothers are at particular risk (23). However, because infants with high birth weight constitute a small fraction of the total births, the proportional contribution of infants with increased birth weight to adult obesity is quite small. Nonetheless, the rising prevalence of type II diabetes mellitus in United States adults makes an increase in the number of infants with high birth weight likely; the proportion of adult obesity attributable to high birth weight will thus also increase. The mechanism responsible for the effect of increased birth weight on subsequent obesity remains uncertain, but it probably is a consequence of endogenous factors entrained by the prenatal experience that affect the individual's susceptibility to later increases in body fat. Such factors might include the effects of increased intrauterine nutrition on the hypothalamic set points for body weight or altered substrate metabolism.

The period of "adiposity" rebound has been used to describe another period of increased risk for the development of obesity in childhood that persists into adulthood (24–26). This period describes the increase in BMI that follows a nadir; and it is apparent between 5 and 6 years of age (Fig. 4.1). Children whose BMI begins to increase early have been described as having early "adiposity" rebound, and they are more likely to have a high BMI in adulthood. The term *adiposity* should be used cautiously because, as yet, no study has demonstrated that the increase in BMI is associated with increased fatness or that the increased BMI observed in adults who had early BMI rebound reflects increased fatness. Furthermore, BMI at the time of rebound may be a better predictor of later BMI than is the timing of the rebound (27). The processes and alterations in body composition that occur at the time of BMI rebound remain uncertain. As a result, the endogenous and exogenous factors that determine the timing of "adiposity" rebound remain unclear.

The third period of risk in childhood is adolescence. Adolescence represents the period of greatest risk of the development of adult obesity (28). Approximately 50% to 75% of obesity present in adolescence persists into adulthood (29). Furthermore, obesity that is present at adolescence appears to carry additional risks for adult morbidity that are independent of the effect of adolescent obesity on adult obesity (30). These effects include early mortality in men but not women; an increased risk of cardiovascular disease, atherosclerosis, and diabetes in both sexes; colorectal cancer and gout in men; and osteoarthritis in women (30) (Table 4.2). The risk of some of these complications may relate to the regional deposition of fat that occurs in adolescence. Increased visceral fat deposition occurs at adolescence, but it is more marked in boys than in girls.

A final observation regarding risk is the fact that early maturation in adolescents appears to increase the risk of adult obesity (31). However, no analyses have yet con-

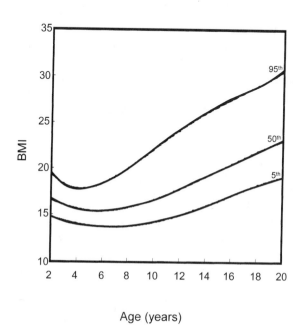

FIG. 4.1. Body mass index (BMI) percentiles for children. Note that the period of BMI rebound occurs after 6 to 7 years of age for children in the 50th percentile, but earlier for children in the 95th percentile. Whether the BMI at rebound is more important than the time at which rebound occurs as a determinant of subsequent BMI is unclear.

TABLE 4.2. *Adult consequences of obesity present in adolescence*

Men	Women
Early mortality	Cardiovascular disease
Cardiovascular disease	Diabetes
Diabetes	Osteoarthritis
Colorectal cancer	Lower education
Gout	Lower rates of marriage
	Lower income

From Must A, Jacques PF, Dallal GE, et al. Long-term morbidity and mortality of overweight adolescents: a follow-up of the Harvard Growth Study of 1922 to 1935. *N Engl J Med* 1992;327:1350–1355; and Gortmaker SL, Must A, Perrin JM, et al. Social and economic consequences of overweight in adolescence and young adulthood. *N Engl J Med* 1993;329:1008–1012, with permission.

trolled the effect of maturational timing for BMI at the time of maturation. Therefore, the subsequent effects of early maturation on later BMI may only reflect increased fatness at the time of maturation.

PATHOPHYSIOLOGY

As Chapter 2 discusses, obesity results from an imbalance of energy intake and expenditure. In the last decade, the availability of techniques such as doubly labeled water has enabled studies of total daily energy expenditure over a 1-week to 2-week period. Because energy expenditure reflects the resting metabolic rate (RMR), the thermic effect of food (TEF), and the energy expended on activity and because the TEF accounts for a small but relatively constant proportion of energy expenditure, the difference between total daily energy expenditure and RMR corrected for the TEF provides an approximation of the energy spent on activity.

As in adults, extensive attention has been focused on physiologic factors in the pediatric age-group that may predispose individuals to obesity. Three of the strategies that are employed to explore factors related to energy expenditure include examining components of energy expenditure in overweight and non-overweight children; comparing individuals with an increased risk of obesity, such as children of obese parents who are at increased risk for weight gain; or employing longitudinal studies to determine whether the risks of excessive weight gain occur in those in whom one or more components of energy expenditure is low.

Comparisons of energy expenditure in overweight and non-overweight children (32) and adolescents (33) have failed to demonstrate significant differences in total energy expenditure, RMR, or the amount of energy spent on activity. Because children of overweight parents have long been recognized as having a higher risk of obesity than do children of normal-weight parents (34), a second strategy has been to compare the energy expenditure of children of obese parents with that of children of nonobese parents. Although early studies based on dietary intake suggested that children of obese parents had lower levels of energy expenditure than did children whose parents were normal weight (35), subsequent studies using measurements of the various components of energy expenditure in infants (36,37) and preschool-aged children (38) have failed to support the studies based on dietary intake.

Longitudinal studies represent the strongest study design for determining whether reduced energy expenditure constitutes a risk factor for the development of obesity. The earliest study of infants or children of overweight and normal-weight mothers suggested that reduced energy expenditure might constitute a risk factor for later weight gain (36). Because metabolic rates did not differ between the groups, these data implied that infants who became overweight at 1 year were less active at the age of 3 months than were those who did not. A subsequent investigation of 33 infants who were studied at 12 weeks of age found no evidence of an effect of parental obesity on any component of energy expenditure (39). In young children, neither total energy expenditure, RMR, nor low-activity–related energy expenditure was inversely related to rates of weight gain (40). In conclusion, the studies of energy expenditure suggest that parental obesity is not associated with low energy expenditure and that low energy expenditure is not associated with an increased risk of weight gain.

Few longitudinal studies have examined the role of physical activity and the genesis of obesity in children and adolescents. Clinical studies have examined limited numbers of children for short periods. In these studies, reduced energy spent on physical activity did not appear to be a risk factor for the later development of obesity (39,40). Difficulties with the accurate measurement of physical activity in epidemiologic studies have contributed to the absence of population-based studies that link changes in physical activity over time with obesity. Nonetheless, several observations support the likelihood that opportunities for physical activity as part of daily life have declined recently and that some of these changes have occurred coincident with the obesity epidemic. For example, the number of schools offering daily physical education in high school declined from 42% of schools in 1991 to 27% of schools in 1998 (41). Fewer than one-third of children within 1 mile of school walk to school. Finally, although 25% of all trips made by children are less than 1 mile in distance, 75% of these trips are by car (42).

COMPLICATIONS

Obesity is associated with a number of adverse social, psychologic, and physical effects. Each of these areas are considered in turn below.

Social Effects

More than 30 years ago, the effects of obesity on the attitudes of children were examined in 10-year-old and 11-year-old children (43). With the help of a series of silhouettes, children were asked which child they liked the best. Alternatives included children who were overweight, missing limbs, or wheelchair bound or those with a disfigured face. Children consistently ranked overweight children as those they liked the least. These individual attitudes appear to be mirrored by the culture. In young women with comparable high school academic records, acceptance rates to a group of elite northeastern colleges were greater in those of normal weight (44). Several studies of young adult women (45,46) indicate that obesity has a significant impact on a variety of socioeconomic factors. Marital rates, years of school completed, and family income levels were lower for overweight women than for women whose weights were normal. However, many of these studies evaluated data collected before the current obesity epidemic. Because obesity has become more common, the discriminatory behaviors observed in the past may no longer be so prevalent.

Psychologic Effects

Although overweight children are widely assumed to have low self-esteem, overweight children and preadolescents tend to have self-images that compare favorably with those of the non-overweight (47,48). Although the earliest studies of self-image were characterized by small samples and the lack of a representative population, these observations were recently confirmed in a large representative sample drawn from the National Longitudinal Survey of Youth (48). However, as adolescence progresses, self-esteem declines slightly, but not significantly, in boys; on the other hand, it declines significantly in white and Hispanic girls. Self-esteem in overweight adolescent girls is not apparently affected (48).

A final area that has not been carefully explored is the role of child abuse and neglect in the development of obesity or the psychologic sequelae that may follow its development. In Europe, child neglect is associated with an increased frequency of obesity in children (49). Furthermore, obesity in adults (BMI $\geq$ 35 kg/m^2) is associated with an increased frequency of retrospective self-reported physical, sexual, or verbal abuse in childhood or a report of household dysfunction (50). The relative contribution of neglect or abuse in childhood to the prevalence or severity of obesity in adults has not yet been carefully assessed.

Physical Effects

Overweight children tend to be taller (51,52), to have an advanced bone age (52), and to mature earlier (31,53) than non-overweight children. The ultimate height expectation for the genetic potential does not appear altered. However, early maturation is associated with increased fatness in adulthood (31,53). The author's clinical experience indicates that another adverse consequence of rapid growth is that the age of overweight children is frequently overestimated by adults, whose expectations of age-appropriate behavior for overweight children cannot be met. Inappropriate expectations may cause an additional frustration for overweight children, but the extent of that frustration has not yet been quantified.

Cardiovascular Risk Factors

As was indicated earlier, more than 60% of overweight children have at least one additional cardiovascular disease risk factor, such as elevated blood pressure or hyperlipidemia; and 25% have two or more (6). The emergence of these factors in childhood in association with obesity emphasizes the long-term cardiovascular risks associated with obesity in childhood. For example, autopsy data on young persons in whom early cardiovascular disease risk factors had been studied in childhood demonstrated an increased risk for fatty streaks and fibrous plaques in the aorta and coronary arteries in the young people with a high BMI; a high systolic and diastolic blood pressure; and high levels of serum total cholesterol, triglycerides, and LDL and HDL cholesterol (54).

Hyperinsulinemia is commonplace (6). In some locations, type II diabetes mellitus, which was rarely seen in adolescents before 1990, now accounts for 8% to 45% of new cases of diabetes (55). In adolescent Native Americans, the prevalence of type II diabetes may be as high as 5%, but, in the general population, the prevalence appears to range from 0.4% to 0.7% (55). The peak age at occurrence is 13 to 14 years; cases occurring in children younger than 10 years of age are uncommon. Acanthosis nigricans, female gender, a positive family history of diabetes, and recent weight loss characterize more than 50% of these patients (55). Signs and symptoms at the time of presentation may mimic type I diabetes insofar as patients may present with ketoacidosis. Type II diabetes may be distinguished from type I by the absence of islet cell antibodies and by elevated insulin and C-peptide concentrations. These findings indicate that fasting insulin levels, lipid profiles, and a urinalysis to exclude glucosuria should be obtained routinely as part of the workup of an overweight child (56).

As in adults, the cardiovascular comorbidities associated with obesity in children and adolescents appear to be associated with central adiposity, which is defined as either truncal or visceral fat. Because central or visceral adiposity can be expected to vary with total body fatness, studies that include total body fat, fat distribution, and obesity-associated comorbidity measures are essential. Few such studies have been done. Two recent studies that included all three types of measurements showed a consistent independent effect of truncal (8) or visceral (9) fat on triglycerides, HDL cholesterol, and systolic blood pressure.

Hepatic

Several clinical studies have suggested that elevated liver enzymes may occur in more than 20% of obese children and adolescents seen in clinics in Japan (57,58) and the United States (WH Dietz, *personal observation*). These observational data have recently been confirmed by a representative study of adolescents in the United States that demonstrated elevated levels of serum alanine aminotransferase (ALT) in 6% of overweight adolescents (BMI at or greater than 85th percentile) and 10% of obese adolescents (BMI at or greater than 95th percentile) (59). Furthermore, more than 60% of adolescents with elevated ALT levels and without evidence of hepatitis B or C were overweight or obese. Elevated ALT levels in overweight adolescents were also associated with an increase in alcohol consumption and a reduction in serum antioxidants (vitamin E, β-carotene, and vitamin C). Although these findings likely reflect steatohepatitis, several massively obese adolescents have had cirrhotic changes with no other explanation than obesity. Clinical experience with those cases indicates that modest weight loss may normalize ALT levels.

OBESITY SEQUELAE THAT REQUIRE AGGRESSIVE THERAPY

Pseudotumor cerebri, type II diabetes mellitus, slipped capital femoral epiphysis, Blount disease, and sleep apnea are all complications of obesity for which urgent and aggressive therapy is required.

Patients with pseudotumor cerebri generally present with a history of headaches (60,61). However, asymptomatic papilledema may also be present. Because blindness or impaired vision may result, aggressive therapy is essential. The pathophysiology of pseudotumor cerebri is unknown.

The two major orthopedic complications of obesity are Blount disease and the slipped femoral capital epiphysis. Both are rare in the general population, but up to 50% of all cases of Blount disease (62) and of slipped capital femoral epiphysis (63) occur in overweight children and adolescents. Both complications are due to the increased stress caused by excess weight on growing bone. Blount disease generally occurs in preadolescents, who present with bowing of the tibia. The pathophysiology of Blount disease is that increased weight bows the tibia, just as downward pressure would bend a green stick. "Beaking" of the medial aspect of the proximal tibial metaphysis is a pathognomonic radiologic sign, and the medial aspect of the tibia thickens in response to the line of weight bearing. Increased bone deposition occurs in response to this stress. Repair requires surgery, but the disease may recur unless sustained weight loss occurs after surgery. Up to 50% of patients with slipped capital femoral epiphysis are obese in early adolescence (63,64). The common presenting symptoms are hip pain, a limp, or both. In this disease, the head of the femur slips on the epiphysis and requires surgical repair. As in patients with Blount disease, weight reduction is essential to prevent the same problem on the contralateral side.

Sleep apnea occurs in fewer than 10% of overweight children, but its frequency may increase with the severity of overweight because peripharyngeal fat may block the airway when the pharyngeal muscles relax during sleep. Snoring or audible apneic episodes are usually present, and multiple episodes of sleep apnea with low oxygen saturation may occur nightly. Daytime somnolence may be the only presenting symptom because the sleep at night is so disturbed; however, neither the severity of overweight nor the history accurately predicts the severity of the sleep apnea (65). Enlarged tonsils frequently accompany sleep apnea, and a tonsillectomy may cure the apnea. However, children with sleep apnea who have tonsillectomies must be carefully monitored after surgery because peripharyngeal swelling may occlude the airway. The high mortality found in published cases of sleep apnea indicates that aggressive therapy is essential. Although no data are available, the author's clinical experience suggests that sleep apnea is far more common in obese children and adolescents than is central hypoventilation.

CONCLUSION

Overweight has become a highly prevalent disease in children and adolescents in the United States. Careful assessment to determine the severity of obesity and its complications is essential. Although obesity clearly has a genetic component, the absence of differences in energy expenditure between obese and nonobese children and the absence of reduced energy expenditure in children who become overweight suggest that the genetic predisposition to obesity may not be associated with a reduction in energy expenditure. Cardiovascular disease risk factors are frequently associated with obesity in children and adolescents. For several additional associated complications, aggressive therapy is warranted. The increased likelihood that obesity that is present in adolescence will persist into adulthood further suggests that vigorous preventive and therapeutic efforts should focus on this age-group.

REFERENCES

1. Himes JH, Dietz WH. Guidelines for overweight in adolescent preventive services: recommendations from an expert committee. *Am J Clin Nutr* 1994;59:307–316.
2. Bellizzi MC, Dietz WH. Workshop on childhood obesity: summary of the discussion. *Am J Clin Nutr* 1999;70: 173S–175S.
3. Cole TJ, Bellizzi MC, Flegal KM, et al. Establishing a standard definition for child overweight and obesity worldwide: international survey. *BMJ* 2000;320:1240–1243.
4. Troiano RP, Flegal KM, Kuczmarski RJ, et al. Overweight prevalence and trends for children and adolescents. *Arch Pediatr Adolesc Med* 1995;149:1085–1091.
5. Nutrition and Physical Activity Communication Team. *Executive summary: healthy weight, physical activity and nutrition: focus group research with African American, Mexican American and white youth.* Atlanta: Centers for Disease Control and Prevention, 2000.
6. Freedman DS, Dietz WH, Srinivasan SR, et al. The relation of overweight to cardiovascular risk factors among children and adolescents: the Bogalusa Heart Study. *Pediatrics* 1999;103:1175–1182.
7. Despres JP, Lemieux I, Prud'homme D. Treatment of obesity: need to focus on high risk abdominally obese patients. *BMJ* 2001;322:716–720.
8. Daniels SR, Morrison JA, Sprecher DL, et al. Association of fat distribution and cardiovascular risk factors in children and adolescents. *Circulation* 1999;99:541–545.
9. Owens S, Gutin B, Barbeau P, et al. Visceral adipose tissue and markers of the insulin resistance syndrome in obese black and white teenagers. *Obes Res* 2000;8:287–293.

10. National Institutes of Health. *Clinical guidelines on the identification, evaluation and treatment of overweight and obesity in adults.* NIH publication no. 98-4083. Washington, D.C.: National Institutes of Health, 1998.
11. Dietz WH. Prevention of childhood obesity: individual, environmental, and policy issues. In: Trowbridge F, Kibbe D, eds. *Childhood obesity: partnerships for research and prevention.* Atlanta, GA: ILSI Center for Health Promotion, 2002.
12. Gillman MW, Rifas-Sherman SL, Frazier AL, et al. Family dinner and diet quality among older children and adolescents. *Arch Fam Med* 2000;9:235–240.
13. Neumark-Sztainer D, Hannan PJ. Weight-related behaviors among adolescent girls and boys. *Arch Pediatr Adolesc Med* 2000;154:569–577.
14. Stice E, Cameron RP, Killen JD, et al. Naturalistic weight-reduction efforts prospectively predict growth in relative weight and onset of obesity among female adolescents. *J Consult Clin Psychol* 1999;67:967–974.
15. Dietz WH, Gortmaker SL. Do we fatten our children at the TV set? Obesity and television viewing in children and adolescents. *Pediatrics* 1985;75:807–812.
16. Gortmaker SL, Must A, Sobol AM, et al. Television viewing as a cause of increasing obesity among children in the United States, 1986–1990. *Arch Pediatr Adolesc Med* 1996;150:356–362.
17. Gortmaker SL, Peterson K, Wiecha J, et al. Reducing obesity via a school-based interdisciplinary intervention among youth: Planet Health. *Arch Pediatr Adolesc Med* 1999:153:409–418.
18. Robinson TN. Reducing children's television viewing to prevent obesity. A randomized controlled trial. *JAMA* 1999;282:1561–1567.
19. Braddon FE, Rodgers B, Wadsworth ME, et al. Onset of obesity in a 36-year birth cohort study. *BMJ* 1986;293:299–303.
20. Rimm IJ, Rimm AA. Association between juvenile onset obesity and severe adult obesity in 73,532 women. *Am J Public Health* 1976;66:479–481.
21. Dietz WH. Critical periods in childhood for the development of obesity. *Am J Clin Nutr* 1994;59:955–959.
22. Whitaker RC, Dietz WH. The role of the prenatal environment in the development of obesity. *J Pediatr* 1998;132:768–776.
23. Curhan GC, Willett WC, Rimm EB, et al. Birth weight and adult hypertension, diabetes mellitus, and obesity in US men. *Circulation* 1996;94:3246–3250.
24. Rolland-Cachera MF, Deheeger M, Guillood-Bataille M, et al. Tracking the development of adiposity from one month of age to adulthood. *Ann Hum Biol* 1987;4:219–229.
25. Siervogel RM, Roche AF, Guo S, et al. Patterns of change in weight/stature^2 from 2 to 18 years: findings from long-term serial data for children in the Fels Longitudinal Growth Study. *Int J Obes* 1991;15:479–485.
26. Whitaker RC, Pepe MS, Wright JA, et al. Early adiposity rebound and the risk of adult obesity. *Pediatrics* 1998;101:E5.
27. Dietz WH. "Adiposity rebound": reality or epiphenomenon? *Lancet* 2000;356:2027–2028.
28. Whitaker RC, Wright JA, Pepe MS, et al. Predicting obesity in young adulthood from childhood and parental obesity. *N Engl J Med* 1997;337:869–873.
29. Clarke WR, Lauer RM. Does obesity track into adulthood? *Crit Rev Food Sci Nutr* 1993;33:423–430.
30. Must A, Jacques PF, Dallal GE, et al. Long-term morbidity and mortality of overweight adolescents: a follow-up of the Harvard Growth Study of 1922 to 1935. *N Engl J Med* 1992;327:1350–1355.
31. van Lenthe FJ, Kemper CG, van Mechelen W. Rapid maturation in adolescence results in greater obesity in adulthood: the Amsterdam Growth and Health Study. *Am J Clin Nutr* 1996;64:18–24.
32. Treuth MS, Figueroa-Colon R, Hunter GR, et al. Energy expenditure and physical fitness in overweight vs non-overweight prepubertal girls. *Int J Obes Relat Metab Disord* 1998;22:440–447.
33. Bandini LG, Schoeller DA, Dietz WH. Energy expenditure in obese and non-obese adolescents. *Pediatr Res* 1990;27:198–203.
34. Garn SM, Clark DC. Trends in fatness and the origins of obesity. *Pediatrics* 1976;57:443–456.
35. Griffiths M, Rivers JP, Payne PR. Energy intake in children at high and low risk of obesity. *Hum Nutr Clin Nutr* 1987;41:425–430.
36. Roberts SB, Savage J, Coward WA, et al. Energy expenditure and intake in infants born to lean and overweight mothers. *N Engl J Med* 1988;318:461–466.
37. Davies PS, Wells JC, Fieldhouse CA, et al. Parental body composition and infant energy expenditure. *Am J Clin Nutr* 1995;61:1026–1029.
38. Goran MI, Carpenter WH, McGloin A, et al. Energy expenditure in children of lean and obese parents. *Am J Physiol* 1995;268:E917–E924.
39. Davies PS, Day JM, Lucas A. Energy expenditure in early infancy and later body fatness. *Int J Obes* 1991;15:727–731.
40. Goran MI, Shewchuk R, Gower BA, et al. Longitudinal changes in fatness in white children: no effect of childhood energy expenditure. *Am J Clin Nutr* 1998;67:309–316.
41. Office of Public Health and Science. *Healthy People 2010 objectives.* Washington, D.C.: United States Department of Health and Human Services, 2000.
42. Koplan JP, Dietz WH. Caloric imbalance and public health policy. *JAMA* 1999;282:1579–1581.
43. Richardson SA, Goodman N, Hastorf AH, et al. Cultural uniformity in reaction to physical disabilities. *Am Sociol Rev* 1961;26:241–247.
44. Canning H, Mayer J. Obesity—its possible effect on college acceptance. *N Engl J Med* 1966;275:1172–1174.

45. Gortmaker SL, Must A, Perrin JM, et al. Social and economic consequences of overweight in adolescence and young adulthood. *N Engl J Med* 1993;329:1008–1012.
46. Sargent JD, Blanchflower DG. Obesity and stature in adolescence and earnings in young adulthood. *Arch Pediatr Adolesc Med* 1994;148:681–687.
47. French SA, Story M, Perry CL. Self-esteem and obesity in children and adolescents: a literature review. *Obes Res* 1995;3:479–490.
48. Strauss RS. Childhood obesity and self-esteem. *Pediatrics* 2000;105:e15.
49. Lissau I, Sorenson TI. Parental neglect during childhood and increased risk of obesity in young adulthood. *Lancet* 1994;343:324–327.
50. Felitti VJ, Anda RF, Nordenberg D, et al. Relationship of childhood abuse and household dysfunction to many of the leading causes of death in adults: the Adverse Childhood Experiences (ACE) Study. *Am J Prev Med* 1998; 14:245–258.
51. Forbes GB. Nutrition and growth. *J Pediatr* 1977;91:40–42.
52. Garn SM, Clark DC. Nutrition, growth, development, and maturation: findings from the Ten-State Nutrition Survey of 1968–1970. *Pediatrics* 1975;56:306–319.
53. Garn SM, LaVelle M, Rosenberg KR, et al. Maturational timing as a factor in female fatness and obesity. *Am J Clin Nutr* 1986;43:879–883.
54. Berenson GS, Srinivasan SR, Bao W. Association between multiple cardiovascular risk factors and atherosclerosis in children and young adults. *N Engl J Med* 1998;338:1650–1656.
55. Fagot-Campagna A, Pettit DJ, Engelgau MM, et al. Type 2 diabetes among North American children and adolescents: an epidemiologic review and public health perspective. *J Pediatr* 2000;136:664–672.
56. Barlow SE, Dietz WH. Assessment and treatment of obesity in children and adolescents: recommendations of an expert committee. *Pediatrics* 1998;102:e29.
57. Tominaga K, Kurata JH, Chen YK, et al. Prevalence of fatty liver in Japanese children and relationship to obesity. *Dig Dis Sci* 1995;40:2002–2009.
58. Tazawa NH, Nishinomiya F, Takada G. Serum alanine aminotransferase activity in obese children. *Acta Paediatr* 1997;86:238–241.
59. Strauss RS, Barlow SE, Dietz WH. Prevalence of abnormal serum aminotransferase values in overweight and obese adolescents. *J Pediatr* 2000;136:727–733.
60. Weisberg LA, Chutorian AM. Pseudotumor cerebri of childhood, *American Journal of Diseases of Children* 1977;131:1243–1248.
61. Grant DN. Benign intracranial hypertension; a review of 79 cases in infancy and childhood. *Arch Dis Child* 1971; 46:651–655.
62. Dietz WH Jr, Gross WL, Kirkpatrick JA Jr. Blount disease (tibia vara): another skeletal disorder associated with childhood obesity. *J Pediatr* 1982;101:735–737.
63. Kelsey JL, Keggi KJ, Southwick WO. The incidence and distribution of slipped femoral epiphysis in Connecticut and southwestern United States. *J Bone Joint Surg Am* 1970;52:1203–1216.
64. Kelsey JL, Acheson RM, Keggi KJ. The body build of patients with slipped femoral capital epiphysis. *American Journal of Diseases of Children* 1972;124:276–281.
65. Mallory GB Jr, Fiser D, Jackson R. Sleep-associated breathing disorders in morbidly obese children and adolescents. *J Pediatr* 1989;115:892–897.

5

Human Body Composition

Daniel J. Hoffman, Rebecca K. Huber-Miller, David B. Allison,
ZiMian Wang, Wei Shen, and Steven B. Heymsfield

The study of human body composition dates back more than a century (1), and today clinical and research applications abound. This chapter reviews the major body components and the current methods used in their measurement. In the first section, these components and their interrelationships are covered. The second section of the chapter discusses methods of evaluating body composition. The third and final section of the chapter presents an overview of body composition method selection.

BODY COMPONENTS

Body mass can be viewed at the following five separate levels: atomic, molecular, cellular, tissue system, and whole body (2). Each of the five levels is distinct, and each level consists of specific components (2), as is shown for the first four levels in Fig. 5.1.

The atomic level consists of the following four major elements: oxygen, carbon, hydrogen, and nitrogen. More than 98% of body mass can be accounted for by nine elements, Fig. 5.1 indicates. All nine of these major elements can be measured *in vivo* by various techniques, including whole-body counting (3) and *in vivo* neutron-activation analysis

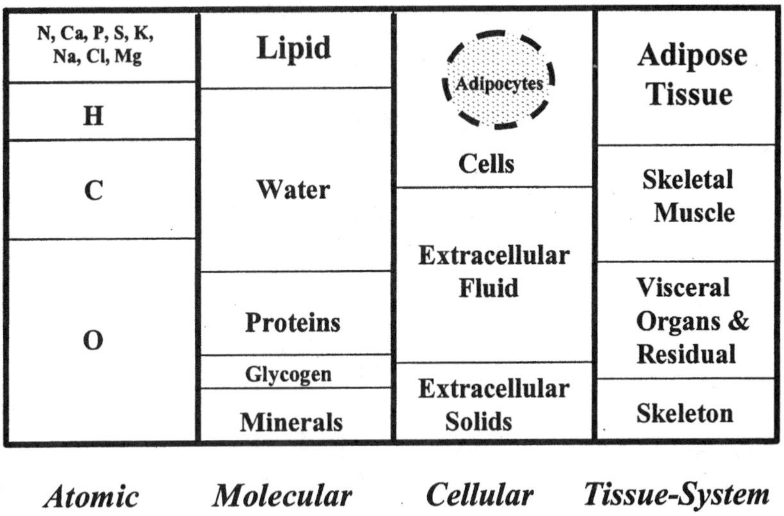

N, Ca, P, S, K, Na, Cl, Mg	Lipid	Adipocytes	Adipose Tissue
H	Water	Cells	Skeletal Muscle
C		Extracellular Fluid	Visceral Organs & Residual
O	Proteins		
	Glycogen	Extracellular Solids	Skeleton
	Minerals		

Atomic   *Molecular*   *Cellular*   *Tissue-System*

FIG. 5.1. The first four body composition levels. The fifth level, whole body, is not shown. (From Wang ZM, Pierson RN Jr, Heymsfield SB. The five level model: a new approach to organizing body composition research. *Am J Clin Nutr* 1992;56:19–28, with permission.)

(4). The significance of elements is their ability to be linked to higher level components. For example, a measurement of total body carbon, nitrogen, and potassium can be used to estimate quantitatively total body fat (5), protein (6), and body cell mass (BCM) (7), respectively.

The molecular level consists of at least the following six major components: lipid, water, protein, glycogen, bone minerals, and soft-tissue minerals. As Fig. 5.2 illustrates, various models of the molecular level that range from two to six components can be created. The two-component model, consisting of fat and fat-free mass (FFM), is the most widely applied model in the body composition methodology area. Models containing three or more components are referred to as *multicomponent models*. FFM is considered the actively metabolizing component at the molecular level of body composition.

Some confusion in terminology exists for molecular level components. The terms *lipid* and *fat* are often used interchangeably, but their meanings can differ widely (2). *Lipid* refers to all of the material extracted with lipid solvents such as ether and chloroform. These lipids include triglycerides, phospholipids, and many other structural lipids that occur in relatively small quantities *in vivo* (8). *Fats,* on the other hand, usually refer to the family of lipids consisting of triglycerides (9). Triglycerides are found almost entirely within adipocytes. Although this terminology system is not uniform, this chapter uses the term *lipid* for all lipids extractable from tissues with ether and chloroform, and the term *fat* is used for triglycerides. Approximately 90% of total body lipid in *reference man* is triglyceride (10), although this fraction differs with various dietary and health conditions. *Reference man* is defined as being between 20 and 30 years of age, weighing 70 kg, measuring 170 cm in height, and living in a climate with an average temperature of 10°C to 20°C. He is white and is a Western European or North American in habitat and custom (10).

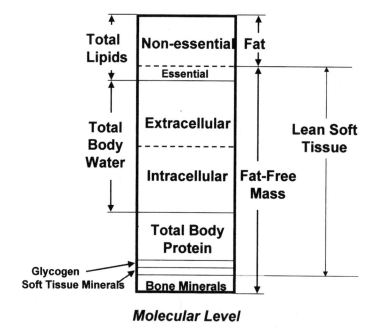

Molecular Level

FIG. 5.2. Main components of the molecular level of body composition. (From Wang ZM, Pierson RN Jr, Heymsfield SB. The five level model: a new approach to organizing body composition research. *Am J Clin Nutr* 1992;56:19–28, with permission.)

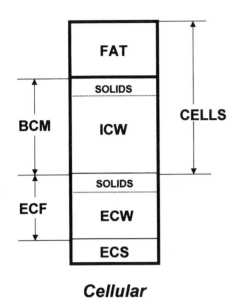

Cellular Level

FIG. 5.3. Main components of the cellular level of body composition. Abbreviations: BCM, body cell mass; ECF, extracellular fluid; ECW, extracellular water; ECS, extracellular solids; ICW, intracellular water. (From Wang ZM, Pierson RN Jr, Heymsfield SB. The five level model: a new approach to organizing body composition research. *Am J Clin Nutr* 1992;56:19–28, with permission.)

The cellular level consists of the following three components: extracellular solids, extracellular fluid (ECF), and cell mass (Fig. 5.3). Cell mass can be additionally partitioned into two further components as follows: fat cell mass and BCM. BCM is the actively metabolizing compartment at the cellular level (7).

As shown in Fig. 5.4, the tissue-system level of body composition consists of major components such as adipose tissue, skeletal muscle, visceral organs, and bone. Adipose

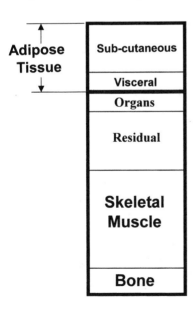

Tissue-System Level

FIG. 5.4. Main components of the tissue-organ level of body composition. (From Wang ZM, Pierson RN Jr, Heymsfield SB. The five level model: a new approach to organizing body composition research. *Am J Clin Nutr* 1992;56:19–28, with permission.)

tissue is composed of adipocytes, ECF, nerves, and blood vessels. Approximately 85% of adipose tissue is fat or triglycerides (10), although this fraction varies with dietary and health conditions. Some tissue-system level components are discrete, such as the brain, heart, liver, and kidneys. Others, such as adipose tissue and skeletal muscle, include many different components dispersed throughout the body. More than 600 individual skeletal muscles and four major adipose-tissue categories exist. The two most important clinically recognized adipose-tissue components are the subcutaneous and organ-surrounding tissue. Subcutaneous adipose tissue is found between the muscles and skin, while organ-surrounding adipose tissue surrounds the organs and may be readily separated at dissection. Adipose tissue is also distributed in the bone marrow compartment and within the interstitium of organs and tissues. Interstitial adipose tissue is interspersed within the cells of a tissue so tightly that it may be included with the tissue/organ at dissection (11). Each anatomic adipose-tissue component has specific metabolic and functional characteristics (12).

Illustrations of the subcutaneous, organ-surrounding (e.g., perirenal and pararenal, mesenteric, and omental), interstitial, and yellow marrow adipose-tissue compartments of the *Visible Man* are shown in Figs. 5.5 and 5.6 for the midabdominal region and leg, respectively. The term *visceral adipose tissue* is often applied to the adipose tissue observed with computed tomography (CT) and magnetic resonance imaging (MRI) scans within the abdominal wall, including intraabdominal and intrapelvic adipose tissue. The compartment is usually entirely encapsulated by the analyst, often at the L4 to L5 level (Fig. 5.7). Thus, omental, mesenteric, perirenal, pararenal, intrahepatic, and many other smaller adipose-tissue components may be included as visceral adipose tis-

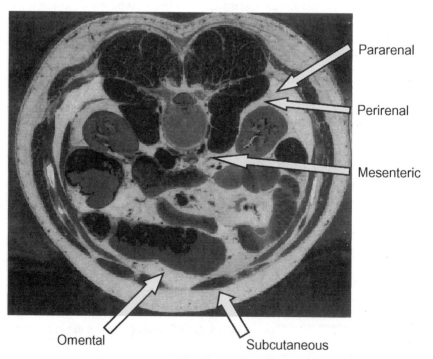

FIG. 5.5. Cross-sectional photograph of Visible Man (National Library of Medicine) at the midabdominal region with identified adipose tissue components.

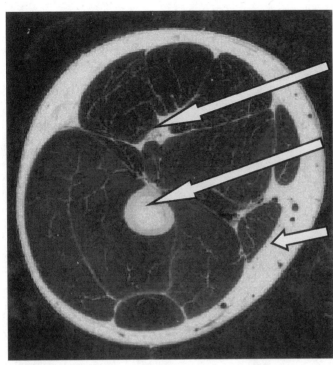

Interstitial

Yellow Marrow

Subcutaneous

FIG. 5.6. Cross-sectional photograph of Visible Man (National Library of Medicine) at the mid-upper arm region with identified adipose tissue components.

sue. Visceral adipose tissue can be further divided into intraperitoneal and retroperitoneal adipose tissue. Intraperitoneal adipose tissue is drained by the portal vein while blood from retroperitoneal adipose tissue empties into the inferior vena cava. Although cross-sectional and prospective studies have reported a positive relationship between the volume or area of visceral adipose tissue and the risk of cardiovascular disease and/or insulin resistance (13,14), the possibility for further localizing these effects to specific depots within the abdominal compartment exists. New CT and MRI sequences and improving image-analysis software make this a likely possibility. Moreover, increasing attention is being directed to the interstitial adipose tissue found within skeletal muscle (15–17), intracellular triglyceride (18), and other adipose-tissue components linked with health and disease.

The fifth and final level of body composition is the whole-body level. The whole body can be divided into regions, such as the appendages, trunk, and head.

Each component at the five composition levels is distinct, and it does not overlap with any of the other respective components. This is important because it prevents confusion when preparing body composition models. No components will overlap with each other, and none will be redundant in the various level and component model equations.

An important concept in the body composition field is that, during periods of stable body weight and energy balance, the components maintain stable relationships with one another. Some of these stable component relationships form the basis of widely used body composition models. An example of these steady-state, or stable, relationships is the hydration of FFM (i.e., about 0.73) (19) and the potassium content of FFM (about

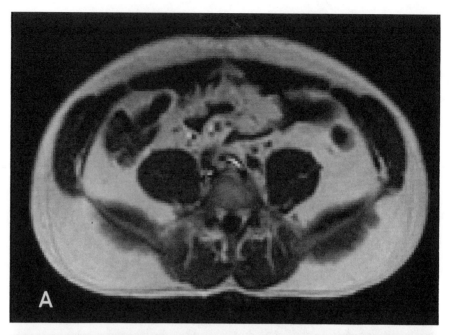

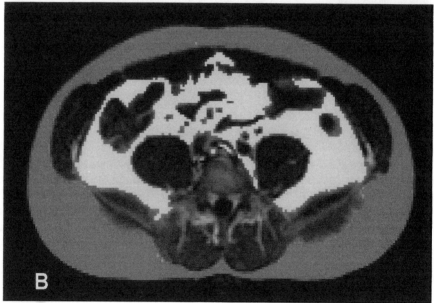

Color	Body Component	Area (cm³)	% of total adipose tissue
	Subcutaneous adipose tissue	167.8	62.1
	Visceral adipose tissue	102.3	37.9
+	Total adipose tissue	270.1	100

FIG. 5.7. Cross-sectional computed tomographic grayscale image at the L4-L5 level **(A)** and the segmented image **(B)**.

68 mmol/kg) (20). Many of these presumed "constants" are incorporated into various body composition models, and their use is described in later sections.

MEASUREMENT METHODS

Potassium-40 Counting

History

Potassium (K) in nature occurs as three isotopes, ^{39}K (93.1%), ^{40}K (0.0118%), and ^{41}K (6.9%) (20). The most abundant forms, ^{39}K and ^{41}K, are nonradioactive, whereas the naturally occurring radioactive potassium isotope ^{40}K ($t_{1/2}$=1.3 × 10^9 years) gives off a 1.46-mega-electron volt gamma ray that can be counted using detectors, such as crystalline sodium iodide (20). The proportion of total potassium found in human tissues as ^{40}K is constant at 0.0118% of the total potassium (20). Thus, by measuring ^{40}K, total body potassium (TBK) can be computed. Furthermore, potassium is distributed almost entirely within the intracellular compartment of FFM. Because the TBK to FFM ratio is relatively stable in adult humans (21), FFM and total body fat can be calculated if TBK is known. In 1961, Forbes et al. (3) were the first to report the measurement of ^{40}K and thus of TBK using a whole-body counter. From measured TBK, Forbes et al. (3) proposed the use of the relatively stable TBK to FFM ratio as a means of estimating FFM and total body fat *in vivo*. For several decades, the whole-body ^{40}K counting method was the reference approach for evaluating total body fat.

Application

The widespread use of whole-body ^{40}K counting as a means of estimating total body fat proliferated for use in humans and animals because the method, once established, is relatively simple to carry out, is safe, and is inexpensive after instrument costs are considered. The measurement approach involves first shielding the subject from naturally occurring radiation in the environment using concrete, lead, or steel (22,23). Once the external radiation is minimized, the subject's natural radiation as ^{40}K is measured using scintillation counters. The ^{40}K counts are quantified over a specified time, and then, using an appropriate calibration standard, the subject's ^{40}K and ultimately TBK levels are estimated. The average adult human has approximately 80 to 150 g of total potassium (10). Although the most common counter type measures the whole body, small regional counters can be constructed for the arms or legs (24). Miniature counters have even been built for small animals (24). The technology for quantifying either regional or whole-body potassium is well developed, and measurements can be completed with a relatively small technical error in the range of 2% to 4% (23).

Although early investigators proposed the use of an assumed stable TBK to FFM ratio as a means of estimating FFM and fat (3), that the TBK to FFM ratio varies as a function of age, sex, and other potential influencing factors is now recognized (23). For this reason, investigators have sought other means of estimating total body fat, and these are described in later sections. However, TBK does offer an important opportunity to estimate two other components, BCM and skeletal muscle mass. Almost all of the potassium is distributed in the intracellular compartment, and the concentration of potassium in the intracellular fluid in mammals remains stable at approximately 150 to 160 mmol per kg (25). TBK is thus frequently used as a measure of BCM and hence of metabolically active tissue (7). Additionally, approximately 60% of TBK is distributed within the skeletal muscle compartment (7). Accordingly, TBK is often used as a surrogate measure of cellular regional and whole-body muscle mass (11). Moreover, recent studies indicate that the relationship between TBK and skeletal muscle in adults is stable across age and sex groups (26). This stable relationship can be exploited as a means of predicting total-body skeletal muscle mass from measured TBK (26).

In summary, estimation of TBK is recognized as a classic method of quantifying total body fat that has been replaced by newer, more accurate approaches, which are described in later sections. Although whole-body counters are extremely costly instruments to install, their operational expenses are relatively small. They systems are simple to operate, and they do have recognized health risks. Because the regional and whole-body counters are extremely heavy, they cannot be used outside of specialized research laboratories dedicated to the study of metabolic diseases and human body composition. Whole-body counters are not widely available; the measurements are sometimes time consuming; and, with some systems, the procedure may be difficult for subjects. Finally, the measurement of potassium offers a means of quantifying both regional and whole-body cell mass and skeletal muscle mass.

In Vivo Neutron-Activation Analysis

History

A chance nuclear accident in the 1950s led to the radiation exposure of several human subjects (20). The subjects were placed inside a whole-body counter, and their radiation exposure was estimated by measuring the decay of specific radioactive nuclei. By extrapolation, the investigators were able to establish each subject's initial radiation dose (20). Anderson et al. (4) later reversed this concept by quantitatively exposing subjects to a neutron radiation source. In this case, the neutron exposure was known beforehand. By counting the subsequent radioactive decay, the investigators were able to estimate the total body amounts of the specific elements present. This classic study gave rise to the group of methods now referred to as *in vivo* neutron-activation analysis (4). The principle of the method is straightforward. Subjects are exposed to a source of neutrons, and these neutrons, in turn, interact with nuclei in organic and inorganic molecules within the tissues. The unstable isotopes decay and, in the process of decay, give off products that can be quantified using scintillation detectors. Today, all of the major elements can be estimated *in vivo* using neutron-activation analysis techniques in combination with whole-body counting (23).

Application

The subject is first placed inside the whole-body counter, and the amount of ^{40}K is measured. This provides an estimate of TBK. The subject is next moved to a neutron-irradiation chamber. The chamber is sealed, and the subject is exposed to a neutron-rich environment via plutonium-beryllium sources. The subject is then removed from the chamber and is moved back into the whole-body counter. The decay products of sodium, chlorine, calcium, phosphorus, and calcium are then counted inside the whole-body counter. This decay process is relatively slow, so the technique is referred to as a "delayed-γ neutron-activation analysis." A typical reaction is that for calcium as follows (27):

$$^{48}\text{Ca} + n \longrightarrow {}^{49}\text{Ca} \overset{+\text{B}^-}{\nearrow} {}^{49}\text{Sc*} \longrightarrow {}^{49}\text{Sc} + \text{E}\gamma \ (3.084 \ \text{MeV}).$$

The expression of this reaction is given as $[^{48}\text{Ca}(n,\gamma)^{49}\text{Sc}]$ for (target nucleus [incident particle, emitted particle] residual nucleus). The 3.084-MeV gamma rays from ^{49}Ca decay are measured in the whole-body counter over 15 minutes.

Delayed-γ neutron-activation analysis provides the unique measurement of total body calcium and, thus, gives an estimate of bone mineral mass. Sodium and chlorine also provide an estimates of the amount of various fluids, particularly ECF. The radiation exposure of delayed-γ neutron-activation analysis is approximately 450 mrem, so children cannot be studied by this approach. The construction of this method is highly costly, and systems are available only at a few centers throughout the world. However, delayed-γ neutron-activation analysis provides the benchmark estimate for bone mineral mass *in vivo,* and this serves as a means of evaluating other less accurate techniques.

A second approach is referred to as prompt-γ neutron-activation analysis (27). Subjects are exposed to a neutron source (e.g., $^{238}\text{PuBe}$), and decay products are counted simultaneously with irradiation. Radioactive thermal neutron capture for ^{14}N produces activated $^{15}\text{N*}$ as follows:

$$^{14}\text{N} + n \overset{\sim 10^{-15} \ \text{s}}{\longrightarrow} {}^{15}\text{N*} \longrightarrow {}^{15}\text{N} \ (\text{stable}) + \text{E}\gamma \ (10.83 \ \text{MeV}).$$

The neutron-activated $^{15}\text{N*}$ decays rapidly, producing stable ^{15}N and releasing a distinct 10.83-MeV gamma ray in the process. The gamma rays produced in the reaction are counted simultaneously with irradiation, and, because their release takes place within about 10^{-15} seconds, the method is referred to as prompt-γ *in vivo* neutron-activation analysis. Sodium iodide detectors quantify the gamma rays that are produced. Two spectral peaks are measured—hydrogen at 2.223 MeV and nitrogen at 10.83 MeV.

A typical head-to-toe scan requires 40 minutes and exposes subjects to about 40 mrem of radiation. Although several elements can be quantified using this approach, the two most important are hydrogen and nitrogen. Hydrogen typically serves as an internal standard, and it is referenced against the amount of hydrogen estimated from measured total body water and other anthropometric dimensions. The measurement of nitrogen is typically used to estimate the amount of total body protein, using the assumption that protein is 16% nitrogen (28). Total body protein then serves as one major molecular level component in neutron-activation multicomponent models for estimating total body fat. As with delayed-γ systems, prompt-γ *in vivo* neutron-activation systems are costly to construct; they require a high level of technical skill to maintain and operate; and they expose subjects to ionizing radiation. Although the use of this approach is limited to specialized laboratories, prompt-γ systems provide the unique opportunity to quantify the metabolically and nutritionally important total body protein component *in vivo.*

The third technique is referred to as *inelastic neutron scattering* (5). The reaction for carbon, the key measured element, is given by the following equation:

$$^{12}\text{C} + n \overset{n'}{\nearrow} \longrightarrow {}^{12}\text{C*} \longrightarrow {}^{12}\text{C} + \text{E}\gamma \ (4.44 \ \text{MeV}).$$

Increasing the energy of the neutrons produced raises the likelihood of inelastic scattering reactions, such as this one for carbon, which have fast neutron thresholds. The

Brookhaven National Laboratory inelastic neutron-scattering system is based on the use of a small deuterium-tritium–sealed tube pulsating (4 to 10 kHz) neutron generator that is fastened beneath the recumbent subject. The 4.44-MeV gamma rays produced by the inelastic scattering of carbon are detected by two bismuth germanate crystals positioned on either side of the subject. The detected counts, which are gathered over a 30-minute time period as the subject moves over the neutron cloud, are converted to total body carbon based on reference phantom calibrations.

Imaging Methods

History

Early workers in the field of clinical nutrition used standard x-ray techniques to examine fat-layer thickness (29). The high radiation exposure and low image contrast limited the research and clinical applicability of this approach. In 1973, Hounsfield (30) introduced the first axial CT system; and, by the early 1980s, CT scanners were installed in hospitals throughout the world. The early CT approach provided cross-sectional images with high contrast, and, by 1979, the first reports of skeletal muscle measurement appeared (31). The first measurements of visceral organ volumes were reported in 1979 (32); this was followed by estimates of visceral adipose tissue in 1981 (33). Several contiguous image slices were assembled into the complete three-dimensional adipose-tissue or organ compartment of interest. Although CT was a major breakthrough in quantifying the volumes of tissues and organs, applicability was limited by radiation exposure. Within a decade, the first reports of MRI of humans appeared; and, in the 1980s, Foster et al. (34) reported the first MRI body composition studies. MRI, like the CT, provides the unique capability of quantifying tissue and organ volumes *in vivo*, but without the radiation hazard. Gradual advances in both CT and MRI capabilities now make single-slice or multiple-slice tissue and organ analysis a reference approach against which other techniques can be compared.

Application

Both CT and MRI provide high-resolution cross-sectional images through selected anatomic regions. At one extreme, the entire body can be imaged, and the volume of all major tissue-system level components can be estimated. Volume estimates can be converted to mass values by assuming specific tissue densities (10). Depending on the selected slice number, whole-body evaluations require scan times ranging from about 20 minutes to several hours. Because CT exposes subjects to radiation, few reports of whole-body CT studies in humans have been made (35–37). Moreover, the use of CT and MRI in phantom and cadaver studies provides similar tissue volume estimates (11); therefore, the trend today is to apply MRI whenever possible. Specific aspects of scanning protocols have been reported in earlier studies (38).

Once images are collected, analyses can take one of several pathways. For CT, pixel intensities are designated in Hounsfield units, and calibrations are similar among all CT scanners. Hounsfield unit ranges differ between tissues; notably, adipose tissue, lean soft tissues, and bone vary sufficiently enough in pixel intensity to allow component separation using designated Hounsfield unit ranges (36). Hounsfield unit ranges for adipose tissue, muscle and organs, and bone, respectively, are as follows: -190 to -30 HU; -30 to $+100$ HU; more than 100 HU.

Selected organs and tissues can also be traced directly on the CT scanner console, and the related areas within each slice may be established. Because CT imaging time is usually rapid, with several seconds per slice, images of moving objects, such as the viscera secondary to peristalsis and respiration, are still relatively sharp, and the boundaries are clear.

Analysis of MRI scans is more complex because pixel intensity varies according to the selected imaging sequence and other factors. Standard pixel "ranges" therefore cannot be set, and analysis is conducted on a scan-by-scan basis. Dedicated image-analysis software is usually applied instead of standard system radiology software. Image-acquisition times for MRI are usually longer than they are for CT, and patients should be instructed to maximize their breath-holds and to maintain a stable position during the scan. Images of the viscera tend to be less sharp than they are for CT, although the new MRI scanning sequences demonstrate improved image clarity (38). For both CT and MRI, training is required for image analysis, and reading times can vary from several minutes for a single slice to several days for the whole body.

Both CT and MRI are uniquely capable of acquiring tissue-organ level volume estimates that include all major organs and tissues, the visceral adipose tissue, and regional estimates. CT and MRI estimates of visceral adipose tissue, whether a single slice or multiple slices, are considered the reference against which other techniques are compared. Cost, instrument access, and the need for trained image-analysis technicians may limit routine imaging method use to specialized research studies and centers. CT and MRI are not appropriate for use in field studies of body composition, although both methods can be used to "calibrate" or validate other simpler, less costly methods.

Although today the focus is still mainly on produced images, rapid growth in magnetic resonance spectroscopy and functional MRI offers great promise in the study of human physiology and metabolism. These new developments carry the potential to add not only to the ability to quantify body composition but also to enhance of the knowledge of closely related metabolic processes.

Hydrometry

History

The following three isotopes of water are recognized in nature: deuterium, tritium, and oxygen-18–labeled water. Schloerb et al. (39) were the first to measure total body water in 1951 using the isotope deuterium. The method's importance greatly increased after the report of Pace and Rathbun in 1945 (19), which indicated that water existed in a relatively stable proportion to FFM—approximately 0.73. This subsequently led to the widespread use of total body water as a means of estimating FFM and total body fat in both animals and humans (40–42).

Application

The method is relatively straightforward and simple to apply. Subjects ingest a known amount of isotope, and, at some later time, the amount of isotope remaining in the body is quantified (43). The water compartment is then resampled through urine, saliva, or blood. Total body water is then calculated using the classic dilution formula (44,45).

Details of the procedure vary depending on the isotope used, the analytical method, and the accuracy desired (42). Deuterium is relatively inexpensive to purchase, is simple to measure in secretions and blood samples, and is safe because the isotope is stable. The isotope tritium is also inexpensive and is easy to measure in blood samples; it does, however, expose the subject to a small amount of radiation (42,45). Today, deuterium is usually favored over tritium as an isotope for water dilution because of the radiation exposure with tritium and the increasing ease with which deuterium can be measured in samples. Oxygen-18–labeled water is relatively expensive, and measurement is possible only in specialized laboratories that have mass spectroscopy equipment (42). Oxygen-18–labeled water is useful for measuring total body water when doubly labeled water studies of energy expenditure are being conducted (46).

Once the dilution space is known from the evaluation protocol, total body water mass must then be calculated. The dilution spaces of deuterium and tritium are slightly larger than the actual total body water because proton exchange with other organic constituents increases the apparent volume of distribution (42). Most investigators assume that the overestimate of total body water by deuterium and tritium is approximately 4% (47). A correction for water density is also required when converting water volume to water mass. Furthermore, the oxygen-18 space is slightly larger than actual total body water by about 1% in most studies (42). Some investigators thus assume that oxygen-18 represents an even more accurate assessment of actual total body water because the oxygen exchange is substantially less than that of the proton exchange for deuterium and tritium.

The technical error of total body water measurement varies with the specific protocol applied. However, most approaches provide reliable measurement of total body water with a technical error in the range of 1% to 3%. With the assumption that subjects are healthy weight-stable adults, the proportion of FFM as total body water is relatively stable at 0.73 (48). Some variability in this ratio is recognized across age-groups and in various disease states (48). The advantage of total body water as a means of estimating FFM and total body fat is that the method is simple, relatively inexpensive, and easy to carry out even in isolated settings. The disadvantages of the method are that dilution protocols often require several hours and that subject conditions can be highly variable depending on the hydration status and the presence of disease or ambient conditions (e.g., environmental temperature). Hydrometry is the only approach capable of measuring extremely large subjects (i.e., those weighing more than several hundred kilograms). Similarly, hydrometry is widely applied in the study of large animals, including whales and other aquatic mammals (48).

Underwater Weighing or Air Plethysmography

History

More than one century ago, investigators sought a means of nondestructively establishing the oil content of fish (49). A novel means was devised whereby the fish-specific gravity was established and oil was then estimated using a two-component model. The model qualitatively assumed that one component was oil with a low specific gravity and that the second component consisted of the remaining tissue, which had a higher specific gravity. In effect, the specific gravity then became a measure of the fish oil content. By the mid-1940s, the technique had been refined and extended by Behnke et al. (50), who devised an underwater weighing system that included correction of specific gravity for residual air trapped in the lungs. Behnke et al. (50) also proposed a quantitative two-compartment model consisting of fat and FFM, each with known and assumed constant densities. Siri (51,52) later refined these densities so that fat was now assumed to have a density of 0.9 g per cm^3 and FFM, a density of 1.1 g per cm^3 at body temperature. With the assumption of these two known and constant densities and given the subject's measured density by underwater weighing, the investigator can then compute the subject's percentage of body weight as fat. The hydrodensitometry, or underwater weighing method, served for at least four decades as the reference technique against which other methods were compared.

Application

The modern technique involves a watertight tank that typically has an electronic scale that is either positioned above the tank or submerged on the floor of the tank (53). The subject exhales, expelling air, and then submerges; the underwater body weight is then recorded. Density is calculated from the subject's weight in air and his or her weight underwater after corrections are made for water temperature. The subject's residual lung volume is also measured either during the underwater weighing procedure or following his or her emergence from the tank. Underwater weighing systems are relatively easy to construct, and they are inexpensive. Accordingly, many systems have been built throughout the world, including in developing countries. The information provided by this technique has contributed significantly to the understanding of human body composition in health and disease.

The two-component model assumes that body weight consists of fat and FFM. The density of fat—approximately 0.9 g per cm^3—is well established in both humans and animals (54). Minimal variation in the density of fat is recognized within and among species. This is because fat, or specifically lipid, is almost entirely triglycerides. On the other hand, FFM is a heterogeneous compartment consisting of at least four major components, including water, protein, glycogen, and minerals. The density of these components varies from a low of 0.994 g per cm^3 for water to a high of 3.04 g per cm^3 for minerals. The assumed density of 1.1 g per cm^3 is based on observations made in a limited number of human cadavers, which suggest relatively stable proportions of water, protein, glycogen, and minerals (55). To the extent that these proportions are changed in any individual subject, corresponding errors in the assumed density of FFM will be introduced. A number of studies suggest that the density of FFM is relatively stable across age-groups and sex groups, although some variation is recognized at the extremes of age (56) and in patients who have underlying medical and surgical conditions. Additionally, race differences in the density of FFM may exist, and variation among special groups, such as body builders or other types of athletic participants, is also seen (57). Thus, although underwater weighing and the two-compartment model have served as a reference technique for several decades, newer approaches without these various assumptions are now replacing hydrodensitometry as the clinical reference method.

The importance of the underwater weighing method is that the measurement systems are relatively inexpensive to construct, they are simple to operate, and the procedure is safe for patients varying widely in age and body weight. The method's disadvantage is that some subjects have concerns about water submersion, and thus they either decline to participate or their measurements are technically inadequate. Underwater weighing is also, by necessity, stationary, and it cannot be moved around for field applications. A reasonable amount of technical skill is required to perform the method, which, under optimal conditions, has a small technical error of about 0.001 g per cm^3 (58). The residual lung volume measurement can also be difficult from some patients; this adds to the measurement error and contributes further to the method's total error.

The main concept of hydrodensitometry, which is that the body consists of two compartments of known and stable density, is quite robust; as mentioned above, it has served investigators well for several decades. However, investigators have searched for alternative means of quantifying body density in humans. A new approach to estimating body volume and body density is referred to as *air plethysmography* (59,60). The air plethysmography technique is based on classic gas laws. Small volume changes are produced within a two-chambered plethysmograph, and the corresponding pressure change is then measured. The subject's body volume is determined by subtraction of the empty chamber volume. Additional corrections are made for body volume based on body surface area and thoracic gas volume. The adjusted value for body volume is used to estimate body density, and fat mass is then calculated from the body weight and the classic Siri equation (51). The available commercial system, BODPOD (Life Measurements Instruments, Concord, CA), has been widely validated in adults and children (59–60a). The system is adequately portable for use in phenotyping in isolated areas, with the assumption that electrical power is available and that ambient conditions, such as temperature and humidity, are adequately controlled and relatively stable. The currently available system is optimized for adults, and smaller systems for use in infants and children are in development. Although many underwater weighing systems can accommodate extremely obese subjects, BODPOD's size is finite and not all obese subjects fit within the fixed chamber volume.

Dual-Energy X-Ray Absorptiometry

History

Anthropologists and health care workers in the field of metabolic bone disease needed a method of quantifying bone mass. The selected approach consisted of exposing one side of the wrist to a photon-emitting radioactive source and positioning a scintillation counter on the other side of the wrist (61). The number of detected counts was related to the amount of attenuating calcium or bone present. The wrist was usually selected for measurement because bone is the main attenuating tissue, unlike the hip or spine, at which soft tissue is also present. Later investigators explored means of evaluating hip and spine because these are clinically important bone areas involved in osteoporosis. The single-photon system evolved to a dual-photon system, which was now based on a filtered x-ray source and was referred to as dual-energy x-ray absorptiometry (DEXA) (62). DEXA systems require information about soft-tissue composition to be able to quantify bone mineral within a soft-tissue–containing pixel. DEXA's capability to quantify the fat and lean soft-tissue content of a pixel evolved such that it takes a central role in modern body composition analysis.

Application

DEXA systems all operate on similar principals, although important technical details may vary (61) (Fig. 5.8). An x-ray source provides a broad photon beam that is usually filtered, yielding two main energy peaks. Some systems produce the two energy peaks by use of a pulsating voltage source. The emitted photons traverse the subject's tissues, and the extent to which they are attenuated is dependent on the tissue's elemental makeup. Low-atomic–weight elements, such as hydrogen, minimally attenuate photons, whereas elements such as calcium are highly attenuating. Additionally, the difference in attenuation between the two energy peaks is characteristic for each element and thus each tissue. The characteristic attenuation signature for fat, lean soft tissue, and bone mineral enables the development of pixel-by-pixel composition estimates using a series of assumptions and reconstruction algorithms (61). Some systems use a simple "pencil-beam" configuration as the patient is scanned, and others have a "fan-beam" configuration for the x-ray source and detector. Fan-beam systems generally are faster, requiring only several minutes for each scan, compared with longer scan times for pencil-beam models. Accuracy

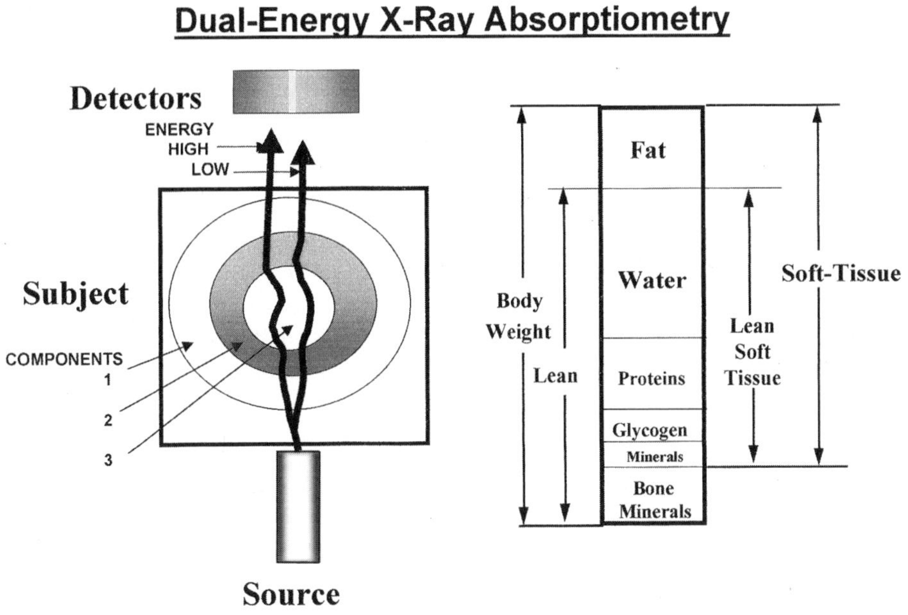

Dual-Energy X-Ray Absorptiometry

FIG. 5.8. Schematic representation of dual-energy x-ray absorptiometry system **(left)** and the three-component model consisting of bone mineral, lean soft tissue, and fat **(right)**. (From Gallagher D, Testolin C, Nuñez C, et al. Anthropometry and methods of body composition measurement for research and field application in the elderly. *Eur J Clin Nutr* 2000;54:S1–S7, with permission.)

varies with system design and software. Calibrations carried out by the manufacturer permit resolution of the three molecular level components—bone mineral, fat, and lean soft tissue. System calibration and function is also carried out once systems are operational on a regular basis. DEXA x-ray exposure is minimal (less than 1 mrem), thus allowing longitudinal studies in children and adults.

Current DEXA systems designed for body composition analysis can provide estimates for the three components of the whole body and for specific regions, such as the arms, legs, and trunk. This unique capability of DEXA creates several important opportunities as follows: (a) regional or total body fat mass can be quantified using standard system settings or at investigator-initiated specific anatomic sites; (b) appendicular lean soft tissue can be quantified and used as a measure of regional or total body skeletal muscle mass (63,64); and (c) acquired bone mineral measurements can be applied not only to the study of osteoporosis but also to the development of more complex multicomponent models (65). DEXA measurements provide valuable insights in longitudinal studies because the measurement precision is quite high. Many studies have now validated DEXA body composition estimates against other reference methods, and they have shown good overall agreement for body fat estimates (66). Some variation in fat and bone mineral estimates is usually observed when different instruments are compared, thus necessitating close scrutiny of the selected instrument for calibration and accuracy (67). Although DEXA provides regional "total" fat estimates, it is not capable of estimating visceral adipose tissue like CT and MRI can.

DEXA systems are increasingly available, they are accurate when properly calibrated and applied, and they are relatively safe to use in most subjects. As a result, DEXA is becoming the method of choice for accurately measuring fat and bone mineral mass at research centers that lack *in vivo* neutron activation (IVNA) systems. Its disadvantages are that it cannot be used in pregnant women, the cost is reasonably high, and very large or obese subjects cannot be easily accommodated on most available systems.

An important feature of DEXA is that it provides investigators with an estimate of bone mineral mass. Combining measured bone mineral with estimates of body volume by underwater weighing and air plethysmography and of total body water by isotope dilution allows the development of "multicomponent" models (47). The best recognized of these is the family of models based on body volume estimates that begins with the classic two-component model (51,55) and then advances to three components with the addition of total body water (51) and to four components with the addition of bone mineral estimates (68). Besides providing more compartmental estimates of biologic interest, the main benefit of multicomponent models is that fewer assumptions are made regarding component relationships that have been assumed to be stable or constant across subjects (e.g., FFM hydration). Accordingly, multicomponent methods are usually considered to be the reference against which other techniques are validated or compared.

Bioimpedance Analysis

History

Bioimpedance analysis (BIA) methods were first conceived and evaluated for use in the study of human physiology during the 1930s by Burger and van Milaan (69) and Barnett (70). Modern BIA methods are all based on a similar principle—resistance to an applied alternating electrical current is a function of tissue composition. By the mid-1980s, technologic improvements permitted the introduction of new and more practical BIA methods for estimating total body water, FFM, and total body fat. These methods proliferated, and, by 1994, the National Institutes of Health organized a watershed conference in which the clinical and research applicability of BIA methods were reviewed in detail (71).

To an extent, all tissues conduct an electrical current. The conductivity of the tissue is dependent on the biologic characteristics of each specific tissue. Tissues with long cylindrical cells and a high fluid and electrolyte content, such as skeletal muscle, impose relatively little resistance to an applied electrical current (72,73). In contrast, tissues with globular cells and a low water content, such as adipose tissue, provide a relatively high resistance to the conductivity of an alternating electrical current. This varying specific tissue resistivity allows the empiric development of body composition prediction models (74). Although advanced methods permit the actual imaging of tissues, current BIA methods usually first make the body component of interest the dependent variable in prediction models. These dependent variables often include total body water as measured by the reference method of isotope dilution and FFM as measured by DEXA or underwater weighing (74). Measured resistance, or the closely related impedance, is then set as the predictor variable in regression models. The electrical measurements are usually adjusted first for path length, typically as $length^2$ or $height^2$. Other predictor variables can also be inserted, such as age, sex, race, and even selected anthropometric measurements. The developed prediction model is then cross-validated before application.

Application

BIA methods vary widely with regard to the nature of the applied electrical current and the selected measurement pathway. The following two system types are available:

single frequency and multiple frequency (72). Single-frequency systems are typically based on a 50-kHz alternating current. These systems provide a measure of impedance, or resistance, at a frequency of 50 kHz, and some may also provide corresponding estimates of reactance and phase angle. The electrical properties are then used in body composition prediction models as was previously described. Electrodes can vary from typical gel electrodes that must be applied first to stainless steel electrodes that maintain pressure contact with the subject (75). More advanced systems are based on multiple frequencies (73). These applied electrical frequencies can vary from as little as 1 kHz to up to 1 MHz. Multiple-frequency systems are applied when measuring fluid compartments, but they offer little advantage to single-frequency systems for the estimation of FFM and total body fat (73).

The measured electrical circuit can also vary, ranging from an isolated region, such as a single leg, to multiple limbs and the whole body (76). The most common approach is the "half-body" pathway, which extends from one arm to the corresponding leg.

An essential feature of BIA methods is the requirement that measurements be taken according to standardized conditions suggested by the manufacturer or developer. Time of day, subject position, room temperature, the level of prior physical activity, and meal ingestion are all variables that should be considered (77,78). When measurements are taken carefully, body composition estimates are usually well correlated with those provided by underwater weighing, DEXA, and other reference methods (79). Consideration should also be given to the quality of the selected instrument and the appropriateness of the instrument's calibration equations for the subjects under evaluation.

Because BIA systems are relatively inexpensive and are simple to operate, they have wide applicability in clinical and field settings. The results will be acceptable if they are properly applied and if calibrated systems are used for evaluating appropriately selected subjects. BIA estimates are suitable for long-term patient monitoring and for phenotyping groups of subjects for genetic studies. BIA body composition estimates are generally not reliable for evaluating short-term changes in body fluid or fat mass, although the newer multiple-frequency systems offer promise as a means of tracking short-term fluid balance (80).

Anthropometry

History

Anthropometric measurements are among the oldest in the body composition field (81). Early workers applied body weight, height, various skinfold thicknesses and circumferences, and other linear dimensions to characterize a subject's fatness and nutritional status. Modern workers have calibrated various anthropometric dimensions against reference body composition estimates to develop specific component prediction models. This calibration approach allows the estimation of total body fat, adipose tissue, skeletal muscle, and other components from various anthropometric estimates. Anthropometric methods are widely available because they are inexpensive, simple to perform, and safe; and they can be used in variety of settings, ranging from the research laboratory to field facilities. Anthropometric methods have limitations, including the need for trained observers, relatively high between-measurement technical error for some measurements, mechanical limitations for the very obese with some instruments, the "errors" in some geometric prediction models produced by the assumption of stable between-subject anatomic proportions, and the population specificity of component prediction formulas (81).

Application

Anthropometric measurements include body weight, height, skinfold measurements, circumferences, and various body diameters. The use of these measurements varies, but, whether used individually or combined, they allow reasonable predictions of body composition in nonobese subjects. For example, weight provides a simple measurement of body mass and thus of total energy content. Skinfold measurements reflect the relative amount of fat for a given body site, and they may be used to describe the regional adiposity. Finally, weight combined with skinfold measurements and body diameters can accurately estimate the amount of FFM and fat mass (82–84). Each of these measurements is discussed in more detail below.

BMI (weight in kilograms divided by height in meters squared) is among the simplest anthropometric expressions that can be applied in body fat estimation (85). The following is a multiple regression formula developed by setting BMI as an independent variable with the percentage of fat as the dependent variable:

$$\% \text{ body fat} = 64.5 - 848\,(1/\text{BMI}) + 0.079\,\text{age} - 16.4\,\text{sex} + 0.05\,\text{sex age} + 39.0\,\text{sex}\,(1/\text{BMI}),$$

where *sex* equals 1 for male and 0 for female (85). Body fat in this study was measured using a four-component model as the reference method. The equation is applicable to whites and African Americans, and a separate equation is available for use in Asian subjects. BMI is limited as a measure of body composition because subjects of the same BMI or body weight may differ widely in fatness (86). Accordingly, BMI is considered a first-level measure of body composition; higher resolution is gained by using other anthropometric estimates.

A large number of anthropometric body fat prediction models based on measured skinfolds and circumferences are reported in the literature (87). These methods vary in the subject populations used to develop the prediction models, as well as in the selected ref-

---

TABLE 5.1. *Durnin–Womersley four-skinfold body fat measurement method*

Calculation of fat and fat-free body mass according Durnin and Womersley method
1. Determine the patient's age and weight (kg).
2. Measure the following skinfolds in mm: biceps, triceps, subscapular, and suprailiac (Tables 56-3 and 56-5).
3. Compute Σ by adding the four skinfolds.
4. Compute the logarithm of Σ.
5. Apply one of the following age-adjusted and sex-adjusted equations to compute body density (D, g/mL)
     Equations for men:
       Age range (yr)
         17–19, $D = 1.1620 - 0.0630 \times (\log \Sigma)$
         20–29, $D = 1.1631 - 0.0632 \times (\log \Sigma)$
         30–39, $D = 1.1422 - 0.0544 \times (\log \Sigma)$
         40–49, $D = 1.1620 - 0.0700 \times (\log \Sigma)$
         50+, $D = 1.1715 - 0.0779 \times (\log \Sigma)$
     Equations for women:
       Age range (yr)
         17–19, $D = 1.1549 - 0.0678 \times (\log \Sigma)$
         20–29, $D = 1.1599 - 0.0717 \times (\log \Sigma)$
         30–39, $D = 1.1423 - 0.0632 \times (\log \Sigma)$
         40–49, $D = 1.1333 - 0.0612 \times (\log \Sigma)$
         50+, $D = 1.1339 - 0.0645 \times (\log \Sigma)$
6. Fat mass is then calculated as fat mass (kg) = body weight (kg) $\times$ [4.95/D − 4.5]
7. Fat-free body mass (FFM) is then calculated as FFM (kg) = body weight (kg) − fat mass (kg)

From Heymsfield, 1984, with permission.

erence methods. Some models rely solely on measured skinfold thickness, while others rely primarily on circumference measurements (83). Geometric models allow the estimation of limb fat areas using a combination of extremity skinfold and circumference measurements (81). A summary of the widely validated and applied four-skinfold method of Durnin and Womersley (84) for estimating total body fat is presented in Table 5.1. Methods of measuring skinfold thicknesses and circumferences and the location of various measurement sites are presented in Table 5.2. Methods of optimizing measurement precision are presented in Table 5.3.

An important feature of anthropometry is the fact that selected skinfold and circumference measurements provide estimates of adipose-tissue distribution (88). In particular, anthropometry allows the estimation of subcutaneous adipose-tissue distribution. For example, the waist circumference measurement provides a well-validated measure of visceral adipose tissue (89). According to the National Institutes of Health guidelines, a waist circumference of 94 cm for men and 80 cm for women should be taken as the cutpoints for limiting weight gain, and a waist circumference of 102 cm for men and 88 cm for women should be taken as the cutpoints for reducing weight (90,91).

Although the waist to hip circumference ratio was once applied as a measure of adipose-tissue distribution, today only the waist circumference is usually measured. The sagittal diameter, measured as the largest body thickness in supine subjects, is also used

TABLE 5.2. *Methods and sites for measuring skinfolds and circumferences*

Skinfolds
1. Arrive at the anatomic site.
2. Lift the skin and fat layer from the underlying tissue by grasping the tissue with the thumb and forefinger.
3. Apply calipers 1 cm distal from the thumb and forefinger and midway between the apex and base of the skinfold.
4. Continue to support the skinfold with the thumb and forefinger for the duration of the measurement.
5. Read skinfold to the nearest 0.5 mm, after 2–3 s of caliper application
6. Perform measures in triplicate until readings agree within ±1.0 mm; then average the results.

Biceps skinfold thickness: Lift the skinfold on the anterior aspect of the upper arm directly above the center of the cubital fossa and at the same level as the triceps skinfold and midarm circumference. The arm should hang relaxed at the patient's side, and the crest of the fold should run parallel to the long axis of the arm.

Triceps skinfold thickness: Grasp the skin and subcutaneous tissue 1 cm above the midpoint between the tip of the acromial process of the scapula and the olecranon process of the ulna. The fold runs parallel to the long axis of the arm. Care should be taken to ensure that the measurement is made in the midline posteriorly and that the arm hangs relaxed and vertical.

Subscapular skinfold: Lift the skin 1 cm under the inferior angle of the scapula with the shoulder and arm relaxed. The fold should run parallel to the natural cleavage lines of the skin; this is usually a line about 45 degrees from the horizontal extending medially upwards.

Suprailiac skinfold: Measure this skinfold 2 cm above the iliac crest in the midaxillary line. The crest of this fold should run horizontally.

Circumferences
1. The tape should be maintained in a horizontal position touching the skin and following the contours of the limb but not compressing underlying tissue.
2. Measurements should be made to the nearest mm in triplicate, as was previously described for skinfolds.

Waist: Perform this measurement using a flexible tape positioned at the narrowest point between the lower rib and the iliac crest. The investigator should be positioned to ensure that the tape is located evenly around the waist of this position.

Hip: Make this measurement in a similar manner to the waist circumference with the tape should positioned at the greatest protuberance of the buttocks. The investigator should ensure that the tape is positioned evenly around the subject.

Modified from Heymsfield. 1992, with permission.

TABLE 5.3. *Methods for optimizing precision*

1. Use skilled professionals to train observers.
2. Use one rather than multiple observers for the same subject over time.
3. Mark the anatomic site of the skinfold and circumferential measurement with indelible ink when repeatedly measuring the same patient over a short time period.
4. Learn the anatomic landmarks, the method of grasping the skinfold, the length of time for compressing the skinfold site, and the proper way to reread the caliper scale.
5. Periodically assess interobserver and between-day measurement differences of different staff members.

Source: Modified from Heymsfield, 1992, with permission.

as a measure of visceral adipose tissue (92), but few studies have provided evidence that this anthropometric dimension is superior to the simpler waist circumference measurement. A major advantage of using anthropometry for assessing visceral adipose tissue is the relative ease with which measurements can be made, although well-trained technicians are an essential requirement. Anthropometric measurements are less costly and easier than the comparable CT and MRI studies, but with these advantages comes a loss of precision and repeatability.

Many validation studies of anthropometric prediction methods have been undertaken, and most published total body fat and adipose-tissue models tend to cross-validate when compared with reference methods. Among the various measurement methods, anthropometric techniques usually demonstrate the largest standard error and the lowest correlation coefficients when compared with other techniques for estimating total body fat, such as DEXA, BIA, or *in vivo* neutron-activation analysis (66). Some technical concerns should also be considered, including the requirement for technician training and the need for special calipers in very obese subjects. Thus, although anthropometric methods are useful in phenotyping subjects for fatness, anthropometry usually is not applied for individual subject evaluations and for examining short-term changes in body fat. Anthropometric methods are important in field studies of nutrition and obesity in which other methods cannot be applied or in which they are impractical in the selected setting.

COMPONENT MEASUREMENT

Adiposity

When Should Adiposity Be Measured?

Body weight or related BMI is correlated with adiposity in populations, but, in some individuals or groups, the possibility of misclassification exists; in other words, a subject may be overweight but not "overfat." Similarly, a subject may have a normal weight but still harbor excess adipose tissue. For example, entry into and retention in the military is based on weight and body fat standards because highly trained muscular men and women may be overweight but not overfat. Increasing attention is also being focused on the relations between adiposity *per se* and health risks, such that most large-scale epidemiologic and clinical trials incorporate body composition measurements into the evaluation protocol. Measuring adipose-tissue distribution also provides additional phenotypic and risk information. Finally, with weight loss treatment, the composition of weight change may vary among individuals according to the level of physical activity, the nature of the ingested diet, or the administered drug. Tracking the composition of weight loss may thus prove enlightening in some situations.

How Should a Method Be Selected?

The available instrumentation, the research question posed, and the subject population determine the appropriate measurement method. Evaluation of large subject populations in field surveys requires simple, practical, and portable methods that can be safely applied. Small-scale studies examining small subject groups or a single individual at one or more times require highly reliable adiposity measurement methods. Methods applied in children, women of childbearing potential, or pregnant women by necessity must meet different safety criteria than those for methods that applied to elderly or ill patients. A summary of some of these considerations is presented for the various methods in Table 5.4. The qualitative summary indicates that methods tend to group by the following characteristics: (a) highly accurate methods tend to be more costly to purchase and operate, they are less practical to apply, and they are often associated with some risk. (b) In contrast, field methods tend to be inexpensive to purchase and operate and to be simple to apply, and they are are usually safe for application in most populations. These various considerations dictate the method selection.

What Is The Patient's Total Body or Regional Adiposity?

Some methods are designed to measure "fat" (e.g., DEXA) and others, "adipose tissue." The posed research or clinical question may dictate which specific component is evaluated. Also, some methods are designed to evaluate whole-body fatness, while others provide regional estimates. Some methods, such as DEXA, CT, and MRI, can provide both regional and whole-body estimates.

Does The Patient Have Normal Total-Body Adiposity?

Several ranges have been published to allow one to establish a subject's or a group's relationship to the "United States population" or to "healthy ranges" (86,93). A growing body of literature exists on this topic, and the present information is particularly limited in certain populations, such as young children.

Is The Patient's Total-Body Adiposity Changing Over Time?

Some methods are more accurate than others in detecting short-term (i.e., days) changes (Table 5.4). Most methods, when carefully applied, are useful in detecting long-term (i.e., weeks and months) changes in adiposity.

TABLE 5.4. *Qualitative characteristics of body composition methods*

Method	Research	Clinical	Cost	Safety	Accessibility[a]
Neutron activation	****	*	****	*	*
WBC	****	*	***	****	*
DXA	***	***	***	***	***
Hydrometry[b]	***	**	**	****	**
UWW-AP	***	**	**	****	**
BIA	**	****	*	****	****
Anthropometry	*	****	*	****	****

Scores range from low (*) to high (****).
[a]Refers to availability of measurement systems.
[b]Assumes stable isotope.
Abbreviations: BIA, bioimpedance analysis; DXA, dual-energy x-ray absorptiometry; UWW-AP, underwater weighing and air plethysmography; WBC, whole body ^{40}K counting.

Adipose-Tissue Distribution: Selecting a Method

Imaging methods, such as CT and MRI, are considered reference methods for quantitating adipose-tissue distribution. Images provided by CT tend to be sharper than those produced by MRI for visceral components, although CT is associated with radiation exposure. The DEXA method provides quantification of regions of interest, such as the abdomen, although no differentiation is provided for subcutaneous and visceral components. Some investigators recommend combining DEXA with anthropometric or ultrasound for partitioning subcutaneous and visceral fat (94). Skinfold measurements and circumferences that are carefully applied provide a simple means of characterizing adipose-tissue distribution. Although sagittal diameter is not widely applied, it is recommended by some as a marker of visceral adiposity (92).

Other Components

The estimation of skeletal muscle, bone mineral, and visceral organs was briefly touched on in this chapter, and extensive discussions are provided in other reports (95). FFM, a metabolically active component, is estimated as the difference between body weight and total body fat. Similarly, adipose-tissue–free mass is the difference between body weight and total body adipose tissue (96). These two components are often used in relation to energy expenditure measurements.

CONCLUSION

Evaluation of adiposity and body composition in general is central to many aspects of studying and treating human weight regulatory disorders. Various methods for quantifying body composition are available and are practical for use in research and clinical settings. These methods provide new opportunities for patient evaluation in research and clinical settings.

ACKNOWLEDGMENTS

This work was supported by grants RR00645 and NIDDK 42618, 51716, 26687 from the National Institutes of Health.

REFERENCES

1. Wang Z, Wang ZM, Heymsfield SB. History of the study of human body composition. *Am J Hum Biol* 1999;11:157–165.
2. Wang ZM, Pierson RN Jr, Heymsfield SB. The five level model: a new approach to organizing body composition research. *Am J Clin Nutr* 1992;56:19–28.
3. Forbes GB, Hirsch J, Gallup J. Estimation of total-body fat from potassium-40 content. *Science* 1961;133:101–102.
4. Anderson J, Osborn SB, Tomlinson RW, et al. Neutron-activation analysis in man in vivo: a new technique in medical investigation. *Lancet* 1964;2:1201–1205.
5. Kehayias JJ, Heymsfield SB, LoMonte AF, et al. *In vivo* determination of body fat by measuring total-body carbon. *Am J Clin Nutr* 1991;53:1339–1344.
6. Cunningham J. N × 6.25: recognizing a bivariate expression for protein balance in hospitalized patients. *Nutrition* 1994;10:124–127.
7. Moore FD, Oleson KH, McMurray JD, et al. *The body cell mass and its supporting environment.* Philadelphia: WB Saunders, 1963.
8. Comizio R, Pietrobelli A, Tan YX, et al. Total-body lipid and triglyceride response to energy deficit: relevance to body composition model. *Am J Physiol* 1998;274:E860–E866.
9. Gurr MI, Harwood JL. *Lipid biochemistry,* 4th ed. London, UK: Chapman and Hall, 1991.

10. Snyder WS, Cook MJ, Nasset ES, et al. *Report of the task group on reference man.* Oxford, UK: Pergamon Press, 1975.
11. Mitsiopoulos N, Baumgartner RN, Heymsfield SB, et al. Cadaver validation of skeletal muscle measurement by magnetic resonance imaging and computerized tomography. *J Appl Physiol* 1998;85:115–122.
12. Pond CM. *The fats of life.* New York: Cambridge University Press, 1998.
13. Gray DS, Fujioka K, Colletti PM, et al. Magnetic-resonance imaging used for determining fat distribution in obesity and diabetes. *Am J Clin Nutr* 1991;54:623–627.
14. Albu JB, Murphy L, Frager DH, et al. Visceral fat and race-dependent health risks in obese nondiabetic premenopausal women. *Diabetes* 1997;46:456–462.
15. He J, Watkins S, Kelley DE. Skeletal muscle lipid content and oxidative enzyme activity in relation to muscle fiber type in type 2 diabetes and obesity. *Diabetes* 2001;50:817–823.
16. Goodpaster BH, Kelley DE, Thaete FL, et al. Skeletal muscle attenuation determined by computed tomography is associated with skeletal muscle lipid content. *J Appl Physiol* 2000;89:104–110.
17. Goodpaster BH, Thaete FL, Kelley DE. Composition of skeletal muscle evaluated with computed tomography. *Ann N Y Acad Sci* 2000;904:18–24.
18. Malenfant P, Tremblay A, Doucet E, et al. Elevated intramyocellular lipid concentration in obese subjects is not reduced after diet and exercise training *Am J Physiol* 2001;280:E632—E639.
19. Pace N, Rathbun EN. Studies on body composition, III: The body water and chemically combined nitrogen content in relation to fat content. *J Biol Chem* 1945;158:685–691.
20. Forbes GB. *Human body composition: growth, aging, nutrition, and activity.* New York: Springer-Verlag New York, 1987.
21. Davies PS, Cole TJ, eds. *Body composition techniques in health and disease.* Cambridge: Cambridge University Press, 1995.
22. Ellis KJ, Eastman JD, eds. *Human body composition: in vivo methods, models, and assessment.* New York: Plenum Publishing, 1993.
23. Ellis KJ. Whole-body counting and neutron activation analysis. In: Roche AF, Heymsfield SB, Lohman TG, eds. *Human body composition.* Champaign, IL: Human Kinetics, 1996:45–62.
24. Spiers FW. Whole-body counting: an introductory review. In: *Symposium on whole-body counting.* Neue Hofburg, Vienna, Austria: International Atomic Energy Agency, 1961.
25. Maffly RH, Pierson RN. In: Brenner BM, Rector FC, eds. *The kidney.* The body fluids: volume, composition, and physical chemistry. Vol. 1. Philadelphia: WB Saunders, 1976:65–103.
26. Wang ZM, Zhu S, Wang J, et al. Whole-body skeletal muscle mass: development and validation of estimates by total body potassium-cellular model. *Am J Clin Nutr (in press).*
27. Heymsfield SB, Ross R, Wang ZM, et al. Imaging techniques of body composition: advantages of measurement and new uses. In: Carlson-Newberry SJ, Costello RB, eds. *Emerging technologies for nutrition research.* New York: National Academic Press, 1997:127–150.
28. Kleiber M. *The fire of life.* Huntington, NY: Krieger, 1975.
29. Garn SM. Roentgenogrammetric determination of body composition. *Hum Biol* 1957;29:337.
30. Hounsfield GN. Computerized transverse axial scanning (tomography). *Br J Radiol* 1973;46:1016–1022.
31. Heymsfield SB, Noel R, Lynn M, et al. Accuracy of soft tissue density predicted by CT. *J Comput Assist Tomogr* 1979;3:859–860.
32. Heymsfield SB, Fulenwider T, Nordlinger B, et al. Accurate measurement of liver, kidney, and spleen volume and mass by computerized axial tomography. *Ann Intern Med* 1979;90:185–187.
33. Heymsfield SB, Noel R. Radiographic analysis of body composition by computerized axial tomography. In: Ellison N, Newell G, eds. *Nutrition and cancer.* New York: Raven Press, 1981:161–172.
34. Foster MA, Fowler PA, Fuller MF, et al. Non-invasive methods for assessment of body composition. *Proc Nutr Soc* 1988;47:375–385.
35. Chowdhury B, Sjostrom L, Alpsten M, et al. A multicompartmental body composition technique based on computerized tomography. *Int J Obes* 1993;18:219–234.
36. Sjöström L. A computer-tomography based multicomponent body composition technique and anthropometric predictions of lean body mass, total and subcutaneous adipose tissue. *Int J Obes* 1991;15:19–30.
37. Wang ZM, Gallagher D, Nelson ME, et al. Total-body skeletal muscle mass: evaluation of 24-h urinary creatinine excretion by computerized axial tomography. *Am J Clin Nutr* 1996;63:863–869.
38. Ross R, Goodpaster B, Kelley D, et al. Magnetic resonance imaging in human body composition research. From quantitative to qualitative tissue measurement. *Ann N Y Acad Sci* 2000;904:12–17.
39. Schloerb PR, Friis-Hansen BJ, Edelman IS, et al. The measurement of deuterium oxide in body fluids by the falling drop method. *J Lab Clin Med* 1951;37:653–662.
40. Annegers J. Total body water in rats and in mice. *Proc Soc Exp Biol Med* 1954;87:454–456.
41. Keys A, Brozek J. Body fat in adult man. *Physiol Rev* 1953;33:245–325.
42. Schoeller DA. Hydrometry. In: Roche AF, Heymsfield SB, Lohman TG, eds. *Human body composition.* Champaign, IL: Human Kinetics, 1996:25–44.
43. Roberts S, Fjeld C, Westerterp K, et al. Use of the doubly labelled water method under difficult circumstances. In: Prentice AM, ed. *The doubly labelled water method for measuring energy expenditure: technical recommendations for use in humans.* Vienna: International Dietary Energy Consultancy Group, 1990:251–263.
44. Fjeld CR, Brown KH, Schoeller DA. Validation of the deuterium oxide methods for measuring average daily milk intake in infants. *Am J Clin Nutr* 1988;48:671–679.

45. Schoeller DA. Isotope dilution methods. In: Bjorntorp P, Brodoff BN, eds. *Obesity.* New York: Lippincott, 1991:80–88.
46. Schoeller DA. Measurement of energy expenditure in free-living humans by using doubly labeled water. *J Nutr* 1988;118:1278–1289.
47. Heymsfield SB, Wang ZM, Withers R. Multicomponent molecular level models of body composition analysis. In: Roche A, Heymsfield SB, Lohman TG, eds. *Human body composition.* Champaign, IL: Human Kinetics, 1996:129–147.
48. Wang ZM, Deurenberg P, Wang W, et al. Hydration of fat-free body mass: new physiological modeling approach. *Am J Physiol* 1999;276:E995–E1003.
49. Heymsfield SB, Wang ZM. Measurement of total body fat by underwater weighing: new insights and uses for an old method. *J Nutr* 1993;9:472–473.
50. Behnke AR, Feen BG, Welham WC. The specific gravity of healthy men. *JAMA* 1942;118:495–498.
51. Siri WE. The gross composition of the body. In: Tobias CA, Lawrence JH, eds. *Advances in biological and medical physics.* New York: Academic Press, 1956:239–280.
52. Siri WE. Body composition from fluid spaces and density: analysis of methods. In: Brozek J, Henschel A, eds. *Techniques for measuring body composition.* Washington, D.C.: National Academy of Sciences National Research Council, 1961:223–244.
53. Going SB. Densitometry. In: Roche AF, Heymsfield SB, Lohman TG, eds. *Human body composition: methods and findings.* Champaign, IL: Human Kinetics, 1996:3–24.
54. Fidanza EF. *Nutritional status assessment.* London: Chapman & Hall, 1991.
55. Brozek J, Grande F, Anderson T, et al. Densitometric analysis of body composition: revisions of some quantitative assumptions. *Ann N Y Acad Sci* 1963;110:113–140.
56. Visser M, Gallagher D, Deurenberg P, et al. Density of fat-free body mass: relationship with race, age, and level of body fatness. *Am J Physiol* 1997;272:781–787.
57. Wagner DR, Heyward VH. Measures of body composition in blacks and whites: a comparative review. *Am J Clin Nutr* 2000;71:1387–1389.
58. Going SB. Densitometry. In: Roche AF, Heymsfield SB, Lohman TG, eds. *Human body composition.* Champaign, IL: Human Kinetics, 1996:3–24.
59. Dempster P, Aitkens S. A new air displacement method for the determination of human body composition. *Med Sci Sports Exerc* 1995;27:1692–1697.
60. McCrory MA, Gomez TD, Bernauer EM, et al. Evaluation of a new air displacement plethysmograph for measuring human body composition. *Med Sci Sports Exerc* 1995;27:1686–1691.
60a. Fields DA, Goran MI, McCrory MA. Body-composition assessment via air-displacement plethysmography in adults and children: a review. *Am J Clin Nutr* 2002;75:453–467.
61. Pietrobelli A, Formica C, Wang ZM, et al. Dual-energy X-ray absorptiometry body composition model: review of physical concepts. *Am J Physiol* 1996;271:941–951.
62. Mazess RB, Barden HS, Bisek JP, et al. Dual-energy x-ray absorptiometry for total-body and regional bone-mineral and soft-tissue composition. *Am J Clin Nutr* 1990;51:1106–1112.
63. Heymsfield SB, Smith R, Aulet M, et al. Appendicular skeletal muscle mass: measurement by dual-photon absorptiometry. *Am J Clin Nutr* 1990;52:214–218.
64. Wang W, Wang ZM, Faith M, et al. Regional skeletal muscle measurement: evaluation of new dual-energy X-ray absorptiometry model. *J Appl Physiol* 1999;87:1163–1171.
65. Baumgartner RN, Heymsfield SB, Lichtman S, et al. Body composition in elderly people: effect of criterion estimates on predictive equations. *Am J Clin Nutr* 1991;53:1345–1353.
66. Wang ZM, Deurenberg P, Guo SS, et al. Six-compartment body composition model: inter-method comparisons of total-body fat measurement. *Int J Obes Relat Metab Disord* 1998;22:329–337.
67. Economos CD, Nelson ME, Fiatarone MA, et al. A multicenter comparison of dual-energy X-ray absorptiometers: in vivo and in vitro measurements of bone mineral content and density. *Am J Clin Nutr* 2000; 71:1392–1402.
68. Selinger A. *The body as a three component system.* Ph.D. Dissertation. Urbana: University of Illinois, 1977.
69. Burger HC, van Milaan JB. Measurements of the specific resistance of the human body to direct current. *Acta Med Scand* 1943;114:584–607.
70. Barnett A. The basic factors in proposed electrical methods for measuring thyroid function. The effect of body size and shape. *West J Surg Obstet Gyn* 1935;45:322–326.
71. Heymsfield SB, Wang ZM, Visser M, et al. Techniques used in the measurement of body composition: an overview with emphasis on bioelectrical impedance analysis. *Am J Clin Nutr* 1996;64:S478–S484.
72. Baumgartner RN, Chumlea WC, Roche AF. Impedance for body composition. In: Pandolf KB, ed. *Exercise and sport science reviews.* Baltimore: Williams & Wilkins, 1990:193–224.
73. Chumlea WC, Siervogel RM, Wu Y, et al. Bioelectrical impedance spectroscopy and body composition. *Ann N Y Acad Sci* 2000;904:210–213.
74. Guo SS, Chumlea WC, Cockram DB. Use of statistical methods to estimate body composition. *Am J Clin Nutr* 1996;64:428S–435S.
75. Nunez C, Gallagher D, Visser M, et al. Bioimpedance analysis: evaluation of leg-to-leg system based on pressure contact foot-pad electrodes. *Med Sci Sports Exerc* 1997;29:524–531.
76. Tan YX, Nunez C, Sun YG, et al. New electrode system for rapid whole body and segmental bioimpedance assessment. *Med Sci Sports Exerc* 1997;29:1269–1273.

77. Kushner RF, deVries PM, Gudivaka R. Use of bioelectrical impedance analysis measurements in the clinical management of patients undergoing dialysis [Review]. *Am J Clin Nutr* 1996;64:503S–509S.
78. Kushner RF, Gudivaka R, Schoeller DA. Clinical characteristics influencing bioelectrical impedance analysis measurements. *Am J Clin Nutr* 1996;64:423S–427S.
79. Houtkooper LB, Lohman TG, Going SB, et al. Why bioelectrical impedance analysis should be used for estimating adiposity. *Am J Clin Nutr* 1996;64:436S–438S.
80. Olde Rikkert MG, Deurenberg P, Jansen RW, et al. Validation of multi-frequency bioelectrical impedance analysis in detecting changes in fluid balance of geriatric patients. *J Am Geriatr Soc* 1997;5:1345–1351.
81. Heymsfield SB, Tighe A, Wang ZM. Nutritional assessment by anthropometric and biochemical methods. In: Shils ME, Olson JA, Shike M, eds. *Modern nutrition in health and disease,* 8th ed. Philadelphia: Lea & Febiger, 1992.
82. Jackson AS, Pollock ML. Factor analysis and multivariate scaling of anthropometric variables for the assessment of body composition. *Med Sci Sports* 1976;8:196–203.
83. Jackson AS, Pollock ML. Steps toward the development of generalized equations for predicting body composition of adults. *Can J Appl Sports Sci* 1982;7:189–196.
84. Durnin JV, Womersley GA. Body fat assessed from total body density and its estimation from skinfold thickness measurements on 481 men and women aged 16 to 72 years. *Br J Nutr* 1974;32:77–97.
85. Gallagher D, Testolin C, Nuñez C, et al. Anthropometry and methods of body composition measurement for research and field application in the elderly. *Eur J Clin Nutr* 2000;54:S1–S7.
86. Gallagher D, Heymsfield SB, Moonseong H, et al. Health percentage body fat ranges: an approach for developing guidelines based on body mass index. *Am J Clin Nutr* 2000;72:694–701.
87. Norton K, Olds T, eds. *Anthropometrica: a textbook of body measurement for sports and health courses,* 1st ed. Sydney, Australia: UNSW Press, 1996.
88. Roche AF, Siervogel RM, Chumlea WC, et al. Grading body fatness from limited anthropometric data. *Am J Clin Nutr* 1981;34:2831–2838.
89. Tornaghi G, Raiteri R, Pozzato C, et al. Anthropometric or ultrasonic measurements in assessment of visceral fat? A comparative study. *Int J Obes Relat Metab Disord* 1994;18:771–775.
90. National Institutes of Health. *The practical guide: identification, evaluation, and treatment of overweight and obesity in adults.* Publication no. 00-4084. Washington, D.C.: United States Department of Health and Human Services, 2000.
91. World Health Organization. *Obesity: preventing and managing the global epidemic.* Geneva: World Health Organization, 1998.
92. Sjöstrom CD, Hakangard AC, Lissner L, et al. Body compartment and subcutaneous adipose tissue distribution—risk factor patterns in obese subjects. *Obes Res* 1995;3:9–22.
93. Shils ME, Olson JA, Shike M, eds. *Modern nutrition in health and disease,* 9th ed. Baltimore: Williams & Wilkins, 1999.
94. Bertin E, Marcus C, Ruiz JC, et al. Measurement of visceral adipose tissue by DXA combined with anthropometry in obese humans. *Int J Obes Relat Metab Disord* 2000;24:263–270.
95. Heymsfield SB, Wang ZM, Baumgartner RN, et al. Human body composition: advances in models and methods. *Annu Rev Nutr* 1997;17:527–558.
96. Wang ZM, Deurenberg P, Wang J, et al. Proportion of adipose tissue-free body mass as skeletal muscle: magnitude and constancy in men. *Am J Hum Biol* 1997;9:487–492.

6

Neuroendocrine Control of Energy Balance

Nicholas A. Tritos and Eleftheria Maratos-Flier

The possible of role of the brain in maintaining energy homeostasis was initially considered more than 50 years ago when investigators noted that lesions affecting the hypothalamus could result in obese or lean animals (1). Surgical lesions in the area of the medial hypothalamus resulted in hyperphagia and obesity in both rats and cats, whereas lesions of the lateral hypothalamus had the opposite effect, leading to hypophagia, hypodipsia, and weight loss (2). Electrical stimulation of these areas had the obverse effects to surgery; stimulation of the medial hypothalamus led to satiety (the process leading to meal termination), while stimulation of the lateral hypothalamus initiated feeding (3,4) (Fig. 6.1). A role for the hypothalamus in appetite regulation in humans was sug-

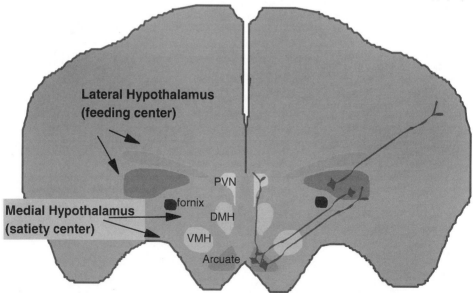

FIG. 6.1. Schematic representation of the hypothalamic areas implicated in mediating feeding behavior. Peptidergic neurons are localized in the arcuate, dorsal medial hypothalamus (DMH), and lateral hypothalamic areas. Secondary effects may be mediated through connections between the various anatomic areas, particularly inputs from the arcuate to the paraventricular nucleus (PVN). Abbreviation: VMH, ventromedial hypothalamus.

gested by the observation that hypothalamic lesions, including craniopharyngiomas, may lead to severe hyperphagia and obesity (5,6).

However, the knowledge of the signaling molecules that might explain the observations was completely lacking; not until the mid-1960s was the presence of monoamine neurotransmitters and, more recently, neuropeptide systems in the brain first appreciated, and an additional interval was required before the actual appetite-regulating role of various peptides could be identified.

Recent data suggest that some cases of morbid obesity in humans are caused by single-gene defects, thus indicating that the role of appetite-regulating molecules discovered in animal studies is similar in humans and suggesting molecular targets for drug development.

PEPTIDERGIC SYSTEMS

A number of peptides that can modify feeding behavior and energy expenditure have been identified. The list of peptides, deriving both from the periphery and the central nervous system (CNS), that have pharmacologic actions on the appetite is long (Table 6.1). The relative importance of these peptides is difficult to determine solely by examination of their pharmacologic effects. In this regard, data from genetic models have proved valuable for determining the relative importance of factors in the modulation in feeding behavior. Some of this information has been derived from the analysis of spontaneous mutations that lead to the alteration of body weight. In some cases, in order to gain increased insight into the potential role of individual peptides, genetic models involving either ablation or overexpression of these peptides have been used.

More than a dozen neuropeptides that are expressed in the CNS are known to regulate eating behavior (Table 6.1). The orexigens include neuropeptide Y (NPY) (7, 8), melanin-concentrating hormone (MCH) (9,10), agouti-related protein (AgRP), and galanin (11–13). Also included in this group are the orexins, which may increase feeding behavior by increasing arousal and activity rather than by having a direct effect on appetite (14,15). The number of CNS peptides that inhibit feeding is rather more extensive, including α-melanocyte–stimulating hormone (α-MSH), corticotropin-releasing hormone (CRH), urocortin, glucagon-like peptide-1 (GLP-1), and cocaine- and amphetamine-

TABLE 6.1. *Appetite-stimulating and appetite-suppressing molecules*

Appetite-stimulating (orexigenic) molecules	Appetite-suppressing (anorectic) molecules
Acetylcholine	Adrenergic receptor stimulation (α_1, β_2)
Adrenergic receptor stimulation (α_2)	α-Melanocyte–stimulating hormone (aMSH)
Agouti-related protein (AgRP)	Bombesin
Dopamine[a]	Cholecystokinin (CCK)
Dynorphin	Cocaine- and amphetamine-regulated transcript (CART)
Galanin	Corticotropin-releasing hormone (CRH)
Ghrelin	Dopamine[a]
Glucocorticoids	Gastrin-releasing peptide (GRP)
Melanin-concentrating hormone (MCH)	Glucagon-like peptide-1 (GLP-1)
Neuropeptide Y (NPY)	Insulin
Orexin A and B	Leptin
Peptide YY (PYY)	Neurotensin
	Serotonin
	Urocortin

[a]Dopamine may have either appetite-stimulating or appetite-suppressing effects.

TABLE 6.2. *Summary of effects of targeted gene ablation or transgenic overexpression on energy homeostasis phenotype of mice*

Peptide	Gene overexpression	Gene ablation	Receptor ablation
NPY	ND	None	Mild obesity, Y1 and Y5 R
MCH	Obese	Lean	Lean
AgRP	Obese	ND	Obese, MC4R, MC3R
Orexin	ND	Narcoleptic	Narcoleptic
Dynorphin	ND	None	—
b-Endorphin	ND	Obesity (POMC)	Obesity
aMSH	—	Obesity (POMC)	Obesity, MC4R, MC3R
Urocortin	—	None	None
CRF	—	None	Decreased anxiety, CRFR1
			Increased anxiety, CRFR2
Neurotensin	—	ND	None, NTR2
CART	—	Increased susceptibility DIO	ND
GLP1	—	ND	None
Serotonin	—	ND	Obesity, epilepsy, 5-HT$_{2c}$

Abbreviations: AgRP, *agouti*-related peptide; aMSH, α-melanocyte-stimulating hormone; CART, cocaine- and amphetamine-regulated transcript; CRF, corticotrophin-releasing factor; CRFR1, CRFR2, CRF receptors-1 and -2; GLP1, glucagon-like peptide-1; 5-HT$_{2c}$, 5-hydroxytryptamine 2C receptor; MC3R, melanocortin-3 receptor; MC4R, melanocortin-4 receptor; MCH, melanin-concentrating hormone; ND, not done; NPY, neuropeptide Y; NTR2, neurotensin receptor-2; POMC, proopiomelanocortin; Y1 R, neuropeptide Y Y1 receptor; Y5 R, neuropeptide Y Y5 receptor.

regulated transcript (CART) (12,16,17). A number of brain–gut peptides also inhibit feeding; these include cholecystokinin (CCK), bombesin, and neurotensin, whereas peptide YY (PYY) and ghrelin stimulate feeding. Insulin also acts to inhibit feeding. Finally, leptin expressed in the adipocyte serves as a potent inhibitor of feeding (9,18).

Many of these effects were initially described pharmacologically, a process which involved injection of the peptide into the rodent lateral ventricle. Subsequent studies have attempted to examine the phenotype of mice that have been genetically altered for ablation or overexpression of these peptides (Table 6.2). These studies showed that the ablation or overexpression of some peptides with pharmacologic effects on feeding and energy homeostasis does not result in a mouse phenotype. For example, mice lacking GLP-1 receptor have no obvious feeding or energy homeostasis phenotype (19,20). When the genetically altered mice lack a phenotype, evaluating the importance of the role of the neuropeptide that has been thus examined is difficult to determine (Table 6.2). However, in some mouse models, the phenotype was predicted by the previously known actions of the peptide under examination. Indeed, successful identification of single-gene mutations leading to obesity in humans has relied partially on screening genes in which the genetics match the pharmacology. Some of these neuropeptides are considered in more detail below.

THE ADIPOCYTE–ARCUATE–HYPOTHALAMIC AXIS

α- Melanocyte–Stimulating Hormone, Agouti-Related Protein, and the Melanocortin Receptor System

The expression of proopiomelanocortin (POMC) in the hypothalamus, particularly in the arcuate nucleus, was reported in 1984 (13,21). However, the role of the POMC product α-MSH in the regulation of feeding behavior was not considered until a few years later. Although the phenomenon of α-MSH–induced inhibition of feeding behavior was reported in 1989 (22,23), the significance of this finding was not appreciated for several years until the molecular explanation for obesity in the Ay mouse was discovered. The Ay mouse is a spontaneously obese, hyperphagic mouse with a vivid yellow coat (24–26). Both the obesity and the coat color result from the ectopic, unregulated expression of a peptide called *agouti* (27). Agouti is normally expressed in hair follicles, and it acts in conjunction with α-MSH on the peripheral MSH receptor, melanocortin-1 receptor (MC1R), to regulate the conversion of pheomelanin, which is yellow, to eumelanin, which is black (28). This receptor is a 7-transmembrane G-protein–coupled receptor, a part of the five-member melanocortin receptor family that also includes the melanocortin-2 receptor (MC2R), the receptor that specifically interacts with adrenocorticotrophic hormone (ACTH). The brown coat results from a mixture of yellow and black melanin in hairs. In the Ay mouse, agouti is overexpressed in hair follicles as well, and it effectively blocks the α-MSH–induced activation of the MC1R (27).

Meanwhile, in this mouse model, agouti is also expressed in the brain, where it blocks the action of α-MSH on the two melanocortin receptors expressed in the CNS, the melanocortin-4 receptor (MC4R) and the melanocortin-3 receptor (MC3R) (29). Hence, the hyperphagia results from the inability of the α-MSH that is expressed in the brain to signal satiety. The obese phenotype of the Ay mouse can be duplicated by ablation of the MC4R (30). Ablation of the MC3R results in mildly increased adiposity and insulin resistance, indicating that MC3R signaling is not as important as MC4R in the mediation of the MSH signals related to anorexia and energy homeostasis (31).

Thus, the melanocortin family of receptors is somewhat unusual in that the receptors respond to a ligand that stimulates the receptor α-MSH and to a second ligand—agouti—that blocks the action of α-MSH. However, agouti is normally not expressed in the brain. This observation opened another avenue of inquiry for agouti-like peptides that might be expressed in the CNS; this ultimately led to the discovery of AgRP (32,33). Pharmacologic administration of AgRP results in prolonged hyperphagia and weight gain. This peptide is expressed exclusively in a subpopulation of neurons in the arcuate hypothalamic nucleus (32,33). Although ablation of AgRP from mice does not yield an obvious phenotype, overexpression of AgRP results in an obese phenotype that is similar to that seen both in Ay mice and in MC4R knockout mice (34).

Although α-MSH and AgRP are both derived from the arcuate neurons, they are expressed in distinct populations without any observed overlap (35). The α-MSH precursor, POMC, may be coexpressed with CART, and most neurons expressing AgRP also express NPY (35–37).

Leptin

The arcuate nucleus appears to be the target of at least one hormone deriving from the periphery, leptin, that acts as a signal from the adipocyte to the brain (38). The discovery of leptin was significant to understanding the regulation of body weight because it confirmed the speculation that signals from the periphery acted on the CNS to regulate body weight and because it firmly established the identity of the adipocyte as an endocrine cell (39).

Speculation regarding the existence of a leptin-like compound dated back to the 1960s. At that time, two spontaneously obese lines of mice were identified in the colonies at Jackson Laboratories in Bar Harbor, Maine. One line was designated *ob/ob*, and the other line, *db/db* (40,41). The phenotype of both of these genetic mutations consisted of severe early onset morbid obesity that was associated with extreme hyperphagia, and it included decreased energy expenditure, cold intolerance, hyperinsulinemia with the ultimate development of diabetes, and infertility associated with hypogonadotrophic hypogonadism (40,41).

These strains could be distinguished only in the parabiosis studies that were performed in the 1960s. When the circulation of an *ob/ob* mouse was parabiosed to the circulation of a normal mouse, the hyperphagia and obese phenotype of the *ob/ob* mouse was corrected (42). In contrast, parabiosis of a normal mouse with a *db/db* mouse led to hypophagia and death by starvation in the normal animal (43). Parabiosis of *ob/ob* and *db/db* mice to each other led to progressive leanness and ultimately death by starvation in the *ob/ob* mouse (42). This led to the speculation that *ob/ob* mice were missing a factor that was produced in normal mice and *db/db* mice (42). In contrast, *db/db* mice produced the factor in excess because of a complete inability to respond to it (42,43).

Although continued study of these mice produced a number of insights into the physiology of obesity and its relationship to insulin-resistant diabetes, the cause of obesity in the *ob/ob* mice was not understood until 1994 when the *ob* gene was identified using positional cloning (39). The product of this gene was soon discovered to be a peptide named leptin. *Ob/ob* mice were discovered to have a premature stop codon in the leptin gene that prevented the transcription of a full-length messenger RNA (mRNA) and thus resulted in a foreshortened, inactive peptide. Treatment of *ob/ob* mice with recombining leptin reversed the phenotype (44–46). Subsequent studies revealed that the *db/db* mice had a mutation in the gene encoding one form of the leptin receptor, the long form, which mediates leptin signaling (47).

Leptin is produced in adipocytes, and it acts on the arcuate neurons to regulate both the expression of POMC, NPY, and AgRP and the polarization state of the neurons (38). Leptin leads to decreases in the expression of NPY and AgRP and acts to increase the expression of POMC. Interestingly, *ob/ob* mice demonstrate increased levels of NPY and AgRP and decreased levels of POMC when compared with wild-type littermates (9,48).

Starvation also regulates the expression of these peptides, and, in normal animals, a significant rise in NPY and AgRP will be seen within 24 to 48 hours of starvation, while POMC levels fall by more than 50% (9,48). Treatment with leptin attenuates these changes, suggesting that leptin is an important regulator of the arcuate neurons. Further evidence for this comes directly from studies visualizing arcuate neurons after the injection of leptin. Leptin treatment leads to the induction of suppressor of cytokine signaling-3 (SOCS-3) (49), and this effect is seen in both NPY and POMC arcuate neurons (38). However, c-Fos is induced only in the POMC neurons, indicating that, although leptin acts on both sets of neurons, only the POMC neurons are activated (38,48). This is confirmed by the findings of patch clamping studies, which indicate that the NPY neurons are hyperpolarized by leptin while the POMC neurons are depolarized (50,51).

Hence, a complete pathway regulating energy homeostasis has been defined (9,18,38). The pathway begins with leptin production in the adipocyte. Leptin is released into the circulation, and it acts on the arcuate nucleus via the long form of the leptin receptor to affect both the POMC-expressing and NPY-expressing neurons. The anorectic action of leptin is mediated by the activation of the POMC neurons, which leads to increased α-MSH levels. At the same time, leptin suppresses NPY and AgRP, which should also contribute to decreased feeding.

This pathway was defined through studies in rodents. However, analysis of single-gene mutations leading to morbid obesity indicates that the same pathway is active in humans so that, as in mice, disruption of the leptin–melanocortin pathway also leads to obesity.

The first indication that a single gene defect would lead to morbid obesity in humans came with the finding that two related children with early onset, severe morbid obesity had exceptionally low leptin levels (52) (Table 6.3). Whereas, in normal animals, leptin appears to inhibit feeding, the obese state is one of leptin resistance; and most obese animals and persons have high systemic leptin levels. Absence of leptin in the circulation of these two children indicated that they might have mutations in the leptin gene; this mutation was identified as a homozygous frameshift mutation that involved the deletion of a single guanine nucleotide in codon 133 (52). The children were cousins, and both were the products of consanguineous marriages. The phenotype of the children overlapped significantly with that of the *ob/ob* mice in that the children were markedly obese and hyperphagic (53). However, their energy expenditure and thyroid function appeared to be normal. After being treated with leptin, the children responded immediately with decreased eating and weight loss; the lost weight consisted entirely of fat body mass (54). The older female child at this time appears to be entering puberty normally. However, over time, increasing doses of leptin have been required to maintain the weight loss (54). This need for an increase has likely been caused by the development of antibodies to leptin.

Subsequent to the description of leptin-deficient children, a family with leptin receptor deficiency was also described (55) (Table 6.3). Members missing both alleles of the *ob* receptor gene were morbidly obese, and they failed to enter puberty. Members missing a single allele were hyperleptinemic but otherwise normal. The mutation was a guanine to adenine substitution in the splice donor site of exon-16, which led to exon-16 skipping and an *ob* receptor protein lacking both the transmembrane and the intracellular domains.

Thus far, multiple mutations in the MC4R have been described (56–59) (Table 6.3). These mutations were discovered studying cohorts of families who had a history of very early onset morbid obesity in at least two generations. Present studies indicate that up to 5% of early onset morbid obesity is caused by mutations in the MC4R (58–61). Thus, mutation in this gene appears to be fairly common in this population. Interestingly, obesity may be caused by a mutation in only one allele. Hence, many of the obesity syndromes seen with MC4R mutation represent "haploinsufficiency." However, in a few mutations, both alleles must be abnormal for the obesity to develop. For example, in a recent report (62), a severely obese woman with a body mass index (BMI) of 62 kilograms per meter squared (kg/m^2) was homozygous for a missense mutation in the second transmembrane domain. Her parents were both heterozygotes for the mutation and had BMIs of 26 and 27. This mutation resulted in no agonist ligand binding.

While no naturally occurring mutations in POMC have been described in rodents, POMC mutations do cause obesity in humans (63) (Table 6.3). Because α-MSH also affects pigmentation in humans, these individuals typically have red hair. Moreover, the

TABLE 6.3. *Monogenic (mendelian) causes of obesity in humans and mice*

Gene product	Human	Mouse
Leptin	Yes	Yes (*ob/ob*)
Leptin receptor	Yes	Yes (*db/db*)
Proopiomelanocortin (POMC)	Yes	Not spontaneous-knockout model[a]
Prohormone convertase-1	Yes	No
Melanocortin-4 receptor (MC4R)	Yes	Not spontaneous-knockout model[a]
Agouti	No	Yes (*lethal yellow, A^y*)
Carboxypeptidase E	No	Yes (*fat/fat*)

[a]Indicates the absence of spontaneous mutations in mice; however, knockout mouse models are obese.

POMC product is processed to produce ACTH and POMC, so the individuals typically present with adrenal insufficiency as children and they quite typically are obese. In one case, the patient was a compound heterozygote with mutations in exon-3 of the POMC gene, which interfered with synthesis of both ACTH and α-MSH. A second patient was found to have a homozygous mutation in exon-2 that abolished the POMC translation (63).

Thus, a pathway important in the regulation of both rodent and human energy homeostasis has been defined (Fig 6.2). This pathway originates with leptin in the adipocyte and ends when leptin acts to stimulate the POMC neurons in the arcuate (Fig. 6.2).

An additional disruption of this pathway can be caused by mutations of the converting enzymes required to process preprohormones. A mutation in prohormone convertase-1 (PC1) leads to a syndrome that includes early onset morbid obesity, hypogonadotrophic hypogonadism, and hypocortisolism in humans (64) (Table 6.3). Only a single patient with this deficiency has been described—a compound heterozygote in which a glycine to arginine substitution at position 483 prevented processing of proPC1 in one allele and an adenosine to cytosine transversion at the other allele at position +4 in the intron-5 donor splice site led to a skip of exon-5 and a loss of 26 residues, creating a frameshift with a premature stop codon. This patient also had elevated plasma proinsulin levels with low insulin levels, as would be expected (64). In the CNS, deletion of this enzyme activity leads to the inability to process a number of neuropeptides, including POMC.

In rodents, point mutation in the coding region of carboxypeptidase E leads to the obese phenotype of the *fat/fat* mouse (65). In addition to low insulin levels, these animals are unable to process neurotensin and promelanin-concentrating hormone appropriately; this defect leads to a decrease in the levels of the anorectic neuropeptide neurotensin and to an increase in the orexigenic peptide MCH (66). As would be expected, the mice also have markedly reduced levels of α-MSH (67).

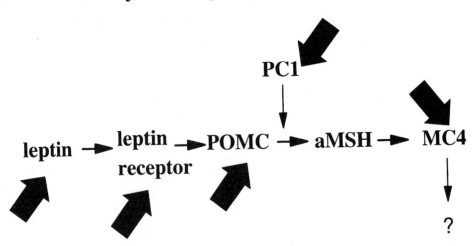

Mutations in Adipocyte to Arcuate Pathway Causing Obesity in Man

FIG. 6.2. The adipocyte–arcuate pathway. Shown is the site (*thick black arrows*) of identified human mutations that lead to obesity. Abbreviations: aMSH, α-melanocyte-stimulating hormone; MC4R, melanocortin-4 receptor; PC1, proconvertase-1; POMC, proopiomelanocortin.

The consistency between mutations causing mouse obesity and human obesity is remarkable (Table 6.3). Clearly, molecules identified as important in regulating energy homeostasis in rodents must be evaluated in humans because a larger percentage of the early onset obesities are likely monogenic. Although they are common, premorbid obesity and "overweight" probably are polygenic, so characterization of additional genetic loci is warranted to direct identification of drug targets.

Leptin Resistance

The absence of leptin signaling is associated with obesity, hyperphagia, and an apparent inability to experience satiety, as well as with neuroendocrine changes, including gonadotropin failure in both mice and humans. Leptin administration corrects the obesity, largely by decreasing feeding (54). Chronic lowering of leptin levels, as is seen with starvation, is associated with a number of neuroendocrine changes, including impairment of fertility, which is mediated through the suppression of gonadotropin-releasing hormone (68). Replacement of leptin during starvation corrects or attenuates the neuroendocrine changes, and treatment with leptin in rodents is associated with early sexual maturation (68,69). This indicates that leptin reliably signals the difference between starvation and sufficient food stores.

In contrast, most obese humans and mice have high leptin levels, and leptin levels, when measured in the fed state, correlate well with total body adiposity (70). Despite increased leptin levels, obese humans and mice are inappropriately hyperphagic, indicating that they are resistant to the appetite inhibitory effects of leptin. This indicates that leptin does not play a significant role in signaling between sufficient stores and excessive stores of fat. The nature and site of leptin resistance is unknown.

Leptin's action on the hypothalamus is to stimulate POMC neurons and POMC expression while inhibiting NPY neurons and NPY expression (36,38,48,50,71,72). As leptin levels fall, POMC levels fall and NPY levels rise. In the obese state, the sensitivity of target neurons in the arcuate changes, and leptin does not signal effectively (72a,72b). However, as the leptin levels rise, NPY is suppressed. This has been reported in diet-induced obesity (73) and in brown-fat–deficient obese mouse (74). One study examined NPY expression in postmortem samples of humans with obesity and found that NPY, as assessed by mRNA expression and immunocytochemistry, was reduced, suggesting that the same phenomenon is seen in humans (75). However, in this human study, AgRP levels were normal. Hence, either leptin resistance is distal to leptin targets in the arcuate or other yet unidentified factors contribute to maintaining excess feeding in obesity.

Other Neuropeptides

NPY is an orexigenic peptide that is widely expressed in the CNS. NPY neurons in the arcuate appear to be a leptin target (38,72) (Fig. 6.3). As has been noted, leptin acts to hyperpolarize and to deactivate these neurons (36).

As a pharmacologic agent, NPY produces a robust and sustained feeding response, and continuous infusion via osmotic pumps leads to obesity (76,77). However, its precise role in energy homeostasis is unclear. Animals made deficient in NPY have an increased susceptibility to seizures, but they do have a normal weight, a normal feeding phenotype, and a normal refeeding response to starvation (78). Crossbreeding of NPY-ablated mice to *ob/ob* mice leads to an attenuation of the obesity phenotype of the *ob/ob* mouse that is secondary to reduced food intake and increased energy expenditure (78,79). Overexpression of NPY leads to mild obesity in mice fed a high-sucrose diet (80). Paradoxically,

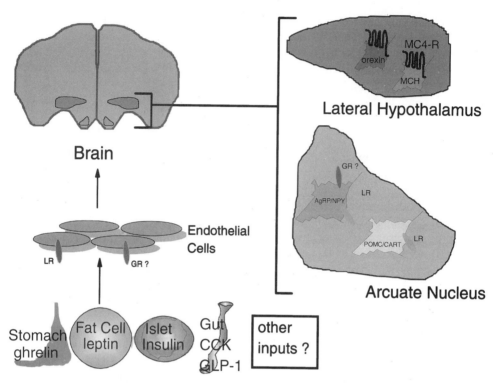

FIG. 6.3. Summary of potential inputs from the periphery into the central nervous system (CNS) that might mediate appetite and energy homeostasis. Peptidergic inputs from the periphery include leptin from adipocytes, ghrelin from the stomach, insulin from the pancreas, and the gut peptides cholecystokinin (CCK) and glucagon-like peptide-1 (GLP-1). Leptin and ghrelin act on the arcuate nucleus. Leptin uptake into the CNS is mediated via specific short-form leptin receptors (LRs). Uptake of other peptides may also be receptor specific. Abbreviations: AgRP, agouti-related peptide; CART, cocaine- and amphetamine-regulated transcript; GR, ghrelin receptor; MC4-R, melanocortin-4 receptor; MCH, melanin-concentrating hormone; NPY, neuropeptide Y; POMC, proopiomelanocortin.

ablation of two of the NPY receptors believed to mediate feeding responses (NPY receptors 1 and 5) leads to mild obesity (81,82).

Information regarding the potential role of NPY in humans is limited. One study reported that, in obese women (BMI =38.3 kg/m^2), circulating NPY levels were decreased compared with levels seen in women with a normal BMI, which is consistent with the lower NPY levels seen in the arcuate in leptin-resistant mice (83).

MCH was originally described as a circulating hormone in fish, where it serves to regulate fish-scale pigmentation (84). In all mammalian species studied, MCH is expressed exclusively in the neurons of the lateral hypothalamus, and studies from mice, rats, and sheep indicate that MCH is an important regulator of body weight (85–87). As a pharmacologic agent, MCH increases feeding acutely (10,68,88–90). Mice with ablation of prepro-MCH are hypophagic and lean (91), whereas mice that overexpress MCH may be susceptible to obesity only on a high-fat diet (when bred on the FVB background) or they may be mildly obese on a standard diet (when bred on the obesity-prone C57Bl/6J background) (92,93). In addition, chronic infusion of MCH into the lateral ventricle of mice leads to mild obesity (94).

In the rodent CNS, MCH acts via a 7-transmembrane receptor, which couples to G_I and G_q. Ablation of this receptor leads to leanness that is secondary to increased activity but not to hypophagia (94). The difference in the phenotype of ablation of the preprohormone and the receptor is probably due to the lack of neuropeptide glutamic acid isoleucine (N-EI) and neuropeptide glycine glutamic acid (N-GE) in the preprohormone knockout animals. The roles of the latter two peptides in energy homeostasis are unknown, but interpretation of the data from the two knockouts suggests that they may be involved in increased motor activity.

Although MCH can be measured in the circulation, plasma MCH in humans does not correlate with BMI (E Maratos-Flier, NA Tritos, *unpublished observations,* 2001). The potential role of MCH in human obesity is not yet understood.

CART is an anorectic peptide that is expressed in a number of regions of the CNS (35,95). It is expressed in the lateral hypothalamus in neurons that make MCH but not orexin (35). In the arcuate, it is coexpressed with neurons that make POMC (35). CART pharmacologically acts as an anorectic agent (95,96). The phenotype of mice with CART ablation appears to be normal. However, these mice gain an excess amount of weight when exposed to a high-fat diet (97).

Although a number of other neuropeptides, including orexin, endorphins, dynorphin, neurotensin, GLP-1, urocortin, and CRH, may affect appetite in a manner similar to the pharmacologic agents, their precise role in either human or rodent obesity is unclear. This remains the subject of continued investigation (12,70).

MONOAMINE NEUROTRANSMITTERS

Norepinephrine And Epinephrine

In rodents and humans, norepinephrine is synthesized by discrete neuronal populations in the brainstem, including the locus ceruleus and the dorsal vagal complex (98). Neuronal fibers from these nuclei reach the cortex, thalamus, and hypothalamus, as well as the spinal cord caudally (98). Similarly, epinephrine-containing neurons are localized in the dorsal vagal complex and the nucleus of the solitary tract, and they project to the hypothalamus and to the spinal cord caudally (98).

Several lines of evidence indicate that norepinephrine-synthesizing and epinephrine-synthesizing neurons have an important role in the regulation of energy homeostasis. Hypothalamic norepinephrine levels are increased in obese leptin-deficient *ob/ob* mice (99). Administration of norepinephrine into the paraventricular hypothalamic nucleus (PVN) leads to an acute increase in food intake, whereas chronic administration leads to weight gain (100). The behavioral effects of central adrenergic stimulation depend on the adrenergic receptor subtype that is being activated (101). Specifically, experimental stimulation of the α_2-adrenergic receptors by selective agonists, such as clonidine, increases food intake (102). In contrast, experimental stimulation of the α_1-adrenergic receptors by selective agonists such as phenylpropanolamine (103) and stimulation of hypothalamic β_2-adrenergic receptors by selective agonists such as terbutaline or salbutamol lead to decreased food intake (11,102) (Table 6.1).

Clinically, many sympathomimetic agents have shown modest short-term efficacy in the treatment of obesity, including drugs that release norepinephrine from synaptic vesicles (e.g., phentermine and diethylpropion), those that inhibit norepinephrine reuptake (e.g., mazindol), or ones that activate α_1-adrenergic receptors (e.g., phenylpropano-lamine) (104). In contrast, weight gain has been observed as a side effect of tricyclic anti-depressants; this may result from activation of the hypothalamic α_2-adrenergic receptors (105).

Dopamine

Dopamine is synthesized by neurons in the substantia nigra and ventral tegmental area that comprise the mesolimbic pathway. Fibers from these neurons project to the nucleus accumbens, striatum (caudate and putamen), olfactory tubercle, and cerebral cortex (106). Other dopamine-synthesizing neurons are located in the arcuate and dorsomedial hypothalamic nuclei, which project to the lateral hypothalamic area (70).

Data on the regulation of hypothalamic dopamine levels by leptin are conflicting. While some (107) suggest that leptin may inhibit dopamine release, other experiments indicate that dopamine levels in the arcuate hypothalamic nucleus are decreased in leptin-deficient *ob/ob* mice (99).

However, several lines of evidence suggest that dopamine has an important role in the regulation of food intake depending on the brain area from which it is released. Experimental data suggest that dopamine release in the lateral hypothalamic area leads to the inhibition of food intake by a decrease in meal size (108). In contrast, other experiments indicate that dopamine release in the nucleus accumbens leads to increased food intake by stimulating the reward aspects of feeding (106).

Genetic disruption of dopamine synthesis leads to the severe suppression of feeding (109). However, because these mice also exhibit motor deficits (109), the interpretation of this finding has been questioned (70).

Clinically, dopamine receptor antagonists, which are used as antipsychotic medications, are associated with significant weight gain that may occur as a result of dopamine-2 (D_2) receptor blockade in the lateral hypothalamic area (110). The so-called "atypical antipsychotic" agents, especially olanzapine, lead to greater weight gain than the older "typical" agents, such as haloperidol (111–113). However, the underlying mechanisms leading to the greater weight gain with the use of atypical agents have not been fully elucidated (114).

Serotonin

Serotonergic neurons are present primarily in the dorsal and medial raphe nuclei, and they send off fibers to the hypothalamus, cortex, and hippocampus (115).

A significant role of serotonin in appetite and body weight regulation is supported by numerous study findings. Increased serotonin release has been documented during feeding, and it may contribute to satiation in rodents (116). Leptin appears to increase serotonin turnover in the hypothalamus by a mechanism involving the inhibition of nitric oxide synthesis (117). Genetic disruption of serotonin signaling through the 5-hydroxytriptamine 2C ($5-HT_{2C}$) serotonin receptor leads to hyperphagia and modest obesity, suggesting that this serotonin receptor isoform has a physiologic role in appetite and body weight regulation (118).

Several pharmacologic agents that facilitate serotonergic neurotransmission lead to decreased food intake and weight loss, including quipazine (acting as $5-HT_{2C}$ and $5-HT_{1B}$ serotonin receptor agonist), fenfluramine and dexfenfluramine (which stimulate serotonin release and inhibit reuptake), and sibutramine and fluoxetine (which inhibit serotonin reuptake) (104). Of these agents, only sibutramine is currently approved by the Food and Drug Administration for the treatment of obesity in humans (104). Fenfluramine and dexfenfluramine are effective in promoting weight reduction, but they have been withdrawn because of their association with significant cardiovascular toxicity (104).

Acetylcholine

Brainstem cholinergic neurons present in the lateral dorsal tegmental nuclei and the pedunculopontine nuclei project to MCH-expressing neurons in the lateral hypothalamic area (119) that coexpress M_3 muscarinic receptors (120). Further data indicate that hypothalamic MCH expression is increased in response to muscarinic stimulation (119).

Genetic disruption of M_3 muscarinic receptor–mediated signaling leads to hypophagia and weight loss despite low hypothalamic MCH expression, thus indicating that the M_3 muscarinic receptor has an important physiologic role in appetite and body weight regulation, acting at least in part through modulation of MCH expression (120).

Although no selective M_3 muscarinic receptor antagonists are available, the future development of such agents may expand the therapeutic options in the treatment of obesity.

OTHER SYSTEMIC HORMONES

Gut Peptides

Cholecystokinin

CCK, secreted from the I cells present in the duodenal and jejunal mucosa, was the first gut peptide implicated in the short-term regulation of energy intake (121,122). It is released in response to the presence of digested fat and protein in the proximal small intestine (123, 124), and it acts on the CCK-A receptors expressed on vagal afferent nerve endings (125).

Several lines of evidence suggest that CCK has an important role as a satiety factor. Administration of CCK to rodents or humans before a meal leads to a dose-dependent decrease in meal size without causing undue malaise or sickness (121,126). Moreover, the administration of specific antibodies or receptor antagonists increases the subsequent meal size, thus indicating that endogenous CCK has a physiologic role as a satiety factor (127,128). In addition, the repeated administration of CCK to experimental animals before each meal leads to decreases in meal size, a compensatory increase in meal number, and no effect on body weight, indicating that CCK is a true satiety factor (129). Central leptin administration potentiates the satiating effects of CCK (130), thus suggesting the presence of physiologic interactions between short-term (CCK) and long-term (leptin) regulators of energy homeostasis.

The satiating effects of CCK will undoubtedly lead to further exploration of the potential therapeutic role of CCK agonists in the treatment of obesity (131).

Gastrin-Releasing Peptide

Gastrin-releasing peptide (GRP), a structural homologue of the amphibian peptide bombesin (not found in mammals), is expressed in the antral and duodenal mucosa. It induces satiety after systemic administration in non-primate mammals and humans (132,133). Although mice lacking the bombesin receptor-3 become obese (134), the plasma GRP levels do not change after meals (135), so the physiologic role of this peptide requires further study.

Glucagon-Like Peptide 1

GLP-1 is expressed in intestinal L cells and in pancreatic islet A cells. It leads to a decrease in meal size after systemic administration in humans (136). However, this finding was not confirmed in a recent study (137), suggesting that the physiologic role of GLP-1 is unclear.

As has been previously discussed, CCK, GRP, and GLP-1 are also expressed in the brain, where they may have an additional role in inducing satiety.

Insulin

Insulin is secreted from the pancreatic beta cells in proportion to an individual's energy intake and adiposity (70), and it is transported across the blood–brain barrier through a saturable transport mechanism (138) (Fig. 6.3). Insulin receptors are widely expressed in the brain, particularly in neurons in the hypothalamus, pituitary, mammillary bodies, lateral septum, amygdala, hippocampus (CA1 region), and the olfactory bulb (139,140). In particular, insulin receptors are present in the arcuate hypothalamic nucleus (140), where insulin has been shown to inhibit NPY expression (141).

Additional experimental data suggest that insulin has a significant role in the regulation of food intake and energy homeostasis. Continuous intraventricular insulin infusion inhibits food intake and leads to weight loss in both rodents (142) and primates without producing sickness (143). Furthermore, central insulin infusion increases the satiating effect of systemic and intraventricular CCK (i.e., CCK-8) (144).

Genetic disruption of insulin signaling by specific ablation of the insulin receptor gene in the brain (145) or the insulin receptor substrate-2 (IRS-2) gene (146) leads to mild hyperphagia and obesity, indicating that insulin signaling in the CNS is physiologically important.

In contrast, both exogenous insulin administration (e.g., diabetic patients) and endogenous insulin hypersecretion (e.g., patients with insulinoma) are frequently associated with weight gain, likely reflecting both the anabolic effects of systemic insulin and the increase in energy intake secondary to hypoglycemia (147).

Ghrelin

This peptide is expressed in both the CNS and the gastrointestinal (GI) tract, and it has recently received increased attention as a potential mediator of hunger in the brain–gut axis. Ghrelin is a 28–amino-acid peptide that was originally identified as the endogenous ligand for the growth hormone secretagogue receptor (GHS-R) (148,149). Ghrelin is primarily expressed in the rodent and human GI tract, including in X/A-like cells in the oxyntic glands of the stomach and enteric endocrine cells (149), as well as in the brain, including the hypothalamic neurons (150). It stimulates growth hormone release *in vivo* (151–153) and *in vitro* (148).

More recently, ghrelin has been implicated in the regulation of appetite and energy homeostasis (Fig. 6.3). Serum ghrelin concentrations are increased by fasting in rodents, and they are decreased with refeeding (154). In humans, serum ghrelin levels decrease with increasing body adiposity (155,156). In addition, serum ghrelin levels increase before meals and decrease postprandially (157).

When ghrelin is centrally administered, it induces NPY and c-Fos expression in arcuate hypothalamic neurons (158) and stimulates feeding in rodents (153,158), which leads to weight gain after long-term administration (158). Central ghrelin also suppresses leptin-induced effects on feeding (158), an result that may be mediated in part by the activation of the hypothalamic NPY-Y Y1 receptor (159). Furthermore, central administration of specific ghrelin antisera suppresses feeding (158), indicating a physiologic role for endogenous ghrelin on the regulation of energy intake. In addition, systemic ghrelin administration leads to weight gain in rodents by decreasing fat use (154). Whether ghrelin induces feeding after systemic administration in rodents has not been conclusively established (153,154).

Recent data suggest that short-term systemic ghrelin administration stimulates appetite and food intake in humans (160). In addition, ghrelin mutations have been associated with obesity, although their functional significance is unclear (161). In summary, increasing evidence suggests a significant role for ghrelin in the regulation of energy homeostasis. However, while it is potentially important in mediating appetite through action in the CNS, the precise physiologic role of ghrelin remains to be determined.

FUTURE DIRECTIONS

During the past decade, the understanding of the mechanisms involved in the regulation of energy homeostasis and body adiposity has rapidly advanced, as has been indicated by the characterization of leptin and hypothalamic appetite-regulating peptides. Clearly, this regulation involves a complex web of signals between the brain and the periphery (Fig. 6.3). However, much remains to be achieved. The neuronal and signaling pathways involved in energy regulation must be fully characterized, and the physiologic role of appetite-regulating hormones and neuropeptides in physiologic and pathophysiologic conditions must be further elucidated.

As the recent characterization of ghrelin indicates, appetite-regulating signals are multiple and diverse, and some may still be unknown. In light of the marked complexity and redundancy exhibited by energy homeostatic systems, multiple molecular targets must be concurrently affected to achieve sustained therapeutic efficacy. The authors anticipate that the plethora of recent discoveries will soon lead to the identification of efficacious, and hopefully safe, therapeutic agents for the treatment of obesity and eating disorders.

REFERENCES

1. Hetherington AW, Ranson SW. Hypothalamic lesions and adiposity in the rat. *Anat Rec* 1940;78:149–172.
2. Anand BK, Brobeck JR. Localization of a "feeding center" in the hypothalamus on the rat. *Proc Soc Exp Biol Med* 1951;77:323–324.
3. Brown FD, Fessler RG, Rachlin JR, et al. Changes in food intake with electrical stimulation of the ventromedial hypothalamus in dogs. *J Neurosurg* 1984;60:1253–1257.
4. Hervey GR, Parameswaran SV, Steffens AB. The effects of lateral hypothalamic stimulation in parabiotic rats [Proceedings]. *J Physiol* 1977;266:64P–65P.
5. Muller HL, Bueb K, Bartels U, et al. Obesity after childhood craniopharyngioma—German multicenter study on pre-operative risk factors and quality of life. *Klin Padiatr* 2001;213:244–249.
6. Roth C, Wilken B, Hanefeld F, et al. Hyperphagia in children with craniopharyngioma is associated with hyperleptinaemia and a failure in the downregulation of appetite. *Eur J Endocrinol* 1998;138:89–91.
7. Clark JT, Sahu A, Kalra PS, et al. Neuropeptide Y (NPY)–induced feeding behaviour in female rats: comparison with human NPY([Met 17]NPY), NPY analog ([norLeu4]NPY) and peptide YY. *Regul Pept* 1987;17: 31–39.
8. Clark JT, Kalra PS, Crowley WR, et al. Neuropeptide Y and human pancreatic polypeptide stimulate feeding behavior in rats. *Endocrinology* 1984;115:427–429.
9. Ahima RS, Saper CB, Flier JS, et al. Leptin regulation of neuroendocrine systems. *Front Neuroendocrinol* 2000;21:263–307.

10. Qu D, Ludwig DS, Gammeltoft S, et al. A role for melanin-concentrating hormone in the central regulation of feeding behaviour. *Nature* 1996;380:243–247.
11. Leibowitz SF. Brain monoamines and peptides: role in the control of eating behavior. *Fed Proc* 1986;45:1396–1403.
12. Flier JS, Maratos-Flier E. Obesity and the hypothalamus: novel peptides for new pathways [see Comments]. *Cell* 1998;92:437–440.
13. Liotta AS, Loudes C, McKelvy JF, et al. Biosynthesis of precursor corticotropin/endorphin-, corticotropin-, alpha-melanotropin-, beta-lipotropin-, and beta-endorphin–like material by cultured neonatal rat hypothalamic neurons. *Proc Natl Acad Sci U S A* 1980;77:1880–1884.
14. Sakurai T, Amemiya A, Ishii M, et al. Orexins and orexin receptors: a family of hypothalamic neuropeptides and G protein–coupled receptors that regulate feeding behavior [see Comments]. *Cell* 1998;92:573–585.
15. Chemelli RM, Willie JT, Sinton CM, et al. Narcolepsy in orexin knockout mice: molecular genetics of sleep regulation [see Comments]. *Cell* 1999;98:437–451.
16. Flier JS. The adipocyte: storage depot or node on the energy information superhighway? *Cell* 1995;80:15–18.
17. Levine AS, Kneip J, Grace M, et al. Effect of centrally administered neurotensin on multiple feeding paradigms. *Pharmacol Biochem Behav* 1983;18:19–23.
18. Ahima RS, Flier JS. Leptin. *Annu Rev Physiol* 2000;62:413–437.
19. Scrocchi LA, Hill ME, Saleh J, et al. Elimination of glucagon-like peptide 1R signaling does not modify weight gain and islet adaptation in mice with combined disruption of leptin and GLP-1 action. *Diabetes* 2000;49:1552–1560.
20. Gallwitz B, Schmidt WE. GLP-1 receptor "knock out" causes glucose intolerance, but no alterations of eating behavior [in German]. *Z Gastroenterol* 1997;35:655–658.
21. Liotta AS, Advis JP, Krause JE, et al. Demonstration of *in vivo* synthesis of pro-opiomelanocortin–, beta-endorphin–, and alpha-melanotropin–like species in the adult rat brain. *J Neurosci* 1984;4:956–965.
22. Poggioli R, Vergoni AV, Bertolini A. ACTH-(1-24) and alpha-MSH antagonize feeding behavior stimulated by kappa opiate agonists. *Peptides* 1986;7:843–848.
23. Tsujii S, Bray GA. Acetylation alters the feeding response to MSH and beta-endorphin. *Brain Res Bull* 1989;23:165–169.
24. Michaud EJ, Bultman SJ, Klebig ML, et al. A molecular model for the genetic and phenotypic characteristics of the mouse lethal yellow (Ay) mutation. *Proc Natl Acad Sci U S A* 1994;91:2562–2566.
25. Bultman SJ, Michaud EJ, Woychik RP. Molecular characterization of the mouse agouti locus. *Cell* 1992;71:1195–1204.
26. Barsh GS, Lovett M, Epstein CJ. Effects of the lethal yellow (Ay) mutation in mouse aggregation chimeras. *Development* 1990;109:683–690.
27. Michaud EJ, Bultman SJ, Klebig ML, et al. A molecular model for the genetic and phenotypic characteristics of the mouse lethal yellow (Ay) mutation. *Proc Natl Acad Sci U S A* 1994;91:2562–2566.
28. Cone RD, Lu D, Koppula S, et al. The melanocortin receptors: agonists, antagonists, and the hormonal control of pigmentation. *Recent Prog Horm Res* 1996;51:287–318.
29. Mountjoy KG, Wong J. Obesity, diabetes and functions for proopiomelanocortin-derived peptides. *Mol Cell Endocrinol* 1997;128:171–177.
30. Huszar D, Lynch CA, Fairchild-Huntress V, et al. Targeted disruption of the melanocortin-4 receptor results in obesity in mice. *Cell* 1997;88:131–141.
31. Chen AS, Marsh DJ, Trumbauer ME, et al. Inactivation of the mouse melanocortin-3 receptor results in increased fat mass and reduced lean body mass. *Nat Genet* 2000;26:97–102.
32. Ollmann MM, Wilson BD, Yang YK, et al. Antagonism of central melanocortin receptors *in vitro* and *in vivo* by agouti-related protein [published erratum appears in *Science* 1998;281:1615]. *Science* 1997;278:135–138.
33. Shutter JR, Graham M, Kinsey AC, et al. Hypothalamic expression of ART, a novel gene related to agouti, is up-regulated in obese and diabetic mutant mice. *Genes Dev* 1997;11:593–602.
34. Graham M, Shutter JR, Sarmiento U, et al. Overexpression of Agrt leads to obesity in transgenic mice [Letter]. *Nat Genet* 1997;17:273–274.
35. Vrang N, Larsen PJ, Clausen JT, et al. Neurochemical characterization of hypothalamic cocaine- amphetamine-regulated transcript neurons. *J Neurosci* 1999;19:RC5.
36. Elias CF, Aschkenasi C, Lee C, et al. Leptin differentially regulates NPY and POMC neurons projecting to the lateral hypothalamic area. *Neuron* 1999;23:775–786.
37. Elias CF, Saper CB, Maratos-Flier E, et al. Chemically defined projections linking the mediobasal hypothalamus and the lateral hypothalamic area. *J Comp Neurol* 1998;402:442–459.
38. Elmquist JK. Hypothalamic pathways underlying the endocrine, autonomic, and behavioral effects of leptin. *Int J Obes Relat Metab Disord* 2001;25:S78–S82.
39. Zhang Y, Proenca R, Maffei M, et al. Positional cloning of the mouse obese gene and its human homologue [published erratum appears in *Nature* 1995;374:479]. *Nature* 1994;372:425–432.
40. Coleman DL, Hummel KP. Physiological and morphological lesions characteristic of diabetes by mutation (db) in mice [in French]. *Journ Annu Diabetol Hotel Dieu* 1968;9:19–30.
41. Coleman DL, Hummel KP. The influence of genetic background on the expression of the obese (Ob) gene in the mouse. *Diabetologia* 1973;9:287–293.
42. Coleman DL. Effects of parabiosis of obese with diabetes and normal mice. *Diabetologia* 1973;9:294–298.

43. Coleman DL, Hummel KP. Effects of parabiosis of normal with genetically diabetic mice. *Am J Physiol* 1969; 217:1298–1304.
44. Halaas JL, Gajiwala KS, Maffei M, et al. Weight-reducing effects of the plasma protein encoded by the obese gene [see Comments]. *Science* 1995;269:543–546.
45. Campfield LA, Smith FJ, Guisez Y, et al. Recombinant mouse OB protein: evidence for a peripheral signal linking adiposity and central neural networks [see Comments]. *Science* 1995;269:546–549.
46. Baringa M. "Obese" protein slims mice. *Science* 1995;269:475–476.
47. Tartaglia LA, Dembski M, Weng X, et al. Identification and expression cloning of a leptin receptor, OB-R. *Cell* 1995;83:1263–1271.
48. Elmquist JK, Maratos-Flier E, Saper CB, et al. Unraveling the central nervous system pathways underlying responses to leptin. *Nat Neurosci* 1998;1:445–450.
49. Bjorbaek C, Elmquist JK, Frantz JD, et al. Identification of SOCS-3 as a potential mediator of central leptin resistance. *Mol Cell* 1998;1:619–625.
50. Cowley MA, Smart JL, Rubinstein M, et al. Leptin activates anorexigenic POMC neurons through a neural network in the arcuate nucleus. *Nature* 2001;411:480–484.
51. Cone RD, Cowley MA, Butler AA, et al. The arcuate nucleus as a conduit for diverse signals relevant to energy homeostasis. *Int J Obes Relat Metab Disord* 2001;25:S63–S67.
52. Montague CT, Farooqi IS, Whitehead JP, et al. Congenital leptin deficiency is associated with severe early-onset obesity in humans. *Nature* 1997;387:903–908.
53. Farooqi S, Rau H, Whitehead J, et al. Ob gene mutations and human obesity. *Proc Nutr Soc* 1998;57:471–475.
54. Farooqi IS, Jebb SA, Langmack G, et al. Effects of recombinant leptin therapy in a child with congenital leptin deficiency. *N Engl J Med* 1999;341:879–884.
55. Clement K, Vaisse C, Lahlou N, et al. A mutation in the human leptin receptor gene causes obesity and pituitary dysfunction [see Comments]. *Nature* 1998;392:398–401.
56. Hinney A, Schmidt A, Nottebom K, et al. Several mutations in the melanocortin-4 receptor gene including a nonsense and a frameshift mutation associated with dominantly inherited obesity in humans. *J Clin Endocrinol Metab* 1999;84:1483–1486.
57. Gu W, Tu Z, Kleyn PW, et al. Identification and functional analysis of novel human melanocortin-4 receptor variants. *Diabetes* 1999;48:635–639.
58. Yeo GS, Farooqi IS, Aminian S, et al. A frameshift mutation in MC4R associated with dominantly inherited human obesity [Letter]. *Nat Genet* 1998;20:111–112.
59. Vaisse C, Clement K, Durand E, et al. Melanocortin-4 receptor mutations are a frequent and heterogeneous cause of morbid obesity. *J Clin Invest* 2000;106:253–262.
60. Vaisse C, Clement K, Guy-Grand B, et al. A frameshift mutation in human MC4R is associated with a dominant form of obesity [Letter]. *Nat Genet* 1998;20:113–114.
61. Froguel P, Guy-Grand B, Clement K. Genetics of obesity: towards the understanding of a complex syndrome [in French]. *Presse Med* 2000;29:564–571.
62. Kobayashi H, Ogawa Y, Shintani M, et al. A novel homozygous missense mutation of melanocortin-4 receptor (MC4R) in a Japanese woman with severe obesity. *Diabetes* 2002;51:243–246.
63. Krude H, Biebermann H, Luck W, et al. Severe early-onset obesity, adrenal insufficiency and red hair pigmentation caused by POMC mutations in humans. *Nat Genet* 1998;19:155–157.
64. Jackson RS, Creemers JW, Ohagi S, et al. Obesity and impaired prohormone processing associated with mutations in the human prohormone convertase 1 gene [see Comments]. *Nat Genet* 1997;16:303–306.
65. Naggert JK, Fricker LD, Varlamov O, et al. Hyperproinsulinaemia in obese fat/fat mice associated with a carboxypeptidase E mutation which reduces enzyme activity. *Nat Genet* 1995;10:135–142.
66. Rovere C, Viale A, Nahon J, et al. Impaired processing of brain pro neurotensin and promelanin-concentrating hormone in obese fat/fat mice. *Endocrinology* 1996;137:2954–2958.
67. Berman Y, Mzhavia N, Polonskaia A, et al. Impaired prohormone convertases in Cpe(fat)/Cpe(fat) mice. *J Biol Chem* 2001;276:1466–1473.
68. Ahima RS, Prabakaran D, Mantzoros C, et al. Role of leptin in the neuroendocrine response to fasting. *Nature* 1996;382:250–252.
69. Ahima RS, Dushay J, Flier SN, et al. Leptin accelerates the onset of puberty in normal female mice. *J Clin Invest* 1997;99:391–395.
70. Schwartz MW, Woods SC, Porte D Jr, et al. Central nervous system control of food intake. *Nature* 2000;404: 661–671.
71. Elmquist JK, Ahima RS, Maratos-Flier E, et al. Leptin activates neurons in ventrobasal hypothalamus and brainstem. *Endocrinology* 1997;138:839–842.
72. Elmquist JK, Elias CF, Saper CB. From lesions to leptin: hypothalamic control of food intake and body weight. *Neuron* 1999;22:221–232.
72a. El-Haschimi K, Pierroz DD, Hileman SM, et al. Two defects contribute to hypothalmic leptin resistance in mice with diet-induced obesity. *J Clin Invest* 2000;105:1827–1832.
72b. Bjorbaek C, El-Haschimi K, Frantz JD, et al. The role of SOCS-3 in leptin resistance. *J Biol Chem* 1999;274: 30059–30065.
73. Bergen HT, Mizuno T, Taylor J, et al. Resistance to diet-induced obesity is associated with increased proopiomelanocortin mRNA and decreased neuropeptide Y mRNA in the hypothalamus. *Brain Res* 1999;851:198–203.

74. Tritos NA, Elmquist JK, Mastaitis JW, et al. Characterization of expression of hypothalamic appetite-regulating peptides in obese hyperleptinemic brown adipose tissue-deficient (uncoupling protein-promoter–driven diphtheria toxin A) mice. *Endocrinology* 1998;139:4634–4641.

75. Goldstone AP, Unmehopa UA, Bloom SR, et al. Hypothalamic NPY and agouti-related protein are increased in human illness but not in Prader–Willi syndrome and other obese subjects. *J Clin Endocrinol Metab* 2002;87: 927–937.

76. Stanley BG, Kyrkouli SE, Lampert S, et al. Neuropeptide Y chronically injected into the hypothalamus: a powerful neurochemical inducer of hyperphagia and obesity. *Peptides* 1986;7:1189–1192.

77. Kalra SP, Dube MG, Pu S, et al. Interacting appetite-regulating pathways in the hypothalamic regulation of body weight. *Endocr Rev* 1999;20:68–100.

78. Erickson JC, Clegg KE, Palmiter RD. Sensitivity to leptin and susceptibility to seizures of mice lacking neuropeptide Y [see Comments]. *Nature* 1996;381:415–421.

79. Erickson JC, Hollopeter G, Palmiter RD. Attenuation of the obesity syndrome of ob/ob mice by the loss of neuropeptide Y [see Comments]. *Science* 1996;274:1704–1707.

80. Kaga T, Inui A, Okita M, et al. Modest overexpression of neuropeptide Y in the brain leads to obesity after high-sucrose feeding. *Diabetes* 2001;50:1206–1210.

81. Marsh DJ, Hollopeter G, Kafer KE, et al. Role of the Y5 neuropeptide Y receptor in feeding and obesity. *Nat Med* 1998;4:718–721.

82. Kushi A, Sasai H, Koizumi H, et al. Obesity and mild hyperinsulinemia found in neuropeptide Y-Y1 receptor–deficient mice. *Proc Natl Acad Sci U S A* 1998;95:15659–15664.

83. Zahorska-Markiewicz B, Obuchowicz E, Waluga M, et al. Neuropeptide Y in obese women during treatment with adrenergic modulation drugs. *Med Sci Monit* 2001;7:403–408.

84. Kawauchi H, Kawazoe I, Tsubokawa M, et al. Characterization of melanin-concentrating hormone in chum salmon pituitaries. *Nature* 1983;305:321–323.

85. Bittencourt JC, Presse F, Arias C, et al. The melanin-concentrating hormone system of the rat brain: an immuno- and hybridization histochemical characterization. *J Comp Neurol* 1992;319:218–245.

86. Bittencourt JC, Frigo L, Rissman RA, et al. The distribution of melanin-concentrating hormone in the monkey brain (Cebus apella). *Brain Res* 1998;804:140–143.

87. Bittencourt JC, Elias CF. Melanin-concentrating hormone and neuropeptide EI projections from the lateral hypothalamic area and zona incerta to the medial septal nucleus and spinal cord: a study using multiple neuronal tracers. *Brain Res* 1998;805:1–19.

88. Ludwig DS, Mountjoy KG, Tatro JB, et al. Melanin-concentrating hormone: a functional melanocortin antagonist in the hypothalamus. *Am J Physiol* 1998;274:E627–E633.

89. Tritos NA, Vicent D, Gillette J, et al. Functional interactions between melanin-concentrating hormone, neuropeptide Y, and anorectic neuropeptides in the rat hypothalamus. *Diabetes* 1998;47:1687–1692.

90. Rossi M, Choi SJ, O'Shea D, et al. Melanin-concentrating hormone acutely stimulates feeding, but chronic administration has no effect on body weight. *Endocrinology* 1997;138:351–355.

91. Shimada M, Tritos NA, Lowell BB, et al. Mice lacking melanin-concentrating hormone are hypophagic and lean. *Nature* 1998;396:670–674.

92. Ludwig DS, Tritos NA, Mastaitis JW, et al. Melanin-concentrating hormone overexpression in transgenic mice leads to obesity and insulin resistance. *J Clin Invest* 2001;107:379–386.

93. Frederich RC, Hamann A, Anderson S, et al. Leptin levels reflect body lipid content in mice: evidence for diet-induced resistance to leptin action. *Nat Med* 1995;1:1311–1314.

94. Marsh DJ, Weingarth DT, Novi DE, et al. Melanin-concentrating hormone 1 receptor-deficient mice are lean, hyperactive, and hyperphagic and have altered metabolism. *Proc Natl Acad Sci U S A* 2002;99:3240–3245.

95. Kristensen P, Judge ME, Thim L, et al. Hypothalamic CART is a new anorectic peptide regulated by leptin. *Nature* 1998;393:72–76.

96. Rohner-Jeanrenaud F, Craft LS, Bridwell J, et al. Chronic central infusion of cocaine- and amphetamine-regulated transcript (CART 55-102): effects on body weight homeostasis in lean and high-fat–fed obese rats. *Int J Obes Relat Metab Disord* 2002;26:143–149.

97. Asnicar MA, Smith DP, Yang DD, et al. Absence of cocaine- and amphetamine-regulated transcript results in obesity in mice fed a high caloric diet. *Endocrinology* 2001;142:4394–4400.

98. Morley JE. Neuropeptide regulation of appetite and weight. *Endocr Rev* 1987;8:256–287.

99. Oltmans GA. Norepinephrine and dopamine levels in hypothalamic nuclei of the genetically obese mouse (ob/ob). *Brain Res* 1983;273:369–373.

100. Leibowitz SF, Roossin P, Rosenn M. Chronic norepinephrine injection into the hypothalamic paraventricular nucleus produces hyperphagia and increased body weight in the rat. *Pharmacol Biochem Behav* 1984;21: 801–808.

101. Leibowitz SF. Hypothalamic neurochemical systems mediate drug effects on food intake. *Clin Neuropharmacol* 1992;15:701A–702A.

102. Tsujii S, Bray GA. Food intake of lean and obese Zucker rats following ventricular infusions of adrenergic agonists. *Brain Res* 1992;587:226–232.

103. Wellman PJ. A review of the physiological bases of the anorexic action of phenylpropanolamine (D,L-norephedrine). *Neurosci Biobehav Rev* 1990;14:339–355.

104. Bray GA. A concise review on the therapeutics of obesity. *Nutrition* 2000;16:953–960.

105. Berken GH, Weinstein DO, Stern WC. Weight gain. A side-effect of tricyclic antidepressants. *J Affect Disord* 1984;7:133–138.
106. Pothos EN, Creese I, Hoebel BG. Restricted eating with weight loss selectively decreases extracellular dopamine in the nucleus accumbens and alters dopamine response to amphetamine, morphine, and food intake. *J Neurosci* 1995;15:6640–6650.
107. Brunetti L, Michelotto B, Orlando G, et al. Leptin inhibits norepinephrine and dopamine release from rat hypothalamic neuronal endings. *Eur J Pharmacol* 1999;372:237–240.
108. Yang ZJ, Meguid MM, Chai JK, et al. Bilateral hypothalamic dopamine infusion in male Zucker rat suppresses feeding due to reduced meal size. *Pharmacol Biochem Behav* 1997;58:631–635.
109. Zhou QY, Palmiter RD. Dopamine-deficient mice are severely hypoactive, adipsic, and aphagic. *Cell* 1995;83: 1197–1209.
110. Blackburn GL. Weight gain and antipsychotic medication. *J Clin Psychiatry* 2000;61:36–42.
111. Basson BR, Kinon BJ, Taylor CC, et al. Factors influencing acute weight change in patients with schizophrenia treated with olanzapine, haloperidol, or risperidone. *J Clin Psychiatry* 2001;62:231–238.
112. Simpson MM, Goetz RR, Devlin MJ, et al. Weight gain and antipsychotic medication: differences between antipsychotic-free and treatment periods. *J Clin Psychiatry* 2001;62:694–700.
113. Jones B, Basson BR, Walker DJ, et al. Weight change and atypical antipsychotic treatment in patients with schizophrenia. *J Clin Psychiatry* 2001;62:41–44.
114. Casey DE, Zorn SH. The pharmacology of weight gain with antipsychotics. *J Clin Psychiatry* 2001;62:4–10.
115. Lauder JM. Ontogeny of the serotonergic system in the rat: serotonin as a developmental signal. *Ann N Y Acad Sci* 1990;600:297–314.
116. Schwartz DH, McClane S, Hernandez L, et al. Feeding increases extracellular serotonin in the lateral hypothalamus of the rat as measured by microdialysis. *Brain Res* 1989;479:349–354.
117. Calapai G, Corica F, Corsonello A, et al. Leptin increases serotonin turnover by inhibition of brain nitric oxide synthesis. *J Clin Invest* 1999;104:975–982.
118. Nonogaki K, Strack AM, Dallman MF, et al. Leptin-independent hyperphagia and type 2 diabetes in mice with a mutated serotonin 5-HT$_{2C}$ receptor gene [see Comments]. *Nat Med* 1998;4:1152–1156.
119. Bayer L, Risold PY, Griffond B, et al. Rat diencephalic neurons producing melanin-concentrating hormone are influenced by ascending cholinergic projections. *Neuroscience* 1999;91:1087–1101.
120. Yamada M, Miyakawa T, Duttaroy A, et al. Mice lacking the M$_3$ muscarinic acetylcholine receptor are hypophagic and lean. *Nature* 2001;410:207–212.
121. Gibbs J, Young RC, Smith GP. Cholecystokinin decreases food intake in rats. *J Comp Physiol Psychol* 1973;84: 488–495.
122. Gibbs J, Young RC, Smith GP. Cholecystokinin elicits satiety in rats with open gastric fistulas. *Nature* 1973; 245:323–325.
123. Liddle RA. Regulation of cholecystokinin secretion by intraluminal releasing factors. *Am J Physiol* 1995;269: G319–G327.
124. Liddle RA. Regulation of cholecystokinin secretion in humans. *J Gastroenterol* 2000;35:181–187.
125. Kopin AS, Mathes WF, McBride EW, et al. The cholecystokinin-A receptor mediates inhibition of food intake yet is not essential for the maintenance of body weight. *J Clin Invest* 1999;103:383–391.
126. Greenough A, Cole G, Lewis J, et al. Untangling the effects of hunger, anxiety, and nausea on energy intake during intravenous cholecystokinin octapeptide (CCK-8) infusion. *Physiol Behav* 1998;65:303–310.
127. Reidelberger RD, O'Rourke MF. Potent cholecystokinin antagonist L 364718 stimulates food intake in rats. *Am J Physiol* 1989;257:R1512–R1518.
128. Matzinger D, Gutzwiller JP, Drewe J, et al. Inhibition of food intake in response to intestinal lipid is mediated by cholecystokinin in humans. *Am J Physiol* 1999;277:R1718–R1724.
129. West DB, Fey D, Woods SC. Cholecystokinin persistently suppresses meal size but not food intake in free-feeding rats. *Am J Physiol* 1984;246:R776–R787.
130. Emond M, Schwartz GJ, Ladenheim EE, et al. Central leptin modulates behavioral and neural responsivity to CCK. *Am J Physiol* 1999;276:R1545–R1549.
131. Pierson ME, Comstock JM, Simmons RD, et al. Synthesis and biological evaluation of potent, selective, hexapeptide CCK-A agonist anorectic agents. *J Med Chem* 1997;40:4302–4307.
132. Stein LJ, Woods SC. Gastrin releasing peptide reduces meal size in rats. *Peptides* 1982;3:833–835.
133. Gutzwiller JP, Drewe J, Hildebrand P, et al. Effect of intravenous human gastrin-releasing peptide on food intake in humans. *Gastroenterology* 1994;106:1168–1173.
134. Ohki-Hamazaki H, Watase K, Yamamoto K, et al. Mice lacking bombesin receptor subtype-3 develop metabolic defects and obesity. *Nature* 1997;390:165–169.
135. Haraguchi Y, Sakamoto A, Yoshida T, et al. Plasma GRP-like immunoreactivity in healthy and diseased subjects. *Gastroenterol Jpn* 1988;23:247–250.
136. Gutzwiller JP, Goke B, Drewe J, et al. Glucagon-like peptide-1: a potent regulator of food intake in humans. *Gut* 1999;44:81–86.
137. Long SJ, Sutton JA, Amaee WB, et al. No effect of glucagon-like peptide-1 on short-term satiety and energy intake in man. *Br J Nutr* 1999;81:273–279.
138. Baura GD, Foster DM, Porte D Jr, et al. Saturable transport of insulin from plasma into the central nervous system of dogs *in vivo*. A mechanism for regulated insulin delivery to the brain. *J Clin Invest* 1993;92:1824–1830.

139. Werther GA, Hogg A, Oldfield BJ, et al. Localization and characterization of insulin receptors in rat brain and pituitary gland using *in vitro* autoradiography and computerized densitometry. *Endocrinology* 1987;121: 1562–1570.
140. Marks JL, Porte D Jr, Stahl WL, et al. Localization of insulin receptor mRNA in rat brain by *in situ* hybridization. *Endocrinology* 1990;127:3234–3236.
141. Schwartz MW, Sipols AJ, Marks JL, et al. Inhibition of hypothalamic neuropeptide Y gene expression by insulin. *Endocrinology* 1992;130:3608–3616.
142. Sipols AJ, Baskin DG, Schwartz MW. Effect of intracerebroventricular insulin infusion on diabetic hyperphagia and hypothalamic neuropeptide gene expression. *Diabetes* 1995;44:147–151.
143. Woods SC, Lotter EC, McKay LD, et al. Chronic intracerebroventricular infusion of insulin reduces food intake and body weight of baboons. *Nature* 1979;282:503–505.
144. Figlewicz DP, Sipols AJ, Seeley RJ, et al. Intraventricular insulin enhances the meal-suppressive efficacy of intraventricular cholecystokinin octapeptide in the baboon. *Behav Neurosci* 1995;109:567–569.
145. Bruning JC, Gautam D, Burks DJ, et al. Role of brain insulin receptor in control of body weight and reproduction. *Science* 2000;289:2122–2125.
146. Burks DJ, de Mora JF, Schubert M, et al. IRS-2 pathways integrate female reproduction and energy homeostasis. *Nature* 2000;407:377–382.
147. The Diabetes Control and Complications Trial Research Group. Weight gain associated with intensive therapy in the diabetes control and complications trial. The DCCT Research Group. *Diabetes Care* 1988;11:567–573.
148. Kojima M, Hosoda H, Date Y, et al. Ghrelin is a growth-hormone–releasing acylated peptide from stomach. *Nature* 1999;402:656–660.
149. Date Y, Kojima M, Hosoda H, et al. Ghrelin, a novel growth hormone–releasing acylated peptide, is synthesized in a distinct endocrine cell type in the gastrointestinal tracts of rats and humans. *Endocrinology* 2000;141: 4255–4261.
150. Shuto Y, Shibasaki T, Wada K, et al. Generation of polyclonal antiserum against the growth hormone secretagogue receptor (GHS-R): evidence that the GHS-R exists in the hypothalamus, pituitary and stomach of rats. *Life Sci* 2001;68:991–996.
151. Takaya K, Ariyasu H, Kanamoto N, et al. Ghrelin strongly stimulates growth hormone release in humans. *J Clin Endocrinol Metab* 2000;85:4908–4911.
152. Date Y, Murakami N, Kojima M, et al. Central effects of a novel acylated peptide, ghrelin, on growth hormone release in rats. *Biochem Biophys Res Commun* 2000;275:477–480.
153. Wren AM, Small CJ, Ward HL, et al. The novel hypothalamic peptide ghrelin stimulates food intake and growth hormone secretion. *Endocrinology* 2000;141:4325–4328.
154. Tschop M, Smiley DL, Heiman ML. Ghrelin induces adiposity in rodents. *Nature* 2000;407:908–913.
155. Tschop M, Weyer C, Tataranni PA, et al. Circulating ghrelin levels are decreased in human obesity. *Diabetes* 2001;50:707–709.
156. Shiiya T, Nakazato M, Mizuta M, et al. Plasma ghrelin levels in lean and obese humans and the effect of glucose on ghrelin secretion. *J Clin Endocrinol Metab* 2002;87:240–244.
157. Cummings DE, Purnell JQ, Frayo RS, et al. A preprandial rise in plasma ghrelin levels suggests a role in meal initiation in humans. *Diabetes* 2001;50:1714–1719.
158. Nakazato M, Murakami N, Date Y, et al. A role for ghrelin in the central regulation of feeding. *Nature* 2001; 409:194–198.
159. Shintani M, Ogawa Y, Ebihara K, et al. Ghrelin, an endogenous growth hormone secretagogue, is a novel orexigenic peptide that antagonizes leptin action through the activation of hypothalamic neuropeptide Y/Y1 receptor pathway. *Diabetes* 2001;50:227–232.
160. Wren AM, Seal LJ, Cohen MA, et al. Ghrelin enhances appetite and increases food intake in humans. *J Clin Endocrinol Metab* 2001;86:5992.
161. Ukkola O, Ravussin E, Jacobson P, et al. Mutations in the preproghrelin/ghrelin gene associated with obesity in humans. *J Clin Endocrinol Metab* 2001;86:3996–3999.

7

Endocrine Control of Fuel Partitioning

Samyah Shadid and Michael D. Jensen

Understanding the regulation of energy balance and nutrient partitioning can potentially facilitate the treatment of obesity. The factors that lead to an imbalance between energy and fat intake and energy expenditure, and thus to the development of obesity, are incompletely understood. For example, some progress has been made in understanding the regulation of nutrient partitioning, the process by which the organism selects fuels for storage (including protein synthesis) or oxidation. Nutrient partitioning may be particularly relevant to the development of obesity as it relates to the hypothesis of Dr. J. P. Flatt (1), who suggests that total food intake increases to meet carbohydrate needs. According to this theory, food intake is regulated, at least in part, to ensure an adequate amount of carbohydrate. Consumption of a high-fat diet requires the intake of excess fat to satisfy carbohydrate needs, leading to obesity under this scenario. The concept of a diet that is "relatively" deficient in carbohydrate becomes important because dysregulation of substrate partitioning could affect the body's sense of what constitutes adequate carbohydrate intake. For example, if fat were preferentially shunted toward storage, more carbohydrate would be required to meet oxidative needs, thereby preventing sufficient repletion of glycogen stores. This is then proposed to generate signals that stimulate appetite. Other examples in which nutrient partitioning relates to obesity and body fat content include the stimulation of lean-tissue synthesis at the expense of fat calories by androgens and growth hormone (GH) and, presumably, the reverse of this process by deficiencies of these hormones.

Endocrine disturbances have long been associated with either the development of obesity or the result of obesity. Examples include Cushing syndrome, thyroid disorders, insulin resistance, and polycystic ovary syndrome. In some cases, endocrine influences may alter fat content and body composition by altering nutrient management without markedly changing either energy intake or expenditure. In other instances, hormones influence body composition by changing energy expenditure (e.g., thyroxine).

Another point of interest is body fat distribution, a determinant of obesity-induced morbidity that is as important as the absolute amount of body fat. Upper-body obesity, which usually connotes visceral obesity, is more strongly associated with insulin resistance, hypertension, coagulation abnormalities, dyslipidemia, and cardiovascular death than obesity *per se* is. Lower-body obesity, in which fat preferentially accumulates in the gluteofemoral region, is less strongly associated with these health hazards. Because endocrine influences may affect fat distribution, these effects are reviewed when information is available.

GENERAL CONSIDERATIONS

When energy intake exceeds energy expenditure, the excess calories are stored. Excess energy intake in sedentary, hormonally stable adults almost inevitably results in the expansion of adipose-tissue triglyceride stores. Circumstances that promote lean-tissue accretion, however, can allow excess energy to be stored as muscle and/or visceral proteins. The most common circumstance resulting in net lean-tissue accretion with excess food intake is increased physical activity, usually in the form of resistance exercise training. The initiation of endurance exercise training in a previously sedentary individual can have similar, albeit less pronounced, effects on lean body mass (LBM). Finally, during the recovery from catabolic illness, repletion of lost body proteins is an important destination for excess energy.

Alterations in nutrient partitioning can also occur at a relatively stable weight. For example, the reduction in protein synthesis and increased fat accumulation with aging can be considered a form of nutrient partitioning. Whether the changes are driven solely by lesser physical activity or are aggravated by other (e.g., hormonal) factors is not clear. Therefore, in summary, ingested nutrients can be directed toward increasing body protein, increasing body fat, or, to a much lesser degree, expanding carbohydrate stores. Various physiologic and cellular events play key roles in determining nutrient partitioning. After examining the regulation of the major pathways of nutrient partitioning, this chapter reviews the specific hormonal regulation of each pathway. The net effects of the major nutrient-partitioning hormones (i.e., insulin, GH, testosterone, and cortisol) are depicted in Fig. 7.1.

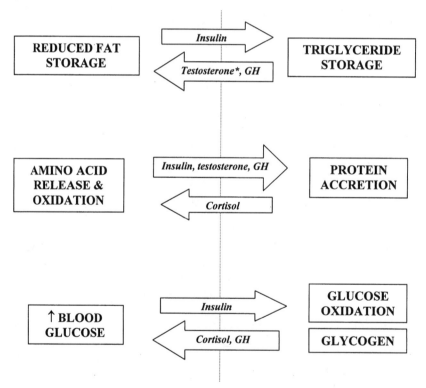

FIG. 7.1. Net effects of hormones on fuel balance. Each hormone affects the net balance between stored and circulating fuel. In some cases, this is achieved by a combination of two opposite actions, one of which dominates the other. Cortisol increases net lipolysis; however, *in vivo,* the concomitant increase in insulin secretion attenuates the rise in plasma free fatty acid, and the appetite-stimulation effects of cortisol promote fat gain. (*Testosterone decreases triglyceride stores by increasing its oxidation rather than by increasing its release into plasma.) Abbreviation: GH, growth hormone.

Processing of Fuel

The main sources of dietary energy are carbohydrates (4 kcal per g), proteins (4 kcal per g), fat (9 kcal per g), and alcohol (7 kcal per g). Alcohol will not be discussed here. Fat, carbohydrates, and protein can serve other functions in addition to fuel provision, and the ultimate fate of these molecules depends on various factors, an important one of which is hormonal influences.

Fat Metabolism

Overview

Dietary triglycerides are transported in chylomicrons for storage or oxidation. The effective use of triglycerides requires the action of lipoprotein lipase (LPL), which is present on the capillary endothelium of many tissues. Adipose tissue and muscle are the major tissues responsible for triglyceride clearance by LPL-mediated fatty acid uptake. Very low density lipoprotein (VLDL), which is secreted by the liver, is the other major form of circulating triglyceride. The fatty acids in these triglycerides are derived largely from plasma free fatty acids (FFAs), as this chapter later describes.

Fat stored in adipocytes is mobilized by the action of hormone-sensitive lipase (HSL), which hydrolyzes the triglyceride, resulting in the release of glycerol and FFA. FFAs circulate bound to albumin, they are present at relatively low concentrations (300 to 600 µmol per L in the postabsorptive state), and they turn over rapidly in the circulation (half-life of about 4 minutes). FFA can be taken up for use as an oxidative substrate (e.g., heart and muscle) or for reesterification (e.g., liver) and subsequent transport in VLDL particles. At rest, FFA release and uptake rates generally exceed fatty acid oxidation rates. Hepatic reesterification of FFA and secretion as a VLDL triglyceride can account for a portion of the FFA that is released in excess of fatty acid oxidation. Substantial portions of VLDL triglyceride fatty acids are thought to be restored in adipose tissue.

Under conditions of grossly excessive carbohydrate intake, glucose can be converted to fatty acids. This process is referred to as *de novo lipogenesis*, and it is thought to take place primarily in the liver. It is energetically inefficient, and it thus accounts for an extremely small fraction of the fatty acids present in VLDL triglyceride under usual conditions.

The availability of FFA in the circulation drives fatty acid oxidation to a significant extent, as the coordinate changes in fatty acid oxidation resulting from artificial elevation and lowering of plasma FFA concentrations demonstrate. Some of the hormones that influence substrate partitioning may do so in large part by altering FFA release from adipose tissue. For example, GH stimulates lipolysis, whereas insulin inhibits lipolysis, which in turn promotes and inhibits fatty acid oxidation. Fatty acid oxidation can also be regulated at other steps, however. Hormones can inhibit or stimulate fatty acid oxidation over and above their effects on FFA availability, thus sparing carbohydrate as an oxidative fuel. Altering the portion of fatty acids that enter the reesterification pathways or altering fatty acid transport into mitochondria could modify fatty acid, and thus glucose, oxidation independent of the availability of circulating FFA.

Regulation of Lipolysis

Because of the importance of FFA availability in determining substrate oxidation, a brief overview of adipose-tissue lipolysis is enclosed. Under overnight postabsorptive conditions, adipose-tissue lipolysis is restrained by the prevailing insulinemia; pharmacologic inhibition of insulin secretion using somatostatin results in an approximate doubling of FFA release rates. Physiologic hyperinsulinemia is capable of suppressing FFA release rates by 80% to 90% from basal levels and of reducing FFA concentrations by more than 90%. Insulin-resistant obese individuals display greater maximal release of FFA during insulin withdrawal and lower suppression of FFA during hyperinsulinemia. Catecholamines are also potent regulators of adipose-tissue lipolysis. For example, epinephrine infusions can increase FFA release by threefold to fourfold. This is similar to the stimulation of lipolysis that occurs during exercise. Catecholamines act through the stimulation of β-adrenergic receptors via a classic G_s protein and cyclic adenosine monophosphate mechanism that activates HSL (2). Other hormonal regulators of lipolysis include GH and cortisol, although these are generally considered to be much less potent than insulin and the catecholamines.

Carbohydrate Metabolism

Most dietary carbohydrate is converted into glucose before storage or oxidation. The liver is the only organ that stores carbohydrate as glycogen for eventual exportation as glucose. The regulation of hepatic glucose export is controlled exquisitely by various hormones, although insulin and glucagon are considered the most potent acute regulators of glucose availability.

A limited capacity for glucose storage as glycogen exists, so increasing carbohydrate intake beyond the usual needs quickly leads to increased carbohydrate oxidation and an attendant reduction in fat oxidation. Increasing carbohydrate intake in the face of unchanging fat intake results in increased fat storage as glucose replaces fat as an oxidative fuel. Massive increases in carbohydrate intake can stimulate *de novo* lipogenesis, although the capacity for this appears to be quite limited in humans, as was discussed above.

Reductions in carbohydrate intake are accompanied by some degree of glycogen depletion and by shifts toward greater fat oxidation. If energy intake is less than energy expenditure, fatty acids from preexisting stores are oxidized, resulting in relatively good preservation of protein stores. The shifts in carbohydrate and fatty acid oxidation that take place with changes in carbohydrate intake appear to be primarily regulated by the changes in insulin secretion that accompany the dietary changes.

Protein Metabolism

Proteins include structural proteins, enzymes, nucleoproteins, oxygen-transporting proteins, contractile proteins, and others. The amino acids in these proteins are part of an interchangeable pool. The daily turnover of amino acids is substantially greater than the amount that is ingested as dietary protein, and only a minor fraction of amino acids are oxidized or converted to glucose or fat.

Mechanical stimuli enhance skeletal muscle contractile protein synthesis, whereas hormonal and other factors determine the synthesis rates of many types of proteins. Given the tremendous variety of proteins in the body, many of which have specific regulatory pathways, this chapter makes only general reference to the hormonal or metabolic regulation of protein metabolism.

Energy Expenditure and Metabolism

Nutrient partitioning may be accompanied by or exaggerated by changes in energy expenditure. Human energy expenditure is usually broken down into the following three components: resting metabolic rate (RMR), the thermic effect of food (TEF), and physical activity. The BMR is determined primarily by LBM, so hormonal effects that increase

TABLE 7.1. *Brief overview of hormones—anabolic, catabolic, body fat distribution, and major importance—and physiologic effects addressing these issues*

Effect	Insulin	Growth hormone	Estrogen	Testosterone	Cortisol
Energy expenditure or fuel mix					
RMR/RQ	↑/↑	↔/↓	↔/↔	↔/↓	↔/↔
TEF/RQ	↑/↑	?/↓	?	?	?
PAEE/RQ	↔/↑	?	?	?	?
Circulating substrate availability					
Fatty acids	↓	↑	↓	↔	↑/↔ (insulin counteracts lipolytic effects of cortisol)
Glucose	↓	↑	↔	↔	↑
Amino acids	↓	↔	↔	↔	↑
Direct intracellular effects					
Fatty acids (oxidation vs. reesterification)	↓	↑	↔	↑	?
Glucose (oxidation vs. glycogen synthesis)	↑	↓	↔	↓	?
Amino acids (protein synthesis)	?	↑	↔	↑	↓
Fat storage	↑	↓	↑	↓	↑
Regional fat storage	?	?	Gluteofemoral	Visceral	↑ (truncal)

Abbreviations: ↑, increased; ↓, decreased; ↔, unchanged; ?, unknown; PAEE, physical activity energy expenditure; RMR, resting metabolic rate, RQ, respiratory quotient; TEF, thermic effect of food.

lean tissue will increase the RMR. The TEF is determined primarily by the amounts of carbohydrate and protein that are ingested, but it may be reduced in insulin-resistant states. Physical activity thermogenesis is a product of the mass of the body moved and the amount of movement. Hormonal effects on energy expenditure and substrate oxidation could theoretically influence either the amount of energy expended in one of these components of energy expenditure or the mix of fuels oxidized. To the extent that hormones influence either energy expenditure or substrate oxidation, these issues are covered below.

A summary of the effects of insulin, GH, cortisol, testosterone, and estrogen on energy expenditure, nutrient availability, and oxidation, as well as fat and regional fat storage is presented in Table 7.1.

ENDOCRINE CONTROL OF FUEL PARTITIONING

Insulin

Physiology

General Considerations on Fuel Partitioning

Insulin is perhaps the prototypical hormone regarding nutrient partitioning. It enhances net energy storage by limiting the release of fuel substrate from tissues into the circulation (Fig. 7.2). This is accompanied by an increase in the cellular uptake of glucose and amino acids. Under usual circumstances, major increases in insulin release occur only after meals when exogenous fuels become available. Thus, insulin's anticatabolic action, which limits lipolysis, glycogenolysis, and proteolysis, takes place under circumstances in which the adverse consequences of hyperinsulinemia, such as hypoglycemia, are avoided. The other important feature of insulin action is the promotion of glucose as the preferred oxidative substrate, which spares amino acids and fatty acids for protein and triglyceride synthesis, respectively.

Much focus has been placed on insulin's glucose metabolic action, although it is an equally important regulator of fat and protein metabolism. Insulin largely controls glucose uptake into most cells and stimulates glucose oxidation and glycogen storage; skeletal muscle is the predominant site of postprandial glucose disposal. Insulin also suppresses endogenous glucose production by inhibiting hepatic glycogenolysis and gluconeogenesis. Thus, insulin largely orchestrates the disposal of meal carbohydrate by simultaneously inhibiting endogenous glucose production and stimulating the uptake and oxidation and/or storage of blood glucose.

As was noted at the beginning of this chapter, insulin also plays a major role in regulating lipolysis, and, probably via its ability to stimulate adipose-tissue LPL synthesis, it facilitates adipose triglyceride uptake. Whether insulin has independent effects on FFA transport into cells is unclear. Insulin's role in stimulating protein synthesis is somewhat controversial, but insulin's inhibition of protein breakdown and the resulting net effect of maintaining lean-tissue mass is well established.

In summary, insulin may be looked at largely as anticatabolic rather than anabolic, although clearly the net effect is to preserve protein and fat stores. Insulin-resistant states are of interest with respect to their common presence in obesity and because resistance to all aspects of insulin action may not appear in different insulin-resistant states.

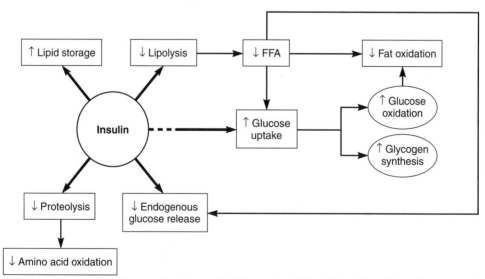

FIG. 7.2. Effects of insulin on substrate availability and oxidation. The effect of insulin on protein synthesis is controversial, and it therefore is not depicted. Abbreviation: FFA, free fatty acid.

Resting Energy Expenditure and the Thermic Effect of Food and Exercise

The issue of whether insulin modulates RMR is puzzling. Insulin deficiency, such as that which occurs with uncontrolled type I or type II diabetes or with brief periods of fasting, is associated with slightly higher (5% to 10%) RMRs, even if the lean-tissue mass is appropriately accounted for. One suggestion that has been made is that the increase in RMR is due to the higher rates of gluconeogenesis, which energetically is an inefficient process. Abrupt increases in insulin concentrations, such as those that occur during euglycemic, hyperinsulinemic clamp studies, also increase RMR coincident with the increased plasma catecholamine concentrations. The increase in RMR in response to hyperinsulinemia may be partly mediated by stimulation of the sympathetic nervous system; adrenergic blockade can inhibit this effect of insulin. The same adrenergically mediated mechanism may be responsible for the much of the insulin-mediated postprandial thermogenesis (3), although not all studies support this notion (4). Insulin resistance and obesity are associated with reduced postprandial thermogenesis (5). This is considered further evidence for the idea that insulin and/or its action modulates at least one, albeit minor, aspect of daily energy expenditure. This effect could have long-term effects on energy balance and nutrient partitioning.

No data address the issue of whether insulin modifies the thermic effect of exercise. Moderate-intensity exercise normally results in a gradual decline in plasma insulin concentrations, which facilitates both glucose and FFA mobilization to provide fuel for exercising muscles. If insulin concentrations do not decline or if they actually increase, carbohydrate oxidation increases above normal, requiring exogenous glucose to prevent hypoglycemia. The limited evidence that is available suggests that individuals with obesity, including more insulin-resistant forms of obesity, have normal substrate oxidation responses to exercise despite somewhat different lipolytic responses. Thus, while insulin could have drastic effects on nutrient partitioning during exercise, the actual magnitude and relative importance of variations in the insulin response to exercise are not well defined.

In summary, the RMR increases in response to both insulin deficiency and hyperinsulinemia, likely via completely different mechanisms. A significant portion of the TEF is mediated by the postprandial insulin response. Whether insulin alters the thermic response to exercise is unknown. Thus, abnormalities in insulin secretion or action can affect nutrient partitioning by altering both the energy expenditure and the tissue selection of substrate oxidation and storage.

Substrate Availability and Oxidation

As has been mentioned, insulin decreases the concentrations of glucose, FFA, and amino acids in the circulation. In the case of FFA, this has direct consequences for substrate use in peripheral tissues, which are then forced to intensify their use of glucose as oxidative fuel. The suppression of adipose-tissue lipolysis with the subsequent decrease in plasma FFA availability makes an important quantitative contribution to insulin's effects on peripheral glucose uptake and oxidation. This has a major impact on nutrient partitioning in that the ineffective suppression of lipolysis after meal ingestion allows more fat and less glucose to be oxidized. This has been proposed as a mechanism by which the insulin resistance of obesity increases fat oxidation, thereby eventually allowing the individual to balance fat oxidation and fat intake.

The concept that failure to suppress fatty acid concentrations in the face of hyperinsulinemia impairs glucose disposal and oxidation has been confirmed. If the fall in FFA concentrations in response to hyperinsulinemia is prevented by the infusion of a lipid emulsion and heparin, glucose disposal and oxidation are not stimulated to the expected degree. In addition, normalizing the suppression of FFA in volunteers with type II diabetes whose lipolysis is normally quite resistant to insulin by administering acipimox, a drug with antilipolytic properties, markedly enhances insulin action with respect to glucose metabolism (6).

Insulin also inhibits the release of amino acids from tissues into the circulation by inhibiting proteolysis. In the context of a mixed meal (i.e., one providing protein and carbohydrate), the plasma amino acid concentrations increase as a consequence of gut delivery of amino acid into the circulation. Increased amino acid availability plays a role in stimulating protein synthesis. If insulin concentrations increase from the ingestion of pure carbohydrate or during intravenous glucose and insulin infusions, plasma amino acid concentrations and protein synthesis rates fall. Thus, the nutrient-partitioning effects of insulin with respect to protein metabolism are strongly influenced by the nutrient content of the challenge.

Intracellular Effects on Nutrient Partitioning

Insulin also promotes glucose oxidation and storage independent of its effects on substrate availability via direct action on intracellular events. Evidence for these effects has been provided by *in vivo* studies whereby FFA concentrations have been maintained via an intravenous lipid and heparin infusion during hyperinsulinemic euglycemic conditions. In these experiments, glucose uptake, storage, and oxidation increase above the basal level in response to insulin, although the rates do not equal those that are seen when FFA concentrations are allowed to fall normally (7). This response is clearly evident in skeletal muscle (7) but not in the liver (8).

These direct intracellular effects of insulin are mediated by a complex signaling cascade that regulates glucose transporter availability at the cell membrane, as well as the activity and synthesis of numerous enzymes. The details of this process are beyond the scope of this chapter. Other direct intracellular effects of insulin include the stimulation of amino acid transport into cells, which should then facilitate protein synthesis.

Tissue Variability in Insulin Action

The effects of insulin on different tissues can vary considerably and in a manner such that nutrient partitioning is influenced. For example, insulin regulation of glucose, protein, and fatty acid metabolism can diverge considerably in fasting. Brief (3 to 4 days) fasting in humans results in insulin resistance with respect to adipose-tissue lipolysis (9) and glucose disposal (10) but in maintenance of insulin's ability to suppress proteolysis (10) and in enhanced suppression of endogenous glucose production (10). This physiologic adaptation allows enhanced mobilization and oxidation of fatty acids while sparing peripheral glucose use and presumably allowing adequate glucose to meet central nervous system needs. It also preserves the protein-sparing effects of insulin, thus minimizing lean-tissue loss. In other insulin-resistant states, such as upper-body obesity, the insulin resistance appears to affect fatty acid, glucose, and protein metabolism (11).

Inherent regional and tissue differences in insulin action that can potentially regulate regional nutrient partitioning are also present. Skeletal muscle protein metabolism is affected differently by insulin than splanchnic protein metabolism is. Under overnight postabsorptive conditions when plasma insulin concentrations are at basal levels, skeletal muscle is a net exporter of amino acids (i.e., protein breakdown exceeds protein synthesis), whereas protein synthesis exceeds protein breakdown in the splanchnic bed (12). Increasing the plasma insulin concentration results in a suppression of muscle protein breakdown without stimulating protein synthesis, but it also suppresses protein synthesis in the splanchnic bed without altering protein breakdown (12). The reduction in splanchnic protein synthesis in response to insulin may be related to the fall in plasma amino acid concentrations that results from isolated hyperinsulinemia. Thus, partitioning of amino acids between skeletal muscle and non-skeletal muscle sources is at least partially regulated by insulin.

Regional differences in the insulin regulation of adipose-tissue lipolysis are also present in humans. Leg adipose-tissue lipolysis is readily suppressed by insulin (13), while upper-body subcutaneous and visceral adipose-tissue FFA release is less well inhibited (13). This is true in both lean and obese humans (13,14). If regional adipose-tissue fatty acid storage were equal in all adipose-tissue beds, a gradual expansion of lower-body fat stores would be expected. Studies of leg, abdominal subcutaneous, and visceral adipose tissue indicate that regional variations in fatty acid uptake proceed in the same direction as regional variations of FFA release (15). Thus, whether regional differences in insulin action contribute to differences in body fat distribution is unknown.

Insulin and Nutrient Partitioning in Obesity

Insulin resistance with respect to glucose and fatty acid metabolism is an exceedingly common feature of obesity that is more severe and more prevalent in upper-body and/or visceral obesity. As has been noted, this insulin resistance with respect to adipose tissue (i.e., less stimulation of LPL synthesis and less suppression of lipolysis) theoretically would act to make more lipid fuel available, thus displacing glucose as an oxidative substrate. If there is a sensing mechanism whereby the internal stimuli for energy intake are modulated by the availability of glucose, the reduced carbohydrate oxidation resulting from insulin resistance could serve to limit excess energy intake. In this regard, insulin resistance has been proposed as a mechanism for limiting weight gain (16).

The development of type II diabetes in obese adults results in a host of nutrient-partitioning changes. The relative insulin deficiency allows further excess mobilization of FFA from adipose tissue, which in theory would further depress glucose uptake and oxidation. The hyperglycemia itself, however, facilitates glucose uptake and oxidation independent of insulin, thereby limiting the extent to which fatty acid oxidation can increase. The loss of the restraining effect of insulin on skeletal muscle protein breakdown results in substantial losses of muscle in uncontrolled diabetes. In addition, glycosuria results in the nonoxidative loss of carbohydrate. This catabolic state with regards to adipose, muscle, and carbohydrate can be reversed with the administration of insulin or insulin secretagogues at the expense of weight gain. This weight gain may well consist of muscle tissue and repletion of glycogen (with its attendant water), with limited adipose accumulation. Thus, the energy deposition that occurs when uncontrolled diabetes is treated is an excellent example of nutrient partitioning into lean tissue.

In summary, insulin to a major extent is involved in virtually every aspect of nutrient partitioning. The primary issue that clinicians face with respect to this hormone and obesity is the weight gain that attends insulin or insulin secretagogue therapy for uncontrolled type II diabetes.

Growth Hormone

Physiology

General Considerations on Fuel Partitioning

GH, a somatotropin, is secreted by the pituitary gland in response to hypothalamic regulation via growth hormone–releasing hormone (GHRH) and somatotropin–inhibitory hormone (SRIH) or a somatostatin. Physiologic stimuli for secretion include starvation, hypoglycemia, exercise, and stress; increased insulin-like growth factor-1 (IGF-1), glucose, and fatty acid concentrations inhibit GH secretion. GH is a major anabolic hormone. Its most important functions consist of fuel redistribution (Fig. 7.3) and the induction of growth in all body cells with growth capacity. The latter is achieved by increasing cell size and number, largely via IGF-1 and in synergism with insulin, which enhances the transport of glucose and amino acids into cells. During puberty, sex hormones substantially increase GH production, thus leading to the growth spurt and the increase in LBM. For the latter, the synergistic interaction with testosterone is responsible for the stimulation of protein synthesis and fat mobilization and oxidation.

The effects of GH on fuel partitioning are directed toward the use of fat as the preferred oxidative substrate, while minimizing the use of protein and carbohydrates for this function. GH stimulates fatty acid release from adipose tissue (17–20); GH-deficient patients are widely reported to have an increased fat mass and a reduced muscle mass that can be reversed back to normal after treatment (17,21–23). Analogously, acromegalic patients have a reduced fat mass and increased LBM (24) that likely result from GH-induced increases in protein synthesis. (See also "Substrate Availability and Oxidation" below.)

GH also increases plasma glucose concentrations, which cannot always be compensated for by increased insulin secretion. Thus, GH is one of the prototypical diabetogenic hormones.

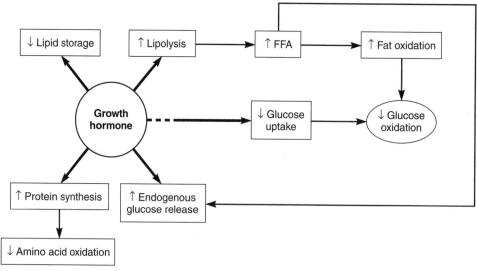

FIG. 7.3. Effects of growth hormone on substrate availability and oxidation. Abbreviations: FFA, free fatty acid.

Insulin-Like Growth Factors

Many GH functions are mediated via IGFs, or somatomedins, of which IGF-1 (somatomedin C) is the most important. These proteins are produced primarily in the liver and, to some extent, in other GH-responsive tissues in which they exert autocrine and paracrine effects.

Although GH is the most important regulator of IGF release, the nutritional status may modulate the response as serum IGF concentrations gradually decrease with fasting and they are consistently low in undernourished states. In obesity, IGF-1 levels are usually normal.

IGF-1 mediates the stimulatory effects of GH on growth, protein synthesis, and whole-body metabolism. Regulation of fat metabolism, however, seems to be IGF-1 independent (17). Adipocytes, in contrast to their abundance of GH receptors, do not appear to possess functional IGF-1 or IGF-2 receptors (25).

IGFs exert a negative feedback on GH secretion at the hypothalamic and pituitary levels.

Resting Energy Expenditure and the Thermic Effect of Food and Exercise

As might be expected, the GH-induced increase in LBM increases the RMR (24,26). This has been confirmed in acromegalic patients (17,27) and in GH-deficient adults and children, as well as in abdominally obese men in whom GH treatment increases RMR (28–30). This effect seems to result from changes in LBM only because, in children, the RMR increases even after correction for fat-free mass (FFM). This adjustment is seen only during the first 2 months of GH administration, after which the RMR stabilizes despite sustained changes in body composition (30). Analogously, in adults, the RMR returns to baseline values after an initial increase in the first 2 weeks of GH treatment (29). This suggests that GH does not influence the RMR independent of changes in LBM.

The thermic response to glucose has been reported as blunted in acromegaly (26). This may be due to the effects of insulin resistance on TEF (see "Insulin" section). Interestingly, TEF increases after GH therapy in GH-deficient children (30), whereas, in GH-deficient adults, no changes are observed (27). No information regarding the potential effects of GH on physical activity thermogenesis is available.

Substrate Availability and Oxidation

The metabolic effects of GH are biphasic. In the first 90 minutes or so after secretion, a transient insulin-like effect is observed and is characterized by accelerated glucose uptake and oxidation (19). The physiologic relevance and mechanism of this phenomenon are unknown; however, once this effect has dissipated, the lipolytic and diabetogenic effects of GH become apparent.

The main effect of GH is to increase FFA and glucose availability to peripheral tissues. Fatty acids are mobilized from adipose tissue via stimulation of hormone-sensitive lipase (HSL) that promotes its action, not its production (20). Some (31,32) have suggested that this is mediated by increased adipocyte responsiveness to catecholamines; however, whether this is entirely responsible for the increased lipolysis is unclear.

In addition, GH inhibits adipose-tissue LPL (18), reportedly at a posttranslational level (18,33). However, an influence on LPL gene expression has not been consistently observed *in vivo* or *in vitro* (18,34). The effect of GH on skeletal muscle LPL is controversial (18,32,34).

In addition to increasing fatty acid availability, GH directly enhances fat oxidation at least partially by stimulating the conversion of fatty acids to long-chain acyl-coenzyme A (acyl-CoA) within responsive cells (35). These actions reduce the need for protein and carbohydrates as energy sources. Thus, cellular uptake and oxidation of glucose diminishes, and glucose that enters the cell is deposited as glycogen (17). In some tissues, GH directly inhibits glucose uptake independent of FFA concentrations (36).

GH also stimulates hepatic glucose production (17). Both acute and prolonged excess GH therefore causes plasma glucose concentrations to rise. This cannot always be compensated for by increased insulin release (17,37).

GH is protein anabolic, meaning that it enhances protein synthesis by increasing cellular amino acid uptake in synergism with insulin (35,38) and by modulating DNA and RNA transcription. Synergistic effects with testosterone make this effect more pronounced in men than in women (35). Although GH influences protein metabolism via IGF-1 (17,35), the presence of both GH and testosterone has a greater effect than that of each one separately (38).

Whether GH also inhibits proteolysis is controversial. Although many studies show no effect of GH on proteolysis (39), 6-hour GH infusions in healthy volunteers indicated that GH suppresses net forearm alanine, phenylalanine, and leucine release (40,41). Whether this merely reflects a decreased amino acid efflux secondary to their increased extraction from the circulation (41) or actually signals a true suppression of proteolysis is unknown. The latter has been demonstrated to be induced by IGF-1 in animal and human studies (38). GH decreases amino acid oxidation by approximately 20%, as may be shown by administering GH to GH-deficient adults (41,42) and children (17).

Regional Fat Storage

When administered to patients with primary GH deficiency, GH redistributes fat from abdominal to peripheral depots. In GH-deficient children and adults, LBM is decreased and visceral fat mass is increased (19). GH treatment has been shown to reverse this centripetal fat deposition, and, in children, it decreases fat cell size in abdominal, as opposed to gluteofemoral, depots (19,22). Cessation of treatment reverses these effects (19).

Analogously, acromegalic patients are found to have a lower total fat mass and increased FFM as a result of both increased total cell mass and increased extracellular fluid (22). After treatment of acromegaly, intraabdominal fat and total body fat increases (19,22). The mechanism of the effect of GH on fat distribution—changes in regional mobilization versus changes in regional storage—has not been investigated using *in vivo* approaches; however, *in vitro* studies offer some possible explanations for the observed effects.

Regional variability in LPL and/or HSL responsiveness to GH exists, and neither has been extensively studied. At this time, only one study, which investigated the effects of GH administration on adipose-tissue LPL of obese women, has examined gluteal and abdominal subcutaneous adipose tissue separately (34). In both regions, GH significantly inhibited LPL activity, an effect that seemed more pronounced in gluteal than in visceral fat. Although this suggests a regional difference in sensitivity to GH inhibition of LPL, the two areas were not statistically compared, so definite conclusions cannot be drawn.

Growth Hormone and Visceral Obesity

The role of GH in obesity is complex and somewhat controversial. Although primary GH deficiency leads to centripetal adiposity, visceral obesity *per se* results in a *secondary* reduction in serum GH concentrations (43). However, the authors view the latter as an adaptation to the state of energy surplus.

The differences in the pathophysiology of the two conditions are exemplified by the different IGF-1 concentrations. IGF-1 is extremely low in primary GH deficiency, but its concentration may be normal, high, or somewhat reduced in obesity. In the last case, IGF-1 concentrations are usually only slightly lower than normal. Moreover, a simultaneous change in the production of IGF-binding proteins (IGFBPs) in central obesity (decreased IGFBP-1 and IGFBP-2 and increased IGFBP-3) may result in free biologically active IGF-1 fractions that exceed those in lean subjects (43). Therefore, IGF-dependent functions of GH, such as the growth ability of children, remain unchanged in obesity (43).

One might reasonably argue that reduced GH may dampen the tendency toward high FFA concentrations in central obesity, thereby preventing further worsening of insulin resistance. Indeed, treatment of centrally obese adults with GH, while resulting in body fat loss, is almost uniformly associated with further increases in FFA and worsening glucose intolerance and/or insulin resistance.

The reasons for this hyposomatotropinism in obesity and its mechanisms have yet to be clarified. Reductions in spontaneous GH secretion, which can be as much as 6% for each unit increase in BMI, and in the half-life of circulating GH have been reported (43). Moreover, the GH response to pharmacologic (e.g., GHRH, L-dopa) and physiologic stimuli, such as sleep, physical exercise, insulin-induced hypoglycemia, and corticosteroids, is impaired in adiposity (43).

Several theories have postulated explanations for the decreased GH concentrations that focus on IGF-1, FFA, peripheral hormones, and the central nervous system. Increased plasma concentrations of FFA and IGF-1 are observed in obesity, and both are known to provide negative feedback control on GH secretion. Thus, each might contribute to the hyposomatotropinism. Indeed, the administration of acipimox, an FFA-lowering nicotinic acid analog, has been proven to increase spontaneous and stimulated GH release in obese subjects, both with acute and chronic application (43). No comparable support exists for the IGF-1 theory, and the quantitative importance of either of these feedback loops in mediating the alterations in GH dynamics in obesity is unknown.

Other hormonal theories explaining the low serum GH in obesity concentrate on leptin and insulin. Because plasma concentrations of leptin rise as a function of percentage of body fat, an inhibiting effect on GH release has been suggested for leptin. However, conflicting *in vitro* evidence, showing both stimulatory and inhibitory effects of leptin on GH release, challenges this theory (43). More likely, altered leptin and GH concentrations are separate reflections of obesity, rather than interrelated phenomena with a cause-and-effect relationship.

The elevated plasma insulin concentrations that are present in visceral obesity have also been proposed as inhibitors to the release of GH from the hypothalamus and pituitary gland, as well as of the peripheral effects of GH. Nevertheless, a central role for insulin in the hyposomatotropinism of obesity has been weakened by the observation of normal GH levels in other hyperinsulinemic disorders, such as hyperprolactinemia (44).

Growth Hormone Administration in Visceral Obesity

The decrease in GH concentrations in obesity, and more specifically in visceral obesity, has led to the experimental administration of this hormone in an attempt to promote weight loss while preserving proteins and improving fat distribution (45–54).

However, no evidence indicates that these goals have been truly reached. Variable amounts of subcutaneous recombinant human GH (rhGH), when given in combination with isoenergetic diets, cause some decrease in total fat that is only slightly more than that observed in placebo controls (45,53). When rhGH is given in combination with an energy-restricted diet, no statistically significant difference has been found between treatment and placebo injection groups (18,54,55).

Fat distribution has been measured using computed tomography (CT) or magnetic resonance imaging (MRI) in a few studies (45,53,56). Although intraabdominal fat decreased with rhGH treatment, well-controlled studies whereby regional fat loss is assessed in patients with equivalent fat loss have not been conducted. Because visceral fat area virtually always decreases disproportionately to subcutaneous fat area, groups must be matched on the amount of total fat loss to be able to assess confidently whether an intervention is "specific" for visceral fat. Even if visceral fat were lost to a greater degree with rhGH therapy, the adverse metabolic consequences associated with its use would argue against a beneficial effect (see later discussion).

Many studies report an increase in FFM with rhGH treatment. Unfortunately, virtually all of these studies are confounded by GH-induced water retention, unless lean tissue is measured using total body potassium. The one study using this technique found no change in FFM after treatment with GH or a placebo (53). Other parameters of changes in muscle mass are nitrogen balance and muscle strength, both of which were studied after a hypocaloric diet in GH-treated versus placebo-treated groups. Muscle strength increased equally in both groups after an exercise program (54), and nitrogen balance was more negative in the placebo group than in the GH group (46,47,49,57). The latter difference, however, was attenuated or even completely lost after 4 and 5 weeks of treatment, respectively (47,48).

When side effects are reported, at least 20% to 40% of the volunteers receiving GH develop reactions such as fluid retention, arthralgias, or carpal tunnel syndrome (45,47, 48,53,54). In children, but not adults, the induction of sleep apnea has been reported (58).

Adverse metabolic effects of rhGH treatment in obesity include decreased high-density lipoprotein (HDL), increased FFA concentrations, and, more importantly, insulin resistance. Despite reassuring claims, in all of the studies available for review, even small amounts of GH (0.025 to 1 mg of rhGH per kilogram of ideal body weight) decreased glucose disposal rates and increased levels of glucose, insulin, and 24-hour C-peptide excretion (18,45–49,53,55,56). This was particularly prominent in, but not limited to, studies in which rhGH was not combined with an energy-restricted diet. In other studies, the adverse effects on glucose metabolism have either not been described (51,54) or, when measured, may not have been statistically significant. However, considering the size of most study populations, the latter should be interpreted with caution, and the clear trends apparent from most studies should be taken seriously.

In summary, no evidence demonstrates substantial beneficial effects of GH administration in visceral obesity. In contrast, in all studies investigating glucose metabolism, insulin resistance was induced to a greater or lesser extent. Other side effects almost invariably included fluid retention, arthralgias, and carpal tunnel syndrome.

Moreover, the rationale of GH administration in obesity is questionable. Low GH levels in most patients with visceral obesity are a consequence not of a primary endocrine deficiency but of an adaptation to an altered physiology. These GH levels return to normal with weight reduction (43). The mechanism of the low GH concentration in obesity is not known with certainty, but high plasma FFA concentrations have been implicated. Instituting a treatment before understanding the mechanism may be disadvantageous rather than beneficial, a belief that has been substantiated by the published reports.

Finally, GH administration does not remove the cause of the problem, thus necessitating supplementation as long as obesity exists. Considering the high costs and the lack of insight into the long-term consequences, the authors do not advise this.

Testosterone

Physiology

General Considerations on Fuel Partitioning

Testosterone is a major anabolic hormone in humans (Fig. 7.4). During male puberty, dramatic increases in skeletal muscle mass and reductions in body fat occur that are mediated by testosterone, which perhaps acts in concert with GH. Testosterone does not exert its effect directly but is converted into dihydrotestosterone (DHT) or estrogens. Both function via nuclear receptors to modify gene transcription.

In addition to being responsible for the development of the primary and secondary sexual characteristics of the male, testosterone markedly influences nutrient partitioning. Its most evident influence is on protein metabolism as it increases the rate of protein formation in target cells, most noticeably myocytes, thus promoting muscle development. This also accounts for the typical lower percentage of body fat in men (about 15%) than in women (about 30%) and their greater RMR, and thus energy expenditure, relative to body weight than that of women. Testosterone also affects body fat distribution and decreases adipose-tissue fatty acid uptake, and it may affect lipolysis in a manner that is perhaps related to its synergistic effects with GH. The abrupt loss of testosterone in males rapidly results in fat gain and the loss of lean tissue and muscle strength (59), thus emphasizing the importance of this hormone in directing substrate partitioning.

Resting Energy Expenditure and the Thermic Effect of Food and Exercise

The redistribution of the body fuel stores toward protein anabolism and away from fat storage results in a greater percentage of the body as lean tissue. These increases in testosterone have not been found to increase RMR beyond levels that may be explained by the increased LBM in healthy men. However, in a small group of men with muscular

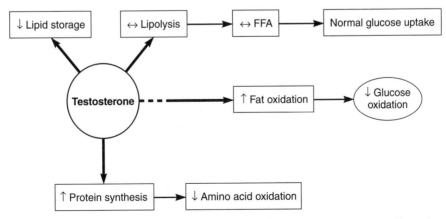

FIG. 7.4. Effects of testosterone on substrate availability and oxidation. The effect of testosterone on lipolysis is somewhat controversial. *In vitro* evidence of increased lipolysis has not been confirmed *in vivo*. Abbreviation: FFA, free fatty acid.

dystrophy, small increases in RMR did seem to occur (60). The effect of testosterone on the other major components of daily energy expenditure (TEF or energy expended on physical activity) has not been well studied.

Substrate Availability and Oxidation

The effects of testosterone on whole-body protein and fat metabolism have been primarily studied using testosterone supplementation in hypogonadal men and adolescents with delayed puberty, as well as by the artificial induction of testosterone deficiency in lean, healthy young men (59,61,62). The latter was achieved via the administration of gonadotropin-releasing hormone (GnRH) analogs. In these experiments in which GH and IGF-1 remained unchanged, a rapid decline in whole-body protein synthesis and proteolysis was observed that resulted in a decrease in FFM and muscle strength (59). Testosterone supplementation studies have confirmed these conclusions, except for the effects on proteolysis, which was found to decline under the influence of testosterone as well.

In all studies, amino acid oxidation rates and plasma amino acid concentrations remained unchanged, suggesting that testosterone amplifies muscle mass by enhancing the intracellular partitioning of amino acids towards protein synthesis, particularly in muscle, rather than by increasing amino acid uptake. The latter has been confirmed in amino acid tracer studies of testosterone administration in healthy young men (63). These studies were conducted in fasted states, and, under physiologic conditions, cellular amino acid availability and uptake are expected to increase as well as a result of postprandial fluctuations in other hormones, such as insulin and GH.

Acute testosterone deficiency diminished the rates of lipid oxidation and the RMR, and it increased body fat mass. This suggests that the testosterone-induced increases in fatty acid oxidation are not entirely due to the greater muscle mass.

To what extent these changes in fat oxidation result from direct effects on intracellular fatty acid trafficking or from changes in FFA availability is not known. Although testosterone increases adipocyte lipolytic responsiveness to catecholamines (e.g., norepinephrine, isoproterenol, and forskolin) in *in vivo* and *in vitro* studies (64,65), the basal lipolytic rates are not influenced. In addition, *in vivo* markers of basal lipolysis have remained unchanged in some testosterone supplementation studies (61).

Fat deposition is greatly influenced by testosterone via its inhibition of LPL (65). (This is further discussed in "Regional Fat Storage" below.)

No evident changes in serum glucose levels or glucose availability have been observed after the induction of hypogonadism in healthy men. Insulin concentrations have a tendency to increase with acute testosterone deficiency (59). Of note is the effect of testosterone treatment in adolescents with delayed puberty; such treatment causes insulin-stimulated oxidative and nonoxidative glucose disposal rates to decline (61). These effects could well be temporary, as is the insulin resistance of puberty; and they may be related to the increased competition caused by greater fatty acid oxidation. In obese men who are known to have lower plasma testosterone levels, testosterone administration increases insulin-stimulated glucose disposal rates (66). Whether this is a direct or an indirect effect that perhaps relates to changes in fat distribution or adipose-tissue function is unclear.

In summary, testosterone increases the oxidation of fatty acids but not of amino acids. The typical protein anabolic effects result from altered intracellular trafficking rather than the increased uptake of amino acids. The reported small effects on glucose metabolism may be the indirect results of fat redistribution.

Regional Fat Storage

Testosterone has distinct effects on body fat distribution, although the androgen and/or fat distribution association varies with gender and stage of development. The increase in testosterone during male puberty is associated with an increase in the portion of intraabdominally stored fat and a concomitant reduction in the relative amount of fat in the lower body. Analogously, adult women with excess androgens demonstrate an increase in intraabdominal fat, and women who develop visceral obesity are found to have increased serum concentrations of free testosterone.

In contrast, adult hypogonadal men also have increased visceral fat that is reduced after testosterone replacement (67), and viscerally obese men have lower serum free testosterone concentrations (68,69). Thus, blanket statements cannot be made about the effects of androgens on regional fat storage.

Testosterone may modify body fat distribution by altering the regional fatty acid uptake or regional lipolysis, and indications that it influences both do exist. Administration of testosterone to hypogonadal men and to viscerally obese men with low serum testosterone concentrations shifts fat deposition from intraabdominal to subcutaneous sites (66). This is associated with concordant changes in regional meal fatty acid uptake as measured with radioactive tracer studies (70). In addition, either 6 weeks or 9 months of testosterone administration decrease LPL activity, a putative mediator of regional fat uptake, in subcutaneous abdominal, but not femoral, fat (65,71,72).

Some evidence also has been found for the regional variability in lipolysis as a result of testosterone "replacement." Testosterone administration decreases the half-life of fatty acids in abdominal, as opposed to femoral, subcutaneous fat in men with lower serum testosterone concentrations (70). Although these radioactive tracer studies suggest that increased lipolysis occurs with testosterone treatment, reductions in uptake that are combined with reductions in regional fat mass may give the same appearance.

Because many studies on the effects of testosterone on regional fat distribution have been conducted in obese subjects in whom the testosterone dynamics are notoriously altered, extrapolation of the above-mentioned results to healthy lean subjects should be done with caution. However, the fact that fat typically accumulates in the upper body in healthy men, an effect that seems to be representative of testosterone, indicates that this extrapolation is justified. Moreover, similar effects of testosterone on fat distribution have been found in physiologic animal studies. Among others, intraabdominal fat depots have been shown to have a higher density of androgen receptors than do subcutaneous depots in rats (73,74).

Testosterone and Visceral Obesity

Testosterone deficiency leads to visceral fat accumulation; however, analogous to GH, visceral obesity as a primary entity is also associated with lower free testosterone levels in men (69). As has been noted, however, visceral obesity in women is associated with increased free testosterone levels (72). A satisfactory explanation for this paradox has not yet been found. Whether the central fat accumulation leads to changed testosterone levels or vice versa is undetermined. In both sexes, weight loss consistently has been found to reverse the abnormalities in testosterone levels (75–78).

Although several theories have postulated that hormones, such as leptin and GH, mediate the observed changes, neither of these is compatible with the changes in testosterone levels that are observed in women (79,80).

Testosterone Administration in Visceral Obesity

Given the known effects of testosterone on nutrient partitioning and the finding that visceral obesity in men is associated with reduced testosterone, testosterone must logically be considered as therapy for obese men. A number of studies have been performed to examine this approach. Intramuscular (250 to 500 mg, one time dose), oral (40 mg four times a day), and transdermal (125 to 250 mg per day) testosterone administration have consistently caused a significant decrease in visceral fat compared with a placebo (65,66,81,82). Somewhat surprisingly, no significant changes were observed in total body fat quantities or LBM.

Testosterone also results in a reduction in waist to hip ratios (WHRs), cholesterol levels (66,82), and, in some studies, serum triglyceride concentrations (82). HDL cholesterol levels remain unchanged (66,82). In addition, testosterone improves insulin action with respect to glucose disposal (66,81,82). The latter is most pronounced in the males who have the lowest testosterone levels before the intervention, and it is thought to be an indirect effect of the reducing visceral fat mass (see "Testosterone and Visceral Obesity"). DHT administration has neither of these effects (81,82). In contrast, lowering androgen concentrations in hyperandrogenic women with GnRH analogs, which also reduce serum estrogen, does not reduce the visceral fat mass (83).

Nevertheless, the practice of administering testosterone to obese men is open to debate. The precise explanation for low free testosterone concentrations in obese men is unknown. Analogous to GH, the low testosterone level may result from adaptations to an altered environment, rather than being the representation of a primary endocrine problem. This is confirmed by the fact that weight loss reverses the abnormalities. For example, testosterone replacement has been reported to create sleep apnea in males (84), and excess endogenous testosterone is associated with sleep apnea in females (85). Another reported side effect in males is prostate hypertrophy.

In summary, testosterone influences protein and fat deposition, and it has major effects on regional adipose-tissue depots. Indications that testosterone replacement may have beneficial effects on fat distribution, lipid profiles, and insulin sensitivity in viscerally obese men with low serum testosterone concentrations do exist. However, routine treatment with testosterone, except in the case of true hypogonadism, is still controversial. Whether the benefits of testosterone replacement in men with modest reductions in serum concentrations outweigh the risks of treatment is unknown.

Estrogens

Physiology

General Considerations

Estrogens are produced primarily in the ovaries and, to some extent, in the adrenals and adipose tissue via conversion of androgens. In humans, the most important estrogen is β-estradiol.

In addition to the role of estrogens in the development of female sex characteristics, they exert mild anabolic effects on fuel partitioning, most noticeably on body fat and its distribution. During female puberty, fat is redistributed onto the gluteofemoral region, an action that is thought to be estrogen mediated. Despite maintaining substantially more body fat (an average of 30% in nonobese women compared with 15% in nonobese men), females have less visceral fat and greater amounts of lower body fat than males do and lower cardiac risk factors (e.g., serum lipids), which perhaps are related to this differing body fat distribution. This gender difference persists throughout the adult reproductive life, but it does begin to reverse after menopause.

Whether estrogens directly influence the moderate anabolic effects and other aspects of fuel partitioning associated with their presence is controversial. Despite the common presence of a physiologic deficiency state (menopause) that should facilitate research into these issues, the interpretation of study results is complicated by several factors.

First, the effects of estrogens on fuel partitioning are subtle compared with, for example, those of testosterone, and therefore they are more difficult to determine. Small changes might be noticeable within individuals, but they may be more difficult to detect in cross-sectional studies. Thus, although longitudinal study approaches are the most suitable for investigations into these issues, cross-sectional studies, which are easier to conduct, are more abundant. The results of these studies are sometimes conflicting.

Other methodologic problems, including the enormous variability in research techniques for measuring similar variables, have added to the difficulty in identifying a nutrient partitioning effect of estrogens. For example, intraabdominal fat accumulation has been assessed by waist circumference, WHR, CT, MRI, and dual-energy x-ray absorptiometry, all of which have different accuracy and reproducibility levels. In addition, in many studies, confounding factors, such as age, have not been taken into account in the analyses.

Finally, estrogens interact with other hormonal systems. In addition to the obvious cyclic and therapeutic interaction with progesterone, estrogens decrease free testosterone concentrations but increase GH production. These contrasting influences on two strongly anabolic hormones may blur the direct measurable effects of estrogens in *in vivo* studies. This is best illustrated by the estrogen-stimulated GH production, which is known to be vital for pubertal growth (59) but which, in adult life, may influence fuel partitioning. Estrogen administration has been found to increase GH production if it is given orally but not if it is dispensed transdermally (86,87). Although the reason for this difference is not completely understood, it may influence the apparent effects of estrogen on fuel partitioning.

To what extent estrogen effects are exerted by interactions—either in synergy or by indirect means—with GH and testosterone is unclear. Although estrogens would appear to have independent nutrient-partitioning effects, the gender differences in fuel partitioning could be argued to result primarily from the difference in testosterone concentrations. This seems unlikely as hypogonadal men have a body fat content and distribution that differs distinctly from that of women. In addition, although aspects of body composition do change in postmenopausal women, they do not have the same nutrient partitioning as men. Therefore, a modest but direct effect on nutrient partitioning seems likely.

Resting Energy Expenditure and the Thermic Effect of Food and Exercise

The RMR has been reported to increase, decrease, or remain unchanged under the influence of estrogen (88–91). However, these conclusions are also mostly based on intramenstrual comparisons or on indirect correlations; one of the few longitudinal studies that has been conducted reported a decrease in RMR of 100 kcal per day after menopause, but this was confounded by lower FFM and physical activity levels in the postmenopausal group (88). Estrogens seem to increase absolute LBM (88,92) and thus RMR (see "Body Composition" below).

The TEF has been found to increase during the follicular phase of the menstrual cycle (91). In obese women, however, glucose-induced thermogenesis is unrelated to estrogen levels when it is corrected for FFM (90). Although studies of menstrual cycle effects and oral contraceptive effects on substrate oxidation during exercise have been conducted, no studies of the thermic effect of exercise or nutrient partitioning during exercise in estrogen-replete versus estrogen-deficient women have been performed. Thus, the effects that estrogen may have on nutrient partitioning during exercise are not known.

Substrate Availability

The influence of estrogens on protein metabolism is controversial, but estrogen appears to have little, if any, effect on the circulating amino acid availability. Estrogen administration to hypogonadal girls (93) and inhibition of estrogen synthesis in young men via the aromatase inhibitor anastrozole (94) do not affect whole-body protein pools, amino acid turnover rates, or amino acid oxidation. In the latter study (94), estrogen inhibition increased testosterone concentrations and decreased IGF levels by 18%, despite unchanged concentrations of GH and IGFBP-3.

That estrogen modulates the synthesis of selected hepatic, endometrial, and other proteins in humans is without question (93). The effects of estrogen on these selected protein pools occur without changing whole-body protein kinetics, however, perhaps because the tissues that are strongly affected account for a relatively minor fraction of total protein synthetic activity.

The effect of estrogens on adipose-tissue fuel export but not that on triglyceride uptake has been examined in humans. Estrogens have been reported to increase or decrease lipolysis or to leave it changed, both in animal and in human studies (73,95). Intervention studies, however, have shown that transdermal estrogen decreases adipose-tissue FFA release in postmenopausal women (96) and that it lowers plasma FFA concentrations in ovariectomized women (97).

Neither glucose production nor insulin-mediated glucose disposal has been shown to be influenced by estrogens in humans. Contrary to the decrease in glucose disposal found in ovariectomized rats and mice (98), insulin sensitivity in postmenopausal women is reported to be unchanged or even increased (98). Longitudinal studies of women going through menopause found unchanged glucose tolerance (99) and increased fasting plasma insulin concentrations, but fasting glucose levels were unchanged (88). Changes in the fasting insulin level in the perimenopausal period are confounded by changes in body fat and body fat distribution that commonly occur at this time of life (88).

The ability to draw unshakable conclusions from the available studies is limited by the variability in insulin-sensitivity measurements ranging from fasting plasma glucose level to insulin clamp techniques, by the methodologic difficulties mentioned, and possibly by the fact that studies may be conducted too early in menopause to observe differences. Nevertheless, estrogen-replacement studies arrive at similar conclusions; therefore, one may safely state that the impact of estrogen on glucose metabolism in humans is too subtle to be clinically significant, if it is present at all.

Substrate Oxidation

Conflicting data about whether estrogen alters the partitioning of fat and glucose toward oxidation are available from human studies. One group reported that combined estrogen and progesterone supplementation of postmenopausal women did not alter basal substrate oxidation, but that, after a mixed meal, carbohydrate oxidation increased at the expense of lipid oxidation (86). This change occurred only at 30 to 60 minutes after meal ingestion and only in the group of women given oral estrogens. Transdermal estrogen administration resulted in an opposite, but nonsignificant, effect. Another study failed to find effects of transdermal estrogen treatment on substrate oxidation under basal, insulin clamp, or adrenergic-stimulation conditions (96). Inhibition of estrogen synthesis in men with an aromatase inhibitor tended (p =0.09) to reduce basal lipid oxidation (94).

In conclusion, estrogens affect FFA availability and perhaps substrate oxidation. Estrogen-deficient women have greater adipose-tissue lipolysis, but not necessarily greater fat oxidation, than do estrogen-replete women. Estrogens selectively increase protein synthesis in some tissues without substantially changing whole-body protein synthesis. Contrary to animal studies, in humans, estrogens appear to have little, if any, influence on insulin-mediated glucose disposal.

Body Composition

Although estrogens clearly appear to increase body fat, this is not true for visceral fat. This issue could be relevant to the reduced cardiovascular health risks in women. The question has been primarily investigated in the menopausal transition, and it appears to be especially subject to the methodologic difficulties described earlier.

The cross-sectional studies have reported that visceral fat either increases after menopause or remains unchanged; no reports of decreased visceral fat have been found (98). Studies using CT and MRI, techniques that have better accuracy and reproducibility, generally report a postmenopausal increase in intraabdominal fat.

The only two longitudinal studies available for review confirmed postmenopausal increases in waist circumference and WHR with an unchanged BMI. The first retrospectively reanalyzed a longitudinal study of 1,462 women (100); and the second monitored a cohort of 35 women for 6 years, a time period during which half of the women experienced menopause. The latter lost more FFM and RMR than the other subjects, but their fasting glucose levels were comparable (88). These postmenopausal women were found to have a decreased level of physical activity, which could have also contributed to the observed changes.

This decrease in FFM after menopause has been confirmed by some, but not all, cross-sectional investigations (98). Intervention studies, however, have found that estrogen and progesterone combination therapy prevents the postmenopausal increase in body fat (101) and that it increases muscle mass and creatinine excretion in postmenopausal women (92). The absence of change in body weight implies a shift in body composition away from fat toward muscle. In an exception to this pattern, one study reported that oral estrogen replacement in postmenopausal women resulted in a significant reduction in lean tissue that was accompanied by a gain in fat tissue; this effect was not seen with transdermal estrogen replacement (86).

In conclusion, despite some conflicting results, longitudinal and interventional studies suggest that estrogen preserves FFM in postmenopausal women. The mechanism, however, remains unclear.

Regional Fat Storage

Many authorities believe the gender-related distribution of body fat can be at least partly attributed to the regional variability in the sensitivity of LPL to estrogens. The inhibitory effect of estrogens on adipose-tissue LPL was first demonstrated in rat adipose tissue (71) and was confirmed *in vivo* in obese women (102). In the latter, a BMI-independent negative correlation was found between plasma estradiol concentrations and LPL activity, both in gluteal adipose tissue and in post–heparin administration plasma. In addition, in lean and obese men, femoral adipose-tissue LPL is more susceptible to suppression by estrogens and testosterone than is its abdominal counterpart (71).

Whether estrogen influences regional variability in other factors that might modulate regional fat distribution, such as adipose-tissue lipolysis, is as yet unknown.

Estrogen-Replacement Therapy and Nutrient Partitioning

The same difficulties encountered in the study of body fat distribution are found in the study of estrogen replacement and its effects on fuel partitioning, and, consequently, results are contradictory (99).

A large metaanalysis concluded that the many available studies provide insufficient evidence for dependable conclusions on the effects of estrogen-replacement therapy on WHR, fat mass, and skinfold thickness (103). Interestingly, this study concluded that neither menopause nor estrogen-replacement therapy affect BMI, regardless of the therapeutic regiment that is chosen.

However, a study of the effects of hormone-replacement therapy (HRT) on body composition and fat distribution in postmenopausal women derives its relevance from the relationship of body fat to cardiovascular risk factors. Although HRT generally has favorable effects on serum lipid concentrations, the effects on insulin resistance and glucose disposal are more difficult to determine—the methodologic problems described earlier are augmented by small sample sizes, a short duration of treatment, and variable and often suboptimal methods for measuring insulin sensitivity.

The gold standard for the last, the hyperinsulinemic euglycemic clamp technique, was used by one crossover study only. This study reported unchanged glucose disposal in postmenopausal women, both after transdermal and oral estrogen monotherapy (87). Transdermal estrogen did, however, lead to greater FFA suppression during the clamp, suggesting an improvement in insulin action on adipose-tissue antilipolysis or increased clearance of FFA. Treatment of women with type II diabetes with estrogen for 6 weeks caused a slight, but significant, decrease in hemoglobin A_{1C} without changing insulin-mediated glucose uptake or plasma FFA concentrations (104).

The concomitant use of progestins clouds the evaluation of estrogen replacement on insulin sensitivity. In animal studies, progestins appear to decrease insulin sensitivity, a result that confirms some, but not all, human studies in which they show a tendency to attenuate the beneficial effects of estrogens on insulin sensitivity (99). The wide variety and dosages of progestins that are used make drawing firm conclusions regarding their effects on substrate partitioning difficult. No strong evidence indicates that HRT—whether combined or with estrogen alone—alters substrate partitioning in a manner that alters the total body fat mass, although the HRT does maintain a female fat distribution. Estrogen administration solely for this purpose does not appear to be indicated, and the decision to provide HRT should be based on traditional clinical considerations, such as osteoporosis, hot flashes, and coagulation risks.

In conclusion, the beneficial effects of postmenopausal estrogen-replacement therapy on serum lipids are well established. However, no proof exists to indicate that this is related to a decrease in intraabdominal fat deposition and that total body fat is not affected. Some evidence demonstrates the modest anabolic effects of estrogen on lean tissue. Despite reports on different influences on fuel partitioning and GH levels, sufficiently convincing evidence does not appear to exist in this regard, nor is recommending a specific route of estrogen administration possible.

Glucocorticoids

Physiology

General Considerations on Fuel Partitioning

The major nutrient-partitioning effects of glucocorticoids, of which 95% of the endogenous glucocorticoid activity is cortisol, are catabolic (Fig. 7.5). Their impact on fuel partitioning is particularly important in physical stress situations and in exogenous (iatrogenic) or pathologic endogenous hypercortisolemia.

Cortisol increases the amount of fuel molecules in the circulation by inhibiting the synthesis of glycogen, fat, and skeletal muscle protein while the increasing breakdown of the last two. In addition, glucocorticoids stimulate appetite, likely via the suppression of corticotropin-releasing hormone (CRH) as discussed below, thus providing the body with additional fuel.

The catabolic qualities of cortisol are far from random. Fat, protein, and carbohydrate supplies are mobilized, restored, and redirected according to their biologic priority in stress situations. For example, protein breakdown is disproportionately increased in many extrahepatic tissues. The amino acids thus derived are used by the liver for enhanced protein synthesis, thereby guaranteeing the production of acute-phase proteins. Immunoglobulin synthesis in lymphocytes also increases.

With prolonged hypercortisolemia, protein catabolism progressively outpaces protein synthesis (105,106). For example, in Cushing syndrome, protein wasting becomes especially evident in the skeletal muscle and skin. Furthermore, the decreased fat deposition in

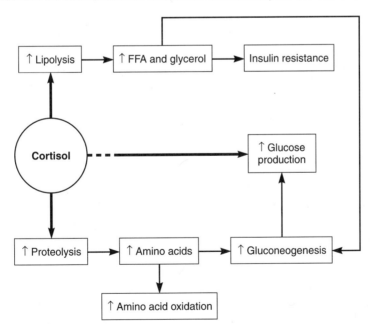

FIG. 7.5. Effects of cortisol on substrate availability and oxidation. All of these effects are counteracted to some extent by an increased insulin secretion, and they can sometimes be offset completely. This is particularly true for lipolytic influences. Abbreviation: FFA, free fatty acid.

the extremities and the increased fat accumulation in the face and trunk lead to the classic fat redistribution of Cushing syndrome despite the presence of greater fat mobilization.

Finally, prolonged and/or extreme corticosteroid excess can induce diabetes. The relative insulin deficiency of the diabetic state further aggravates the protein catabolic effects of hypercortisolemia. Thus, the combination of corticosteroid excess and uncontrolled diabetes is particularly disadvantageous with respect to nutrient partitioning (107).

Cortisol and the Hypothalamic–Pituitary–Adrenal Axis

The interaction between the hypothalamus (CRH), the pituitary (adrenocorticotropic hormone [ACTH]), and the adrenals (glucocorticoids) provides the basic endocrine regulatory system; however, numerous modulating factors may be superimposed on this system and thus may alter cortisol secretion. These internal and external conditions include illness and injury; hypoglycemia; psychologic depression; and environmental factors, such as excess alcohol or nicotine and temperature differences (108). Hypothalamic nuclei integrate the various impulses (109).

In addition, the regulation of the hypothalamic–pituitary–adrenal (HPA) axis is intertwined with food intake and energy balance. Most types of hypercortisolemia increase appetite (110), an effect that is thought to be mediated by feedback inhibition of corticosteroids on CRH release.

CRH is a potent anorectic peptide that, in rodent models, reduces the body weight threshold for food-hoarding behavior (111). It is therefore thought to mediate the anorexia of primary adrenal insufficiency. In addition, obesity has been proposed to be a CRH-deficient state, a suggestion that is discussed below.

Resting Energy Expenditure and the Thermic Effect of Food and Exercise

RMR is reported to increase by 9% to 15% following hydrocortisone infusions at physiologic and supraphysiologic infusion levels (80 and 200 μg per kg per h, respectively) (105,112). Another report indicates that the administration of oral prednisone for 1 week does not increase RMR (105); however, many methodologic factors complicate the comparison of this study to the former. To the authors' knowledge, no information on the effects of cortisol on the thermic effects of food or exercise is available.

Substrate Availability and Oxidation

Hypercortisolemia increases plasma concentrations of glucose, amino acids, and fatty acids. In stress situations, this facilitates the delivery of fuel and substrate supplies to tissues that are dependent on these compounds to mount a host defense.

This is particularly evident in protein and fat metabolism, in which whole-body catabolic effects of hypercortisolemia dominate the isolated selective anabolic effects (105). In acute hypercortisolemia, the well-demonstrated increase in whole-body proteolysis (105,112,113) is accompanied by a decrease in whole-body protein synthesis (38). However, as has been mentioned, the synthesis of some hepatic and lymphocyte proteins is selectively stimulated (106). Overall, amino acid oxidation increases (105,114). With chronic hypercortisolemia, whole-body protein synthesis has been shown to decrease, but the effects on proteolysis are controversial (38,107).

Analogously, acute hypercortisolemia has been demonstrated to have a net whole-body lipolytic effect and to result in increased FFA concentrations and a trend toward increased fat oxidation (105) despite the simultaneous, perhaps localized, stimulation of LPL (115).

Cortisol has been demonstrated to facilitate catecholamine-induced lipolysis *in vivo,* despite conflicting *in vitro* evidence (116–118). However, the subsequent FFA release is largely counteracted by concomitant insulin overproduction (119). In chronic hypercortisolemia, a net increase in fat mass and body weight is observed (120).

Some *in vitro* studies of human adipose tissue have also shown that cortisol increases LPL activity and fat uptake (115). These investigators suggested that small amounts of insulin are needed for LPL enhancement (115), which may be important given the insulin resistance and hyperinsulinemia that are induced by excess glucocorticoids.

One suggestion is that regional stimulation of LPL might contribute to the redistribution of fat by cortisol, similar to its role in protein metabolism. Fat may be broken down in one region but stored in another under conditions of excess glucocorticoid availability—although lipolysis supplies increased amounts of FFA to peripheral tissue, circulating triglycerides (VLDL and chylomicrons), which are derived from increased food intake, may be preferentially stored in truncal fat as is discussed below.

The increased FFA supply stimulates fatty acid oxidation, as both indirect calorimetric measurements (decrease in the respiratory quotient) (105) and the appearance of ketone bodies (112) demonstrate. Whether cortisol also increases fat oxidation via direct intracellular effects is unclear.

Glucose levels are almost invariably reported to increase during both acute and chronic hypercortisolemia, an effect that is only partially attenuated by the simultaneous increase in insulin levels (113,121,122). The decrease in insulin-stimulated glucose uptake (35,104,112) in response to hypercortisolism may be due to the increased circulating FFA level. As would be expected, the whole-body glucose oxidation diminishes (105). Glucose overproduction can be, in part, attributed to the increased gluconeogenesis that is induced by the increased supply of amino acids, especially alanine, and glycerol, derived from protein and fat mobilization (35,122).

The combination of increased circulating glucose and peripheral insulin resistance likely also reflects the redistribution of fuel. The peripheral organs thus are forced to derive their energy from fat, perhaps to spare glucose for use by the brain.

Regional Fat Storage

The central fat accumulation characteristic of chronic hypercortisolemia is likely due to regional differences in cortisol effects on either the adipocyte fatty acid uptake or lipolysis. Alternatively, regional differences in fat cell proliferation, differentiation, or apoptosis in response to excess cortisol could play a role in the fat redistribution of Cushing syndrome. Cortisol affects abdominal adipose tissue more than gluteofemoral adipose tissue. In women with Cushing syndrome, subcutaneous abdominal adipose-tissue LPL activity increases threefold, whereas lipolytic rates were 50% less than those found in lean control subjects and lower-body obese women (118). In contrast, in the femoral region, lipolytic rates and LPL activity are similar in these three groups and in upper-body obese women.

The net response of intraabdominal adipose tissue to cortisol is similar to that of subcutaneous abdominal fat; treatment of Cushing syndrome in women results in a clear redistribution of fat from the visceral depots to the legs (120).

The physiologic mediator of the regional difference in fat accumulation in response to excess cortisol has not been definitely determined. The density of glucocorticoid receptors in visceral adipose tissue has been shown to be higher than that in other tissues (120), which could contribute to the observed effects. Unfortunately, the analyses of these studies are complicated by the lack of information that is given regarding the site from which fat was taken. When the data are reported, many times different sites are pooled for analysis, thus preventing firm conclusions from being drawn.

The Hypothalamic–Pituitary–Adrenal Axis and Obesity

Visceral obesity shares many characteristics with Cushing syndrome. Both conditions are associated with large abdominal subcutaneous fat cells with high lipolytic qualities, insulin resistance, hypertension, and even buccal fat accumulation (123,124). Because neither of these is typical of lower-body obesity, visceral adiposity has been suggested to be associated with changes in the HPA axis or cortisol receptors. One glucocorticoid receptor polymorphism is associated with visceral obesity (125); however, how common or physiologically relevant these types of gene polymorphisms are in visceral obesity is unclear.

Several changes in the HPA axis have been found in obesity, and they are more prevalent in the visceral, rather than the gluteofemoral, type (108). The secretory rates of cortisol are elevated in most, but not all studies, even when corrected for body surface area, although the plasma concentrations of cortisol remain normal or they are slightly lowered (108,109). This is thought to be a result of increased plasma cortisol clearance rates. Indeed, many, but not all, human studies report increased urinary cortisol excretion rates in obesity (124). In addition, the urinary excretion of 5-reductase cortisol metabolites is positively correlated with waist circumference in nonobese men and postmenopausal women, which suggests that fat accumulation in the upper body is associated with increased cortisol turnover (126).

To the extent that cortisol production is increased in upper-body obesity, an idea that is not uniformly accepted, indications that components of the HPA axis might be hyperactive do exist. The adrenal sensitivity to ACTH; the responsiveness of ACTH and cortisol to CRH; and several adrenal stimulation tests, such as postprandial HPA activation, have all been reported to be increased in obesity (124). However, these parameters have been unchanged in other investigations. Absolute ACTH levels were comparable in obese and lean individuals in most studies (124).

Thus, in obesity, the HPA axis is reported to be hyperactive or normal. This somewhat contradicts the concept of obesity as a CRH-deficient state. This theory of obesity as a CRH-deficient state, which has been substantiated by rat and molecular experiments, has further been challenged by the finding of either normal or only slightly lowered cerebrospinal CRH levels in obese humans (124).

The study of the HPA axis in visceral obesity is complicated by several obstacles that likely account for some of the inconsistent findings. For example, earlier investigations have studied different obesity phenotypes as one entity. This may have confounded the results considerably, because central obesity with its cushingoid fat distribution may be associated with entirely different dynamics of the HPA axis than are those of peripheral obesity. Another difficulty is the complexity of the regulation of the HPA axis, which is influenced by many heterogeneous and often uncontrollable variables, thus complicating standardization for research purposes and the subsequent interpretation of the results.

Finally, the latter is additionally complicated by the intertwined relationship between food intake, energy balance, and the HPA axis. For example, changes in body weight trigger counterregulatory mechanisms whose aim is to maintain the steady state that is thought to be mediated by the HPA axis. Thus, compensatory mechanisms blur the effect of weight change, a fact that is reflected by the observation that both overfeeding and starvation experiments have been found to amplify cortisol production (108).

In summary, an intertwined and complex relationship exists between energy balance, food intake, and several components of the HPA axis. In visceral, and to a much lesser extent gluteofemoral, obesity, increased cortisol secretion and clearance rates result in normal or decreased plasma concentrations. No evidence indicates an increased exposure of cells and tissues to cortisol in visceral obesity, despite its similarities with Cushing syndrome. Whether changes on an intracellular or receptor level are involved is currently unknown.

Managing Glucocorticoid Therapy in Obese Patients

Considering the adverse effects of corticosteroids on muscle mass, body fat, and insulin sensitivity, counteracting their side effects in long-term therapeutic use would be beneficial. This is particularly relevant in obese patients. One approach has been to coadminister protein anabolic hormones with corticosteroids; this has met with only limited success. GH has been shown to counteract the whole-body protein catabolic effects of acute hypercortisolemia, but the aggravation of glucose intolerance precludes its therapeutic use (113). Testosterone therapy after long-term steroid treatment in asthmatic patients slightly increases FFM (0.9 kg), decreases body fat, and improves bone density (127). However, HDL levels also decrease, and whether these and other perhaps as yet undiscovered side effects outweigh the minor improvements in body composition is unclear.

Therefore, the preferred approach to maintain skeletal muscle mass and limit fat gain during corticosteroid therapy is physical activity and resistance exercise, particularly considering its additional beneficial effects for reducing fat mass.

CONCLUSION

The balance between energy intake and energy expenditure may greatly influence human health and obesity, as may the trafficking of different nutrients within the body and cells. The latter process in which the organism selects fuels for storage or oxidation is known as nutrient partitioning. It may be influenced by several variables, some of which are hormones. These exert influence at several different levels, including their effects on the mobilization of FFA, glucose, and amino acids, as well as their subsequent fates within tissues. This chapter first reviewed fuel (i.e., carbohydrate, fat, and protein) processing and then discussed the effects of insulin, GH, testosterone, estrogens, and glucocorticoids on several aspects of nutrient partitioning. These facets include RMR, TEF, and the energy expended on physical activity (e.g., exercise); substrate availability and oxidation; regional fat storage; and the pathophysiologic changes found in obesity. The therapeutic administration of these hormones in visceral obesity has been discussed where it is applicable.

REFERENCES

1. Flatt JP. Carbohydrate balance and food intake regulation. *Am J Clin Nutr* 1995;62:155–157.
2. Kelley DE, Mandarino LJ. Hyperglycemia normalizes insulin-stimulated skeletal muscle glucose oxidation and storage in non–insulin-dependent diabetes mellitus. *J Clin Invest* 1990;86:1999–2007.
3. Acheson KJ, Ravussin E, Wahren J, et al. Thermic effect of glucose in man. Obligatory and facultative thermogenesis. *J Clin Invest* 1984;74:1572–1580.
4. Morgan JB, York DA, Wilkin TJ. Influence of propranolol on the acute thermic effect of feeding in man. *Ann Nutr Metab* 1986;30:386–392.
5. Segal KR, Albu J, Chun A, et al. Independent effects of obesity and insulin resistance on postprandial thermogenesis in men. *J Clin Invest* 1992;89:824–833.
6. Saloranta C, Franssila-Kallunki A, Ekstrand A, et al. Modulation of hepatic glucose production by non-esterified fatty acids in type 2 (non–insulin-dependent) diabetes mellitus. *Diabetologia* 1991;34:409–415.
7. Kelley DE, Mokan M, Simoneau JA, et al. Interaction between glucose and free fatty acid metabolism in human skeletal muscle. *J Clin Invest* 1993;92:91–98.
8. Rigalleau V, Binnert C, Minehira K, et al. In normal men, free fatty acids reduce peripheral but not splanchnic glucose uptake. *Diabetes* 2001;50:727–732.

9. Jensen MD, Haymond MW, Gerich JE, et al. Lipolysis during fasting. Decreased suppression by insulin and increased stimulation by epinephrine. *J Clin Invest* 1987;79:207–213.
10. Jensen MD, Miles JM, Gerich JE, et al. Preservation of insulin effects on glucose production and proteolysis during fasting. *Am J Physiol* 1988;254:E700–E707.
11. Jensen MD, Haymond MW. Protein metabolism in obesity: effects of body fat distribution and hyperinsulinemia on leucine turnover. *Am J Clin Nutr* 1991;53:172–176.
12. Meek S, Persson M, Ford GC, et al. Differential regulation of amino acid exchange and protein dynamics across splanchnic and skeletal muscle beds by insulin in healthy human subjects. *Diabetes* 1998;47:1824–1835.
13. Meek S, Nair KS, Jensen MD. Insulin regulation of regional free fatty acid metabolism. *Diabetes* 1999;48:10–14.
14. Guo ZK, Hensrud DD, Johnson CM, et al. Regional postprandial fatty acid metabolism in different obesity phenotypes. *Diabetes* 1999;48:1586–1592.
15. Romanski SA, Nelson R, Jensen MD. Meal fatty acid uptake in adipose tissue: gender effects in non-obese humans. *Am J Physiol Endocrinol Metab* 2000;279:E455–E462.
16. Eckel RH. Insulin resistance: an adaptation for weight maintenance. *Lancet* 1992;340:1452–1453.
17. Mauras N, O'Brien KO, Welch S, et al. Insulin-like growth factor I and growth hormone (GH) treatment in GH-deficient humans: differential effects on protein, glucose, lipid, and calcium metabolism. *J Clin Endocrinol Metab* 2000;85:1686–1694.
18. Richelsen B, Pedersen SB, Kristensen K, et al. Regulation of lipoprotein lipase and hormone-sensitive lipase activity and gene expression in adipose and muscle tissue by growth hormone treatment during weight loss in obese patients. *Metabolism* 2000;49:906–911.
19. Bengtsson BA, Brummer RJ, Edén S, et al. Effects of growth hormone on fat mass and fat distribution. *Acta Paediatr* 1992;383:62–65.
20. Slavin BG, Ong JM, Kern PA. Hormonal regulation of hormone-sensitive lipase activity and mRNA levels in isolated rat adipocytes. *J Lipid Res* 1994;35:1535–1541.
21. Biller BM, Sesmilo G, Baum HB, et al. Withdrawal of long-term physiological growth hormone (GH) administration: differential effects on bone density and body composition in men with adult-onset GH deficiency. *J Clin Endocrinol Metab* 2000;85:970–976.
22. Brummer RJ. Effects of growth hormone treatment on visceral adipose tissue. *Growth Horm IGF Res* 1998;8:19–23.
23. Russell-Jones DL, Bowes SB, Rees SE, et al. Effect of growth hormone treatment on postprandial protein metabolism in growth hormone-deficient adults. *Am J Physiol* 1998;274:E1050–E1056.
24. O'Sullivan AJ, Kelly JJ, Hoffman DM, et al. Body composition and energy expenditure in acromegaly. *J Clin Endocrinol Metab* 1994;78:381–386.
25. DiGirolamo M, Edén S, Enberg G, et al. Specific binding of human growth hormone but not insulin-like growth factors by human adipocytes. *FEBS Lett* 1986;205:15–19.
26. O'Sullivan AJ, Kelly JJ, Hoffman DM, et al. Energy metabolism and substrate oxidation in acromegaly. *J Clin Endocrinol Metab* 1995;80:486–491.
27. Hoffman DM, O'Sullivan AJ, Freund J, et al. Adults with growth hormone deficiency have abnormal body composition but normal energy metabolism. *J Clin Endocrinol Metab* 1995;80:72–77.
28. Salomon F, Cuneo RC, Hesp R, et al. The effects of treatment with recombinant human growth hormone on body composition and metabolism in adults with growth hormone deficiency. *N Engl J Med* 1989;321:1797–1803.
29. Karlsson C, Stenlof K, Johannsson G, et al. Effects of growth hormone treatment on the leptin system and on energy expenditure in abdominally obese men. *Eur J Endocrinol* 1998;138:408–414.
30. Vaisman N, Zadik Z, Akivias A, et al. Changes in body composition, resting energy expenditure, and thermic effect of food in short children on growth hormone therapy. *Metabolism* 1994;43:1543–1548.
31. Bjorgell P, Rosberg S, Isaksson O, et al. The antilipolytic, insulin-like effect of growth hormone is caused by a net decrease of hormone-sensitive lipase phosphorylation. *Endocrinology* 1984;115:1151–1156.
32. Oscarsson J, Ottosson M, Vikman-Adolfsson K, et al. GH but not IGF-I or insulin increases lipoprotein lipase activity in muscle tissues of hypophysectomized rats. *J Endocrinol* 1999;160:247–255.
33. Ottosson M, Vikman-Adolfsson K, Enerback S, et al. Growth hormone inhibits lipoprotein lipase activity in human adipose tissue. *J Clin Endocrinol Metab* 1995;80:936–941.
34. Richelsen B. Effect of growth hormone on adipose tissue and skeletal muscle lipoprotein lipase activity in humans. *J Endocrinol Invest* 1999;22:10–15.
35. Guyton AC, Hall JE. *Textbook of medical physiology.* Philadelphia: WB Saunders, 2000.
36. Goodman HM. Effects of growth hormone on glucose utilization in diaphragm muscle in the absence of increased lipolysis. *Endocrinology* 1967;81:1099–1103.
37. Seng G, Galgoti C, Louisy P, et al. Metabolic effects of a single administration of growth hormone on lipid and carbohydrate metabolism in normal-weight and obese subjects. *Am J Clin Nutr* 1989;50:1348–1354.
38. Umpleby AM, Russell-Jones DL. The hormonal control of protein metabolism. *Baillieres Clin Endocrinol Metab* 1996;10:551–570.
39. Garlick PJ, McNurlan MA, Bark T, et al. Hormonal regulation of protein metabolism in relation to nutrition and disease. *J Nutr* 1998;128:356S–359S.
40. Moller N, Jorgensen JO, Alberti KG, et al. Short-term effects of growth hormone on fuel oxidation and regional substrate metabolism in normal man. *J Clin Endocrinol Metab* 1990;70:1179–1186.

41. Fryburg DA, Barrett EJ. Growth hormone acutely stimulates skeletal muscle but not whole-body protein synthesis in humans. *Metabolism* 1993;42:1223–1227.
42. Lucidi P, Lauteri M, Laureti S, et al. A dose–response study of growth hormone (GH) replacement on whole body protein and lipid kinetics in GH-deficient adults. *J Clin Endocrinol Metab* 1998;83:353–357.
43. Scacchi M, Pincelli AI, Cavagnini F. Growth hormone in obesity. *Int J Obes Relat Metab Disord* 1999;23: 260–271.
44. Maccario M, Grottoli S, Procopio M, et al. The GH/IGF-I axis in obesity: influence of neuro-endocrine and metabolic factors. *Int J Obes Relat Metab Disord* 2000;24:S96–S99.
45. Richelsen B, Pedersen SB, Børglum JD, et al. Growth hormone treatment of obese women for 5 wk: effect on body composition and adipose tissue LPL activity. *Am J Physiol* 1994;266:E211–E216.
46. Tagliaferri M, Scacchi M, Pincelli AI, et al. Metabolic effects of biosynthetic growth hormone treatment in severely energy-restricted obese women. *Int J Obes Relat Metab Disord* 1998;22:836–841.
47. Snyder DK, Clemmons DR, Underwood LE. Treatment of obese, diet-restricted subjects with growth hormone for 11 weeks: effects on anabolism, lipolysis, and body composition. *J Clin Endocrinol Metab* 1988;67:54–61.
48. Snyder DK, Underwood LE, Clemmons DR. Persistent lipolytic effect of exogenous growth hormone during caloric restriction. *Am J Med* 1995;98:129–134.
49. Drent ML, Wever LD, Adèr HJ, et al. Growth hormone administration in addition to a very low calorie diet and an exercise program in obese subjects. *Eur J Endocrinol* 1995;132:565–572.
50. Snyder DK, Underwood LE, Clemmons DR. Anabolic effects of growth hormone in obese diet-restricted subjects are dose dependent. *Am J Clin Nutr* 1990;52:431–437.
51. Skaggs SR, Crist DM. Exogenous human growth hormone reduces body fat in obese women. *Horm Res* 1991; 35:19–24.
52. Kim KR, Nam SY, Song YD, et al. Low-dose growth hormone treatment with diet restriction accelerates body fat loss, exerts anabolic effect and improves growth hormone secretory dysfunction in obese adults. *Horm Res* 1999;51:78–84.
53. Johannsson G, Mårin P, Lönn L, et al. Growth hormone treatment of abdominally obese men reduces abdominal fat mass, improves glucose and lipoprotein metabolism, and reduces diastolic blood pressure. *J Clin Endocrinol Metab* 1997;82:727–734.
54. Thompson JL, Butterfield GE, Gylfadottir UK, et al. Effects of human growth hormone, insulin-like growth factor I, and diet and exercise on body composition of obese postmenopausal women. *J Clin Endocrinol Metab* 1998;83:1477–1484.
55. Norrelund H, Borglum J, Jorgensen JO, et al. Effects of growth hormone administration on protein dynamics and substrate metabolism during 4 weeks of dietary restriction in obese women. *Clin Endocrinol (Oxf)* 2000; 52:305–312.
56. Nam SY, Kim KR, Cha BS, et al. Low-dose growth hormone treatment combined with diet restriction decreases insulin resistance by reducing visceral fat and increasing muscle mass in obese type 2 diabetic patients. *Int J Obes Relat Metab Disord* 2001;25:1101–1107.
57. Snyder DK, Clemmons DR, Underwood LE. Dietary carbohydrate content determines responsiveness to growth hormone in energy-restricted humans. *J Clin Endocrinol Metab* 1989;69: 745–752.
58. Gerard JM, Garibaldi L, Myers SE, et al. Sleep apnea in patients receiving growth hormone. *Clin Pediatr* 1997; 36:321–326.
59. Mauras N, Hayes V, Welch S, et al. Testosterone deficiency in young men: marked alterations in whole body protein kinetics, strength, and adiposity. *J Clin Endocrinol Metab* 1998;83:1886–1892.
60. Welle S, Jozefowicz R, Forbes G, et al. Effect of testosterone on metabolic rate and body composition in normal men and men with muscular dystrophy. *J Clin Endocrinol Metab* 1992;74:332–335.
61. Arslanian S, Suprasongsin C. Testosterone treatment in adolescents with delayed puberty: changes in body composition, protein, fat, and glucose metabolism. *J Clin Endocrinol Metab* 1997;82:3213–3220.
62. Buchter D, Behre HM, Kliesch S, et al. Effects of testosterone suppression in young men by the gonadotropin releasing hormone antagonist cetrorelix on plasma lipids, lipolytic enzymes, lipid transfer proteins, insulin, and leptin. *Exp Clin Endocrinol Diabetes* 1999;107:522–529.
63. Ferrando AA, Tipton KD, Doyle D, et al. Testosterone injection stimulates net protein synthesis but not tissue amino acid transport. *Am J Physiol Endocrinol Metab* 1998;275:E864–E871.
64. Xu X, De Pergola G, Björntorp P. The effects of androgens on the regulation of lipolysis in adipose precursor cells. *Endocrinology* 1990;126:1229–1234.
65. Rebuffe-Scrive M, Mårin P, Björntorp P. Effect of testosterone on abdominal adipose tissue in men. *Int J Obes* 1991;15:791–795.
66. Mårin P, Holmang S, Jonsson L, et al. The effects of testosterone treatment on body composition and metabolism in middle-aged obese men. *Int J Obes Relat Metab Disord* 1992;16:991–997.
67. Bhasin S, Storer TW, Berman N, et al. Testosterone replacement increases fat-free mass and muscle size in hypogonadal men. *J Clin Endocrinol Metab* 1997;82:407–413.
68. Seidell JC, Björntorp P, Sjostrom L, et al. Visceral fat accumulation in men is positively associated with insulin, glucose, and C-peptide levels, but negatively with testosterone levels. *Metabolism* 1990;39:897–901.
69. Couillard C, Gagnon J, Bergeron J, et al. Contribution of body fatness and adipose tissue distribution to the age variation in plasma steroid hormone concentrations in men: the HERITAGE Family Study. *J Clin Endocrinol Metab* 2000;85:1026–1031.

70. Mårin P, Oden B, Olbe L, et al. Assimilation of triglycerides in subcutaneous and intraabdominal adipose tissues *in vivo* in men: effects of testosterone. *J Clin Endocrinol Metab* 1996;81:1018–1022.
71. Ramirez ME, McMurry MP, Wiebke GA, et al. Evidence for sex steroid inhibition of lipoprotein lipase in men: comparison of abdominal and femoral adipose tissue. *Metabolism* 1997;46:179–185.
72. Jensen MD. Androgen effect on body composition and fat metabolism. *Mayo Clin Proc* 2000;75:S65–S69.
73. Lafontan M, Berlan M. Fat cell α₂-adrenoceptors: the regulation of fat cell function and lipolysis. *Endocr Rev* 1995;16:716–738.
74. Björntorp P. Hormonal regulation of visceral adipose tissue. *Growth Horm IGF Res* 1998;8:15–17.
75. Lima N, Cavaliere H, Knobel M, et al. Decreased androgen levels in massively obese men may be associated with impaired function of the gonadostat. *Int J Obes Relat Metab Disord* 2000;24:1433–1437.
76. Kraemer WJ, Volek JS, Clark KL, et al. Influence of exercise training on physiological and performance changes with weight loss in men. *Med Sci Sports Exerc* 1999;31:1320–1329.
77. Turcato E, Zamboni M, De Pergola G, et al. Interrelationships between weight loss, body fat distribution and sex hormones in pre- and postmenopausal obese women. *J Intern Med* 1997;241:363–372.
78. Wabitsch M, Hauner H, Heinze E, et al. Body fat distribution and steroid hormone concentrations in obese adolescent girls before and after weight reduction. *J Clin Endocrinol Metab* 1995;80:3469–3475.
79. Isidori AM, Caprio M, Strollo F, et al. Leptin and androgens in male obesity: evidence for leptin contribution to reduced androgen levels. *J Clin Endocrinol Metab* 1999;84:3673–3680.
80. Vermeulen A, Goemaere S, Kaufman JM. Testosterone, body composition and aging. *J Endocrinol Invest* 1999;22:110–116.
81. Mårin P, Krotkiewski M, Björntorp P. Androgen treatment of middle-aged, obese men: effects on metabolism, muscle and adipose tissue. *Eur J Med* 1992;1:329–336.
82. Mårin P, Holmang S, Gustafsson C, et al. Androgen treatment of abdominally obese men. *Obes Res* 1993;1:245–251.
83. Dumesic DA, Abbott DH, Eisner JR, et al. Pituitary desensitization to gonadotropin releasing hormone increases abdominal adiposity in hyperadrenogenic anovulatory women. *Fertil Steril* 1998;70:94–101.
84. Matsumoto AM, Sandblom RE, Schoene RB, et al. Testosterone replacement in hypogonadal men: effects on obstructive sleep apnea, respiratory drives, and sleep. *Clin Endocrinol (Oxf)* 1985;22:713–721.
85. Schneider BK, Pickett CK, Zwillich CW, et al. Influence of testosterone on breathing during sleep. *J Appl Physiol* 1986;61:618–623.
86. O'Sullivan AJ, Crampton LJ, Freund J, et al. The route of estrogen replacement therapy confers divergent effects on substrate oxidation and body composition in postmenopausal women. *J Clin Invest* 1998;102:1035–1040.
87. O'Sullivan AJ, Ho KK. A comparison of the effects of oral and transdermal estrogen replacement on insulin sensitivity in postmenopausal women. *J Clin Endocrinol Metab* 1995;80:1783–1788.
88. Poehlman ET, Toth MJ, Gardner AW. Changes in energy balance and body composition at menopause: a controlled longitudinal study. *Ann Intern Med* 1995;123:673–675.
89. Paolisso G, Rizzo MR, Mazziotti G, et al. Lack of association between changes in plasma leptin concentration and in food intake during the menstrual cycle. *Eur J Clin Invest* 1999;29:490–495.
90. Van Gaal LF, Vanuytsel JL, Vansant GA, et al. Sex hormones, body fat distribution, resting metabolic rate and glucose-induced thermogenesis in premenopausal obese women. *Int J Obes Relat Metab Disord* 1994;18:333–338.
91. Piers LS, Diggavi SN, Rijskamp J, et al. Resting metabolic rate and thermic effect of a meal in the follicular and luteal phases of the menstrual cycle in well-nourished Indian women. *Am J Clin Nutr* 1995;61:296–302.
92. Jensen J, Christiansen C, Rodbro P. Oestrogen-progestogen replacement therapy changes body composition in early post-menopausal women. *Maturitas* 1986;8:209–216.
93. Mauras N. Estrogens do not affect whole-body protein metabolism in the prepubertal female. *J Clin Endocrinol Metab* 1995;80:2842–2845.
94. Mauras N, O'Brien KO, Klein KO, et al. Estrogen suppression in males: metabolic effects. *J Clin Endocrinol Metab* 2000;85:2370–2377.
95. Mauriege P, Imbeault P, Prud'Homme D, et al. Subcutaneous adipose tissue metabolism at menopause: importance of body fatness and regional fat distribution. *J Clin Endocrinol Metab* 2000;85:2446–2454.
96. Jensen MD, Martin ML, Cryer PE, et al. Effects of estrogen on free fatty acid metabolism in humans. *Am J Physiol* 1994;266:E914–E920.
97. Pansini F, Bonaccorsi G, Genovesi F, et al. Influence of estrogens on serum free fatty acid levels in women. *J Clin Endocrinol Metab* 1990;71:1387–1389.
98. Toth MJ, Sites CK, Eltabbakh GH, et al. Effect of menopausal status on insulin-stimulated glucose disposal: comparison of middle-aged premenopausal and early postmenopausal women. *Diabetes Care* 2000;23:801–806.
99. Tchernof A, Calles-Escandon J, Sites CK, et al. Menopause, central body fatness, and insulin resistance: effects of hormone-replacement therapy. *Coron Artery Dis* 1998;9:503–511.
100. Bjorkelund C, Lissner L, Andersson S, et al. Reproductive history in relation to relative weight and fat distribution. *Int J Obes Relat Metab Disord* 1996;20:213–219.
101. Hassager C, Christiansen C. Estrogen/gestagen therapy changes soft tissue body composition in postmenopausal women. *Metabolism* 1989;38:662–665.
102. Iverius PH, Brunzell JD. Relationship between lipoprotein lipase activity and plasma sex steroid level in obese women. *J Clin Invest* 1988;82:1106–1112.

103. Norman RJ, Flight IH, Rees MC. Oestrogen and progestogen hormone replacement therapy for peri-menopausal and post-menopausal women: weight and body fat distribution. *Cochrane Database System Review* 2000;2:CD001018.
104. Brussaard HE, Leuven JA, Frölich M, et al. Short-term oestrogen replacement therapy improves insulin resistance, lipids and fibrinolysis in postmenopausal women with NIDDM. *Diabetologia* 1997;40:843–849.
105. Brillon DJ, Zheng B, Campbell RG, et al. Effect of cortisol on energy expenditure and amino acid metabolism in humans. *Am J Physiol Endocrinol Metab* 1995;268:E501–E513.
106. Putignano P, Kaltsas GA, Korbonits M, et al. Alterations in serum protein levels in patients with Cushing's syndrome before and after successful treatment. *J Clin Endocrinol Metab* 2000;85:3309–3312.
107. De Feo P. Hormonal regulation of human protein metabolism. *Eur J Endocrinol* 1996;135:7–18.
108. Björntorp P, Rosmond R. Obesity and cortisol. *Nutrition* 2000;16:924–936.
109. Björntorp P, Rosmond R. Neuroendocrine abnormalities in visceral obesity. *Int J Obes Relat Metab Disord* 2000;24:S80–S85.
110. Castonguay TW. Glucocorticoids as modulators in the control of feeding. *Brain Res Bull* 1991;27:423–428.
111. Richard D, Huang Q, Timofeeva E. The corticotropin-releasing hormone system in the regulation of energy balance in obesity. *Int J Obes Relat Metab Disord* 2000;24:S36–S39.
112. Shamoon H, Soman V, Sherwin RS. The influence of acute physiological increments of cortisol on fuel metabolism and insulin binding to monocytes in normal humans. *J Clin Endocrinol Metab* 1980;50:495–501.
113. Horber FF, Haymond MW. Human growth hormone prevents the protein catabolic side effects of prednisone in humans. *J Clin Invest* 1990;86:265–272.
114. Haymond MW, Horber FF. The effects of human growth hormone and prednisone on whole body estimates of protein metabolism. *Horm Res* 1992;38:44–46.
115. Ottosson M, Vikman-Adolfsson K, Enerbäck S, et al. The effects of cortisol on the regulation of lipoprotein lipase activity in human adipose tissue. *J Clin Endocrinol Metab* 1994;79:820–825.
116. Ottosson M, Lönnroth P, Björntorp P, et al. Effects of cortisol and growth hormone on lipolysis in human adipose tissue. *J Clin Endocrinol Metab* 2000;85:799–803.
117. Slavin BG, Ong JM, Kern PA. Hormonal regulation of hormone-sensitive lipase activity and mRNA levels in isolated rat adipocytes. *J Lipid Res* 1994;35:1535–1541.
118. Rebuffe-Scrive M, Krotkiewski M, Elfverson J, et al. Muscle and adipose tissue morphology and metabolism in Cushing's syndrome. *J Clin Endocrinol Metab* 1988;67:1122–1128.
119. Divertie GD, Jensen MD, Miles JM. Stimulation of lipolysis in humans by physiological hypercortisolemia. *Diabetes* 1991;40:1228–1232.
120. Lönn L, Kvist H, Sjostrom L. Changes in body composition and adipose tissue distribution after treatment of women with Cushing's syndrome. *Metabolism* 1994;43:1517–1522.
121. Krotkiewski M, Björntorp P, Smith U. The effect of long-term dexamethasone treatment on lipoprotein lipase activity in rat fat cells. *Horm Metab Res* 1976;8:245–246.
122. Gelfand RA, Matthews DE, Bier DM, et al. Role of counterregulatory hormones in the catabolic response to stress. *J Clin Invest* 1984;74:2238–2248.
123. Levine JA. Relation between chubby cheeks and visceral fat. *N Engl J Med* 1998;339:1946–1947.
124. Pasquali R, Vicennati V. Activity of the hypothalamic–pituitary–adrenal axis in different obesity phenotypes. *Int J Obes Relat Metab Disord* 2000;24:S47–S49.
125. Buemann B, Vohl MC, Chagnon M, et al. Abdominal visceral fat is associated with a BclI restriction fragment length polymorphism at the glucocorticoid receptor gene locus. *Obes Res* 1997;5:186–192.
126. Andrew R, Phillips DI, Walker BR. Influence of gender and body composition on glucocorticoid metabolism in middle-aged humans. *Int J Obes Relat Metab Disord* 2000;24:S144–S145.
127. Reid IR, Wattie DJ, Evans MC, et al. Testosterone therapy in glucocorticoid-treated men. *Arch Intern Med* 1996; 156:1173–1177.

PART II

Comorbidities

8

Heart Disease

Paul Poirier and Martin A. Alpert

As the previous chapters have discussed, people of industrialized countries have and continue to become more overweight because of changes in lifestyle; therefore, obesity may well become the most common health problem of the twenty-first century. Obesity is associated with an increased risk of heart disease, stroke, hypertension, dyslipidemia, type II diabetes mellitus, deep venous thrombosis, pulmonary embolism, and sleep apnea (1–5). Moreover, obesity is associated with reduced life expectancy (6). This chapter discusses the influence of obesity from a cardiac evaluation perspective and structural viewpoint, and it covers the impact of obesity on modern cardiology.

ADIPOSE TISSUE AS AN ENDOCRINE ORGAN

Adipose tissue is not simply a passive storehouse for fat but rather is an endocrine organ that is capable of synthesizing and releasing into the bloodstream various peptides and nonpeptide compounds that may play a central role in cardiovascular homeostasis. Adipose tissue is an important source of tumor necrosis factor α (TNF-α), interleukin-6 (IL-6), plasminogen activator inhibitor-1 (PAI-1), resistin, lipoprotein lipase, acylation-stimulating protein, cholesteryl-ester transfer protein, retinal-binding protein, estrogens (through cytochrome P450 aromatase activity), leptin, angiotensinogen, adiponectin, insulin-like growth factor-1 (IGF-1), insulin-like growth factor–binding protein-3, and monobutyrin (7–11). Clinically, circulating concentrations of PAI-1, angiotensin II (AT-II), C-reactive protein (CRP), fibrinogen, and TNF-α are all related to body mass index (BMI) (12,13). *In vivo*, about 30% of the total circulating concentrations of IL-6 have been estimated to originate from adipose tissue, which is important because IL-6 modulates CRP production in the liver and CRP may be a marker of a chronic inflammatory state that predisposes the individual to acute coronary syndromes (12,14,15). Tchernof et al. (16) recently reported that plasma CRP levels are positively associated with total fatness, visceral obesity, and triglyceride levels and are negatively related to insulin sensitivity and that weight loss reduces CRP levels significantly. In addition, cytokines have been implicated in endothelial cell dysfunction, as well as in increases in AT-II levels that may contribute to hypertension and heart failure.

THE CARDIOVASCULAR IMPACT OF INCREASED ADIPOSE TISSUE MASS

Adipose-Tissue Circulation

An extensive capillary network surrounds adipose tissue, and adipocytes are located close to vessels with the highest permeability, the lowest hydrostatic pressure, and the shortest distance for transport of molecules from the adipocytes (17–19). Resting blood flow usually ranges from 2 to 3 mL per minute per 100 g of adipose tissue, and it can

TABLE 8.1. *Tissue blood flow during experimental hypovolemia*

Tissue	Percent of resting blood flow (approximate)
Subcutaneous adipose tissue	10%
Renal cortical flow	40%
Skeletal muscle	60%
Liver	60%
Myocardium	60%
Hypothalamus	60%

increase about tenfold. However, this increment is still half (20 to 30 mL per minute per 100 g) of that which is seen in skeletal muscle (50 to 75 mL per minute per 100 g) (20–22). Adipose tissue comprises a substantial fraction of body weight. This implies that a substantial quantity of fluid is present in the interstitial space of adipose tissue, as the interstitial space represents approximately 10% of the tissue wet weight (23). This could be important in the regulation of blood volume if this third space volume is mobilized into the circulation. Excess fluid that may be present in this compartment may have important repercussions in obese individuals with heart failure if this extra volume is redistributed into the circulation. However, regulation of blood flow in adipose tissue prevents this from occurring in most stressful situations. The decrease in blood flow in response to hypovolemia (hemorrhagic shock) is most important in adipose tissue when compared to other tissues (Table 8.1). Indeed, the increase in epinephrine levels decreases blood flow much more in adipose tissue than it does in skeletal muscle because the β-adrenergic receptors that mediate vasodilation in adipose tissue are mainly β_1-receptors, unlike those of skeletal muscle, which are mainly β_2-receptors (19).

Extensive adrenergic innervation that finely regulates the perfusion of vessels is present in adipose tissue. Although cardiac output increases with total fat mass, the perfusion per unit of adipose tissue decreases by about 35% with increasing obesity in patients who have 15% to 26% body fat compared to those who have more than 36% body fat (21). Accordingly, the increase in systemic blood flow encountered in obesity cannot be solely explained by increased requirements caused by adipose-tissue perfusion because the enlarged vascular bed of adipose tissue is less vascularized than that of other tissue. Basal adipocyte blood flow remains relatively constant as cells increase in size during lipid deposition. Most likely, the concomitant increase in lean body mass (LBM) in these individuals may account for some of the increased cardiac output (24).

Central Hemodynamics

Because of the increased metabolic demand induced by excess body weight, obesity produces an incremental increase in total blood volume and cardiac output (25,26). Thus, at any given level of activity, the cardiac workload is greater for obese subjects compared with lean subjects; for example, walking has been demonstrated to be an exercise of moderate to high intensity for most obese individuals (27,28). Obese subjects are known to have higher cardiac outputs and a lower total peripheral resistance than lean individuals. The increased cardiac output is attributable to increased stroke volume, because the heart rate usually remains unchanged (29,30). For any given level of arterial pressure, the cardiac output is higher and the peripheral vascular resistance is lower in an obese individual compared with a nonobese individual. Both stroke volume and cardiac output are higher in men than in women (about 10%) and in overweight, than in normal-weight, individuals (about 9%) (24). These differences are eliminated by normalization for fat-free mass (FFM) or body surface area (BSA) (24). Moreover, in obesity, the Frank–Starling curve (left ventricular function) is shifted to the left as a result of incremental increases in left ventricular filling pressure and volume that, over time, produce chamber dilation. Ventricular chamber dilation increase wall stress, which predisposes the individual to increasing myocardial mass in an attempt to normalize wall stress. This results in left ventricular hypertrophy (LVH), which, characteristically, is of the eccentric type (31,32). Left atrial enlargement is also present in normotensive obese individuals, and it is associated with increased left ventricular mass. Left atrial enlargement is not necessarily mediated through left ventricular diastolic function impairment, and it may simply reflect a physiologic adaptation to the expanded blood volume (33). Obese subjects with systemic hypertension are confronted with a double burden—increased preload and afterload (high blood pressure). This may contribute to premature heart failure (Fig. 8.1).

Using right-sided heart catheterization, Backman et al. (34,35) have shown that surgically induced weight loss produces a decrease in resting oxygen consumption and cardiac output proportional to the magnitude of weight loss. Stroke volume falls parallel to the decrease in blood volume and heart volume. Systemic arterial pressure declines, but sys-

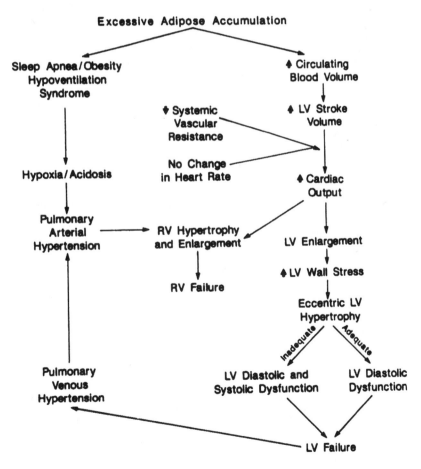

FIG. 8.1. Pathophysiology of obesity-related cardiomyopathy. (From Alpert MA, Hashimi MW. Obesity and the heart. *Am J Med Sci* 1993;306:117–123, with permission.)

temic arterial resistance changes by little, if at all. Left ventricular stroke work diminishes. Pulmonary capillary wedge pressures tend to decrease, but they are still higher, relative to cardiac output, in obese subjects than in normal-weight subjects. Left ventricular dysfunction persists, as is evidenced by reduced myocardial wall compliance, most strikingly during exercise (34). At any given cardiac output, all right-sided heart pressures tend to be higher in obese subjects than in normal-weight subjects, with related increases in left ventricular end-diastolic pressure (29,34).

Obesity is associated with a persistence of elevated cardiac filling pressures during exercise (34,36). Cardiac output is able to increase adequately enough to accommodate mild to moderate exercise workloads. Increased cardiac output during exercise is typically accompanied by an increase in left ventricular filling pressure that often exceeds 20 mm Hg. Therefore, the average left ventricular filling pressure is often within the upper limits of normal at rest, but it increases disproportionately with increased venous return or during exercise (29). This is consistent with a high-pressure system, and, accordingly, obese patients may demonstrate higher right-sided heart filling pressures, systolic pressure, cardiac output, and pulmonary vascular resistance index (26). The last may reflect intrinsic pulmonary disease; abnormal left ventricular function; or undiagnosed causes of pulmonary hypertension, such as sleep apnea. With increased venous return, small incremental increases of central blood volume are associated with a significant increase in left ventricular end-diastolic pressure. A decrease in central blood volume accompanies weight reduction, and, when edema and dyspnea are present, a relief of these may accompany this improvement (29). However, abnormal ventricular compliance characterized by left ventricular diastolic dysfunction during exercise does not always improve with weight loss.

Alterations in Cardiac Morphology

Before the advent of echocardiography, the cardiac status of obese individuals was difficult to assess. Nevertheless, transthoracic echocardiography can be technically difficult in obese patients (37,38). Differentiating between subepicardial adipose tissue and pericardial effusion can be difficult in obese patients (38). Epicardial adipose tissue is known to be a common cause of pseudopericardial effusion, and this adipose-tissue depot may cause an underestimation of the amount of pericardial fluid (39). The presence of an anterior echo-free space in the absence of a posterior clear space has generally been attributed to pericardial fat. Another concern is the presence of fat within the heart. The site of predilection tends to be the interatrial septum. From necropsy descriptions, the definition of the lipomatous hypertrophy of the interatrial septum corresponds to a maximal transverse dimension of interatrial fat of more than 20 mm (40,41). Thus, lipomatous hypertrophy of the interatrial septum, a finding associated with obesity and advancing age, consists of the accumulation of adipose tissue, including fetal adipose tissue, in the interatrial septum cephalad and caudal to the fossa ovalis, but it always spares the fossa, thus imparting a "dumbbell" shape on the two-dimensional echocardiogram (42,43). This accumulation of fat projects toward the right atrium.

In the echocardiographic evaluation of LVH, the left ventricular mass is customarily corrected for BSA. Although indexing left ventricular mass to BSA is appropriate for nonobese subjects, such indexing in obese individuals may underestimate obesity as a predictor of increased left ventricular mass. This may be especially true in children (44). Thus, some investigators have proposed that adjusting left ventricular mass for height, height[2.13], or height[2.7] is preferable (45,46). This may reduce the left ventricular mass variability that is associated with body size and gender. Indices using height[2.13] or height[2.7] may be more appropriate for the evaluation of left ventricular mass in obese persons than is normalization for BSA or even for height (47,48). Another potential way to normalize the left ventricular mass is with LBM (44,49). Interestingly, after indexing using LBM, no gender differences on left ventricular mass have been seen, and the relative effects of adiposity and blood pressure on left ventricular mass were of similar magnitude (49). This finding was underscored recently by the results of the Strong Heart Study cohort, which showed that stroke volume and cardiac output are more strongly related to FFM than to other variables in both normal-weight and overweight individuals (24). Undoubtedly, the adiposity status has an impact on the heart size, but the optimal indexing criteria for definition of LVH after an echocardiographic study in an obese individuals remains to be refined and confirmed.

Effects on Ventricular Function

Eccentric LVH, which is commonly present in morbidly obese patients, is often associated with left ventricular diastolic dysfunction. Moreover, as with left ventricular mass, longer durations of obesity are associated with poorer left ventricular systolic function and greater impairment of left ventricular diastolic function (Figs. 8.2 and 8.3) (50). Although numerous indices of left ventricular diastolic filling are derived from echocardiography or

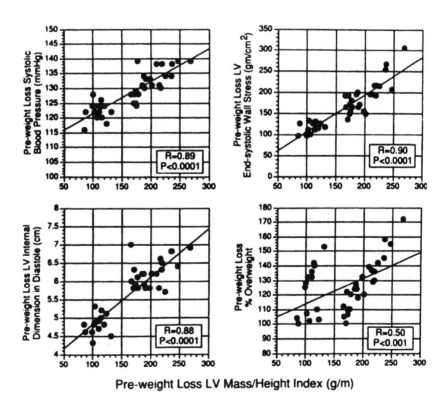

FIG. 8.2. Relationship among left ventricular mass to height index before weight loss, percentage overweight, left ventricular dimension in diastole, systolic blood pressure, and left ventricular end-systolic wall stress in morbidly obese subjects. (From Alpert MA, Lambert CR, Terry BE, et al. Effect of weight loss on left ventricular mass in non-hypertensive morbidly obese patients. *Am J Cardiol* 1994;73:918–921, with permission.)

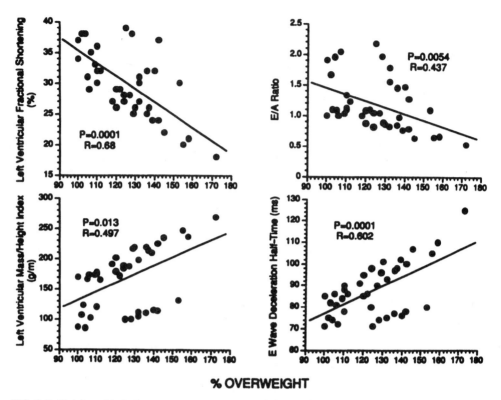

FIG. 8.3. Relationship between percentage overweight and left ventricular mass to height index, left ventricular fractional shortening, transmitral E/A wave ratio and transmitral E-wave deceleration half-time in morbidly obese subjects. (From Alpert MA, Lambert CR, Terry BE, et al. Interrelationship of left ventricular mass, systolic function and diastolic filling in normotensive morbidly obese patients. *Int J Obes Relat Metab Disord* 1995;19:550–557, with permission.)

cardiac Doppler evaluation, the increased intravascular volume in obesity may mask the Doppler-derived abnormalities of diastolic filling. Of particular interest are the abnormal filling patterns that are present in obese subjects despite hemodynamics that are unfavorable for detection. Because of the presence of nonspecific symptoms, the evaluation of the presence of left ventricular diastolic dysfunction is clinically important in obese subjects (1,51–53). Pulmonary venous Doppler evaluation may be used, but, if it is not technically accessible, transmitral Doppler imaging with the use of the Valsalva maneuver may properly evaluate the presence of left ventricular diastolic dysfunction (54–57). Left ventricular diastolic dysfunction is most likely to occur in those with increased left ventricular mass. This group of subjects experiences improvement in left ventricular diastolic filling after weight loss (53,58). Although antihypertensive drugs favorably influence the arterial blood pressure, they may be less important than weight loss for decreasing the left ventricular mass. In hypertensive obese subjects, weight loss is associated with greater decreases in ventricular and posterior wall thickness and left ventricular mass than in subjects treated with metoprolol, suggesting that changes in weight, independent of changes in blood pressure, are directly associated with changes in left ventricular mass (59).

Impairment of left ventricular systolic function is not consistently present in obese individuals. Several factors that may adversely affect left ventricular systolic function in obese subjects have been identified. After years of obesity, cardiac adaptation to obesity may result in cardiac hypertrophy of the concentric or, more commonly, the eccentric type (60–62). Necropsy studies have demonstrated a relationship between heart weight and body weight, and echocardiographic studies have shown that left ventricular end-diastolic dimension and septal and posterior wall dimensions are greater in obese subjects than in lean subjects (32,60,63). Obesity associated with hypertension results in myocardial hypertrophy with left ventricular dilation, and this combination increases the frequency of premature ventricular complexes at a rate that is 30 times higher in obese patients with eccentric LVH than that seen in lean subjects (30,62). Even if weight loss produces a reduction in left ventricular mass, only 14% to 25% of the reduction in left ventricular mass can be explained solely by the change in body weight (59,64). Perhaps the most important variable in weight loss–induced reduction of left ventricular mass is the drop in blood pressure and associated neurohormones. The combination of obesity and hypertension burdens the heart with high preload and high afterload, thereby greatly enhancing the risk of congestive heart failure (CHF).

Sympathetic mechanisms have been implicated in the development of LVH, and weight reduction in obese subjects reduces the indices of sympathetic activity, including plasma norepinephrine levels and urinary norepinephrine excretion (65). The renin–angiotensin system may also be involved in the pathogenesis of LVH, and weight reduction may decrease plasma renin activity and aldosterone levels (66). The improvement in hyperinsulinemia may also contribute to the reduction in left ventricular mass in hypertensive obese subjects because insulin resistance is an important independent contributing factor to left ventricular mass in normotensive, nondiabetic obese subjects (67). The exact mechanism explaining the association between LVH and insulin resistance is not known, but one may speculate that hyperinsulinemia plays a role as a growth factor because septal hypertrophy of the heart is found more frequently in newborn infants of mothers with diabetes (68). Nevertheless, the role of all of these neurohumoral factors in the regression of cardiac hypertrophy associated with weight reduction deserves further investigation.

CLINICAL AND LABORATORY ASSESSMENT OF OBESE INDIVIDUALS

History and Physical Examination

Symptoms potentially attributable to cardiac involvement (e.g., progressive dyspnea with exertion and lower extremity edema) are often nonspecific in obesity (28,51). The physical examination and electrocardiogram (ECG) of obese patients often underestimate the presence and extent of cardiac dysfunction. However, signs and symptoms of obesity-related cardiomyopathy most commonly occur in patients with a relative weight that is more than or equal to 175% of ideal body weight or a BMI of more than or equal to 40 kilograms per meter squared (kg/m^2) (25). On physical examination, jugular venous distention and the hepatojugular reflux are often not seen, and the heart sounds are usually distant. Although no reports are available, the use of electronic stethoscopes may help the clinician assess heart sounds in severely obese individuals. A common finding in massive obesity is pedal edema, which may be partly a consequence of elevated ventricular filling pressure despite the elevation in cardiac output (69,70). However, in patients with circadian venous edemas, high-volume lymphatic overload (dynamic insufficiency) and the increased intravascular volume that is associated with the decreased mobility encountered in obese individuals, which thus reduces the pumping function of calf and leg muscles, may result in reflux of blood in the leg veins as a result of valvular incompetence

(71,72). Nonetheless, in patients with lipedema characteristic of obesity, no scintigraphic alteration in lymphatic transport is seen (71).

Obese individuals may also experience increased demand for ventilation and breathing workload, particularly in the supine position. Because hypertension is six times more common in obese subjects than in nonobese subjects, accurate blood pressure measurement is fundamental, and a small cuff size can cause considerable artifactual increases in blood pressure (73,74). According to one study, this could result in a misclassification of up to 35% of normotensive individuals as hypertensive in the presence of obesity (74). In the very obese patient, the symptoms of *cor pulmonale* are often nonspecific, but the clinician should carefully search for its presence when examining an obese individual who snores and complains of daytime somnolence (see Chapter 9). In most individuals, the splitting of the S_2 is most often heard at the second or third left interspace parasternally, but, in obese patients, the split S_2 is either inaudible or is very poorly defined in the second interspace; it is often best heard at the first left interspace (75). The difficulty in the bedside evaluation of heart sounds may obscure an incremental increase in the intensity of P_2 that is suggestive of pulmonary hypertension.

Cardiomyopathy of Obesity (*Adipositas Cordis*)

Obesity-related cardiomyopathy occurs when cardiac structural (left ventricular dilation) and hemodynamic (increased left ventricular wall stress) adaptations result in CHF. Right ventricular structure and function may be similarly affected. Usually, the cardiomyopathy of obesity is found in individuals with severe and long-standing obesity (76). This pathology was recognized as early as 1818 (77). This case, which was described by Cheyne (77), is historically interesting not only because it is a carefully recorded documentation of a fatty heart but also because it is considered the first reported case in which a specific type of respiration, now recognized as Cheyne–Stokes respiration, was portrayed. Subsequently, others have described excess epicardial fat and fatty infiltration of the myocardium that may interfere with cardiac function in the hearts of obese subjects (63,78). Typically, in the cardiomyopathy of obesity, the thickness of the atrial septum is increased (lipomatous hypertrophy), but myocardial fatty infiltration without any relationship to obesity has also been depicted (79).

Myocardial fat infiltration, which is more prevalent in women than men, is an uncommon autopsy finding, with an incidence of approximately 3% (80,81). In obesity, the presence of excess adipose tissue on the surface of the right ventricle represents an exaggeration of the normal architecture. Initially, the fatty heart is probably not an infiltrative process but is most likely a metaplastic phenomenon (80). Gradually, the cords of fat cells infiltrate between the muscle fibers and result in myocyte degeneration, thus resulting in cardiac conduction defects (82,83). These cords of fat cells frequently emanate from the epicardial fat (80). Along with the fat infiltration of the right ventricle, the sinus node musculature, the atrioventricular (AV) node, and the right bundle branch can be infiltrated (82), and the entire myocardium of the AV region may be replaced by fat (83). Another rare feature of *adipositas cordis* is a pattern of restrictive cardiomyopathy (79,84). Necropsy study has shown that small irregular aggregates and bands of adipose tissue separating the myocardial cells, thus reducing the diameter of the myocardial fibers, may be the result of pressure-induced atrophy from the intervening fat (84). An alternative explanation resides in the lipotoxicity of the myocardium that is induced by free fatty acid (FFA) metabolism (85). When lipids overaccumulate in nonadipose tissues, fatty acids enter a deleterious pathway, causing apoptosis of lipid-laden cells such as cardiomyocytes (85). In general, the right ventricle is more likely to be involved than the left ventricle, and the anterior wall is involved to a greater extent than is the posterior. In individuals in whom uncomplicated fatty infiltration occurred, the pathology consisted of areas of fat surrounded by fibrosis that was unattached to epicardial fat (25). In most cases, however, cardiac hypertrophy is a direct reflection of BMI, and this hypertrophy results from myocyte change and not from excessive fat infiltration or fibrosis (86). Although the limitations of endomyocardial biopsy are well known (87), structural myocardial biopsy findings that seek a specific cause of CHF may be disappointing in obesity and may provide fewer histologic diagnoses than in lean patients (26). Idiopathic dilated cardiomyopathy has been found in 77% of obese subjects but in only 36% of lean subjects. Not surprisingly, the most common finding on endomyocardial biopsy in the obese group is mild myocyte hypertrophy (26).

The Electrocardiogram

The ECG is influenced by the morphologic changes induced by obesity, including (a) the displacement of the heart that is caused by elevation of the diaphragm in the supine position, (b) an increased cardiac workload with associated cardiac hypertrophy, (c) an increase in the distance between the heart and the recording electrodes that is induced by the accumulation of adipose tissue in the subcutaneous tissue of the chest wall (and possibly increased epicardial fat), and (d) the associated chronic lung disease secondary to the sleep apnea–hypoventilation syndrome.

ECG parameters in obese patients should be expected to change after weight loss. The impact of weight loss in obese patients on the QRS voltage is not consistent; some studies report a decrease (88–90), no change (91), or an increase in the QRS amplitude after weight reduction (92–94). Importantly, weight loss with decreased amount of fat mass may counterbalance a real decrease in left ventricular mass, and low QRS voltage after drastic weight loss could be secondary to lean mass loss and myocardial atrophy (90,95,96). These opposite vectors may negate the resultant QRS amplitudes.

Table 8.2 describes the ECG changes with increasing obesity. About 8% of patients display a corrected QT (QTc) interval of more than 0.44 seconds, and about 2% show a QTc of more than 0.46 seconds (97). Prolongation of the QTc interval has been shown to be associated with visceral obesity in healthy premenopausal women, as assessed by computed tomography (CT) imaging, independent of obesity and other risk factors (98). Beyond the QRS voltage and trends toward left-axis deviation, the most alterations seen are the nonspecific flattening of the T wave in the inferolateral leads, which is attributed to the horizontal displacement of the heart, and ECG criteria for left atrial abnormality

TABLE 8.2. *Electrocardiographic changes with progressive obesity*

↑ Heart rate
↑ PR interval
↑ QRS interval
↑ or ↓ QRS voltage
↑ QTc interval
↑ QT dispersion
↑ Signal-averaged electrocardiogram (late potentials)
Left axis deviation
Flattening of the T wave (inferolateral leads)
Left atrial abnormalities
False-positive criteria for inferior myocardial infarction

(94,99,100). These left atrial abnormalities may well indicate the presence of left ventricular diastolic dysfunction (101).

Weight loss induces a rightward shift of the QRS axis (92,93), but the conduction intervals—duration of the P wave, QRS complex, and PQ interval—are not affected by weight loss (93) because they often are not clinically different from those of lean subjects (99). Also, a less negative P-terminal force in V_1 and decreased T-wave flattening in the inferolateral leads have been reported after weight loss. Although weight loss has been associated with a reduction in ECG criteria of left atrial dilation, it has not been related to a significant decrease in left atrial dimension when evaluated by echocardiography (92). Clinically, one must emphasize the fact that an increased incidence of false-positive criteria for inferior myocardial infarction has been reported in both obese individuals and women in the final trimester of pregnancy. This is presumably because of diaphragmatic elevation (102).

LVH is strongly associated with cardiac morbidity and mortality (65). Multiple ECG criteria for LVH are present more regularly in those with morbid obesity compared to lean individuals, but they occur less frequently than might be expected based on the high prevalence of echocardiographic evidence of LVH in such patients (99). Therefore, LVH is underdiagnosed by usual ECG criteria in morbidly obese individuals. One recent study reported a low frequency for various ECG criteria for the detection of LVH in morbid obesity, in which LVH may be demonstrated in two-thirds of the obese subjects (76,99, 103). As left ventricular mass increases, the electrical forces usually become more posteriorly oriented and the S wave in lead V_3 may be the most representative voltage for evaluating posterior forces. With LVH, the heart is oriented more horizontally in the mediastinum, which may explain the usefulness of the R wave in aVL. In obesity, the heart is shifted horizontally, presumably from the restricted diaphragmatic expansion that results from the abdominal pannus. Thus, one proposal is that, for men at all ages, LVH can be considered present by QRS voltage alone when the amplitude of the R wave in lead aVL and that of the S wave in lead V_3 are more than 35 mm. For women at all ages, the same criteria should be used, but with amplitudes of more than 25 mm, not 35 mm (104). When these ECG voltage criteria are compared with the left ventricular mass estimated by echocardiography, a sensitivity of 49%, a specificity of 93%, and an overall accuracy of 76% are found. These percentages are higher than those of the most widely used criteria (Romhilt–Estes point score and Sokolow–Lyon voltage) (Table 8.3). Therefore, Sokolow–Lyon voltage criteria should be avoided in obese hypertensive patients and

TABLE 8.3. *Detection of left ventricular hypertrophy by QRS voltage in obesity*

	Sensitivity in obesity (%)	Specificity in obesity (%)	Accuracy in obesity (%)
Sokolow–Lyon	20	93	65
Romhilt–Estes Point score ≥4	31	83	63
Cornell	49	93	76

Sokolow–Lyon voltage criteria: R in V_5 or V_6 + S in V_1 > 35 mm.
Romhilt–Estes point score from Romhilt DW, Estes EN Jr. A point-score system for the ECG diagnosis of left ventricular hypertrophy. *Am Heart J* 1968;75:752–758.
Cornell voltage criteria: R in aVL + S in V_3 >28 mm in men, >20 mm in women.
Adapted from Casale PN, Devereux RB, Kligfield P, et al. Electrocardiographic detection of left ventricular hypertrophy: development and prospective validation of improved criteria. *J Am Coll Cardiol* 1985;6: 572–580, with permission.

should be replaced by the Cornell voltage criteria, which seems to be less influenced by the presence of obesity (105).

Alpert et al. (92) demonstrated that substantial weight loss in morbidly obese patients results in a decrease in voltage, making the ECG criteria less reliant on the precordial voltage (R wave in lead aVL). Meanwhile, an increase in the frequency of LVH that was diagnosed using precordial voltage ($SV_1 + RV_5$ or V_6) was observed. Accordingly, regression of LVH after weight loss should be evaluated with ECG criteria that are less influenced by anterior chest wall fat.

Malignant Arrhythmias

Hippocrates is believed to have stated, "Sudden death is more common in those who are naturally fat than in the lean" (1). Stable-weight obese subjects have an increased risk of arrhythmias and sudden death, even in the absence of cardiac dysfunction (30,106); and the risk of sudden cardiac death with increasing weight is seen in both sexes (107). In the Framingham study, the risk of sudden cardiac death with increasing weight was encountered in both genders (107), and the annual sudden cardiac mortality rate in obese men and women was estimated to be about 40 times higher than the rate of unexplained cardiac arrest in a matched nonobese population (108). Specifically, in severely obese men, a 6-fold to 12-fold excess mortality rate was demonstrated (6).

A prolonged QT interval reflects the delayed cardiac repolarization and refractory period, and it is a known risk factor for ventricular arrhythmias and sudden death. A correlation exists between BMI and QTc, with longer intervals being observed in obese subjects (109). Although the relationship between fatness and the QTc interval is not consistent (110), it does remain even after adjusting the absolute QT intervals for heart rate using different formulas (e.g., Bazett, Framingham, and Fridericia formulas) and with multiple regression analysis (109). Hence, a prolonged QT interval is observed in a relatively high percentage of obese subjects, and the association between abnormal QTc and BMI is most evident in the severely obese (91,109). Although an abnormal QTc has been shown in other insulin-resistant states that are often associated with obesity, such as hypertension and diabetes (111), no reports describe specific ECG abnormalities in the lipodystrophy or the polycystic ovary syndromes, both of which are also characterized by insulin resistance and higher levels of FFAs but differing degrees of obesity. QT dispersion represents a functional substrate of arrhythmias because this variable may imply an inhomogeneous ventricular repolarization and refractory period. QT dispersion has been reported to be increased in obesity and to be without improvement after weight loss, unlike the QTc interval (110). In contrast, the QT dispersion is comparable to age-matched and sex-matched controls when the obese subjects are not afflicted by the comorbidities that are often associated with obesity (112).

The occurrence of small high-frequency ECG potentials (1 to 20 V), which cannot be determined using the routine 12-lead ECG, that can be seen at the end of the QRS complex and into the ST segment is also associated with an increased risk of ventricular arrhythmias and sudden cardiac death (113). The evaluation of these "late potentials" can be conducted with signal-averaged ECG (SAECG), a computer-assisted technique that allows the detection of occult abnormal electrical potentials occurring during ventricular repolarization. The occurrence of late potentials in a group of obese individuals without clinical heart disease was evaluated using SAECG (114). The prevalence and number of abnormalities increased with increasing BMI. In the subgroup with a BMI of 31 to 40 kg/m², 35% of the subjects had abnormal late potentials, whereas in the subgroup with a BMI of 41 to 50 kg/m^2 and in that with a BMI of more than 50 kg/m^2, 86% and 100% of the subjects, respectively, had abnormalities (114). These abnormalities were found in obese patients both with and without hypertension or diabetes. The presence of these late potentials may be facilitated by the pathologic myocardial changes associated with obesity, such as myocyte hypertrophy, focal myocardial disarray, fibrosis, and fat and mononuclear cell infiltration.

The mechanisms involved and, in particular, the clinical significance of obesity-associated QT prolongation remain speculative (1). However, of interest from a metabolic viewpoint is the idea that elevated FFA levels, which are associated with obesity, may affect cardiac repolarization, secondary in part to increased plasma catecholamines (115). Clinically, a correlation between the levels of long-chain saturated fatty acids and the occurrence of ventricular arrhythmias in patients with myocardial infarction have been reported in a univariate analysis (116). Although the QTc interval may not be extremely increased (about 440 msec) in the obese population (97,110), screening for prolonged QT in obesity may suffer from customary criteria because a prolongation of the QTc interval of more than 420 msec may be predictive of increased mortality in a healthy population that is followed for 15 years (117). Moreover, because extremely obese patients often have a dilated cardiomyopathy, fatal arrhythmias may be the most frequent cause of death (30,62).

Coronary Artery Disease

Atherosclerosis in human arteries develops over decades from an asymptomatic phase to manifest disease. The process begins in childhood as deposits of cholesterol and its esters settle in the intima of large muscular arteries (118). The initial lesion of atherosclerosis is referred to as "the fatty streak." Fatty streaks begin to appear in the coronary arteries 5 to 10 years later than in the aorta (118,119). In adults, obesity is associated with advanced atherosclerosis. Examination of arteries and tissue from autopsied young individuals (15 to 34 years) who have died from accidental injury, homicide, or suicide demonstrates that fatty streaks and raised lesions (fibrous plaques and plaques with calcification or ulceration) in the right coronary artery and the abdominal aorta are associated with obesity (120–123). More specifically, the Pathobiological Determinants of Atherosclerosis in Youth study demonstrated that both the thickness of the adipose pannus and an increased BMI were associated with more extensive fatty streaks and raised lesions in the right coronary artery (123). Moreover, after a follow-up of 26 years, the Framingham Heart Study and the Manitoba Study have documented that obesity represents an independent predictor of cardiovascular disease, particularly in women (107, 124). This association is more pronounced in individuals less than 50 years of age, reinforcing the contention that obesity leads to premature atherosclerosis; however, the association between obesity and ischemic heart disease may be evident only after 2 decades of follow-up (107).

Evidence indicates that dyslipidemia, smoking, obesity, and hyperglycemia are closely related to fatty streaks in the second decade of life, and the same risk factors, along with hypertension, are associated with plaques in the third decade of life (120). These data have led the American Heart Association to state that obesity is a major modifiable risk factor for cardiovascular disease (125,126). A high BMI is significantly associated with myocardial infarction, coronary insufficiency, and sudden death; the association is stronger with sudden death (107). Although obesity *per se* is considered a major modifiable risk factor for ischemic heart disease (8), one must remember that a remarkable heterogeneity exists among obese subjects and that the presence of visceral obesity generally worsens "the metabolic portrait," which is associated with a cluster of traditional and nontraditional risk factors—dyslipidemia, hypertension, type II diabetes mellitus, prothrombotic state, hyperinsulinemia, hypertriglyceridemia, and elevated apolipoprotein B—that are all potentially synergic and deleterious (127). Because not all obese individuals have an increased risk of coronary heart disease (CHD), the challenge for the clinician is to screen the obese patients who are "at risk," in other words, those who have obesity associated with the insulin-resistance syndrome.

Ample evidence suggests that the presence of excess fat in the abdomen in proportion to total body fat is an independent predictor of CHD (128–130). Only recently, however, has prospective evidence been provided that shows that abdominal obesity is associated with the accelerated progression of carotid atherosclerosis in men, independent of overall obesity and other risk factors and after only 4 years of follow-up (131). This relationship is significant in subjects with abdominal obesity and low-density lipoprotein (LDL) cholesterol levels of more than or equal to 3.8 mmol per L or serum apolipoprotein B levels of more than or equal to 1.01 g per L (131). Carotid thickening is considered a valid indicator of generalized atherosclerosis (132). Additionally, disturbances in lipoprotein metabolism and plasma insulin–glucose homeostasis, as well as elevations of blood pressure, which are risk factors for heart disease, have been reported in subjects with an excessive deposition of adipose tissue in the abdomen (13,133). Moreover, the abdominal distribution of body fat is associated with increased plasma levels of fibrinogen and factor VII, greater factor VIII:C coagulant activities, an elevated tissue plasminogen activator antigen level, and higher plasminogen activator inhibitor-1 antigen levels and activity (13,133–135). This hypercoagulable state that accompanies excessive central fat deposition may also be associated with left ventricular dysfunction (135) and impaired endothelial function (136,137).

Although the waist to hip ratio or waist circumference are somewhat less reproducible measures of obesity than BMI because of the larger extent of measurement variability (138), waist circumference positively correlates with abdominal fat content, and it may represent the most practical anthropometric measurement for the clinician for assessing a patient's abdominal fat content (139). This could further refine the screening of the obese individual "at risk." Lemieux et al. (140) reported that identification of men with a waist circumference of more than 90 cm and triglyceride levels of more than 2.0 mmol per L may allow detection of as many as 80% of the subjects with the insulin-resistance syndrome, which is associated with a cluster of risk factors for CHD. However, the waist circumference cutoff loses predictive power in patients with a BMI of more than or equal to 35 kg/m^2 (5).

Significant clinical coronary artery disease may be adequately assessed in obese subjects with nuclear cardiology imaging techniques (141–143). Because of obvious mechanical and physiologic limitations to stress testing (28), a dipyridamole thallium-201 or technetium-99m perfusion scan may be used for the evaluation of the presence of ischemic heart disease in lieu of exercise testing in very obese patients. Prolonged transmission scanning with thallium-201 in obese patients, as opposed to lean patients, is not required if one corrects for the attenuation factor resulting from obesity (144), and triple-head simultaneous emission transmission tomography using technetium-99m is also accurate in obesity (145). However, obese individuals may have several limitations because the examination table for nuclear medicine or catheterization usually does not accommodate subjects weighing more than 160 kg. In the catheterization laboratory, vascular access to the femoral vein and artery may be problematic and technically difficult, and bleeding may be difficult to control after catheter removal. Femoral access may not be ideal, not only because of the volume of adipose tissue but also because of the presence of intertrigo. The percutaneous radial approach has numerous advantages in the very obese patient because the frequency of complications using the percutaneous radial technique is very low (146).

The insulin-resistance syndrome generally should be treated aggressively after reperfusion therapy. Abnormal glucose tolerance may be an important determinant for long-term prognosis after coronary angioplasty (147) and after coronary artery bypass graft (CABG) surgery, as the components of the insulin-resistance syndrome are associated with the angiographic progression of atherosclerosis in nongrafted coronary arteries (148).

Surgeons often rightfully quote obesity as a risk factor for perioperative morbidity and mortality. The presence of comorbidities, such as hypertension, coronary artery disease, dyslipidemia, and type II diabetes mellitus, as well as the technical difficulties inherent to the surgical and postsurgical care of the obese patients, likely contributes to this perception. Obese patients have been shown to have a higher incidence of postoperative thromboembolic disease in noncardiac surgery, and the high risk of thromboembolic disease in obese patients may necessitate an aggressive position with regard to deep venous thrombosis prophylaxis (149). However, in contrast to frequent beliefs, obesity is not associated with increased mortality or postoperative cerebrovascular accidents after CABG surgery except for an increased incidence of sternal and superficial wound infection, saphenous vein harvest site infection, and atrial dysrhythmias (150,151). Possible explanations are that the large, poorly vascularized pannus is associated with a higher incidence of perioperative hyperglycemia in the obese and that the difficulty in wound surveillance may predispose these individuals to wound infections (151). These findings have been confirmed by another study in which obesity, which was defined by a BMI greater than 30 kg/m^2, was not associated with an increase risk of operative mortality, stroke, renal failure, acquired respiratory distress syndrome, prolonged mechanical ventilation, pneumonia, sepsis, pulmonary embolism, or ventricular arrhythmias (150). Notably, despite numerous alterations in respiratory physiology in obese patients, including the increased breathing workload, respiratory muscle inefficiency, the decreased functional reserve capacity and expiratory reserve volume, and closure of peripheral lung units, the rate of pulmonary complications is comparable to those seen in nonobese patients after CABG surgery (150,151). This discrepancy may reflect different treatment attitudes from staff in the late postoperative period, including performance of a more vigorous pulmonary toilet or more vigilance in enforcing the postoperative use of incentive spirometry and early ambulation in patients undergoing cardiac surgery. However, a study in the immediate postoperative period that included more than 24,000 patients reported infrequent, major unanticipated problems with ventilation in the postanesthesia period; obesity, along with diabetes, renal dysfunction, male sex, and an age greater than 60 years, was a risk factor for this complication (152).

Benefits of Weight Reduction on the Cardiovascular System

Thus, weight gain and obesity are associated with deleterious adaptations imposed on the cardiovascular system. Although weight loss may not represent a panacea for remedying all alterations to the heart, it remains a simple treatment for alleviating the numerous abnormalities encountered. Although different systems are affected by weight loss

TABLE 8.4. *Benefits of weight reduction on the cardiovascular system*

↓ Blood volume
↓ Stroke volume
↓ Cardiac output
↓ Pulmonary capillary wedge pressure
↓ Left ventricular mass
Improvement of left ventricular diastolic dysfunction

(e.g., neuroendocrine, articular, pulmonary, and digestive), Table 8.4 shows some beneficial effects of weight loss on the cardiovascular system.

Cardiopulmonary Complications of Weight Reduction Therapy

Weight loss through different modalities such as starvation (88,90), liquid protein diets (95,96), very low calorie diets, and even obesity-reduction surgery (61) has been associated with prolongation of the QTc interval. The prolongation of the QTc interval occurs independent of the biologic and nutritional value of the constituent protein or of the addition of mineral and trace supplements in the diet (95). Most importantly, liquid protein diets have been associated with potentially life-threatening arrhythmias that were only discovered after a 24-hour Holter recording with an associated normal routine ECG (153). Ventricular tachycardia (*torsade de pointes*) and fibrillation refractory to lidocaine, propranolol, phenytoin, mexiletine, disopyramide, and procainamide have been documented in subjects who have died under observation (88,95,154). Even alternative treatments, such as the infusion of potassium, calcium, magnesium, bicarbonate, glucagon, and even ventricular overdrive pacing or open chest cardiac massage have been ineffective in controlling the refractory arrhythmia (61,95).

Fenfluramine and dexfenfluramine, which reduce appetite by enhancing serotonin at nerve terminals in the hypothalamus, were removed from the United States marketplace in 1997 after reports of cardiac valve disorders (155), particularly aortic and mitral valve insufficiency. Valve involvement in these patients is histopathologically similar to that noted in the carcinoid syndrome or ergotamine-induced valve disease (156,157). The development of valvulopathy correlated strongly with the duration of exposure (158). An increased risk of primary pulmonary hypertension has also been documented (159–162). Of interest is the fact that no cases of cardiac valve abnormalities have been associated with the use of phentermine alone (163), and regression of valvular disease after the cessation of fenfluramine or dexfenfluramine has been described (164–166). Moreover, after the discontinuation of therapy, development or progression of valvular regurgitation is uncommon (164,165). Because improvement in valvular regurgitation may occur, surgical referral for valve repair and/or replacement may be delayed.

Sibutramine hydrochloride, a centrally acting drug that has been approved for long-term use, has not been associated with valve abnormalities (167). The prevalence of cardiac valve dysfunction was not increased in 133 obese patients treated with sibutramine for an average of 7.6 months (168). However, increases in blood pressure and heart rate may occur with the use of this drug (169), and, like phentermine, sibutramine should not be used in patients with untreated hypertension, coronary heart disease, CHF, arrhythmias, or stroke (167). Not surprisingly, because no significant systemic absorption occurs, no studies report orlistat-induced valve abnormalities.

CONCLUSION

Obesity is a chronic metabolic disorder associated with cardiovascular disease and increased morbidity and mortality. A variety of adaptations and alterations in cardiac structure and function occur as excessive adipose tissue accumulates, even in the absence of systemic hypertension or underlying organic heart disease. To meet increased metabolic needs, circulating blood volume, plasma volume, and cardiac output all increase in obesity. The increase in blood volume in turn increases venous return to the right and left ventricles, eventually producing dilation of these cardiac cavities and increasing wall tension. This leads to LVH, which is accompanied by a decrease in diastolic chamber compliance, eventually resulting in an increase in left ventricular filling pressure and left ventricular enlargement. As long as the LVH adapts to left ventricular chamber enlargement, systolic function is preserved. When the LVH fails to keep pace with progressive left ventricular dilation, the wall tension increases even further and systolic dysfunction may ensue. Systemic hypertension, pulmonary hypertension (left ventricular failure, chronic hypoxia), and coronary artery disease all occur with disproportionately high frequency in obese individuals, and these may cause or contribute to alterations in cardiac structure and function. An increased risk of sudden cardiac death also exists in obesity.

Although no prospective studies demonstrate that weight loss increases survival, strong evidence indicates that weight loss in overweight and obese individuals reduces risk factors for diabetes and cardiovascular disease.

REFERENCES

1. Poirier P, Eckel RH. The heart and obesity. In: Fuster V, Alexander RW, King S, et al., eds. *Hurst's the heart.* New York: McGraw-Hill, 2000:2289–2303.
2. Calle EE, Thun MJ, Petrelli JM, et al. Body-mass index and mortality in a prospective cohort of U.S. adults. *N Engl J Med* 1999;341:1097–1105.
3. Goldhaber SZ, Grodstein F, Stampfer MJ, et al. A prospective study of risk factors for pulmonary embolism in women. *JAMA* 1997;277:642–645.
4. Hansson PO, Eriksson H, Welin L, et al. Smoking and abdominal obesity: risk factors for venous thromboembolism among middle-aged men: "the study of men born in 1913." *Arch Intern Med* 1999;159:1886–1890.
5. National Institutes of Health. Clinical guidelines on the identification, evaluation, and treatment of overweight and obesity in adults—the evidence report. *Obes Res* 1998;6:51S–209S.
6. Drenick EJ, Bale GS, Seltzer F, et al. Excessive mortality and causes of death in morbidly obese men. *JAMA* 1980;243:443–445.
7. Kern PA, Saghizadeh M, Ong JM, et al. The expression of tumor necrosis factor in human adipose tissue. Regulation by obesity, weight loss, and relationship to lipoprotein lipase. *J Clin Invest* 1995;95:2111–2119.
8. Hotamisligil GS, Arner P, Caro JF, et al. Increased adipose tissue expression of tumor necrosis factor-alpha in human obesity and insulin resistance. *J Clin Invest* 1995;95:2409–2415.
9. Lundgren CH, Brown SL, Nordt TK, et al. Elaboration of type-1 plasminogen activator inhibitor from adipocytes. A potential pathogenetic link between obesity and cardiovascular disease. *Circulation* 1996;93:106–110.
10. Steppan CM, Bailey ST, Bhat S, et al. The hormone resistin links obesity to diabetes. *Nature* 2001;409:307–312.
11. Wajchenberg BL. Subcutaneous and visceral adipose tissue: their relation to the metabolic syndrome. *Endocr Rev* 2000;21:697–738.
12. Yudkin JS, Stehouwer CD, Emeis JJ, et al. C-reactive protein in healthy subjects: associations with obesity, insulin resistance, and endothelial dysfunction: a potential role for cytokines originating from adipose tissue? *Arterioscler Thromb Vasc Biol* 1999;19:972–978.
13. Cigolini M, Targher G, Bergamo AI, et al. Visceral fat accumulation and its relation to plasma hemostatic factors in healthy men. *Arterioscler Thromb Vasc Biol* 1996;16:368–374.
14. Mohamed-Ali V, Goodrick S, Rawesh A, et al. Subcutaneous adipose tissue releases interleukin-6, but not tumor necrosis factor-alpha, *in vivo. J Clin Endocrinol Metab* 1997;82:4196–4200.
15. Ridker PM. Novel risk factors and markers for coronary disease. *Adv Intern Med* 2000;45:391–418.
16. Tchernof A, Nolan A, Sites CK, et al. Weight loss reduces C-reactive protein levels in obese postmenopausal women. *Circulation* 2002;105:564–569.

17. Christian HA. Some newer aspects of the pathology of fat and fatty infiltration. *Bulletin of the Johns Hopkins Hospital* 1905;16:1–6.
18. Crandall DL, Hausman GJ, Kral JG. A review of the microcirculation of adipose tissue: anatomic, metabolic, and angiogenic perspectives. *Microcirculation* 1997;4:211–232.
19. Rosell S, Belfrage E. Blood circulation in adipose tissue. *Physiol Rev* 1979;59:1078–1104.
20. Larsen OA, Lassen NA, Quaade F. Blood flow through human adipose tissue determined with radioactive xenon. *Acta Physiol Scand* 1966;66:337–345.
21. Lesser GT, Deutsch S. Measurement of adipose tissue blood flow and perfusion in man by uptake of ^{85}Kr. *J Appl Physiol* 1967;23:621–630.
22. Oberg B, Rosell S. Sympathetic control of consecutive vascular sections in canine subcutaneous adipose tissue. *Acta Physiol Scand* 1967;71:47–56.
23. Linde B, Chisolm G. The interstitial space of adipose tissue as determined by single injection and equilibration techniques. *Acta Physiol Scand* 1975;95:383–390.
24. Collis T, Devereux RB, Roman MJ, et al. Relations of stroke volume and cardiac output to body composition: the Strong Heart Study. *Circulation* 2001;103:820–825.
25. Alpert MA. Obesity cardiomyopathy; pathophysiology and evolution of the clinical syndrome. *Am J Med Sci* 2001;321:225–236.
26. Kasper EK, Hruban RH, Baughman KL. Cardiomyopathy of obesity: a clinicopathologic evaluation of 43 obese patients with heart failure. *Am J Cardiol* 1992;70:921–924.
27. Mattsson E, Larsson UE, Rossner S. Is walking for exercise too exhausting for obese women? *Int J Obes Relat Metab Disord* 1997;21:380–386.
28. Poirier P, Després JP. Exercise in the management of obesity. *Cardiol Clin* 2001;19:459–470.
29. Kaltman AJ, Goldring RM. Role of circulatory congestion in the cardiorespiratory failure of obesity. *Am J Med* 1976;60:645–653.
30. Messerli FH, Nunez BD, Ventura HO, et al. Overweight and sudden death. Increased ventricular ectopy in cardiopathy of obesity. *Arch Intern Med* 1987;147:1725–1728.
31. Messerli FH. Cardiopathy of obesity—a not-so-Victorian disease. *N Engl J Med* 1986;314:378–380.
32. Ku CS, Lin SL, Wang DJ, et al. Left ventricular filling in young normotensive obese adults. *Am J Cardiol* 1994;73:613–615.
33. Sasson Z, Rasooly Y, Gupta R, et al. Left atrial enlargement in healthy obese: prevalence and relation to left ventricular mass and diastolic function. *Can J Cardiol* 1996;12:257–263.
34. Backman L, Freyschuss U, Hallberg D, et al. Reversibility of cardiovascular changes in extreme obesity. Effects of weight reduction through jejunoileostomy. *Acta Med Scand* 1979;205:367–373.
35. Backman L, Freyschuss U, Hallberg D, et al. Cardiovascular function in extreme obesity. *Acta Med Scand* 1973;193:437–446.
36. Alexander JK, Peterson KL. Cardiovascular effects of weight reduction. *Circulation* 1972;45:310–318.
37. Alpert MA, Lambert CR, Terry BE, et al. Effect of weight loss on left ventricular mass in nonhypertensive morbidly obese patients. *Am J Cardiol* 1994;73:918–921.
38. Alpert MA, Kelly DL. Value and limitations of echocardiography assessment of obese patients. *Echocardiography* 1986;3:261–272.
39. House AA, Walley VM. Right heart failure due to ventricular adiposity: "adipositas cordis"—an old diagnosis revisited. *Can J Cardiol* 1996;12:485–489.
40. Prior JT. Lipomatous hypertrophy of the cardiac interatrial septum. A lesion resembling hibernoma, lipoblastomatosis and infiltrating lipoma. *Arch Pathol* 1964;78:11.
41. Page DL. Lipomatous hypertrophy of the cardiac interatrial septum: its development and probable clinical significance. *Hum Pathol* 1970;1:151–163.
42. Isner JM, Swan CS, Mikus JP, et al. Lipomatous hypertrophy of the interatrial septum: *in vivo* diagnosis. *Circulation* 1982;66:470–473.
43. Jornet A, Batalla J, Uson M, et al. Lipomatous hypertrophy of the interatrial septum. *Echocardiography* 1992;9:501–503.
44. Daniels SR, Kimball TR, Morrison JA, et al. Effect of lean body mass, fat mass, blood pressure, and sexual maturation on left ventricular mass in children and adolescents. Statistical, biological, and clinical significance. *Circulation* 1995;92:3249–3254.
45. Levy D, Savage DD, Garrison RJ, et al. Echocardiographic criteria for left ventricular hypertrophy: the Framingham Heart Study. *Am J Cardiol* 1987;59:956–960.
46. Levy D, Anderson KM, Savage DD, et al. Echocardiographically detected left ventricular hypertrophy: prevalence and risk factors. The Framingham Heart Study. *Ann Intern Med* 1988;108:7–13.
47. de Simone G, Daniels SR, Devereux RB, et al. Left ventricular mass and body size in normotensive children and adults: assessment of allometric relations and impact of overweight. *J Am Coll Cardiol* 1992;20:1251–1260.
48. Lauer MS, Anderson KM, Larson MG, et al. A new method for indexing left ventricular mass for differences in body size. *Am J Cardiol* 1994;74:487–491.
49. Hense HW, Gneiting B, Muscholl M, et al. The associations of body size and body composition with left ventricular mass: impacts for indexation in adults. *J Am Coll Cardiol* 1998;32:451–457.
50. Alpert MA, Lambert CR, Panayiotou H, et al. Relation of duration of morbid obesity to left ventricular mass, systolic function, and diastolic filling, and effect of weight loss. *Am J Cardiol* 1995;76:1194–1197.

51. Karason K, Lindroos AK, Stenlof K, et al. Relief of cardiorespiratory symptoms and increased physical activity after surgically induced weight loss. Results from the Swedish Obese Subjects Study. *Arch Intern Med* 2000; 160:1797–1802.

52. Chakko S, Mayor M, Allison MD, et al. Abnormal left ventricular diastolic filling in eccentric left ventricular hypertrophy of obesity. *Am J Cardiol* 1991;68:95–98.

53. Alpert MA, Lambert CR, Terry BE, et al. Effect of weight loss on left ventricular diastolic filling in morbid obesity. *Am J Cardiol* 1995;76:1198–1201.

54. Poirier P, Bogaty P, Garneau C, et al. Diastolic dysfunction in type 2 diabetes men without hypertension or coronary artery disease: importance of the Valsalva maneuver in screening patients. *Diabetes Care* 2001;24:5–10.

55. Rakowski H, Appleton C, Chan KL, et al. Canadian consensus recommendations for the measurement and reporting of diastolic dysfunction by echocardiography: from the Investigators of Consensus on Diastolic Dysfunction by Echocardiography. *J Am Soc Echocardiogr* 1996;9:736–760.

56. Dumesnil JG, Gaudreault G, Honos GN, et al. Use of Valsalva maneuver to unmask left ventricular diastolic function abnormalities by Doppler echocardiography in patients with coronary artery disease or systemic hypertension. *Am J Cardiol* 1991;68:515–519.

57. Paquette C, Marceau P, Biron S, et al. Importance of maneuvers in echocardiographic screening for preclinical left ventricular diastolic dysfunction in morbidly obese subjects with type 2 diabetes. *Circulation* 2001;102: 793.

58. Caviezel F, Margonato A, Slaviero G, et al. Early improvement of left ventricular function during caloric restriction in obesity. *Int J Obes* 1986;10:421–426.

59. MacMahon SW, Wilcken DE, Macdonald GJ. The effect of weight reduction on left ventricular mass. A randomized controlled trial in young, overweight hypertensive patients. *N Engl J Med* 1986;314:334–339.

60. Amad KH, Brennan JC, Alexander JK. The cardiac pathology of chronic exogenous obesity. *Circulation* 1965; 32:740–745.

61. Drenick EJ, Fisler JS. Sudden cardiac arrest in morbidly obese surgical patients unexplained after autopsy. *Am J Surg* 1988;155:720–726.

62. Messerli FH, Sundgaard-Riise K, Reisin ED, et al. Dimorphic cardiac adaptation to obesity and arterial hypertension. *Ann Intern Med* 1983;99:757–761.

63. Smith HL, Willius FA. Adiposity of the heart: a clinical and pathologic study of one hundred and thirty-six obese patients. *Arch Intern Med* 1933;52:911–931.

64. Himeno E, Nishino K, Nakashima Y, et al. Weight reduction regresses left ventricular mass regardless of blood pressure level in obese subjects. *Am Heart J* 1996;131:313–319.

65. Benjamin EJ, Levy D. Why is left ventricular hypertrophy so predictive of morbidity and mortality? *Am J Med Sci* 1999;317:168–175.

66. Tuck ML, Sowers J, Dornfeld L, et al. The effect of weight reduction on blood pressure, plasma renin activity, and plasma aldosterone levels in obese patients. *N Engl J Med* 1981;304:930–933.

67. Sasson Z, Rasooly Y, Bhesania T, et al. Insulin resistance is an important determinant of left ventricular mass in the obese. *Circulation* 1993;88:1431–1436.

68. Vela-Huerta MM, Vargas-Origel A, Olvera-Lopez A. Asymmetrical septal hypertrophy in newborn infants of diabetic mothers. *Am J Perinatol* 2000;17:89–94.

69. de Divitiis O, Fazio S, Petitto M, et al. Obesity and cardiac function. *Circulation* 1981;64:477–482.

70. Nakajima T, Fujioka S, Tokunaga K, et al. Correlation of intraabdominal fat accumulation and left ventricular performance in obesity. *Am J Cardiol* 1989;64:369–373.

71. Brautigam P, Foldi E, Schaiper I, et al. Analysis of lymphatic drainage in various forms of leg edema using two compartment lymphoscintigraphy. *Lymphology* 1998;31:43–55.

72. Fowkes FG, Lee AJ, Evans CJ, et al. Lifestyle risk factors for lower limb venous reflux in the general population: Edinburgh Vein Study. *Int J Epidemiol* 2001;30:846–852.

73. Stamler R, Stamler J, Riedlinger WF, et al. Weight and blood pressure. Findings in hypertension screening of 1 million Americans. *JAMA* 1978;240:1607–1610.

74. Maxwell MH, Waks AU, Schroth PC, et al. Error in blood-pressure measurement due to incorrect cuff size in obese patients. *Lancet* 1982;2:33–36.

75. Nelson WP, North RL. Splitting of the second heart sound in adults forty years and older. *Am J Med Sci* 1967; 254:805–807.

76. Alpert MA, Alexander JK. *The heart and lung in obesity.* Armonk: Futura Publishing, 1998.

77. Cheyne J. A case of apoplexy in which the fleshy part of the heart was converted into fat. *Dublin Hosp Rep* 1818;2:216–223.

78. Roberts WC, Roberts JD. The floating heart or the heart too fat to sink: analysis of 55 necropsy patients. *Am J Cardiol* 1983;52:1286–1289.

79. De Scheerder I, Cuvelier C, Verhaaren R, et al. Restrictive cardiomyopathy caused by adipositas cordis. *Eur Heart J* 1987;8:661–663.

80. Carpenter CL. Myocardial fat infiltration. *Am Heart J* 1962;63:491–496.

81. Saphir O, Corrigan M. Fatty infiltration of the myocardium. *Arch Intern Med* 1933;52:410–428.

82. Balsaver AM, Morales AR, Whitehouse FW. Fat infiltration of myocardium as a cause of cardiac conduction defect. *Am J Cardiol* 1967;19:261–265.

83. Spain DM, Cathcart RT. Heart block caused by fat infiltration of the inter-ventricular septum (cor adiposum). *Am Heart J* 1946;32:659–664.

84. Dervan JP, Ilercil A, Kane PB, et al. Fatty infiltration: another restrictive cardiomyopathic pattern. *Catheter Cardiovasc Diagn* 1991;22:184–189.
85. Unger RH. Lipotoxic diseases. *Annu Rev Med* 2002;53:319–336.
86. Duflou J, Virmani R, Rabin I, et al. Sudden death as a result of heart disease in morbid obesity. *Am Heart J* 1995;130:306–313.
87. Mason JW, O'Connell JB. Clinical merit of endomyocardial biopsy. *Circulation* 1989;79:971–979.
88. Pringle TH, Scobie IN, Murray RG, et al. Prolongation of the QT interval during therapeutic starvation: a substrate for malignant arrhythmias. *Int J Obes* 1983;7:253–261.
89. Sandhofer F, Dienstl F, Bolzano K, et al. Severe cardiovascular complication associated with prolonged starvation. *BMJ* 1973;1:462–463.
90. Garnett ES, Barnard DL, Ford J, et al. Gross fragmentation of cardiac myofibrils after therapeutic starvation for obesity. *Lancet* 1969;1:914–916.
91. Rasmussen LH, Andersen T. The relationship between QTc changes and nutrition during weight loss after gastroplasty. *Acta Med Scand* 1985;217:271–275.
92. Alpert MA, Terry BE, Hamm CR, et al. Effect of weight loss on the ECG of normotensive morbidly obese patients. *Chest* 2001;119:507–510.
93. Pidlich J, Pfeffel F, Zwiauer K, et al. The effect of weight reduction on the surface electrocardiogram: a prospective trial in obese children and adolescents. *Int J Obes Relat Metab Disord* 1997;21:1018–1023.
94. Eisenstein I, Edelstein J, Sarma R, et al. The electrocardiogram in obesity. *J Electrocardiol* 1982;15:115–118.
95. Sours HE, Frattali VP, Brand CD, et al. Sudden death associated with very low calorie weight reduction regimens. *Am J Clin Nutr* 1981;34:453–461.
96. Isner JM, Sours HE, Paris AL, et al. Sudden, unexpected death in avid dieters using the liquid-protein–modified fast diet. Observations in 17 patients and the role of the prolonged QT interval. *Circulation* 1979;60:1401–1412.
97. Frank S, Colliver JA, Frank A. The electrocardiogram in obesity: statistical analysis of 1,029 patients. *J Am Coll Cardiol* 1986;7:295–299.
98. Peiris AN, Thakur RK, Sothmann MS, et al. Relationship of regional fat distribution and obesity to electrocardiographic parameters in healthy premenopausal women. *South Med J* 1991;84:961–965.
99. Alpert MA, Terry BE, Cohen MV, et al. The electrocardiogram in morbid obesity. *Am J Cardiol* 2000;85:908–910.
100. Master AM, Oppenheimer ET. A study of obesity: circulatory, roentgen-ray and electrocardiographic investigations. *JAMA* 1929;92:1652–1656.
101. Lavie CJ, Amodeo C, Ventura HO, et al. Left atrial abnormalities indicating diastolic ventricular dysfunction in cardiopathy of obesity. *Chest* 1987;92:1042–1046.
102. Starr JW, Wagner GS, Behar VS, et al. Vectorcardiographic criteria for the diagnosis of inferior myocardial infarction. *Circulation* 1974;49:829–836.
103. Nath A, Alpert MA, Terry BE, et al. Sensitivity and specificity of electrocardiographic criteria for left and right ventricular hypertrophy in morbid obesity. *Am J Cardiol* 1988;62:126–130.
104. Casale PN, Devereux RB, Kligfield P, et al. Electrocardiographic detection of left ventricular hypertrophy: development and prospective validation of improved criteria. *J Am Coll Cardiol* 1985;6:572–580.
105. Abergel E, Tase M, Menard J, et al. Influence of obesity on the diagnostic value of electrocardiographic criteria for detecting left ventricular hypertrophy. *Am J Cardiol* 1996;77:739–744.
106. Kannel WB, Plehn JF, Cupples LA. Cardiac failure and sudden death in the Framingham Study. *Am Heart J* 1988;115:869–875.
107. Rabkin SW, Mathewson FA, Hsu PH. Relation of body weight to development of ischemic heart disease in a cohort of young North American men after a 26 year observation period: the Manitoba Study. *Am J Cardiol* 1977;39:452–458.
108. Alexander JK. The cardiomyopathy of obesity. *Prog Cardiovasc Dis* 1985;27:325–334.
109. el-Gamal A, Gallagher D, Nawras A, et al. Effects of obesity on QT, RR, and QTc intervals. *Am J Cardiol* 1995;75:956–959.
110. Mshui ME, Saikawa T, Ito K, et al. QT interval and QT dispersion before and after diet therapy in patients with simple obesity. *Proc Soc Exp Biol Med* 1999;220:133–138.
111. Festa A, D'Agostino R Jr, Rautaharju P, et al. Relation of systemic blood pressure, left ventricular mass, insulin sensitivity, and coronary artery disease to QT interval duration in nondiabetic and type 2 diabetic subjects. *Am J Cardiol* 2000;86:1117–1122.
112. Girola A, Enrini R, Garbetta F, et al. QT dispersion in uncomplicated human obesity. *Obes Res* 2001;9:71–77.
113. Signal-averaged electrocardiography. *J Am Coll Cardiol* 1996;27:238–249.
114. Lalani AP, Kanna B, John J, et al. Abnormal signal-averaged electrocardiogram (SAECG) in obesity. *Obes Res* 2000;8:20–28.
115. Marfella R, De Angelis L, Nappo F, et al. Elevated plasma fatty acid concentrations prolong cardiac repolarization in healthy subjects. *Am J Clin Nutr* 2001;73:27–30.
116. Abraham R, Riemersma RA, Wood D, et al. Adipose fatty acid composition and the risk of serious ventricular arrhythmias in acute myocardial infarction. *Am J Cardiol* 1989;63:269–272.
117. Schouten EG, Dekker JM, Meppelink P, et al. QT interval prolongation predicts cardiovascular mortality in an apparently healthy population. *Circulation* 1991;84:1516–1523.
118. McGill HC. Fatty streaks in the coronary arteries and aorta. *Lab Invest* 1968;18:560–564.

119. Strong JP, McGill HC Jr. The natural history of coronary atherosclerosis. *Am J Pathol* 1962;40:37–49.
120. McGill HC Jr, McMahan CA, Herderick EE, et al. Origin of atherosclerosis in childhood and adolescence. *Am J Clin Nutr* 2000;72:1307S–1315S.
121. Berenson GS. Bogalusa Heart Study: a long-term community study of a rural biracial (black/white) population. *Am J Med Sci* 2001;322:293–300.
122. Enos WF, Holmes RH, Beyer J. Coronary disease among United States soldiers killed in action in Korea. *JAMA* 1953;152:1090–1093.
123. McGill HC, McMahan CA, Malcom GT, et al. Relation of glycohemoglobin and adiposity to atherosclerosis in youth. Pathobiological Determinants of Atherosclerosis in Youth (PDAY) Research Group. *Arterioscler Thromb Vasc Biol* 1995;15:431–440.
124. Hubert HB, Feinleib M, McNamara PM, et al. Obesity as an independent risk factor for cardiovascular disease: a 26-year follow-up of participants in the Framingham Heart Study. *Circulation* 1983;67:968–977.
125. Eckel RH. Obesity and heart disease: a statement for healthcare professionals from the Nutrition Committee, American Heart Association. *Circulation* 1997;96:3248–3250.
126. Eckel RH, Krauss RM. American Heart Association call to action: obesity as a major risk factor for coronary heart disease. AHA Nutrition Committee. *Circulation* 1998;97:2099–2100.
127. Després JP. Health consequences of visceral obesity. *Ann Med* 2001;33:534–541.
128. Larsson B, Svardsudd K, Welin L, et al. Abdominal adipose tissue distribution, obesity, and risk of cardiovascular disease and death: 13 year follow up of participants in the study of men born in 1913. *BMJ* 1984;288: 1401–1404.
129. Folsom AR, Kaye SA, Sellers TA, et al. Body fat distribution and 5-year risk of death in older women. *JAMA* 1993;269:483–487.
130. Rexrode KM, Carey VJ, Hennekens CH, et al. Abdominal adiposity and coronary heart disease in women. *JAMA* 1998;280:1843–1848.
131. Lakka TA, Lakka HM, Salonen R, et al. Abdominal obesity is associated with accelerated progression of carotid atherosclerosis in men. *Atherosclerosis* 2001;154:497–504.
132. O'Leary DH, Polak JF, Kronmal RA, et al. Carotid-artery intima and media thickness as a risk factor for myocardial infarction and stroke in older adults. Cardiovascular Health Study Collaborative Research Group. *N Engl J Med* 1999;340:14–22.
133. Svendsen OL, Hassager C, Christiansen C, et al. Plasminogen activator inhibitor-1, tissue-type plasminogen activator, and fibrinogen: effect of dieting with or without exercise in overweight postmenopausal women. *Arterioscler Thromb Vasc Biol* 1996;16:381–385.
134. Folsom AR, Qamhieh HT, Wing RR, et al. Impact of weight loss on plasminogen activator inhibitor (PAI-1), factor VII, and other hemostatic factors in moderately overweight adults. *Arterioscler Thromb* 1993;13: 162–169.
135. Licata G, Scaglione R, Avellone G, et al. Hemostatic function in young subjects with central obesity: relationship with left ventricular function. *Metabolism* 1995;44:1417–1421.
136. Steinberg HO, Chaker H, Leaming R, et al. Obesity/insulin resistance is associated with endothelial dysfunction. Implications for the syndrome of insulin resistance. *J Clin Invest* 1996;97:2601–2610.
137. Hashimoto M, Akishita M, Eto M, et al. The impairment of flow-mediated vasodilatation in obese men with visceral fat accumulation. *Int J Obes Relat Metab Disord* 1998;22:477–484.
138. Williams SR, Jones E, Bell W, et al. Body habitus and coronary heart disease in men. A review with reference to methods of body habitus assessment. *Eur Heart J* 1997;18:376–393.
139. Pouliot MC, Després JP, Lemieux S, et al. Waist circumference and abdominal sagittal diameter: best simple anthropometric indexes of abdominal visceral adipose tissue accumulation and related cardiovascular risk in men and women. *Am J Cardiol* 1994;73:460–468.
140. Lemieux I, Pascot A, Couillard C, et al. Hypertriglyceridemic waist. A marker of the atherogenic metabolic triad (hyperinsulinemia; hyperapolipoprotein B; small, dense LDL) in men? *Circulation* 2000;102:179–184.
141. Alaud-din A, Meterissian S, Lisbona R, et al. Assessment of cardiac function in patients who were morbidly obese. *Surgery* 1990;108:809–818.
142. Gal RA, Gunasekera J, Massardo T, et al. Long-term prognostic value of a normal dipyridamole thallium-201 perfusion scan. *Clin Cardiol* 1991;14:971–974.
143. Ferraro S, Perrone-Filardi P, Desiderio A, et al. Left ventricular systolic and diastolic function in severe obesity: a radionuclide study. *Cardiology* 1996;87:347–353.
144. Prvulovich EM, Lonn AH, Bomanji JB, et al. Transmission scanning for attenuation correction of myocardial ^{201}Tl images in obese patients. *Nucl Med Commun* 1997;18:207–218.
145. Barnden LR, Ong PL, Rowe CC. Simultaneous emission transmission tomography using technetium-99m for both emission and transmission. *Eur J Nucl Med* 1997;24:1390–1397.
146. Barbeau GR, Gleeton O, Juneau C, et al. Transradial approach for coronary angiography and interventions: procedural results and vascular complications from a series of 7049 procedures. *Circulation* 1999;100:I306.
147. Otsuka Y, Miyazaki S, Okumura H, et al. Abnormal glucose tolerance, not small vessel diameter, is a determinant of long-term prognosis in patients treated with balloon coronary angioplasty. *Eur Heart J* 2000;21: 1790–1796.
148. Korpilahti K, Syvanne M, Engblom E, et al. Components of the insulin resistance syndrome are associated with progression of atherosclerosis in non-grafted arteries 5 years after coronary artery bypass surgery. *Eur Heart J* 1998;19:711–719.

149. Marik P, Varon J. The obese patient in the ICU. *Chest* 1998;113:492–498.

150. Moulton MJ, Creswell LL, Mackey ME, et al. Obesity is not a risk factor for significant adverse outcomes after cardiac surgery. *Circulation* 1996;94:II87–II92.

151. Birkmeyer NJ, Charlesworth DC, Hernandez F, et al. Obesity and risk of adverse outcomes associated with coronary artery bypass surgery. Northern New England Cardiovascular Disease Study Group. *Circulation* 1998;97:1689–1694.

152. Rose DK, Cohen MM, Wigglesworth DF, et al. Critical respiratory events in the postanesthesia care unit. Patient, surgical, and anesthetic factors. *Anesthesiology* 1994;81:410–418.

153. Lantigua RA, Amatruda JM, Biddle TL, et al. Cardiac arrhythmias associated with a liquid protein diet for the treatment of obesity. *N Engl J Med* 1980;303:735–738.

154. Singh BN, Gaarder TD, Kanegae T, et al. Liquid protein diets and torsade de pointes. *JAMA* 1978;240:115–119.

155. Centers for Disease Control and Prevention. Cardiac valvulopathy associated with exposure to fenfluramine or dexfenfluramine: US Department of Health and Human Services interim public health recommendations. *JAMA* 1997;278:1729–1731.

156. Robiolio PA, Rigolin VH, Wilson JS, et al. Carcinoid heart disease. Correlation of high serotonin levels with valvular abnormalities detected by cardiac catheterization and echocardiography. *Circulation* 1995;92: 790–795.

157. Redfield MM, Nicholson WJ, Edwards WD, et al. Valve disease associated with ergot alkaloid use: echocardiographic and pathologic correlations. *Ann Intern Med* 1992;117:50–52.

158. Ryan DH, Bray GA, Helmcke F, et al. Serial echocardiographic and clinical evaluation of valvular regurgitation before, during, and after treatment with fenfluramine or dexfenfluramine and mazindol or phentermine. *Obes Res* 1999;7:313–322.

159. Connolly HM, Crary JL, McGoon MD, et al. Valvular heart disease associated with fenfluramine-phentermine. *N Engl J Med* 1997;337:581–588.

160. Weissman NJ, Tighe JF Jr., Gottdiener JS, et al. An assessment of heart-valve abnormalities in obese patients taking dexfenfluramine, sustained-release dexfenfluramine, or placebo. Sustained-Release Dexfenfluramine Study Group. *N Engl J Med* 1998;339:725–732.

161. Khan MA, Herzog CA, St Peter JV, et al. The prevalence of cardiac valvular insufficiency assessed by transthoracic echocardiography in obese patients treated with appetite-suppressant drugs. *N Engl J Med* 1998;339: 713–718.

162. Abenhaim L, Moride Y, Brenot F, et al. Appetite-suppressant drugs and the risk of primary pulmonary hypertension. International Primary Pulmonary Hypertension Study Group. *N Engl J Med* 1996;335:609–616.

163. Jick H, Vasilakis C, Weinrauch LA, et al. A population-based study of appetite-suppressant drugs and the risk of cardiac-valve regurgitation. *N Engl J Med* 1998;339:719–724.

164. Weissman NJ, Panza JA, Tighe JF, et al. Natural history of valvular regurgitation 1 year after discontinuation of dexfenfluramine therapy. A randomized, double-blind, placebo-controlled trial. *Ann Intern Med* 2001;134: 267–273.

165. Mast ST, Jollis JG, Ryan T, et al. The progression of fenfluramine-associated valvular heart disease assessed by echocardiography. *Ann Intern Med* 2001;134:261–266.

166. Cannistra LB, Cannistra AJ. Regression of multivalvular regurgitation after the cessation of fenfluramine and phentermine treatment. *N Engl J Med* 1998;339:771.

167. McNeely W, Goa KL. Sibutramine. A review of its contribution to the management of obesity. *Drugs* 1998;56: 1093–1124.

168. Bach DS, Rissanen AM, Mendel CM, et al. Absence of cardiac valve dysfunction in obese patients treated with sibutramine. *Obes Res* 1999;7:363–369.

169. Atkinson RL. Use of drugs in the treatment of obesity. *Annu Rev Nutr* 1997;17:383–403.

9

Sleep-Disordered Breathing

Tracey D. Robinson and Ronald R. Grunstein

PATHOGENESIS

Physiology of Sleep

To sleep physiologists, humans exist in the following three states: wakefulness, nonrapid eye movement (NREM) sleep, and rapid eye movement (REM or dreaming) sleep. These states exhibit marked differences in many aspects of physiology. Sleep has profound effects on breathing, and these effects are usually greatest during REM sleep. Moreover, sleep can amplify the effects of drugs such as alcohol and opiates on breathing.

In normal subjects, sleep is associated with a fall in minute ventilation that is primarily caused by a drop in tidal volume. As a result, a small rise occurs in arterial blood carbon dioxide tension ($PaCO_2$), and a small fall occurs in arterial blood oxygen tension (PaO_2). During NREM sleep, the hypoxic drive to breathe is reduced, and the ventilatory response to hypercapnia is diminished. This depression of chemosensitivity is greatest during REM sleep. Sleep is also associated with a reduction in tone of the upper-airway dilator muscles with a resulting increase in resistance to airflow. REM sleep is characterized by postural muscle atonia with bursts of eye movements and associated peripheral muscle twitches (phasic REM). Phasic REM is associated with marked breathing irregularity. The loss of postural muscle tone during REM sleep leaves humans largely reliant on the diaphragm, a nonpostural muscle, to maintain ventilation. An individual with abnormal diaphragm function resulting from either neuromuscular disease or mechanical disadvantage (e.g., kyphoscoliosis, lung disease, or obesity) will have impaired breathing in sleep, particularly during REM sleep. An individual with a combination of these factors (e.g., an obese patient with lung disease) will have an even greater risk of developing sleep-related respiratory failure.

Definitions

Sleep-disordered breathing is defined by the loss of a normal pattern of breathing during sleep, and it ranges from snoring to profound nocturnal hypoventilation and respiratory failure during sleep. Intermittent snoring with no associated sleep fragmentation (so-called "simple snoring") is common, and it is generally not considered part of the spectrum of sleep-disordered breathing. On the other hand, heavy snoring can result in arousals from sleep with accompanying sleep disruption, and it should be considered part of the disease state (1).

Obstructive sleep apnea (OSA) is characterized by repetitive episodes of a complete cessation of airflow (apnea) during sleep that result from collapse of the upper airway, generally at the level of the pharynx (2). During an apnea, continued respiratory efforts occur against the closed airway (Table 9.1), resulting in hypoxemia until the apnea is terminated by arousal from sleep with restoration of upper-airway patency. Typically, after a few deep breaths, this cycle is repeated, often hundreds of times through the night (Fig. 9.1). The recurrent arousals cause sleep fragmentation, resulting in daytime sleepiness (3).

Significant upper-airway obstruction can occur in the absence of complete collapse of the upper airway. Increased airway resistance can produce a measurable reduction in airflow (hypopnea) that has the same consequences—hypoxemia and arousal—as an apnea. Even extremely minor increases in airway resistance without detectable reductions in airflow can produce recurrent arousals and excessive daytime sleepiness (EDS)—the "upper-airway resistance syndrome" (1).

Patients with impaired daytime respiratory function, whatever the cause, will have abnormal breathing and will often develop impaired gas exchange during sleep. These patients may have prolonged periods of hypoxemia that last minutes, usually because of reduced ventilation—hypoventilation—although worsening ventilation and/or perfusion mismatches may also contribute. Hypercapnia also develops during sleep as a result of hypoventilation. These prolonged episodes of sleep-related hypercapnic hypoxia can lead to a "resetting" of chemoreceptors with subsequent blunted daytime chemosensitivity and the development or worsening of daytime hypercapnic respiratory failure. In addition, the prolonged exposure to hypoxemia and hypercapnia may lead to pulmonary hypertension (PHT) and right-sided heart failure, which is known as *cor pulmonale*. Patients with these severe forms of respiratory failure in sleep include patients with many types of chronic lung disease, respiratory muscle failure resulting from neuromuscular disorders, and, significantly, the obesity-hypoventilation syndrome (OHS) (see"Obesity-Hypoventilation Syndrome" below).

Central apnea refers to the cessation of airflow with no detectable respiratory effort, which contrasts with obstructive apneas in which breathing efforts are often vigorous. Some confusion surrounds this term because it has been used to describe the patterns of breathing in patients in whom hypoventilation is the predominant pathology. The pattern of breathing that tends to occur in patients with awake hypercapnia and reduced respiratory drive should be differentiated from the "true" central apneas that classically occur as part of the periodic breathing seen in patients with cardiac failure (also called Cheyne–Stokes breathing) (4). In this breathing pattern, ventilation waxes and wanes

TABLE 9.1. *Terms used to describe sleep-disordered breathing*

Term	Definition
Apnea	Complete cessation of airflow for at least 10 sec
Hypopnea	Reduction in airflow for at least 10 sec ending with an arousal or associated with oxygen desaturation of at least 3%
Obstructive event	Continued respiratory effort occurs despite reduced airflow, as above
Central event	Respiratory effort is absent, with absent airflow
Periodic breathing (Cheyne–Stokes respiration)	Respiration that waxes and wanes, alternating between hyperventilation and central apnea—seen in patients with heart failure or neurologic disease
Hypoventilation	An abnormal rise in $Paco_2$ during sleep that is usually associated with oxygen desaturation with or without discrete respiratory events
Apnea-hypopnea index (respiratory disturbance index)	Number of apneic and hypopneic episodes per hr of sleep; more than five is usually considered abnormal

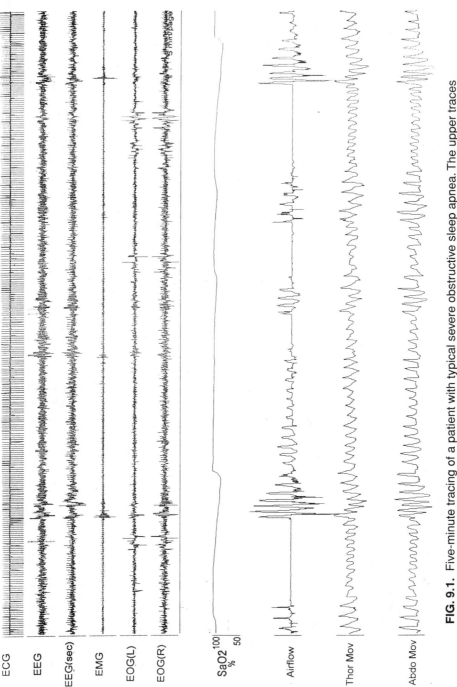

FIG. 9.1. Five-minute tracing of a patient with typical severe obstructive sleep apnea. The upper traces show the variables used for sleep staging and indicate that this patient is in rapid eye movement sleep. The apneas are indicated by intermittent cessation of airflow (*Airflow*, nasal airflow), and they are obstructive in nature, as continued respiratory effort is seen when airflow is absent (*Abdo Mov*, abdominal movement or effort; *Thor Mov*, thoracic movement or effort). Repetitive falls in oxygen saturation (Sao$_2$) are seen after each apnea. Abbreviations: *ECG*, electrocardiogram; *EEG*, electroencephalogram; *EMG*, electromyogram; *EOG*, electrooculogram.

from hyperventilation to central apnea. Periodic breathing can also occur in patients with neurologic disease caused by strokes or rarely as an idiopathic form. Sporadic central apneas may also occur in patients with severe OSA, and these usually disappear when the OSA is treated. The etiology of central apnea in the patient with cardiac failure is complex, involving interplay between circulation time, a brisk chemoreceptor drive, and upper-airway narrowing (4).

Pathogenesis of Obstructive Sleep Apnea

General

Upper-airway collapse occurs when the negative (or suction) pressure applied to the upper airway during inspiration is greater than the dilating forces applied by the upper-airway muscles, such as the genioglossus (2,5). Collapse of the upper airway usually occurs in the retropalatal or retroglossal areas, and most patients have more than one site of collapse. Less frequently, upper-airway collapse can occur at the epiglottis or glottis (4). The determinants of the site of collapse in individual patients are unclear. Any factors that reduce airway size, decrease airway muscle tone, increase upper-airway compliance, or lead to the generation of a greater inspiratory pressure will predispose a patient to the development of OSA (5). Muscle tone and suction pressure are influenced by sleep stage and the relative respiratory drive to the diaphragm versus that to the upper-airway dilator muscles.

Several studies have shown that the pharyngeal airway is smaller in patients with OSA than in normal subjects (6,7). When the airway size is reduced, a greater suction pressure is required during inspiration. In the awake state, patients with OSA have increased upper-airway dilator muscle activity that normalizes airflow resistance despite the anatomically smaller airway (8,9). This compensatory increased upper-airway muscle activity is lost during sleep, particularly in the genioglossus, thus resulting in airway closure (2). However, although the increased waking genioglossus activity is seen in some patients with OSA, some patients have genioglossus muscle activity values similar to those of control subjects (9). Compensatory muscle activity may be increased in other muscle groups, or other mechanisms may be important in such patients.

Patients with OSA may also have defects in the sensory mechanisms that normally protect the upper airway from closure (10). However, determining whether identified defects in sensory control, which are based on both clinical and histopathologic changes in patients with OSA, have a role in the genesis of OSA or if they are due to chronic airway vibration from snoring is difficult.

Role of Obesity

Obesity is one of the strongest risk factors for OSA. Obesity can reduce upper-airway size in a number of ways and can therefore predispose the upper airway to collapse. External neck circumference is increased in patients with OSA; this measurement may explain a portion of the link between obesity and sleep apnea (11,12). Neck circumference is an index of neck fat deposition, particularly in the lateral pharyngeal fat pads, and this fat deposition may lead to airway narrowing and OSA (13). Imaging studies have shown that these fat pads are larger in obese patients with OSA (14). However, excess fat deposition around the airway is not a universal finding in obese patients with OSA, and well-matched controls are often difficult to obtain (15). Other studies have shown that obese patients with sleep apnea have larger tongues (16) and smaller upper-airway volumes (6) than nonobese patients. Obesity may predispose these individuals to OSA by enlarging the upper-airway soft-tissue structures, although the cause of this increase is unknown. Soft-tissue edema may be present from the repeated vibration of snoring and apnea. Human upper-airway pathologic studies have been described infrequently in sleep apnea, although, in one report, more fat and muscle was observed in the uvula of patient with sleep apnea (17).

Although neck size in morbidly obese patients is a better predictor of sleep apnea than are other body anthropomorphic measurements, in a wide weight range of patients that were being seen in sleep apnea clinics, the authors observed that waist measurement provided either similar or better statistical correlations with sleep apnea (18,19). Abdominal obesity may reduce lung volumes, particularly in the supine posture, and may thus reduce upper-airway size. Lung volume directly influences upper-airway size during respiration. Thoracic inspiratory activity produces caudal traction on the trachea, thus increasing the pharyngeal cross-sectional area (20). This effect may be reduced in obese patients since impaired respiratory muscle force has been noted in obese patients (21). Cephalad movement of the trachea, as would occur with a decrease in lung volume, decreases upper-airway size and increases pharyngeal resistance (22). Passive inflation of the lung, producing an increase in end-expiratory lung volume, increases the size of the retropalatal airway (23).

Obesity likely promotes sleep apnea through a variety of mechanisms. In some patients, subcutaneous neck fat may be the critical "load" that tips the balance in favor of upper-airway closure in sleep. In other patients, abdominal fat loading may be important. In addition, more speculatively, the central obesity–sleep apnea link may be related to abnormal upper-airway muscle function. Obesity is associated with changes in relative muscle fiber composition in skeletal muscle (24). Some studies of patients with sleep apnea before and after weight loss have demonstrated changes in the upper-airway function rather than the structure, supporting the hypothesis of abnormal upper-airway muscle function in obese patients with sleep apnea (25).

Obesity-Hypoventilation Syndrome

Most patients with OSA have normal $PaCO_2$ tensions when awake. The term *OHS* describes those patients with obesity and daytime hypercapnia (and usually hypoxemia) in the absence of lung or muscle disease. This association between obesity, hypersomnolence, and hypercapnia has been recognized for many years, and it was labeled *pickwickian syndrome* in honor of Joe, the fat boy in Dickens' *Pickwick Papers*. However the pathogenesis of the condition was poorly understood, and the link with OSA was not recognized. Early theories surmised that obesity produced a load to breathing, which together with depressed chemosensitivity produced OHS. The subsequent recognition that sleep apnea is present in these patients and that relief of upper-airway obstruction by tracheostomy effectively treats the respiratory failure altered the understanding of OHS. Upper-airway obstruction is a crucial factor in the pathogenesis of OHS (5). However, most patients with OSA do not have hypercapnia when awake, so the upper-airway obstruction alone is not enough to produce OHS. In addition, most patients with obesity and eucapnia have normal resting ventilation and occlusion pressures and normal or increased responses to hypoxia and hypercapnia.

No longitudinal studies on the development of OHS are available, but almost certainly OHS starts out as heavy snoring, and then OSA and sleep-induced respiratory abnormalities occur before the development of daytime respiratory failure. During an apneic period, the $Paco_2$ level rises acutely and the Pao_2 falls (Fig. 9.2). When the apnea is terminated by an arousal, the ventilation increases and the oxygen and carbon dioxide levels can return to normal. If arousal responses *or* ventilatory responses to hypoxia or hypercapnia are depressed, the apneic periods will be longer, the degree of blood gas derangement greater, and the normalization of blood gases in the period after arousal compromised (5). In patients who are able to compensate for the loss of ventilation during apneic periods by increased ventilation between events, overall eucapnia will be maintained. In contrast, if the compensatory mechanisms are poor, then the overall ventilation will be reduced during sleep, followed by the development of persistent hypercapnia and hypoxia during sleep. This will result in the resetting of the chemoreceptors and the progression to daytime carbon dioxide retention (26). Sleep fragmentation as a result of repetitive arousals will also depress the arousal responses. Arousal responses can be further impaired in patients who are prescribed sedatives or hypnotics to improve "insomnia" or opiate analgesics to ease musculoskeletal pain or with consumption of alcohol. The term *pickwickian syndrome* should be replaced by *OHS* or *OSA with awake respiratory failure,* terms which better describe the syndrome within the spectrum of sleep-disordered breathing.

The development of OHS is likely multifactorial, with the key elements being a combination of obesity, which causes increased upper-airway loading and reduced lung vol-

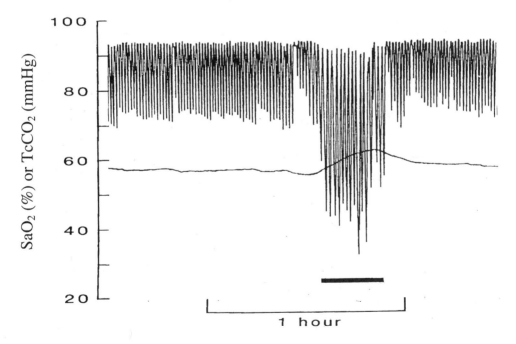

FIG. 9.2. Two-hour oximetry recording, with transcutaneous (tc) CO_2 monitoring in a patient with severe obstructive sleep apnea and obesity-hypoventilation syndrome. A period of rapid eye movement (REM) sleep (*black bar*) is also shown. Repetitive arterial oxygen desaturations, with profound hypoxemia in REM sleep, are associated with a marked rise in $tcCO_2$, indicating hypoventilation.

umes; OSA; poor chemoreceptor function, particularly defective arousal responses to hypoxia; and possibly alcohol consumption, which reduces upper-airway tone and arousal responses to asphyxia (5). Assessment of chemoreceptor function in this patient group is made difficult by the fact that prolonged hypoxia and hypercapnia alter ventilatory responses, but studies in other diseases have shown familial clustering in the level of chemosensitivity, thus suggesting a genetic component (27). The fact that awake hypercapnia can occur in obese patients in the absence of any smoking history or lung or muscle disease must be stressed (28). The prevalence of OHS in the obese population is unknown, but the condition is probably underdiagnosed. A recent study found that 31% of obese patients (body mass index [BMI] greater than 35 kg/m^2) admitted to medical wards had OHS (29).

EPIDEMIOLOGY

The General Community

Studies examining prevalence in the area of sleep-disordered breathing have largely concentrated on self-reported estimates of snoring and daytime sleepiness. These symptoms are commonly reported in the general community, which includes obese subjects; and sleepiness may have many causes (Table 9.2). In addition, snoring may be underestimated if history from a bed partner is unavailable. Therefore, questionnaire estimates of OSA are difficult to interpret, and they have limited usefulness.

The Wisconsin Sleep Cohort Study (30) is the largest reported prevalence study in which sleep studies were performed. This group found an apnea index of more than five events per hour in 9% of female and 24% of male middle-aged public servants. The "OSA syndrome" (daytime sleepiness and an apnea index of more than five per hour) was found in 2% of women and 4% of men. An apnea index of more than 15 events per hour was found in 4% of women and 9% of men. The authors' group has found a similar prevalence of OSA in an Australian rural community using home monitoring of breathing (31).

Even where sleep studies are performed, the estimates of prevalence are made difficult by the varying definitions of OSA. In the past, researchers have used an apnea index of more than five events per hour to define OSA. However, given that hypopneas and even increased upper-airway resistance can produce the OSA syndrome, that definition is probably inadequate. Other measurements, such as the arousal index or changes in heart rate and blood pressure through the night, may be important. In addition, more recent work (see "Hypertension" under "Chronic Effects" in "Clinical Aspects") has suggested that an apnea index of as few as one to five events per hour may influence the development of hypertension (32).

TABLE 9.2. *Sleepiness in the obese patient*

Problem	Possible causes
Inadequate amounts of sleep	Lifestyle (especially shift work and commercial drivers)
	Insomnia
Drugs (causing sleepiness or disrupting sleep)	Hypnotics
	Alcohol
	Drug abuse
Disorders disrupting sleep	Obstructive sleep apnea
	Periodic limb movement disorder
Primary brain disorders	Narcolepsy
	Idiopathic hypersomnolence

The Obese Population

Multiple investigations have consistently shown that obesity, particularly central obesity, is strongly associated with sleep-disordered breathing in adults (19,30,31). Measurements of central obesity, such as waist or neck measurements, are closely linked to OSA in sleep clinic populations, and this association remains tight in the general population, although it is not as strong as that seen in sleep clinic cohorts (19). In the Busselton Sleep Survey (31), a strong effect of BMI in increasing the risk of sleep-disordered breathing in the community was observed (Fig. 9.3).

Limited data exist on the prevalence of sleep apnea in the obese population. The Swedish Obese Subjects study, which examined 3,034 subjects with BMIs of more than 35 kilograms per meter squared (kg/m^2), found that more than 50% of obese men reported habitual loud snoring, compared to the 15% reported by age-matched, gender-matched nonobese subjects (33). Similarly, 33% of the men and 12% of the women in this study reported a history of frequent witnessed apneas. Questionnaires tend to underestimate the prevalence of OSA. The exact prevalence of the spectrum of sleep-breathing disorders in the obese is unknown, but OSA and related conditions clearly occur in quite a high proportion of obese subjects.

BMI as a Predictor of Sleep-Disordered Breathing

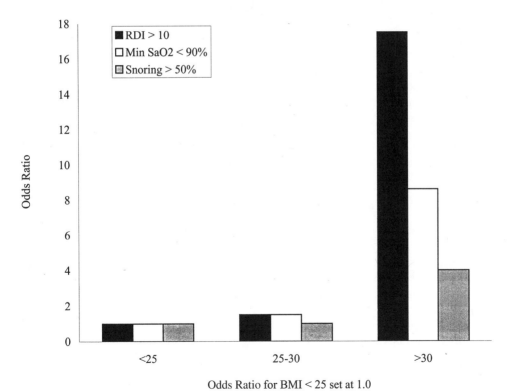

Odds Ratio for BMI < 25 set at 1.0

FIG. 9.3. Obesity (measured by body mass index [BMI]) is an important predictor of obstructive sleep apnea (OSA) in the Busselton Sleep Survey. With the odds ratio for a BMI of less than 25 set at 1.0, a BMI of more than 30 increased the odds ratio of either OSA (respiratory disturbance index >10), desaturation during the night (minimal SaO_2 <90%), or heavy snoring (snoring for >50% of the night) by 4 to 18 times, depending on the variable.

More recent longitudinal studies have demonstrated a strong association between weight gain and the development of sleep-disordered breathing. The Wisconsin group prospectively evaluated 690 randomly selected local residents twice at 4-year intervals for the presence of sleep-disordered breathing (34). They found that weight gain of 10% predicted an approximate 32% increase in the apnea-hypopnea index (AHI), and, similarly, weight loss of 10% predicted a 26% fall in the AHI. Therefore, even relatively small changes in baseline weight have a powerful impact on the degree of sleep-disordered breathing.

Other Risk Factors for Obstructive Sleep Apnea

Age

The prevalence of OSA increases with age (31). Some of this association may be due to increased central fat deposition with age, but other factors, such as changes in tissue elasticity, ventilatory control, and cardiopulmonary and neurologic comorbidity, may be important.

Gender

In the middle-aged population, the risk of OSA is three to four times greater in men than in women (30,34). The prevalence of OSA increases in women after menopause, suggesting a protective role for female hormones or an OSA-promoting role for male hormones. These effects may be due to hormonal influences on the ventilatory control and mechanical behavior of the upper airway or on the patterns of body fat deposition (35).

The redistribution of fat from peripheral to central sites that occurs with menopause may lead to an increased prevalence of sleep apnea resulting from the upper-airway mass loading. Alternatively, the change in hormonal status may affect the arousal of ventilatory responses to blood gas changes during sleep. Finally, after menopause, the female airway may be more "collapsible" because of changes in upper-airway mechanical properties that are caused by lowered female hormone levels.

Familial, Genetic, and Maxillofacial Factors

Familial clustering of OSA, independent of age and obesity, has been noted. This association is probably due to similarities in the facial structure that affect the upper-airway dynamics during sleep. Certain maxillofacial appearances, such as class II malocclusion and the retroposed mandible, are strongly linked to OSA in nonobese subjects (36). In obese patients, certain familial maxillofacial structures further increase the likelihood of OSA.

Some congenital conditions are linked to OSA. The Pierre Robin syndrome is strongly associated with OSA because of mandibular shortening. Patients with Down syndrome are predisposed to OSA because of oropharyngeal crowding and obesity. Nearly two-thirds of patients with Marfan syndrome have OSA, despite a thin body habitus, because of the abnormal compliance of their upper-airway tissue (37).

Any conditions causing narrowing of the upper airway, such as tonsillar and adenoidal hypertrophy, macroglossia, and high-arched palates, predispose an individual to the development of OSA. Nasal obstruction is also a significant risk factor for OSA (38). Again, the presence of these abnormalities interacts with obesity to produce a greater risk for OSA (39).

Comorbid Conditions

Many endocrine abnormalities are associated with an increased prevalence of OSA. Hypothyroidism reduces chemosensitivity and promotes airway narrowing by upper-airway myopathy and myxedematous infiltration (40). More than 50% of patients with acromegaly have OSA, and an increased prevalence of central sleep apnea has been associated with increased disease activity, as assessed by biochemical markers (41). Cushing disease is also associated with OSA (42).

Cardiac failure, no matter what the cause, is associated with a high incidence of sleep-disordered breathing. In a recent study of 450 patients with cardiac failure who were referred to a sleep laboratory, either with sleep symptoms or with persistent dyspnea, 72% had more than ten apnea-hypopnea episodes per hour (43). Patients had OSA or central sleep apnea (Cheyne–Stokes respiration), with OSA being more common in those patients with a BMI of more than 35 kg/m^2.

Cerebrovascular disease is associated with the presence of sleep-disordered breathing. A recent report examined patients in both the acute and the convalescent stage of a first-ever stroke, whether hemorrhagic or ischemic (44). In the acute phase, 71% of the patients had an AHI of more than 10, with an AHI of more than 30 seen in 28%. Cheyne–Stokes breathing was observed in 26%. In the convalescent phase (i.e., 3 months later), the overall AHI and the amount of Cheyne–Stokes breathing had fallen, but the obstructive apnea index was unchanged. Some patients had persistent central apneas after their stroke.

CLINICAL ASPECTS

Signs and Symptoms

The history and physical examination have fairly poor sensitivity and specificity for the detection of sleep-disordered breathing (45). The typical symptoms associated with OSA are heavy snoring and EDS. The reporting of witnessed apneas is a relatively specific symptom, but it is also relatively insensitive. Other symptoms are listed in Table 9.3. Nocturnal symptoms include those related to the breathing disorder, such as choking and gasping, nocturia, and nocturnal gastroesophageal reflux. The daytime symptoms are related to the effects of sleep fragmentation, and they can include morning headaches, fatigue, poor memory and concentration, alteration in mood, and impotence (3). Of note is the fact that the arousal responses to upper-airway narrowing during sleep can be so brisk that some patients, particularly women, can present with symptoms such as insomnia, restless sleep, or anxiety (46).

TABLE 9.3. *Symptoms of sleep-disordered breathing*

Snoring
Daytime sleepiness
Disrupted sleep
Choking or gasping during sleep
Dry throat and/or mouth in morning
Morning headaches
Nocturia
Heartburn
Poor memory and/or concentration
Fatigue
Impotence
Altered mood and/or irritability

These symptoms emphasize the importance of obtaining a confirmatory history from a spouse, bed partner, and/or other family members. Few people are aware that they snore or stop breathing during sleep. The initial consultation is often precipitated by the bed partner's concerns about snoring and apnea. Excessive sleepiness may be recognized by the patient, but this may be underreported if patients are unaware that their sleepiness is abnormal or if they are afraid of the potential consequences of EDS (e.g., the loss of their driver's license or work).

Examination of the upper airway may be important. Obvious pharyngeal crowding and tonsillar enlargement suggest upper-airway obstruction (47). The vibration of soft tissues from heavy snoring can lead to a reddened and edematous uvula and soft palate. Systemic hypertension is commonly associated with OSA. Detailed cephalometric measurements as predictors for OSA appear to be more useful in the nonobese populations (45).

Diagnosis

The gold standard approach for the investigation of sleep-disordered breathing is an overnight in-laboratory sleep study (polysomnography [PSG]). Sleep stage, sleep architecture, and arousals from sleep are monitored during a full sleep study by two electroencephalogram (EEG) channels, two electrooculogram (EOG) channels, and one electromyogram (EMG) channel. Breathing during sleep is usually monitored qualitatively with a measure of airflow at the nose and/or mouth; usually two measures of respiratory effort, such as a diaphragm EMG and chest wall and abdominal movement; and oxygen saturation. Other variables that may be measured include electrocardiogram, leg EMG, the transcutaneous carbon dioxide level, the body position, and snoring. A sleep study should be scored manually, and, at a minimum, the report should include the total amount of sleep and the proportions of different sleep stages, the number of respiratory events seen (i.e., apneas and hypopneas per hour both in REM and NREM sleep), the degree of oxygen desaturation recorded, the number of EEG arousals, and the presence or absence of periodic limb movements. Definitions of events are not standard across all sleep laboratories, and different methods for measuring airflow and other respiratory variables have differing sensitivities.

In the area of sleep-disordered breathing, the definitions of normal and abnormal sleep are under constant revision. In general, an AHI of less than 5 events per hour is considered normal, and an AHI of more than 15 events per hour is regarded as at least moderate disease. An AHI of 5 to 15 events per hour is considered mild disease, but significant individual variability in the symptoms related to this mild degree of OSA exists. If a patient is symptomatic, a trial of treatment is warranted. However, more recent studies have suggested that even an AHI between one and five may significantly increase the risk of developing hypertension, regardless of symptoms (32).

Although PSG is considered the best available test for the diagnosis of OSA, patients with OSA can have significant night-to-night variability in the severity of their disease, thus having the potential for false-negative study results (Table 9.4). A negative PSG result with high clinical suspicion warrants further review and often even a second sleep study.

The expense and inconvenience of PSG has led to a search for alternative tools for the diagnosis of OSA. Overnight oximetry can detect the repetitive oxygen desaturations that are seen in OSA (Fig. 9.4), and thus it can be diagnostic in some patients (48). However, not all apneic events produce significant desaturation, so a normal oximetry study result does not exclude OSA. Similarly, limited portable or "at-home" systems have had some success in the diagnosis of OSA, but these again do not exclude the diagnosis if the

TABLE 9.4. *Reasons for false-negative sleep study results*

Poor sleep efficiency (laboratory effect)
Little or no REM sleep seen
Usual sedatives or alcohol not taken
Patient not sleeping in usual position (especially supine)
Occurrence of "subcriterion events"
Night-to-night variability in the severity of obstructive sleep apnea
  (significant in milder disease)

Abbreviation: REM, rapid eye movement.

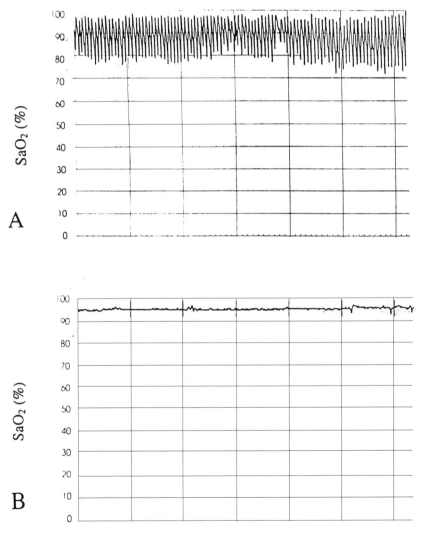

FIG. 9.4. A: One-hour oximetry recording during sleep in a patient with severe obstructive sleep apnea showing typical repetitive arterial oxygen desaturations. **B:** One-hour oximetry recording during sleep in the same patient during treatment with nasal continuous positive airway pressure, with desaturations abolished and oxygen saturation (SaO_2) maintained above 90%.

results are negative. Currently, they are probably most useful in patients with whom clinical suspicion is high or in those who cannot readily be studied in a laboratory, such as the immobile or medically unstable patient.

Consequences

Psychosocial Effects

EDS is characteristic of sleep apnea. However, sleepiness and fatigue are commonly reported symptoms in the general community, particularly in the obese population. The sleepiness seen in patients with OSA is predominantly related to the repetitive arousal and sleep fragmentation, but it may also be a direct effect of hypoxemia (49). However, OSA is characterized by a range of EDS, and a relatively poor correlation exists between the markers of severity of OSA, such as AHI, and daytime sleepiness. People probably vary in their susceptibility to the effects of sleep fragmentation and sleep deprivation, and no simple tests exist that can quantify daytime sleepiness accurately. Sleepiness may lead to impaired work performance and driving (50). Patients with untreated OSA form an important risk group for motor-vehicle accidents. Driving performance on various simulators is impaired in patients with OSA (51). Treatment with nasal continuous positive airway pressure (CPAP) dramatically improves daytime sleepiness and driving simulator performance (52,53).

Many studies have found that patients with OSA perform poorly on psychometric tests when compared to controls. With nasal CPAP, patients have shown a variable degree of improvement (49). The detrimental effects of OSA have other social implications, with data from the Swedish Obese Subjects study showing that, in equally obese men and women, OSA is associated with impaired work performance, increased sick leave, and a higher divorce rate (33).

Cardiovascular Effects

Acute Effects

The acute cardiovascular effects seen during obstructive events have been well characterized, with marked changes seen in both the systemic and pulmonary arterial blood pressure. As a patient's obstructive apnea progresses, he or she experiences increasing swings in pleural pressure, worsening hypoxemia, vagally mediated bradycardia, and increased sympathetic nerve activity. As the apnea is terminated by arousal and increased ventilation, the heart rate increases and both the systolic and diastolic blood pressure increase markedly, often by more than 100 mm Hg (Fig. 9.5). These profound hemody-

FIG. 9.5. Five-minute tracing of a patient with typical severe obstructive sleep apnea. The upper traces show the variables used for sleep staging and indicate that this patient is in rapid eye movement sleep. The apneas are indicated by intermittent cessation of airflow (*Autoflow,* nasal airflow), and they are obstructive in nature as continued respiratory effort is seen when airflow is absent (*Thor Res,* thoracic movement or effort; *EMG/dia,* diaphragm electromyogram). Repetitive falls in oxygen saturation (SaO_2) are seen after each apnea. The lowest trace is a noninvasive recording of blood pressure (*BP*) showing an increase in both systolic (>50 mm Hg) and diastolic (>25 mm Hg) BP at the end of an apnea. Abbreviations: *ECG,* electrocardiogram; *EEG,* electroencephalogram; *EMG,* submental electromyogram; *EOG,* electrooculogram; *Leg,* leg electromyogram.

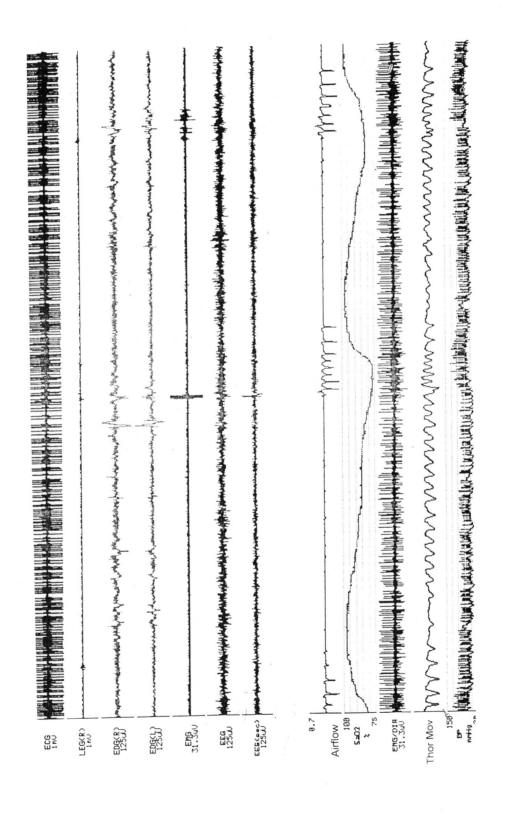

namic fluctuations are largely due to surges in sympathetic nerve activity that result from the combination of the blood gas derangement, the large swings in intrathoracic pressure, and the arousals. Patients with OSA demonstrate increased sympathetic activity through the night, with persistence of this increased activity into wakefulness (54). In addition, these patients have a potent pressor response to hypoxia compared to normal subjects, possibly as a result of repetitive nocturnal hypoxia (55). Studies using an elegant canine model of OSA have shown that sustained hypertension develops after 1 to 3 months of OSA (56). Studies in rats have found that intermittent hypoxia induces a persistent increase in diurnal blood pressure that is mediated through renal sympathetic nerve activity and the renin–angiotensin system (57).

Chronic Effects

Hypertension. Sleep apnea is a common finding among patients in hypertension clinics, and many patients with OSA have hypertension (58,59). A cross-sectional study of 1,400 patients referred for a sleep study showed that the degree of OSA was an independent predictor of morning blood pressure (19). With the use of echocardiography, left ventricular hypertrophy, which is an important outcome of hypertension, was shown to be increased in normotensive patients with OSA in comparison to matched controls without OSA (60). Studies of blood pressure, as measured by either intraarterial monitoring, automated daytime blood pressure readings, or 24-hour ambulatory blood pressure, have demonstrated a decrease in blood pressures after CPAP treatment (61). Despite these studies, a causal link between OSA with hypertension has been disputed because of the presence of important confounders, such as obesity and age. However, more recently published data from two large epidemiologic studies have convincingly demonstrated that OSA is an independent risk factor for hypertension, regardless of obesity. Data from the Sleep Heart Health Study, a large cross-sectional community-based study with more than 6,000 subjects, found that AHI and the percentage of sleep time with an oxygen saturation of less than 90% were significantly associated with systemic hypertension, independent of anthropomorphic variables, such as BMI, waist to hip ratio, and neck circumference (62). Similarly, prospective data from the Wisconsin Sleep Cohort study (32), which followed more than 700 subjects for over 4 to 8 years, have shown a dose–response association between sleep-disordered breathing and hypertension that was independent of measures of obesity. In this study, an AHI of less than 4.9 events per hour had an odds ratio for hypertension at follow-up of 1.42, with odds ratios of 2.03 and 2.89 for an AHI of 5.0 to 14.9 and of more than 15, respectively. The mechanisms of the relationship between apnea and hypertension are unknown, but they may involve the effects of nocturnal blood gas abnormalities on chemoreceptors, of acute blood pressure changes during apneas on baroreflexes, and of the above and the recurrent arousals on sympathetic activity.

Cardiovascular Disease and Mortality. As with hypertension, the cause-and-effect relationships between OSA and other cardiovascular endpoints are difficult to establish. A number of groups have reported an increased risk of myocardial infarction and stroke in patients with sleep apnea (63,64). Recent data from the Sleep Heart Health Study (65) have demonstrated a relationship between AHI and prevalent cardiovascular disease, which was defined by various manifestations of ischemic heart disease, heart failure, and stroke. The odds ratios were fairly modest, and surprisingly a dose to response ratio did not appear to exist with an AHI higher than 10. However, this study has been criticized for the mean age of the group (65 years). Prior work had suggested that the effects of

OSA on cardiovascular disease, including mortality, are most marked in those patients younger than 50 years of age. A prospective study of more than 1,600 patients found that age, BMI, hypertension, and the apnea index were independent predictors of death (66). He et al. (67) observed an increased cumulative mortality in untreated patients with an apnea index greater than 20 compared to those with an apnea index of less than 20 that again was most marked in patients younger than 50 years of age. Treatment with CPAP or tracheostomy reduced the mortality. Snoring is a strong risk factor for sleep-related strokes, while sleep apnea symptoms—snoring plus reported apneas or EDS—increase the risk of cerebral infarction, with an odds ratio of 8.0. Mechanisms other than increased blood pressure and sympathetic activity may be involved. Tests have demonstrated increased platelet aggregation overnight in a group of patients with OSA when compared to control subjects in whom platelet aggregation decreased overnight (68). Treatment with CPAP decreased the nighttime level of platelet aggregability and reversed the overnight increases that were seen before treatment. Other studies of vascular responsiveness have demonstrated impaired vasodilation in patients with OSA, whether hypertension was or was not present (69). These findings have implications in the analysis of data linking obesity and cardiac disease. More difficult still is the issue of treating patients with OSA who do not have significant sleepiness, in order to prevent the effects of sleep-disordered breathing on cardiovascular outcomes.

Pulmonary Hypertension and Lung Disease. Obstructive apneas can produce PHT acutely, largely because of hypoxic pulmonary vasoconstriction, although hypercapnia may also play a role. A number of studies have found a relationship between OSA and the development of daytime PHT, with the prevalence of PHT ranging from 10% to 70% in patients presenting with OSA (70–72). Some of these studies have included patients with lung disease, particularly chronic obstructive pulmonary disease (COPD), as well as OSA, possibly confounding the results. However, several studies carefully excluded patients with any lung disease and found PHT in 10% to 40% of patients with OSA (72,73). Individual variation in the response of the pulmonary vasculature to hypoxia seemingly accounts for the development of PHT in some patients with OSA. Sleep-disordered breathing should therefore be considered in any patient who develops PHT.

The "overlap syndrome" describes patients with both OSA and lung disease, particularly COPD. The combination of these diseases results in a greater degree of PHT and blood gas abnormality than that which would expected for either disease alone. In general, patients with COPD develop daytime hypercapnia only when their lung function falls to less than 30% of their predicted level. However, patients with only moderate COPD (i.e., lung function greater than 40% of the predicted) can develop significant awake hypercapnic-hypoxic respiratory failure if they also have OSA. The hypercapnia is due to hypoventilation secondary to changes in ventilatory control, and it can be partially or fully reversed with effective treatment of the sleep apnea.

Endocrine Abnormalities. Impaired growth hormone (GH) secretion in adults can lead to central obesity and reduced bone and muscle mass, and individuals with obesity have low levels of GH. Men with OSA have a defect in both GH and testosterone secretion that can be reversed with CPAP treatment, independent of any weight change (74,75). The low GH levels in patients with OSA may add to the already low levels that are seen in obesity, but whether the changes in GH and testosterone in OSA result in any measurable changes in body composition or body fat distribution is still unknown.

In a group of patients with a high likelihood of OSA based on questionnaire data, plasma insulin levels were found to be increased, independent of obesity, in both men and women (18). Another study examined patients with type II diabetes mellitus and OSA and found an improvement in insulin sensitivity after treatment with CPAP (76). This improvement again was independent of any changes in weight or other treatment. Grunstein et al. (74) also reported normalization of low testosterone levels with treatment of OSA. These data suggest that OSA has an effect on insulin resistance, possibly through increased sympathetic nerve activity. Some of the hormonal abnormalities in central obesity may be attributable to OSA.

More recently, leptin has been implicated in sleep-disordered breathing in obese subjects. In obese leptin-deficient mice with OHS, leptin replacement resulted in an increase in minute ventilation while both awake and asleep and in increased chemosensitivity to carbon dioxide during sleep (77). These changes were independent of food intake, weight, and carbon dioxide production. Patients with OSA have higher leptin levels than do subjects with similar obesity but without OSA (78). Leptin levels fell significantly in a group of 22 patients with OSA after 4 days of treatment with CPAP, possibly because of reduced sympathetic activity (79). OSA may well be a confounder in some of the hormonal associations that are observed in central obesity, and it may possibly be associated with resistance to the weight-reducing effects of leptin. In this context, hypoleptinemia and accelerated weight gain appear to be closely associated with the worsening of sleep apnea (78).

TREATMENT

The approach to any treatment should be tailored to suit the individual patient, and, in sleep-disordered breathing, it will be determined primarily by the severity of symptoms and the severity of the OSA. A secondary consideration is the presence or absence of cardiovascular risk factors. The question about whether patients should be treated for this reason alone, regardless of symptoms, remains unanswered, and this debate is made more difficult by the fact that compliance with the most successful form of treatment available (i.e., CPAP) is related to the relief of symptoms. However, patient denial of symptoms, either conscious or not, may produce an "asymptomatic" patient, and, if possible, family input should be sought when a patient with a highly positive study result denies having symptoms. Patient occupation may also influence the decision to treat, particularly given data regarding motor-vehicle accidents and OSA, as well as the fact that sleep deprivation, which is common among commercial drivers, may act synergistically with even mild OSA to increase daytime sleepiness.

Weight Loss

Weight loss is an important part of any treatment regimen when the disease is related to obesity. Weight loss by either caloric restriction or bariatric surgery significantly reduces the severity of OSA (Table 9.5) (80–82). Even moderate weight loss (i.e., 10%) can decrease the AHI and can improve daytime alertness. As detailed above, recently published longitudinal data on 690 subjects that were followed over 8 years with sleep studies show that a 10% weight gain predicts an increase in the AHI of around 32% and a 10% weight loss produces a decrease of 26% in the AHI (83). In a group of 313 patients with a BMI of more than 35 kg/m² who were assessed by questionnaire 1 year after bariatric surgery, marked improvements were seen in habitual snoring (82% preoperatively to 14% at follow-up), observed sleep apnea (33% to 2%), and daytime sleepiness (39% to 4%) (84). This group lost an average of 48% of their excess weight. However,

TABLE 9.5. *Effects of weight change on severity of obstructive sleep apnea*

Study	Baseline	Follow-up	Comment
Smith et al., 1985 (80)	AHI: 55 ± 8 Weight: 106 ± 7 kg	AHI: 29 ± 7 Weight: 97 ± 6 kg	Dietary means (15 patients)
Pasquali et al., 1990 (82)	AHI: 67 ± 23	AHI: 33 ± 26	Mean weight loss: 19 ± 15 kg (23 patients)
Suratt et al., 1992 (81)	AHI: 90 ± 32 BMI: 54 ± 13 kg/m²	AHI: 62 ± 49 BMI: 46 ± 10 kg/m²	Very low calorie diet (eight patients); six of eight patients improved
Pillar et al. 1994 (85)	AHI: 40 ± 29 BMI: 45 ± 7 kg/m²	AHI: 11 ± 16 BMI: 33 ± 8 kg/m²	Bariatric surgery (14 patients) Initial results at 3 mo
		AHI: 24 ± 23 BMI: 35 ± 6 kg/m²	Same group at follow-up at 7 yr; nonsignificant change in weight but significantly worse OSA
Sampol et al., 1998 (86) Group I (67 patients)	AHI: 52 ± 23 BMI: 32 ± 5 kg/m²	AHI: 44 ± 26 BMI: 26 ± 3 kg/m²	Weight loss of more than 10% by dietary means in each group (follow-up time 11 mo): cure in 34 patients in Group II
Group II (34 patients)	AHI: 44 ± 28 BMI: 33 ± 5 kg/m²	AHI: 3 ± 3 BMI: 27 ± 3 kg/m²	At long-term follow-up (94 mo) in Group II, AHI increased to 40 ± 24 in six patients with no change in weight

Abbreviations: AHI, apnea-hypopnea index; BMI, body mass index; OSA, obstructive sleep apnea.

the effects of weight loss on OSA are variable, as a complete cure of all sleep-disordered breathing after weight loss is rare, and many patients have significant residual disease that warrants further treatment. In addition, OSA has been reported to recur despite the maintenance of weight loss (85,86). For these reasons, patients should be reassessed after weight loss.

Other General Measures

Alcohol and sedatives such as benzodiazepines should be avoided in patients with sleep-disordered breathing because these drugs can reduce pharyngeal muscle tone and can depress arousal responses, resulting in more and longer apneas during sleep. Similarly, sleep deprivation can impair upper-airway muscle tone and can increase the arousal thresholds, thus increasing any tendency to OSA. Smoking cessation can reduce self-reported snoring, possibly by eliminating the effects of smoke on airway inflammation and, as always, this should be encouraged. Some patients have predominantly positional apnea that is related to the supine posture, and attempts to avoid this position during sleep may help reduce the severity of OSA. However, positional therapy is often poorly tolerated, and this type of apnea is unusual in obese patients. Nasal obstruction will worsen any tendency to snoring and OSA, and thus it should be treated, usually by pharmacologic means; little evidence exists to indicate that nasal surgery is useful in the treatment of OSA. The effects of external nasal dilator strips on snoring are variable, with some studies reporting success (87). These strips, however, have no effect on OSA. Although drugs have been tried for the treatment of both OSA and OHS, no evidence that any available drugs are effective exists at this time (88).

Devices

Continuous Positive Airway Pressure

The application of nasal CPAP for the treatment of OSA was first described by Sullivan et al. (89) in 1981, and it revolutionized the field of sleep-disordered breathing. Nasal CPAP is the most effective treatment available for OSA. A CPAP machine works by delivering positive pressure to the upper airway via a nose or face mask, thus providing a pneumatic splint that prevents upper-airway closure. The pressure is usually generated by an electromechanical blower that delivers airflow through wide-bore tubing to a nasal mask with a fixed expiratory resistance. Adjusting the airflow allows different pressures to be delivered at the nares. The optimal pressure required to prevent upper-airway closure is determined by a sleep study. The required pressure can vary from 4 to 20 cm H_2O. Many patients show a rebound phenomenon during these treatment nights that includes markedly increased amounts of REM and slow-wave sleep.

Treatment with nasal CPAP normalizes sleep architecture (Fig. 9.4), decreases upper-airway edema, and significantly improves daytime sleepiness both subjectively and objectively (90). Studies have shown that CPAP improves daytime alertness, cognitive function, mood, and quality of life in patients with OSA of all degrees of severity, ranging from mild (including "upper-airway resistance syndrome") to severe (91–95). These studies include carefully controlled trials with either placebo tablets or subtherapeutic CPAP (92,96). Evidence also indicates that treatment with CPAP reduces the incidence of actual and near-miss traffic accidents in patients with OSA (52,97). As has been discussed previously, CPAP treatment reverses many of the adverse effects of OSA on blood pressure, PHT, and various hormonal levels, including leptin, and reduces mortality. CPAP does not cure OSA. When treatment with CPAP is stopped, OSA recurs and the symptoms return. However, regular use of CPAP may lead to a reduction in the underlying severity of OSA, as assessed by sleep studies performed after a period of treatment. This reduction in severity is probably due to the effects of CPAP in reducing upper-airway edema and treating sleep deprivation.

The main problem limiting the efficacy of CPAP has been long-term compliance (98). Various reports of compliance indicate that somewhere between 40% and 70% of patients have difficulties with compliance (98,99). On the whole, centers that provide more intensive initial (i.e., within the first few weeks of treatment) assistance to patients have better long-term compliance than others; compliance with treatment in this initial period predicts long-term compliance. In addition, patients who have the greatest symptomatic improvement with CPAP are, not surprisingly, more compliant. The CPAP machine and mask remain fairly cumbersome and inconvenient. Side effects related to the patient–mask interface are the most common, and, although they are often minor, they can have a major impact on patient tolerance and use of the treatment. Poorly fitting masks can cause skin irritation and even ulceration. More importantly, a poor mask fit can result in air leaks either around the mask or through the mouth. Because the high airflow generated by the CPAP machine, leaks can produce major effects on the mouth and nose, including dryness of the mouth and nasal congestion and rhinorrhea. These problems can be effectively treated either by improving mask fit, providing a chin strap to prevent mouth opening, or humidifying and warming the air with humidifiers built into the circuit. The technology of mask and machine is constantly improving, with machines that are now able to ramp pressure up slowly at sleep onset and that also can continuously adjust the required pressure through the night. These modifications may improve compliance in some patients. Those patients who require higher pressures or who have milder disease are less likely to be compliant. Obese patients with OSA generally require higher pressures than do patients who are not obese. Despite these problems, CPAP remains highly effective for the treatment of all symptoms related to all degrees of OSA, and it should not be abandoned without intensive attempts to improve an individual's tolerance and compliance.

Mandibular Advancement Devices

Mandibular advancement devices (MADs) are intraoral orthodontic devices designed to displace the mandible anteriorly, thus increasing the anteroposterior diameter of the upper airway and reducing upper-airway closure and collapse when they are worn at night. These devices are demonstrated to be effective at reducing snoring, when assessed both objectively and subjectively (100). The effects of these devices on OSA are less clear. A number of uncontrolled studies have demonstrated significant reductions in the AHI with MADs, but many patients have had significant residual apnea and some patients have actually had increased AHIs with these devices (101,102). Controlled trials comparing MADs with CPAP have confirmed that MADs reduce the AHI by around 50% in some, but not all, patients with mild to moderate OSA and that they significantly reduce daytime sleepiness (103). However, CPAP treatment results in a lower AHI, and it is successful in more patients. These devices require careful orthodontic attention to ensure that adequate anterior displacement of the mandible is achieved. The efficacy of these devices is likely to be reduced in more obese patients because skeletal factors and maxillofacial abnormalities are less important in the genesis of upper-airway obstruction in this group. In general, these devices tend to be less effective in those patients with more severe OSA. However, if a patient is intolerant of CPAP, a trial of a MAD may be worthwhile. Few data are available on compliance. Side effects related to the temporomandibular joint are common, and the effects of long-term use on teeth, occlusion, and the jaw are unknown.

Surgery

Tracheostomy

Before the advent of CPAP, tracheostomy was the only effective treatment for OSA (104). This operation is invasive with significant morbidity, particularly in obese subjects, and it is only partially effective in treating OHS. It should be reserved for those patients with very severe OSA who are completely intolerant of any other treatment. Before any surgery, the patient should be reviewed in a specialist sleep center with intensive attempts to introduce nasal CPAP, including customized masks; humidification of inspired air; and even ear, nose, and throat review and/or intervention to facilitate CPAP usage. With skillful surgery and close follow-up, tracheostomy may be a "last-resort" therapeutic option in some patients.

Uvulopalatopharyngoplasty and Other Upper-airway Surgery

Uvulopalatopharyngoplasty (UPPP) was originally described in Japan in the 1950s for the treatment of heavy snoring; it involves a careful surgical removal of the uvula and part of the soft palate, either with or without tonsillectomy. The operation was introduced to the United States for the treatment of OSA in the early 1980s and was greeted with some enthusiasm. However, the efficacy of UPPP in the treatment of OSA is limited (105). If treatment success is defined as a reduction in AHI of only 50%, a successful result is seen in fewer than 50% of patients. No preoperative tests satisfactorily predict the response to surgery, and a significant morbidity and even mortality are observed. Excessive removal of palatal tissue can lead to velopharyngeal incompetence with nasal regurgitation and speech changes. Subsequent use of CPAP may be more difficult after UPPP. Not surprisingly, many studies report particularly poor results in obese patients. Current guidelines state that the efficacy of UPPP is variable and that it should be considered only after non-surgical therapies have failed (104).

More recently, modifications of UPPP have been introduced; in these, either a surgical laser is used to resect the palate (laser-assisted uvulopalatoplasty [LAUP]) or high-frequency radio waves ("somnoplasty") are used in an attempt to stiffen palatal tissue. The treatment response is variable and unpredictable. Ryan and Love (106) studied 44 patients at baseline and 3 months after LAUP and reported worsening of OSA (AHI increased by more than 100%) in 30% of their patient group, with an extremely poor relationship between subjective and objective measures of efficacy. Clearly, a "placebo" effect, which has also been demonstrated in other forms of surgical intervention, is observed following surgery for snoring.

More complex maxillofacial surgery, which is usually performed in two phases, has been used with some success in the treatment of OSA The first phase involves a UPPP with genioglossus advancement, via a mandibular osteotomy and hyoid myotomy. The Stanford group has reported overall success rates of around 60% with this procedure, but they had less success in those patients with more severe disease (more than 60 events per hour and desaturation to 70%) and in the morbidly obese (107). The second phase involves bimaxillary advancement, which has been reported to be as successful as CPAP in treating a group of patients with severe OSA (AHI of 68 events per hour) and a mean BMI of 31 kg/m² (108). In contrast, Bettega et al. (109) found that phase I surgery was generally ineffective in OSA, with successful results in only 22% of patients. In their study, phase II surgery was successful in 75% of patients, but the morbidity was significant. These complex surgical procedures are highly specialized, and they are not widely available.

Pharmacologic Treatment

No placebo-controlled studies show a constant efficacy of any medication in OSA or OHS (110). Obviously, weight-lowering drugs may be beneficial through weight loss, but no drug has been found to alter the collapsibility of the upper airway during sleep.

Management of Obstructive Sleep Apnea with Daytime Respiratory Failure, Including Obesity Hypoventilation Syndrome

Patients with OSA and daytime respiratory failure should be managed in a specialist sleep and respiratory failure center, and, depending on the chronicity and the severity of their condition, the best management for many is a brief period of hospitalization. A wide range in the degree of hypercapnic-hypoxic respiratory failure is associated with the combination of OSA and obesity, and the management of these patients should be individualized. For example, the obese patient with severe OSA and a daytime $Paco_2$ level of 48 mm Hg, normal pH level, and a Pao_2 level of 72 mm Hg can usually be managed with CPAP alone; when the OSA is adequately treated, the daytime blood gases will improve.

Many of these patients come to medical attention with acute-on-chronic respiratory failure resulting from a superimposed condition, such as a respiratory tract infection, or even postanesthetic for an unrelated surgical procedure. In these decompensated patients, oxygen therapy alone should be used with caution and with very close monitoring of hypercapnia; moreover, because the main pathology in these patients is impaired respiratory drive, sedatives or hypnotics should be avoided. Until recently, the only treatments available for these decompensated patients and for those patients with severe chronic respiratory failure from OHS were very-high CPAP pressures; CPAP plus added oxygen; or, for the most unwell or obtunded patients, a short period of intubation and mechanical ventilation (90,111,112).

New devices that are modifications of CPAP are available for the treatment of respiratory failure (Fig. 9.6). These devices can deliver either volume-cycled ventilation or positive pressure ventilation to the upper airway via a nose or face mask, thus effectively providing mechanical ventilation without the need for intubation. These devices can either provide support to the patient's spontaneous respiratory efforts or deliver a set number of breaths as a backup if the patient's inspiratory efforts are inadequate to trigger the machine. These devices are extremely effective in the treatment of both acute and chronic respiratory failure resulting from hypoventilation related to obesity and OSA, and they are well tolerated by the patients (113,114).

When the acutely unwell patient has been stabilized, sleep studies can be performed to determine whether home use of noninvasive positive pressure ventilation (NIPPV) is required; if so, at what pressures; and whether added oxygen is needed. A similar approach is used in the treatment of patients with chronic severe OHS. After a period of treatment with NIPPV (months), some of these patients can be treated with CPAP alone. A specialist sleep unit is the best option for managing these patients because of its expertise in the long-term management of sleep-related respiratory failure.

CONCLUSION

Obesity can produce a measurable reduction in lung function that is very strongly associated with breathing disorders in sleep, such as OSA and hypoventilation.

Moderate to severe degrees of obesity can lead to a restrictive abnormality in lung function because of the mechanical effects of central body fat. Obese subjects may have reduced lung volumes and an increased work of breathing. Central fat deposition is also linked to upper-airway collapsibility in sleep, and epidemiologic data have identified obesity as a crucial risk factor in the development of OSA. Sleep-disordered breathing has a number of clinical consequences, including excess cardiovascular morbidity. The combination of obesity-induced reduced pulmonary function and sleep-disordered breathing can lead to progressive respiratory failure during sleep, finally resulting in awake hypercapnic respiratory failure (i.e., OHS, central hypoventilation). This respiratory failure can occur without any intrinsic lung disease. Weight reduction can improve lung function and can reduce the severity of sleep apnea and OHS. Treatment of sleep-breathing disorders has been greatly advanced by the use of positive airway pressure devices, and OHS can be reversed with the use of these devices.

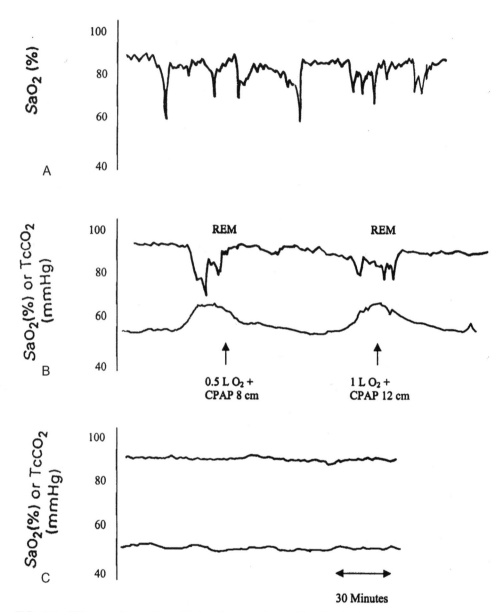

FIG. 9.6. Efficacy of nasal ventilation in a patient with obesity-hypoventilation syndrome.
A: Recordings of oxygen saturation (SaO_2, %) show marked decreases in oxygen level during
sleep. **B:** Addition of continuous positive airway pressure and low-flow oxygen (*0.5 L*, 0.5 L/min
of supplemental oxygen; *1L*, 1 L/min) results in normal oxygen saturation in nonrapid eye
movement sleep but in persisting hypoxemia in rapid eye movement (REM) sleep. **C:** Use of
nasal ventilation, either pressure support or volume cycled, will prevent oxygen desaturation
in REM sleep, as well as increases in transcutaneous CO_2 ($tcCO_2$) levels.

REFERENCES

1. Guilleminault C, Stoohs R, Clerk A, et al. From obstructive sleep apnea syndrome to upper airway resistance syndrome: consistency of daytime sleepiness. *Sleep* 1992;15:S13–S16.
2. Remmers JE, deGroot WJ, Sauerland EK, et al. Pathogenesis of upper airway occlusion during sleep. *J Appl Physiol* 1978;44:931–938.
3. McNamara SG, Grunstein RR, Sullivan CE. Obstructive sleep apnoea. *Thorax* 1993;48:754–764.
4. Rubinstein I, Bradley TD, Zamel N, et al. Glottic and cervical tracheal narrowing in patients with obstructive sleep apnea. *J Appl Physiol* 1989;67:2427–2431.
5. Sullivan CE, Grunstein RR, Marrone O, Berthon-Jones M. Sleep apnea—pathophysiology: upper airway and control of breathing. In: Guilleminault C, Partinen M, eds. *Obstructive sleep apnea syndrome: clinical research and treatment.* New York: Raven Press, 1990:274–316.
6. Fleetham JA. Upper airway imaging in relation to obstructive sleep apnea. *Clin Chest Med* 1992;13:399–416.
7. Schwab RJ, Gefter WB, Hoffman EA, et al. Dynamic upper airway imaging during awake respiration in normal subjects and patients with sleep disordered breathing. *Am Rev Respir Dis* 1993;148:1385–1400.
8. Horner RL, Innes JA, Murphy K, et al. Evidence for reflex upper airway dilator muscle activation by sudden negative airway pressure in man. *J Physiol* 1991;436:15–29.
9. Mezzanotte WS, Tangel DJ, White DP. Waking genioglossal electromyogram in sleep apnea patients versus normal controls (a neuromuscular compensatory mechanism). *J Clin Invest* 1992;89:1571–1579.
10. Larsson H, Carlsson-Nordlander B, Lindblad LE, et al. Temperature thresholds in the oropharynx of patients with obstructive sleep apnea syndrome. *Am Rev Respir Dis* 1992;146:1246–1249.
11. Katz I, Stradling J, Slutsky AS, et al. Do patients with obstructive sleep apnea have thick necks? *Am Rev Respir Dis* 1990;141:1228–1231.
12. Davies RJ, Stradling JR. The relationship between neck circumference, radiographic pharyngeal anatomy, and the obstructive sleep apnoea syndrome. *Eur Respir J* 1990;3:509–514.
13. Koenig JS, Thach BT. Effects of mass loading on the upper airway. *J Appl Physiol* 1988;64:2294–2299.
14. Horner RL, Mohiaddin RH, Lowell DG, et al. Sites and sizes of fat deposits around the pharynx in obese patients with obstructive sleep apnoea and weight matched controls. *Eur Respir J* 1989;2:613–622.
15. Schwab RJ, Gupta KB, Gefter WB, et al. Upper airway and soft tissue anatomy in normal subjects and patients with sleep-disordered breathing. Significance of the lateral pharyngeal walls. *Am J Respir Crit Care Med* 1995;152:1673–1689.
16. Ryan CF, Lowe AA, Li D, et al. Three-dimensional upper airway computed tomography in obstructive sleep apnea. A prospective study in patients treated by uvulopalatopharyngoplasty. *Am Rev Respir Dis* 1991;144:428–432.
17. Stauffer JL, Buick MK, Bixler EO, et al. Morphology of the uvula in obstructive sleep apnea. *Am Rev Respir Dis* 1989;140:724–728.
18. Grunstein RR, Stenlof K, Hedner J, et al. Impact of obstructive sleep apnea and sleepiness on metabolic and cardiovascular risk factors in the Swedish Obese Subjects (SOS) Study. *Int J Obes Relat Metab Disord* 1995;19:410–418.
19. Grunstein R, Wilcox I, Yang TS, et al. Snoring and sleep apnoea in men: association with central obesity and hypertension. *Int J Obes Relat Metab Disord* 1993;17:533–540.
20. Van de Graaff WB. Thoracic influence on upper airway patency. *J Appl Physiol* 1988;65:2124–2131.
21. Lopata M, Onal E. Mass loading, sleep apnea, and the pathogenesis of obesity hypoventilation. *Am Rev Respir Dis* 1982;126:640–645.
22. Series F, Cormier Y, Desmeules M. Influence of passive changes of lung volume on upper airways. *J Appl Physiol* 1990;68:2159–2164.
23. Begle RL, Badr S, Skatrud JB, et al. Effect of lung inflation on pulmonary resistance during NREM sleep. *Am Rev Respir Dis* 1990;141:854–860.
24. Wade AJ, Marbut MM, Round JM. Muscle fibre type and aetiology of obesity. *Lancet* 1990;335:805–808.
25. Rubinstein I, Colapinto N, Rotstein LE, et al. Improvement in upper airway function after weight loss in patients with obstructive sleep apnea. *Am Rev Respir Dis* 1988;138:1192–1195.
26. Berthon-Jones M, Sullivan CE. Time course of change in ventilatory response to CO_2 with long-term CPAP therapy for obstructive sleep apnea. *Am Rev Respir Dis* 1987;135:144–147.
27. Fleetham JA, Arnup ME, Anthonisen NR. Familial aspects of ventilatory control in patients with chronic obstructive pulmonary disease. *Am Rev Respir Dis* 1984;129:3–7.
28. Leech JA, Onal E, Baer P, et al. Determinants of hypercapnia in occlusive sleep apnea syndrome. *Chest* 1987;92:807–813.
29. Nowbar S, Burkart KM, Zwillich CW. Hypoventilation among obese patients: a common and under-diagnosed problem. *Am J Respir Crit Care Med* 2000;161:A890.
30. Young T, Palta M, Dempsey J, et al. The occurrence of sleep-disordered breathing among middle-aged adults. *N Engl J Med* 1993;328:1230–1235.
31. Bearpark H, Elliott L, Grunstein R, et al. Snoring and sleep apnea. A population study in Australian men. *Am J Respir Crit Care Med* 1995;151:1459–1465.
32. Peppard PE, Young T, Palta M, et al. Prospective study of the association between sleep-disordered breathing and hypertension. *N Engl J Med* 2000;342:1378–1384.

33. Grunstein RR, Stenlof K, Hedner JA, et al. Impact of self-reported sleep-breathing disturbances on psychosocial performance in the Swedish Obese Subjects (SOS) study. *Sleep* 1995;18:635–643.
34. Redline S, Kump K, Tishler PV, et al. Gender differences in sleep disordered breathing in a community-based sample. *Am J Respir Crit Care Med* 1994;149:722–726.
35. Brooks LJ, Strohl KP. Size and mechanical properties of the pharynx in healthy men and women. *Am Rev Respir Dis* 1992;146:1394–1397.
36. Nelson S, Hans M. Contribution of craniofacial risk factors in increasing apneic activity among obese and nonobese habitual snorers. *Chest* 1997;111:154–162.
37. Cistulli PA, Sullivan CE. Sleep apnea in Marfan's syndrome. Increased upper airway collapsibility during sleep. *Chest* 1995;108:631–635.
38. Lofaso F, Coste A, d'Ortho MP, et al. Nasal obstruction as a risk factor for sleep apnoea syndrome. *Eur Respir J* 2000;16:639–643.
39. Ferguson KA, Ono T, Lowe AA, et al. The relationship between obesity and craniofacial structure in obstructive sleep apnea. *Chest* 1995;108:375–381.
40. Grunstein RR, Sullivan CE. Sleep apnea and hypothyroidism: mechanisms and management. *Am J Med* 1988;85:775–779.
41. Grunstein RR, Ho KY, Sullivan CE. Sleep apnea in acromegaly. *Ann Intern Med* 1991;115:527–532.
42. Rosenow F, McCarthey V, Caruso AC. Sleep apnoea in endocrine diseases. *J Sleep Res* 1998;7:3–11.
43. Sin DD, Fitzgerald F, Parker JD, et al. Risk factors for central and obstructive sleep apnea in 450 men and women with congestive heart failure. *Am J Respir Crit Care Med* 1999;160:1101–1106.
44. Parra O, Arboix A, Bechich S, et al. Time course of sleep-related breathing disorders in first-ever stroke or transient ischemic attack. *Am J Respir Crit Care Med* 2000;161:375–380.
45. Redline S, Strohl KP. Recognition and consequences of obstructive sleep apnea hypopnea syndrome. *Clin Chest Med* 1998;19:1–19.
46. Ambrogetti A, Olson LG, Saunders NA. Differences in the symptoms of men and women with obstructive sleep apnoea. *Aust N Z J Med* 1991;21:863–866.
47. Hoffstein V, Szalai JP. Predictive value of clinical features in diagnosing obstructive sleep apnea. *Sleep* 1993;16: 118–122.
48. Gyulay S, Olson LG, Hensley MJ, et al. A comparison of clinical assessment and home oximetry in the diagnosis of obstructive sleep apnea. *Am Rev Respir Dis* 1993;147:50–53.
49. Montplaisir J, Bedard MA, Richer F, Rouleau I. Neurobehavioral manifestations in obstructive sleep apnea syndrome before and after treatment with continuous positive airway pressure. *Sleep* 1992;15:S17–S19.
50. Findley LJ, Fabrizio MJ, Knight H, et al. Driving simulator performance in patients with sleep apnea. *Am Rev Respir Dis* 1989;140:529–530.
51. Juniper M, Hack MA, George CF, et al. Steering simulation performance in patients with obstructive sleep apnoea and matched control subjects. *Eur Respir J* 2000;15:590–595.
52. Findley L, Smith C, Hooper J, et al. Treatment with nasal CPAP decreases automobile accidents in patients with sleep apnea. *Am J Respir Crit Care Med* 2000;161:857–859.
53. George CF, Boudreau AC, Smiley A. Effects of nasal CPAP on simulated driving performance in patients with obstructive sleep apnoea. *Thorax* 1997;52:648–653.
54. Carlson JT, Hedner J, Elam M, et al. Augmented resting sympathetic activity in awake patients with obstructive sleep apnea. *Chest* 1993;103:1763–1768.
55. Hedner JA, Wilcox I, Laks L, et al. A specific and potent pressor effect of hypoxia in patients with sleep apnea. *Am Rev Respir Dis* 1992;146:1240–1245.
56. Brooks D, Horner RL, Kozar LF, et al. Obstructive sleep apnea as a cause of systemic hypertension. Evidence from a canine model. *J Clin Invest* 1997;99:106–109.
57. Fletcher EC, Bao G, Li R. Renin activity and blood pressure in response to chronic episodic hypoxia. *Hypertension* 1999;34:309–314.
58. Worsnop CJ, Naughton MT, Barter CE, et al. The prevalence of obstructive sleep apnea in hypertensives. *Am J Respir Crit Care Med* 1998;157:111–115.
59. Stradling JR, Crosby JH. Predictors and prevalence of obstructive sleep apnoea and snoring in 1001 middle aged men. *Thorax* 1991;46:85–90.
60. Hedner J, Ejnell H, Caidahl K. Left ventricular hypertrophy independent of hypertension in patients with obstructive sleep apnoea. *J Hypertens* 1990;8:941–946.
61. Obstructive sleep apnea and blood pressure elevation: what is the relationship? Working Group on OSA and Hypertension. *Blood Press* 1993;2:166–182.
62. Nieto FJ, Young TB, Lind BK, et al. Association of sleep-disordered breathing, sleep apnea, and hypertension in a large community-based study. Sleep Heart Health Study. *JAMA* 2000;283:1829–1836.
63. Hung J, Whitford EG, Parsons RW, et al. Association of sleep apnoea with myocardial infarction in men. *Lancet* 1990;336:261–264.
64. Palomaki H, Partinen M, Erkinjuntti T, et al. Snoring, sleep apnea syndrome, and stroke. *Neurology* 1992;42: 75–82.
65. Shahar E, Whitney CW, Redline S, et al. Sleep-disordered breathing and cardiovascular disease cross sectional results of the Sleep Heart Health Study. *Am J Respir Crit Care Med* 2001;163:19–25.

66. Lavie P, Herer P, Peled R, et al. Mortality in sleep apnea patients: a multivariate analysis of risk factors. *Sleep* 1995;18:149–157.
67. He J, Kryger MH, Zorick FJ, et al. Mortality and apnea index in obstructive sleep apnea. Experience in 385 male patients. *Chest* 1988;94:9–14.
68. Sanner BM, Konermann M, Tepel M, et al. Platelet function in patients with obstructive sleep apnoea syndrome. *Eur Respir J* 2000;16:648–652.
69. Carlson JT, Rangemark C, Hedner JA. Attenuated endothelium-dependent vascular relaxation in patients with sleep apnoea. *J Hypertens* 1996;14:577–584.
70. Weitzenblum E, Krieger J, Apprill M, et al. Daytime pulmonary hypertension in patients with obstructive sleep apnea syndrome. *Am Rev Respir Dis* 1988;138:345–349.
71. Sajkov D, Cowie RJ, Thornton AT, et al. Pulmonary hypertension and hypoxemia in obstructive sleep apnea syndrome. *Am J Respir Crit Care Med* 1994;149:416–422.
72. Sajkov D, Wang T, Saunders NA, et al. Daytime pulmonary hemodynamics in patients with obstructive sleep apnea without lung disease. *Am J Respir Crit Care Med* 1999;159:1518–1526.
73. Bady E, Achkar A, Pascal S, et al. Pulmonary arterial hypertension in patients with sleep apnoea syndrome. *Thorax* 2000;55:934–939.
74. Grunstein RR, Handelsman DJ, Lawrence SJ, et al. Neuroendocrine dysfunction in sleep apnea: reversal by continuous positive airways pressure therapy. *J Clin Endocrinol Metab* 1989;68:352–358.
75. Grunstein RR, Handelsman DJ, Stewart DA, Sullivan CE. Growth hormone secretion is increased by nasal CPAP treatment of sleep apnoea. *Am Rev Respir Dis* 1993;147:A686.
76. Brooks B, Cistulli PA, Borkman M, et al. Obstructive sleep apnea in obese noninsulin-dependent diabetic patients: effect of continuous positive airway pressure treatment on insulin responsiveness. *J Clin Endocrinol Metab* 1994;79:1681–1685.
77. O'Donnell CP, Schaub CD, Haines AS, et al. Leptin prevents respiratory depression in obesity. *Am J Respir Crit Care Med* 1999;159:1477–1484.
78. Phillips BG, Kato M, Narkiewicz K, et al. Increases in leptin levels, sympathetic drive, and weight gain in obstructive sleep apnea. *Am J Physiol Heart Circ Physiol* 2000;279:H234–H237.
79. Chin K, Shimizu K, Nakamura T, et al. Changes in intra-abdominal visceral fat and serum leptin levels in patients with obstructive sleep apnea syndrome following nasal continuous positive airway pressure therapy. *Circulation* 1999;100:706–712.
80. Smith PL, Gold AR, Meyers DA, et al. Weight loss in mildly to moderately obese patients with obstructive sleep apnea. *Ann Intern Med* 1985;103:850–855.
81. Suratt PM, McTier RF, Findley LJ, et al. Effect of very-low-calorie diets with weight loss on obstructive sleep apnea. *Am J Clin Nutr* 1992;56:182S–184S.
82. Pasquali R, Colella P, Cirignotta F, et al. Treatment of obese patients with obstructive sleep apnea syndrome (OSAS): effect of weight loss and interference of otorhinolaryngoiatric pathology. *Int J Obes* 1990;14:207–217.
83. Peppard PE, Young T, Palta M, et al. Longitudinal study of moderate weight change and sleep-disordered breathing. *JAMA* 2000;284:3015–3021.
84. Dixon JB, Schachter LM, O'Brien PE. Sleep disturbance and obesity: changes following surgically induced weight loss. *Arch Intern Med* 2001;161:102–106.
85. Pillar G, Peled R, Lavie P. Recurrence of sleep apnea without concomitant weight increase 7.5 years after weight reduction surgery. *Chest* 1994;106:1702–1704.
86. Sampol G, Munoz X, Sagales MT, et al. Long-term efficacy of dietary weight loss in sleep apnoea/hypopnoea syndrome. *Eur Respir J* 1998;12:1156–1159.
87. Pevernagie D, Hamans E, Van Cauwenberge P, et al. External nasal dilation reduces snoring in chronic rhinitis patients: a randomized controlled trial. *Eur Respir J* 2000;15:996–1000.
88. Hudgel DW, Thanakitcharu S. Pharmacologic treatment of sleep-disordered breathing. *Am J Respir Crit Care Med* 1998;158:691–699.
89. Sullivan CE, Issa FG, Berthon-Jones M, et al. Reversal of obstructive sleep apnoea by continuous positive airway pressure applied through the nares. *Lancet* 1981;1:862–865.
90. Sullivan CE, Grunstein RR. Continuous positive airway pressure in sleep disordered breathing. In: Kryger MH, Dement WC, Roth TP, eds. *Principles and practice of sleep medicine.* Philadelphia: WB Saunders, 1994:559–570.
91. Engleman HM, Kingshott RN, Wraith PK, et al. Randomized placebo-controlled crossover trial of continuous positive airway pressure for mild sleep apnea/hypopnea syndrome. *Am J Respir Crit Care Med* 1999;159:461–467.
92. Engleman HM, Martin SE, Kingshott RN, et al. Randomised placebo controlled trial of daytime function after continuous positive airway pressure (CPAP) therapy for the sleep apnoea/hypopnoea syndrome. *Thorax* 1998;53:341–345.
93. Jenkinson C, Stradling J, Petersen S. Comparison of three measures of quality of life outcome in the evaluation of continuous positive airways pressure therapy for sleep apnoea. *J Sleep Res* 1997;6:199–204.
94. Ballester E, Badia JR, Hernandez L, et al. Evidence of the effectiveness of continuous positive airway pressure in the treatment of sleep apnea/hypopnea syndrome. *Am J Respir Crit Care Med* 1999;159:495–501.
95. Engleman HM, Martin SE, Deary IJ, et al. Effect of continuous positive airway pressure treatment on daytime function in sleep apnoea/hypopnoea syndrome. *Lancet* 1994;343:572–575.

96. Jenkinson C, Davies RJ, Mullins R, et al. Comparison of therapeutic and subtherapeutic nasal continuous positive airway pressure for obstructive sleep apnoea: a randomised prospective parallel trial. *Lancet* 1999;353: 2100–2105.

97. Krieger J, Meslier N, Lebrun T, et al. Accidents in obstructive sleep apnea patients treated with nasal continuous positive airway pressure: a prospective study. The Working Group ANTADIR, Paris and CRESGE, Lille, France. Association Nationale de Traitement a Domicile des Insuffisants Respiratoires. *Chest* 1997;112: 1561–1566.

98. Grunstein RR. Sleep-related breathing disorders, V. Nasal continuous positive airway pressure treatment for obstructive sleep apnoea. *Thorax* 1995;50:1106–1113.

99. Krieger J. Long-term compliance with nasal continuous positive airway pressure (CPAP) in obstructive sleep apnea patients and nonapneic snorers. *Sleep* 1992;15:S42–S46.

100. Clark GT, Blumenfeld I, Yoffe N, et al. A crossover study comparing the efficacy of continuous positive airway pressure with anterior mandibular positioning devices on patients with obstructive sleep apnea. *Chest* 1996;109:1477–1483.

101. Schmidt-Nowara W, Lowe A, Wiegand L, et al. Oral appliances for the treatment of snoring and obstructive sleep apnea: a review. *Sleep* 1995;18:501–510.

102. O'Sullivan RA, Hillman DR, Mateljan R, et al. Mandibular advancement splint: an appliance to treat snoring and obstructive sleep apnea. *Am J Respir Crit Care Med* 1995;151:194–198.

103. Ferguson KA, Ono T, Lowe AA, et al. A randomized crossover study of an oral appliance vs nasal-continuous positive airway pressure in the treatment of mild-moderate obstructive sleep apnea. *Chest* 1996;109: 1269–1275.

104. Standards of Practice Committee for the American Sleep Disorders Association. Practice parameters for the treatment of obstructive sleep apnea in adults: the efficacy of surgical modifications of the upper airway. Report of the American Sleep Disorders Association. *Sleep* 1996;19:152–155.

105. Rodenstein DO. Assessment of uvulopalatopharyngoplasty for the treatment of sleep apnea syndrome. *Sleep* 1992;15:S56–S62.

106. Ryan CF, Love LL. Unpredictable results of laser assisted uvulopalatoplasty in the treatment of obstructive sleep apnoea. *Thorax* 2000;55:399–404.

107. Powell NB, Riley RW, Robinson A. Surgical management of obstructive sleep apnea syndrome. *Clin Chest Med* 1998;19:77–86.

108. Riley RW, Powell NB, Guilleminault C. Obstructive sleep apnea syndrome: a review of 306 consecutively treated surgical patients. *Otolaryngol Head Neck Surg* 1993;108:117–125.

109. Bettega G, Pepin JL, Veale D, et al. Obstructive sleep apnea syndrome. fifty-one consecutive patients treated by maxillofacial surgery. *Am J Respir Crit Care Med* 2000;162:641–649.

110. Hedner J, Grote L. Pharmacological therapy in sleep apnea. In: McNicholas WT, Phillipson EA, eds. *Breathing disorders in sleep.* London: WB Saunders, 2002:149–156.

111. Piper AJ, Sullivan CE. Effects of long-term nocturnal nasal ventilation on spontaneous breathing during sleep in neuromuscular and chest wall disorders. *Eur Respir J* 1996;9:1515–1522.

112. Sullivan CE, Berthon-Jones M, Issa FG. Remission of severe obesity-hypoventilation syndrome after short-term treatment during sleep with nasal continuous positive airway pressure. *Am Rev Respir Dis* 1983;128: 177–181.

113. Piper AJ, Sullivan CE. Effects of short-term NIPPV in the treatment of patients with severe obstructive sleep apnea and hypercapnia. *Chest* 1994;105:434–440.

114. Piper AJ, Laks L, Sullivan CE. Effectiveness of short-term NIPPV in the management of patients with severe OSA and REM hypoventilation. *Sleep* 1993;16:S115–S117.

10

Obesity and Type II Diabetes Mellitus

Robert R. Henry and Sunder Mudaliar

Obesity is closely associated with type II diabetes in populations across the world. Indeed, abdominal (or visceral) obesity in humans is a genetically controlled phenotype that constitutes a major risk factor for the development of type II diabetes (1). Worldwide, the prevalence of both obesity and type II diabetes are dramatically increasing, and the global epidemic of obesity and type II diabetes, which could more aptly be termed "diobesity," will undoubtedly lead to a major global public health problem.

In the United States today, nearly 16 million people have type II diabetes, and 90% of these are overweight or obese (2). However, not all individuals with type II diabetes are obese, and, furthermore, most obese individuals will not develop type II diabetes (3). Since type II diabetes is genetically heterogeneous, the presumption is that an obese individual must inherit additional mutations producing dysregulation of normal glucose homeostasis in order to be susceptible to obesity-induced diabetes (4). This chapter reviews the association between obesity and type II diabetes; discusses the pathophysiologic basis of type II diabetes and its association with obesity; evaluates the role of nutrition therapy and exercise therapy in promoting weight loss and glucose control in type II diabetes; and elaborates on the effects of pharmacologic antidiabetic agents, antiobesity agents, and bariatric surgery on glycemic control and body weight in obese patients with type II diabetes.

ASSOCIATION BETWEEN TYPE II DIABETES AND OBESITY

Type II diabetes is a metabolic syndrome associated with hyperglycemia, hyperlipidemia, hypertension, and a hypercoagulable state, among other abnormalities. The following three major defects are found in type II diabetes: impaired insulin secretion; diminished insulin action (insulin resistance) in skeletal muscle, liver, and adipose tissue; and excessive hepatic glucose production (HGP), secondary to hepatic insulin resistance (5) (Fig. 10.1). Of these abnormalities, insulin resistance is a characteristic feature that is commonly seen in both type II diabetes and obesity. Approximately 90% of type II diabetics are obese, and a strong association has been found between obesity and type II diabetes (4). In a study of ten different populations across the world, West et al. (6) noted a strong correlation between the prevalence of increased body weight and the prevalence of diabetes. An increased risk of diabetes has also been documented in several prospective studies (4). In one recent study, Resnick et al. (7) followed a cohort of 1,929 overweight nondiabetic adults for 10 years. Over this period, 251 subjects developed diabetes. The age-adjusted cumulative incidence of diabetes increased by 9.6% for patients with a body mass index (BMI) of less than 29 kilograms per meter squared (kg/m^2) and by 26. 2% for those with a BMI of more than or equal to 37 kg/m^2. Furthermore, in comparison to overweight people with stable weight, each kilogram of weight gained annually over 10 years

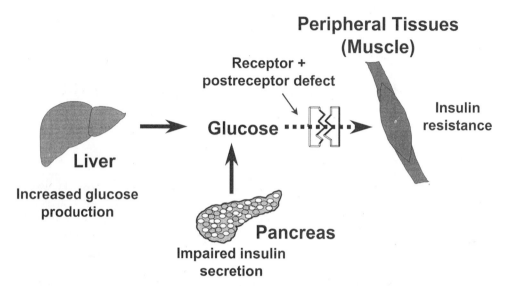

FIG. 10.1. The major sites of defects leading to hyperglycemia in type II diabetes.

in the study was associated with a 49% increase in the individual's risk of developing diabetes in the subsequent 10 years. Similarly, each kilogram of weight lost annually over 10 years was associated with a 33% lower risk of diabetes in that individual in the subsequent 10 years. Evidence also suggests that increasing duration of obesity significantly increases the risk of developing diabetes (8). In Pima Indians, the risk of diabetes in those who have been obese for more than 10 years is twice that of those who have been obese for fewer than 5 years. In a recent study of 6,916 middle-aged British men followed for

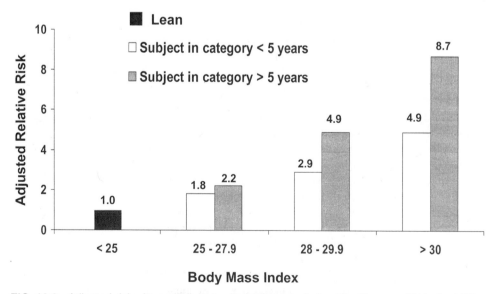

FIG. 10.2. Adjusted risk of type II diabetes by body mass index after 5 years. (Data from Wannamethee SG, Shaper GA. Weight change and duration of overweight and obesity in the incidence of type 2 diabetes. *Diabetes Care* 1999;22:1266–1272, with permission.)

a mean of 12 years, Wannamethee et al. (9) found that the risk of type II diabetes increased progressively and significantly with increasing levels of initial BMI and with the duration of overweight and obesity (Fig. 10.2).

Recently, the location of excess body fat has become the focus of major research. Growing evidence implicates upper-body or central (visceral) distribution of body fat as a major risk factor for type II diabetes, independent of the absolute level of obesity (10–14). Unlike subcutaneous fat, an association between increased visceral fat and increased HGP and reduced glucose disposal has been demonstrated (15) (Fig. 10.3). This association is independent of the methodology used to assess insulin sensitivity in humans (14). Although visceral fat is a strong predictor of insulin resistance in obese subjects, the same relationship is not maintained in normal-weight individuals, suggesting that the association might occur only beyond a certain threshold of visceral fat amount (16). Several prospective and cross-sectional studies have shown a higher risk of diabetes in association with greater abdominal obesity (17–20). Indeed, increased visceral obesity may be a very early abnormality in individuals destined to become diabetic. In a recent prospective study among Japanese Americans, Boyko et al. (21) observed that greater visceral adiposity, as measured by computed tomographic (CT) scan, precedes the devel-

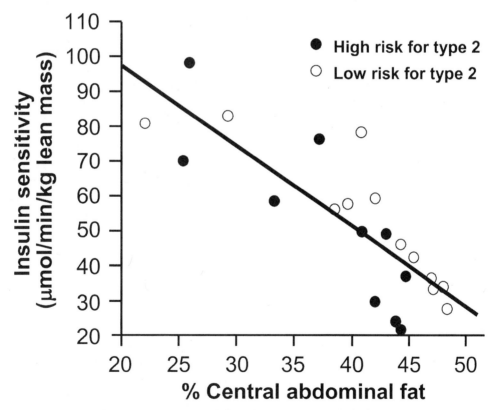

FIG. 10.3. Relationship between central abdominal fat and insulin sensitivity as measured by the glucose clamp technique in women with a body mass index (BMI) of greater than 25 kg/m² (•) and women with a BMI less than or equal to 25 kg/m² (○). (From Carey DG, Jenkins AB, Campbell LV, et al. Abdominal fat and insulin resistance in normal and overweight women: direct measurements reveal a strong relationship in subjects at both low and high risk of NIDDM. *Diabetes* 1996;45:633–638, with permission.)

opment of type II diabetes; this effect was independent of the fasting insulin level, insulin secretion, total and regional adiposity, and even the family history of diabetes. In an earlier prospective study, Lilloja et al. (12) analyzed the relative roles of obesity, body fat distribution, insulin sensitivity, insulin secretion, and HGP in the development of type II diabetes in a Pima Indian population. In this study, in a univariate analysis, insulin resistance, as measured by the glucose clamp technique, was the strongest predictor of type II diabetes. In multivariate analyses, insulin resistance and insulin secretory dysfunction, but not HGP, had independent and cumulative effects on the development of type II diabetes. Furthermore, the degree of obesity, which was measured anthropometrically, had little effect in predicting diabetes when insulin resistance was considered, thus suggesting that insulin resistance may be the major mechanism involved in the association of obesity with an increased risk of type II diabetes.

Although substantial evidence exists to indicate that visceral obesity is accompanied by abnormalities of fatty acid (FA) metabolism that may cause insulin resistance, data from other studies suggest that the sequence may be reversed. Skeletal muscle is the largest tissue in the body, and it is responsible for the majority of lipid oxidation and insulin-stimulated glucose utilization. Colberg et al. (22) studied free fatty acid (FFA) and glucose utilization during basal and insulin-stimulated conditions in the skeletal muscle of 17 healthy lean and obese premenopausal women whose the cross-sectional area of visceral fat ranged from 18 to 180 cm^2. Using leg balance studies and muscle biopsy studies, they demonstrated that defects in basal FA uptake and insulin-stimulated glucose storage coexist in muscle and that these could contribute to the development of visceral obesity. By this scenario, FAs that cannot be taken up by muscle would be stored in visceral fat depots, and thus the initial lesion for both visceral obesity and type II diabetes may well begin in skeletal muscle (22).

Regardless of whether visceral obesity is a consequence of insulin resistance or precedes it, not all obese individuals develop type II diabetes. An obese individual must inherit additional defects producing impairment of pancreatic beta-cell function to be susceptible to type II diabetes. Moreover, the exact mechanisms by which excess adiposity and/or its hormonal milieu impairs or worsens insulin sensitivity and insulin secretion and results in the diabetic state still remain to be determined. The relative roles of insulin resistance, insulin secretion, and HGP in the pathophysiology of type II diabetes, as well as their interaction with obesity, is discussed.

PATHOPHYSIOLOGY OF TYPE II DIABETES

Insulin Resistance in Type II Diabetes and Obesity

Insulin normally increases the uptake, phosphorylation, storage, and oxidation of glucose, primarily in skeletal muscle. The binding of insulin to its receptor results in a series of phosphorylation or dephosphorylation reactions that activate or inhibit several intracellular molecules or pathways and that result in the uptake and storage or oxidation of glucose. In patients with type II diabetes, insulin resistance has been primarily associated with decreased stimulation of muscle glycogen synthesis by insulin (23,24). Several defects have been implicated in the reduced rate of glycogen synthesis, including defects in glycogen synthase (25–27), hexokinase (28–32), and glucose transport activity (31–34). Using nuclear magnetic resonance imaging (MRI) studies, Shulman et al. (24) identified glucose transport as a primary site at which insulin action fails in patients with type II diabetes. Because glucose transport is crucial for glycogen synthesis, this impaired glucose transport is believed to lead to a secondary reduction in glycogen synthesis in muscle.

For many years, the Randle glucose FA cycle has been invoked to explain insulin resistance in skeletal muscle of patients with type II diabetes or obesity. According to the hypothesis put forward by Randle et al. (35), the increased availability of FAs and the consequent increase in fat oxidation result in substrate competition and reduced glucose metabolism. Indeed, several investigations have shown that artificially increasing fat oxidation by providing excess lipid does decrease glucose oxidation in the whole body. However, results from human studies that have more directly examined muscle fuel metabolism have shown that, with insulin resistance under basal conditions, there is increased, rather than decreased, skeletal muscle glucose oxidation, as well as impaired fat oxidation (36). On the other hand, under insulin-stimulated circumstances, decreased glucose oxidation and impaired suppression of fat oxidation are observed, thereby producing a state of "metabolic inflexibility" (36). Thus, insulin-resistant skeletal muscle in individuals with obesity and type II diabetes has a reduced capacity for fat oxidation and a tendency toward increased lipid storage (36). Several investigators have shown that an excess accumulation of skeletal muscle lipid is associated with insulin resistance in human obesity (37).

Free Fatty Acids and Insulin Resistance

FFAs appear to be an important link between obesity, insulin resistance, and type II diabetes (38) (Fig. 10.4). FFAs are produced by hydrolysis of triglycerides stored in adipose tissue, and they can inhibit glucose use by peripheral tissues (39). Plasma FFA levels are elevated in most obese and diabetic subjects, and strong evidence indicates that

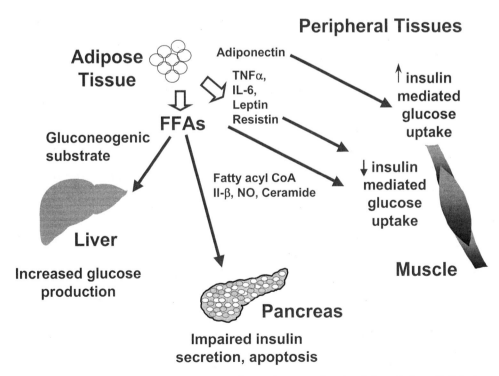

FIG. 10.4. Molecular mechanisms linking adipose tissue and major defects in type II diabetes. Abbreviations: CoA, coenzyme A; FFA, free fatty acid; IN-6, interleukin-6 necrosis factor; NO, nitrous oxide; TNF-α, tumor necrosis factor α.

physiologic elevations in plasma FFA concentrations cause insulin resistance (38). Furthermore, lowering of FFA levels both acutely and chronically improves insulin sensitivity (39–41). Boden et al. (38) showed that lipid and heparin infusions inhibit insulin-stimulated peripheral glucose uptake in a dose-dependent manner both in normal controls and in patients with type II diabetes. This inhibition occurs initially through a fat-related inhibition of glucose transport and/or phosphorylation, which appears after 3 to 4 hours of fat infusion, and later through a decrease in muscle glycogen synthase activity, which develops after 4 to 6 hours of lipid infusion. The exact molecular mechanisms by which FFAs affect insulin signaling and glucose transport are still unknown. Some evidence indicates that long-chain acyl-coenzyme A (LCAC), the activated form of FFAs that can be transported across the mitochondrial membrane for oxidation, modulates protein kinase C activity and thereby inhibits insulin-mediated glycogen synthesis (43). Evidence also suggests that LCACs are intimately involved in the regulation of glucose transporter-4 (GLUT-4) translocation (44–46). Another potential mechanism for the induction of insulin resistance is through uridine 5′-diphosphate (UDP)-*N*-acetylglucosamine, which is the end product of the hexosamine pathway. Stimulation of this pathway by hyperglycemia, infusion of glucosamine, or the increased availability of FFAs has been shown to cause muscle insulin resistance (47).

Besides FFAs, several other molecules secreted by adipose tissue could contribute to the insulin resistance associated with obesity and type II diabetes. These include leptin; tumor necrosis factor α (TNF-α); interleukin-6 (IL-6); and the recently described adipocyte hormones, resistin and adiponectin (Fig. 10.4).

Adipocyte-Secreted Hormones and Insulin Resistance

Until recently, the adipocyte has been regarded as a fat storage organ. However, it is increasingly becoming clear that adipose tissue operates as an endocrine organ and that it releases several hormones that modulate metabolic processes and influence insulin sensitivity. These hormones, which are also termed *adipokines*, include leptin, TNF-α, IL-6, resistin, and adiponectin. Of these, adiponectin is unique because, unlike the other adipokines, it is associated with increased insulin sensitivity.

Leptin

Leptin is produced by adipocytes, and, as with FFAs, leptin levels are also elevated in animals and humans in direct proportion to the degree of obesity (48–50). Leptin has been shown to have both central nervous system and peripheral effects (51–54) (Fig. 10.5). In mouse myotubes and Hep-G2 cells, leptin has been shown to inhibit insulin receptor substrate-1 (IRS-1) phosphorylation and thereby to impair insulin-mediated glucose uptake (55,56). In human cell lines derived from the liver, lung, and kidney, Cohen et al. (57) demonstrated that exposure to leptin at concentrations comparable to those present in obese individuals causes attenuation of several insulin-induced activities, including tyrosine phosphorylation of the IRS-1, association of the adapter molecule growth factor receptor-bound protein-2 with IRS-1, and downregulation of gluconeogenesis. In addition, *in vitro* evidence shows that leptin suppresses insulin release in *ob/ob* mouse and human islet cells, thereby potentially affecting insulin secretion and insulin sensitivity (58,59). However, in contrast to *in vitro* data, in intact animal models of diabetes and obesity, leptin administration actually improves glucose metabolism (60–63). In human studies, subcutaneous leptin administration for 24 weeks is associated with a dose–response relationship to weight and fat loss in both lean and obese subjects (64). In this study, no evidence was found to indicate that leptin administration worsened glucose

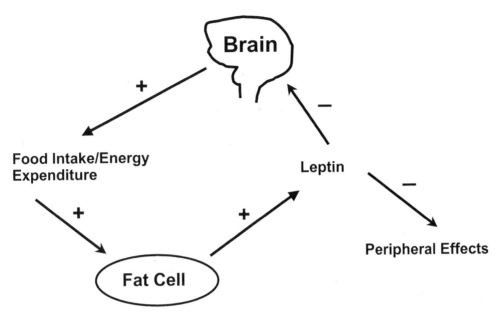

FIG. 10.5. Central nervous system and peripheral effects of leptin in animal studies.

tolerance in nondiabetic individuals. Thus, the relationship between leptin and its influence on glucose metabolism in obesity and type II diabetes remains to be fully elucidated.

Tumor Necrosis Factor α

TNF-α is a cytokine that is produced in significant quantities in adipose tissue, and it is increasingly being implicated in the insulin resistance of obesity and type II diabetes. Like leptin, TNF-α expression is elevated in association with obesity in both animals and humans (65,66). A pivotal role for TNF-α in the pathogenesis of peripheral insulin resistance in obesity is suggested by the observation that TNF-α is overexpressed in the adipose tissue of both obese insulin-resistant rodents and humans. Furthermore, in *in vitro* studies, TNF-α has been shown to impair insulin signaling by decreasing IRS-1 phosphorylation and GLUT-4 expression (67,68). On the other hand, neutralization of TNF-α in *fa/fa* Zucker rats decreases insulin resistance and increases insulin receptor tyrosine kinase activity in adipose tissue and muscle (69). However, in a recent study in humans, neutralization of TNF-α with an antibody over a 4-week period had no effect on insulin sensitivity in obese patients with type II diabetes (70).

Since TNF-α levels in the circulation are extremely low, its effect may not be endocrine, but rather paracrine, in nature, or it may possibly even be mediated indirectly through another factor that is released into the circulation, thus inhibiting insulin action on muscle. The most likely candidate for this role are FFAs because TNF-α has been shown to increase lipolysis. Hence, the effect of TNF-α on glucose uptake may be direct, or it may be mediated, at least in part, by FFAs. Indeed, the infusion of TNF-α in humans has been shown to increase plasma FFA levels (71). In animal studies, the neutralization of TNF-α in Zucker rats is associated not only with an increase in insulin sensitivity but also with a decrease in plasma FFA levels (72). Thus, like leptin, TNF-α plays a complex role in the link between human obesity and insulin resistance. Further research is clearly needed to clarify this relationship.

Interleukin-6

Similar to TNF-α, IL-6 is a proinflammatory cytokine that is expressed and secreted by adipose tissue (73). Levels of IL-6 have been shown to be increased in obesity (74). In human studies, IL-6 has been found to induce the release of glucagon and cortisol and to increase hepatic glucose release (75). In a recent study, Bastard et al. (76) evaluated the potential role of adipose cytokines in obesity-associated insulin resistance. They compared the serum concentrations of IL-6, TNF-α, and leptin in eight healthy lean female control patients and in centrally obese female patients both without (number of subjects [n] = 14) and with (n = 7) type II diabetes. Compared to the lean controls, both the non-diabetic and diabetic obese patients were more insulin resistant and they had higher levels of leptin, IL-6, TNF-α, and C-reactive protein. In the group as a whole, IL-6 values were more closely related to the insulin resistance than to the leptin or TNF-α values. They also measured the levels of these cytokines both in the serum and in the subcutaneous adipose tissue in the 14 obese nondiabetic women before and after 3 weeks of a very low calorie diet (VLCD). A VLCD resulted in weight loss of approximately 3 kg and decreased the body fat mass. After weight loss, insulin sensitivity was improved with no significant change in both the serum and adipose tissue TNF-α levels. In contrast, weight loss with a VLCD induced significant decreases in IL-6 and leptin levels in both the adipose tissue and serum. The authors concluded that, like leptin, circulating IL-6 concentrations reflect, at least in part, adipose tissue production. Furthermore, the reduced production and serum concentrations of IL-6 after weight loss might have contributed to the improved sensitivity to insulin that was seen in these patients.

In another recent study, Vozarova et al. (77) examined whether a relationship existed between circulating plasma IL-6 concentrations and direct measures of insulin resistance and insulin secretory dysfunction in Pima Indians, a population with high rates of obesity and type II diabetes. In this population of 58 Pima Indians without diabetes (24 women, 34 men), fasting plasma IL-6 concentrations were positively correlated with percentage of body fat (correlation coefficient $[r] = 0.26$, probability $[p] = 0.049$) and were negatively correlated with insulin sensitivity ($r = -0.28$, $p = 0.031$) but were not related to acute insulin response ($r = 0.13$, $p = 0.339$). After adjusting for percentage of body fat, however, the plasma IL-6 level was not related to insulin sensitivity (partial $r = -0.23$, $p = 0.089$). The authors concluded that fasting plasma IL-6 concentrations are positively related to adiposity and are negatively related to insulin action in Pima Indians and that the relationship between IL-6 and insulin action seems to be mediated through adiposity.

Resistin

In a recent report, Lazar et al. (78) identified a new signaling molecule (messenger RNA), which they termed "resistin" (for resistance to insulin). Resistin is secreted by adipocytes, and its levels are increased in diet-induced obesity and in genetic forms of obesity in mice and are decreased by the antidiabetic drug rosiglitazone, a peroxisome proliferator-activated receptor γ (PPARγ) agonist. Moreover, administration of antiresistin antibody improves blood sugar levels and insulin action in mice with diet-induced obesity. The authors postulate that resistin may be a hormone that could potentially link obesity to diabetes.

Adiponectin

Perhaps the most exciting recent development has been the identification and characterization of adiponectin, which is a novel adipocyte-derived hormone (also called apM1 [adipose most abundant gene transcript 1] and acrp30 or adipoQ for the murine homologue) (79,80). With a concentration of about 5 μg per mL in human plasma, adiponectin represents one of the most abundant circulating proteins, and, in contrast to previously discussed peptide hormones released from adipocytes, adiponectin seems to protect from insulin resistance and type II diabetes. In a recent study, Weyer et al. (81) found that plasma adiponectin levels are significantly decreased in both Pima Indians and white subjects. Furthermore, adiponectin concentrations positively correlate with insulin sensitivity and are significantly decreased with deteriorating glucose tolerance (81). In other studies in humans, circulating adiponectin levels have been shown to increase significantly after both weight reduction and treatment with rosiglitazone, a PPARγ agonist (82,83). In animal studies, intravenous administration of recombinant adiponectin to rodent models of insulin resistance restores normal insulin sensitivity (84). Several mechanisms by which adiponectin improves insulin sensitivity have been postulated. These include increases in muscle lipid metabolism through increased expression of genes encoding CD36, acyl-coenzyme A (CoA) oxidase, and uncoupling protein-2 (UCP-2) with consequent increases in FA transport, fat combustion, and heat dissipation (85). Interestingly, there is also data indicating that adiponectin depresses the inflammatory response that accompanies atherosclerosis (86). Thus, adiponectin appears to be a crucial link between obesity and insulin resistance, and adiponectin or perhaps its putative receptor represents an exciting target for the development of drugs for diabetes or even obesity (85).

Peroxisome Proliferator–Activated Receptors and Insulin Resistance

PPARs are a family of nuclear receptors that include the following three subtypes: PPARα, PPARγ, and PPARβ (previously termed PPARδ, FAAR, or NUC-1) (87). PPARγ receptors are found in key target tissues for insulin action, such as adipose tissue, skeletal muscle, and liver. Evidence shows that these receptors are important regulators of lipid homeostasis, adipocyte differentiation, and insulin action, and thus, they may play

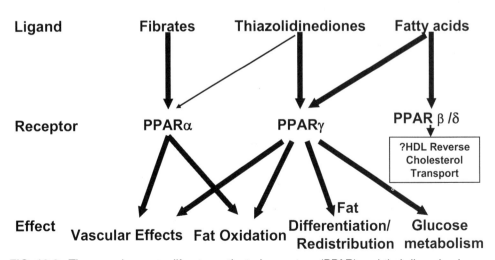

FIG. 10.6. The peroxisome proliferator-activated receptors (PPAR) and their ligands play an important role in lipid and carbohydrate metabolism. Abbreviation: HDL, high density lipoprotein. (From Saltiel AR, Olefsky JM. Thiazolidinediones in the treatment of insulin resistance in type 2 diabetes. *Diabetes* 1996;45:1661–1669, with permission.)

an important role in the pathogenesis of obesity, insulin resistance, and type II diabetes (87) (Fig. 10.6). Indeed, PPARγ agonists comprise one of the classes of oral agents used to treat type II diabetes. Through their action on PPARγ, the thiazolidinediones (glitazones) appear to enhance insulin action without directly stimulating insulin secretion. Treatment with thiazolidinediones restores the ability of insulin to suppress HGP and to increase peripheral glucose disposal in human and animal models of insulin resistance These metabolic effects are accompanied by a dramatic improvement in insulin sensitivity in isolated fat and muscle tissue and by a reduction in glucose and insulin levels (88).

There is now some evidence that mutations in PPARγ may play a role in human disease. Recently, Barroso et al. (89) reported two different heterozygous loss-of-function mutations in three subjects who had severe insulin resistance, early onset diabetes, and hypertension. Surprisingly, these subjects were not obese (BMI about 25 kilograms per meter squared [kg/m^2]). On the other hand, Kahn et al. (90) reported a heterozygous mutation in PPARγ in three unrelated subjects who were obese. These subjects, however, had normal insulin sensitivity. Further research is clearly needed to advance knowledge in this field.

Insulin-Secretory Defects in Type II Diabetes and Obesity

Along with diminished insulin sensitivity and increased HGP, impaired pancreatic beta-cell function with abnormal insulin secretion is a key defect in patients with type II diabetes. Indeed, the beta cell can compensate for defects in insulin sensitivity and for increased HGP by increasing insulin secretion, which thereby decreases or even prevents hyperglycemia. On the other hand, abnormalities in beta-cell function cannot be compensated for by changes in insulin sensitivity or HGP.

As with insulin resistance, FFAs appear to be an important link between obesity, insulin secretion, and type II diabetes (Fig. 10.4). Plasma FFA levels are elevated in most obese subjects, and physiologic elevations of FFAs have been shown not only to inhibit insulin-stimulated glucose uptake into muscle but also to stimulate insulin secretion acutely (38,91). Insulin-secretory rates both basally and after meals have been demonstrated to correlate strongly with BMI in obese subjects (92,93). Most evidence suggests that this hyperinsulinemia represents an adaptive response by the beta cell to the coexisting insulin resistance (38). In the long term, however, exposure to FFAs appears to have deleterious effects on pancreatic beta-cell function and insulin secretion in both human and animal studies (94–96). Thus, hypersecretion in the early phases of type II diabetes is followed by declining insulin secretion as the disease progresses and by relative, and later absolute, insulinopenia in the later stages. An attractive hypothesis has been postulated by Boden (38), who speculates that, in normal obese subjects, increased plasma FFA concentrations stimulate insulin secretion in amounts that are sufficient or nearly sufficient to compensate for the FFA-induced insulin resistance. Hence, these individuals have either no deficit or only a small deficit between FFA-mediated insulin resistance and insulin secretion. In contrast, obese subjects who are genetically predisposed to develop type II diabetes gradually fail to secrete appropriate amounts of insulin in response to FFAs, and therefore they develop increasingly larger FFA-induced insulin resistance and/or secretion deficits (38).

Data to support this hypothesis are available in rodent models (39). In the ZDF (*fa/fa*) rat, the onset of obesity occurs at about 4 weeks of age, and the pattern of beta-cell response to this lipid overload is biphasic. Initially, with the nearly tenfold increase in intraislet lipid content, there is a fourfold increase in beta-cell mass and increased secretion of insulin to compensate for insulin resistance. Later, however, as the intraislet lipid content rises even further, there is a marked increase in apoptosis, a net loss of beta cells, and a decline in insulin production to below the levels required to compensate for insulin resistance. Unger and Zhou (39) link this beta-cell "lipotoxicity" to a failure of normal leptin function. They speculate that one of the functions of leptin is to protect nonadipose tissues from the nonoxidative metabolic products of long-chain FAs during periods of overnutrition by increasing the beta-oxidative metabolism of surplus FAs and thereby reducing lipogenesis. When this protective system fails, as is seen in leptin-deficient and leptin-resistant obese animals, harmful products of nonoxidative metabolism, such as ceramide, increase in nonadipose tissues, including the pancreatic islets, and cause nitric oxide–mediated lipotoxicity and lipoapoptosis. In normal animal tissue, even when the caloric intake is excessive, compensatory FFA-induced upregulation of oxidation prevents overaccumulation. However, if leptin is deficient or if leptin receptors are nonfunctional, this autoregulatory system does not operate and the triacylglycerol content rises in nonadipose tissues. This provides a source of excess FFAs that then enter potentially toxic pathways of nonoxidative metabolism leading to apoptosis of certain tissues; in pancreatic islets, it causes beta-cell dysfunction, apoptosis, and diabetes (39).

In addition to quantitative changes in insulin secretion, qualitative changes in beta-cell function have also been described in patients with type II diabetes. This defect is characterized by an absent first-phase insulin response to an intravenous glucose load and a decreased second-phase response. Delayed and blunted secretory responses to mixed meals and alterations in ultradian oscillations and pulsatile insulin secretion are also seen (97).

The exact mechanism by which FFAs cause initial insulin hypersecretion is not fully known. However, data from *in vitro* studies provide evidence that long-chain fatty acyl-CoA mediates a rise in phosphofructikinase activity that, in turn, lowers the glucose 6-phosphate levels. This leads to an attenuation of inhibition of hexokinase, thereby causing basal insulin hypersecretion (98). To explain the beta-cell defect in the later stages, several candidate molecules that might mediate the "lipotoxic effect" of FFAs on the beta cell have been identified. They include interleukin-1β, nitrous oxide, and ceramide, which causes accelerated apoptosis in fat-laden beta cells (Fig. 10.4) (99–100). Other than "lipotoxicity" (38,39), there is also evidence that chronic hyperglycemia may itself be toxic to the beta cell (101). This "glucose toxicity" may be responsible for initially reversible and later irreversible defects in beta-cell function resulting from the chronic exposure of the beta cell to supraphysiologic glucose concentrations (102).

Hepatic Glucose Production in Type II Diabetes and Obesity

Increased HGP is a characteristic abnormality in subjects with type II diabetes (Fig. 10.7). Of the three major abnormalities present in individuals with type II diabetes—insulin resistance, insulin secretory dysfunction, and increased HGP—only increased HGP is not found in obese nondiabetic subjects (103). In type II diabetes, basal HGP is increased or is inappropriately suppressed despite fasting hyperglycemia and hyperinsulinemia. Several studies have demonstrated a strong relationship between fasting glucose levels and HGP, although some investigators argue that the basal HGP is normal in patients with type II diabetes. They attribute increases in HGP to methodologic problems with the use of tritiated glucose as a tracer to estimate HGP (104). Despite this assertion, HGP is clearly abnormal in obese type II diabetics because even normal HGP in the presence of elevated fasting glucose and insulin levels reflects abnormal liver metabolism in type II diabetes.

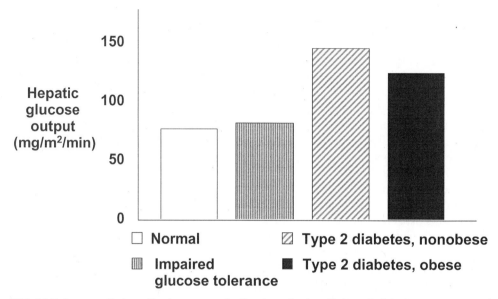

FIG. 10.7. Increase in hepatic glucose production in patients with type II diabetes as compared with nondiabetic controls. (From Kolterman OG, Gray RS, Griffin J, et al. Increase in hepatic glucose production (HGP) in patients with type 2 diabetes as compared to non-diabetic controls. *J Clin Invest* 1981;68:957–969, with permission.)

As with insulin resistance and insulin secretion, FFAs again appear to be the common link between type II diabetes and obesity. Under basal circumstances, insulin exerts an inhibitory effect on HGP. Studies in normal controls or in patients with type II diabetes have demonstrated that, when plasma FFA levels are raised during euglycemic and/or hyperinsulinemic or hyperglycemic and/or hyperinsulinemic clamp conditions, the effect of insulin to suppress HGP is partially inhibited (105–106). Other studies have documented the stimulatory effect of FFAs on HGP. Plasma glucose levels and HGP rise dramatically when plasma FFA levels are raised by the infusion of triglycerides and heparin into normal volunteers after an overnight fast and under basal insulin conditions (obtained through the infusion of somatostatin and basal insulin replacement) (107). On balance, the available human data suggest that FFAs increase HGP, but that the extent of the increase is determined by the FFA-mediated stimulation of insulin secretion.

The cause of the abnormal HGP in diabetes has been attributed primarily to increased gluconeogenesis (108). Good *in vitro* evidence shows that FFAs promote gluconeogenesis (38,109). The proposed mechanisms include the increased production of adenosine triphosphate (ATP) and NADH and the activation of pyruvate carboxylase by the acetyl-CoA that is generated via FA oxidation (38,110). Thus, in the presence of increased gluconeogenic precursor substrate availability, elevated FFA concentrations provide the necessary source of intracellular energy via FA oxidation to drive the gluconeogenic process (38). Recent *in vitro* studies with human hepatocytes have also demonstrated that the efficiency of conversion of gluconeogenic substrates to glucose is increased in diabetes (104). Surprisingly, in this study, the biochemical mechanisms for this were not entirely clear as no increase was seen in any of the following three gluconeogenic enzymes: phosphoenolpyruvate carboxykinase, fructose-2,6-diphosphatase, and glucose 6-phosphatase. In contrast, glucokinase activity has been shown to be markedly decreased in the livers of patients with type II diabetes. Because increased substrate flux through glucokinase is required for glucose-induced inhibition of HGP, defective hepatic glucokinase might conceivably impair the ability of hyperglycemia to suppress HGP in type II diabetes (106).

Thus, FFAs appear to play an important role in all of the three major abnormalities in type II diabetes—insulin resistance, defective insulin secretion, and increased HGP. Physiologic elevations of plasma FFAs inhibit insulin-stimulated glucose uptake into muscle, chronic exposure to FFAs has deleterious effects on pancreatic beta-cell function, and good *in vitro* evidence shows that FFAs promote gluconeogenesis. As postulated by Boden (38), FFAs may initially stimulate insulin secretion in obese nondiabetic individuals. Some of this insulin in the peripheral circulation may compensate for FFA-mediated peripheral insulin resistance. However, FFA-mediated portal hyperinsulinemia counteracts the stimulation of FFAs on HGP and thus prevents hepatic glucose overproduction. Conversely, in obese individuals who are genetically predisposed to develop type II diabetes, FFAs eventually fail to promote insulin secretion, and the stimulatory effect of FFAs on HGP is then no longer checked, thus resulting in hyperglycemia. Therefore, continuously elevated levels of plasma FFAs may play a key role in the pathogenesis of type II diabetes in predisposed individuals by impairing peripheral glucose utilization and promoting hepatic glucose overproduction.

The exact sequence in which the major abnormalities characteristic of type II diabetes develop and their relative importance in the development of glucose intolerance are still not fully understood. In a recent longitudinal study, Weyer et al. (111) measured insulin action, insulin secretion, and HGP in a Pima Indian population over 5 years. In this study, transition from normal glucose tolerance (NGT) to impaired glucose tolerance (IGT) was associated with an increase in body weight, a decline in insulin-stimulated glucose disposal, and a decrease in the acute insulin-secretory response (AIR) to intravenous glucose, but no change in HGP. Further progression from IGT to diabetes was accompanied by a greater increase in body weight, further decreases in insulin-stimulated glucose disposal and AIR, and an increase in basal HGP. Thirty-one subjects who retained NGT over a similar period also gained weight, but their AIR increased with decreasing insulin-stimulated glucose disposal.

In this study, development of type II diabetes was accompanied by a marked increase in body weight that was significantly higher than in the nonprogressors. The greater weight gain in the progressors was accounted for by larger increases in both fat mass and fat-free mass relative to the nonprogressors. In contrast, changes in percentage of body fat and waist to thigh ratio did not differ between groups, which suggests that the absolute amount of weight gain, rather than the specific changes in body composition or body fat distribution, is important in the development of type II diabetes. These results also indicate that defects in both insulin secretion and insulin action occur early and that they contribute to the decline in glucose tolerance as people transition from NGT to IGT and finally to type II diabetes. Increases in endogenous glucose output, in contrast, occur only during the transition from IGT to type II diabetes.

MANAGEMENT OF TYPE II DIABETES

The cornerstone of management in obese patients with type II diabetes is the recommendation to lose weight through lifestyle measures, including diet and exercise (112). As was described earlier, type II diabetes is characterized by insulin resistance and insulin-secretory defects, and the presence of obesity not only aids and abets the development of diabetes but also increases insulin resistance and glucose intolerance and exacerbates the metabolic abnormalities of hyperglycemia, hyperinsulinemia, and dyslipi-

TABLE 10.1. *Goals for glycemic control*

Biochemical index	Normal	Goal	Action suggested
Fasting and/or preprandial plasma glucose (mg/dL)	<110	80–120	<80 or >140
Bedtime plasma glucose (mg/dL)	<120	100–140	<100 or >160
Glycosylated hemoglobin (%) (normal range 4–6)	<6	<7	>8

From American Diabetes Association. Clinical practice recommendations 2002. *Diabetes Care* 2002;25: S1–S147, with permission.

demia (5). Moreover, the coexistence of obesity and type II diabetes increases the risk of developing hypertension and cardiovascular disease, and it significantly increases morbidity and mortality (4). On the other hand, weight loss through diet and exercise in obese patients with type II diabetes is accompanied by improvements in insulin sensitivity and by concurrent improvements in glycemia, dyslipidemia, and blood pressure, as well as reductions in medication costs (4). Observational evidence now indicates that intentional weight loss is also associated with substantial reductions in mortality in overweight patients with type II diabetes (113).

However, over the long term, obese patients show poor compliance with nutrition and exercise recommendations, and most obese patients with type II diabetes will need to be started on pharmacologic agents to achieve glycemic goals (Table 10.1). If patients with type II diabetes attain and maintain these goals, microvascular, and possibly macrovascular, complications may be retarded or prevented (114,115). To help patients achieve

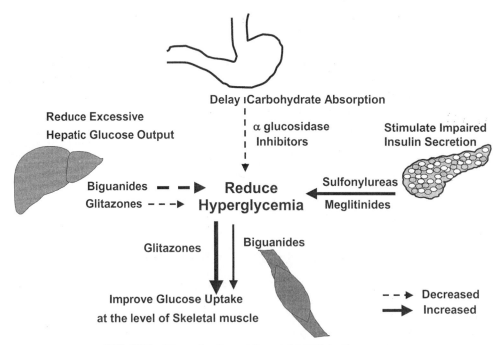

FIG. 10.8. Sites of action of the oral antidiabetic agents.

TABLE 10.2. *Oral antidiabetic agents as initial monotherapy*

Agent	Major mechanism(s) of action	Most suitable patient profile	Glycemic benefit
Insulin secretagogues			
Sulfonylureas	↑↑ Day-long pancreatic insulin secretion	Lean and/or insulinopenic	Fasting and postprandial glycemia
Meglitinides	↑↑ Postprandial pancreatic insulin secretion	Lean and/or insulinopenic	Postprandial glycemia
Biguanide (metformin)	↓↓ Hepatic glucose production ↑ Peripheral glucose utilization	Obese and/or insulin resistant	Fasting and postprandial glycemia
α-Glucosidase inhibitors (acarbose and miglitol)	↓ Postprandial carbohydrate absorption	Lean and/or insulinopenic or obese and/or insulin resistant	Postprandial glycemia
Thiazolidinediones or glitazones (rosiglitazone and or pioglitazone)	↑↑ Peripheral glucose utilization ↓ Hepatic glucose production	Obese and/or insulin resistant	Fasting and postprandial glycemia

↓, decreased; ↑, increased. Number of arrows indicates degree of increase or decrease.
See references 161, 171, 181, and 188 for more information.

glycemic goals, a wide array of pharmacologic agents are now available. They include insulin and the following four major classes of oral agents: insulin secretagogues (sulfonylureas [SUs], meglitinides), biguanides, α-glucosidase inhibitors, and thiazolidinediones. Each class varies in its mechanism of action, primary use (Fig. 10.8 and Table 10.2), and efficacy (Table 10.3). With the exception of metformin and the α-glucosidase inhibitors, all the other antidiabetic agents, including insulin, are associated with increasing body weight (Table 10.4). To counter this increase in weight, particularly when lifestyle recommendations are not successful, two pharmacologic antiobesity agents, sibutramine and orlistat, are now available for use. Growing evidence points to the efficacy of these agents not only to reduce weight but also to improve glycemia and other metabolic abnormalities. Finally, in morbidly obese patients with type II diabetes and comorbid conditions, when intensive lifestyle measures and oral agents fail to reduce weight, bariatric surgery represents a viable option in selected patients.

TABLE 10.3. *Relative efficacy of oral antidiabetic agents as monotherapy (change from placebo)*

Agent	Reduction in fasting plasma glucose (mg/dL)	Reduction in HbA$_{1C}$ (%)	Reduction in postprandial plasma glucose (mg/dL)
Insulin secretagogues			
Sulfonylureas (various agents/doses)	54–70	1.5–2.0	92
Repaglinide	61	17	104
Nateglinide	21	08	—
Metformin (2,550 mg/d)	59–78	1.5–2.0	83
Rosiglitazone (8 mg/d)	62–76	1.5	—
Pioglitazone (45 mg/d)	59–80	1.4–2.6	—
Acarbose (300 mg/d)	20–30	0.5–1.0	40–50
Miglitol (300 mg/d)	—	0.5–0.8	40–60

See references 161, 171, 181, and 188 for more information.

TABLE 10.4. *Metabolic effects of oral antidiabetic agents as monotherapy*

	Sulfonylureas and meglitinides	Acarbose	Metformin	Rosiglitazone and pioglitazone
Weight	↑	↔	↓ or ↔	↑
Low density-lipoprotein cholesterol	↔	↔	↓	↔ or ↑
High-density lipoprotein cholesterol	↔	↔	↑ or ↔	↑↑
Triglycerides	↔	↔	↓	↔ or ↓

↓, decreased; ↑, increased; ↔, no change. Number of arrows indicates degree of change. See references 161, 171, 181, and 188 for more information.

Role of Nutrition Therapy in Type II Diabetes

Several lifestyle factors affect the incidence of type II diabetes. Obesity and weight gain dramatically increase the risk, and physical inactivity further elevates the risk, independent of obesity (116). Hence, diet and exercise remain the cornerstone of therapy in obese patients with type II diabetes. The most recent position statement on nutrition from the American Diabetes Association (ADA) recommends an individualized approach to nutrition based on a nutritional assessment and the desired outcomes in each patient (112). These recommendations should consider patient preferences and the control of hyperglycemia and dyslipidemia. While prescribing a weight loss regime for obese patients with type II diabetes, the clinician should pay attention to both calorie content and macronutrient composition.

With moderate caloric restriction, individuals on a hypocaloric diet (1,000 to 1,500 kcal per day) generally lose about 10% of their initial body weight (4,117). Even short-term weight loss improves insulin sensitivity (Fig. 10.9), and modest weight loss, if maintained over the long term, has been shown to produce important glycemic, metabolic, and even survival benefits. In one study evaluating the effect of a long-term weight loss program on glycemic control, patients who lost more than 6.9 kg (or more than 5% of baseline body weight) experienced significant long-term improvements in glycemia (117). In another retrospective review of 263 obese patients with type II diabetes or IGT, an average weight loss of 1 kg was associated with an increased survival of 3 to 4 months, and, in this analysis, it was estimated that a weight loss of only 10 kg could restore approximately 35% of the reduction in life expectancy in obese type II diabetics (118). However, the rate of recidivism with nutrition and lifestyle measures in obese patients—both diabetic and nondiabetic—is extremely high. About one-third of the lost weight is usually regained in the first year after treatment, and almost all of the lost weight is regained

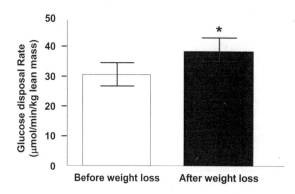

FIG. 10.9. Short-term weight loss improves insulin sensitivity. Insulin sensitivity was measured by the insulin/glucose clamp technique. $p < 0.05$ at before and after weight loss. (From Fransila-Kalkunki A, Rissanen A, Ekstrand A, et al. Effects of weight loss on substrate oxidation, energy expenditure, and insulin sensitivity in obese individuals. *Am J Clin Nutr* 1992;55: 356–361, with permission.)

within 5 years (119). Further research is needed into what measures are required to prevent weight regain in these subjects.

One of the options to accelerate weight loss in obese patients with type II diabetes is the use of VLCDs. In contrast to standard low-calorie diets of 1,000 to 1,500 kcal per day that produce an average weight loss of 8.5 kg in 20 to 24 weeks, VLCDs produce weight losses of 15 to 20 kg in 12 weeks (120). VLCDs are usually consumed over a 12-week to 16-week period, and they contain 400 to 800 kcal per day, with at least 70 g of high-quality protein to conserve lean body mass (4). In obese patients with type II diabetes, treatment with VLCDs has generally been associated with large, statistically significant improvements in body weight and metabolic control (4). The improvement in metabolic control is rapid, and it occurs in the first 1 to 2 weeks of treatment, before any significant weight loss (121). Thus, caloric restriction *per se,* rather than weight loss, may be the major factor underlying the glucose-lowering effects observed with VLCDs. However, although treatment with a VLCD generally results in an initial large weight loss and an improvement in glycemic control, these effects seldom are maintained on a long-term basis and weight regain is almost inevitable.

Apart from calories, the macronutrient composition of the diets for weight loss in type II diabetes is important, but the ideal composition remains a matter of controversy (122). Until recently, dietary recommendations for patients with diabetes emphasized the reduction of calories from total and saturated fat and their replacement with calories from starches (123). The rationale underlying this approach is that lower fat diets will reduce the risk of coronary artery disease by reducing total and low-density lipoprotein (LDL) cholesterol levels. However, in patients with type II diabetes, the substitution of carbohydrate for fat in the diet may impair glucose tolerance, increase hypertriglyceridemia, and reduce high-density lipoprotein (HDL) cholesterol levels (122–124). These potential deleterious effects of high-carbohydrate diets in some patients with type II diabetes have prompted the investigation of diets enriched with monounsaturated FAs (MUFAs) (125). Short-term studies show some evidence indicating that such diets are associated with better glycemic control and lower triglyceride levels than are high-carbohydrate diets (126,127). A concern in the longer term is that the increased fat content of such diets may promote weight gain and thus may impair glycemic control through increased insulin resistance (128). However, a recent metaanalysis of various studies comparing low-saturated fat, high-carbohydrate diets or a high MUFA diet in patients with type II diabetes revealed that high-MUFA diets improve lipoprotein profiles and glycemic control (125). High-MUFA diets were shown to reduce fasting plasma triglyceride levels and very low density lipoprotein cholesterol concentrations by 19% and 22%, respectively, and to cause a modest increase in HDL cholesterol concentrations without adversely affecting the LDL cholesterol concentrations. Furthermore, the metaanalysis revealed no evidence showing that high-MUFA diets induce weight gain in patients with diabetes mellitus, provided that energy intake is controlled.

Recently, awareness of the role of dietary fiber in weight loss diets has increased. In a recent study, Chandalia et al. (129) observed that a high intake of dietary fiber (50 g per day), particularly of the soluble type (25 g per day), above the level recommended by the ADA, not only improves glycemic control and decreases hyperinsulinemia but also lowers plasma lipid concentrations in patients with type II diabetes. The mechanisms of the improved glycemic control associated with high fiber intake remain undefined. Whether this effect is due to an increase in soluble fiber, insoluble fiber, or both is unclear. Besides causing increased fecal excretion of bile acids, dietary fiber may cause the malabsorption of fat. However, in this study, the patients' weight did not change with the high-fiber diet, which suggests that the degree of reduction in the absorption of fat was insignificant. Dietary fiber also may improve glycemic control by reducing or delaying the absorption of carbohydrates.

Apart from the caloric content and macronutrient composition of the diet and dietary fiber, a "Western" diet, with its higher consumption of red meat, processed meat, French fries, high-fat dairy products, refined grains, and sweets and desserts, may *per se* predispose individuals to type II diabetes. During 12 years of follow-up in the Health Professionals Study, a "Western dietary pattern" was associated with a substantially increased risk of type II diabetes in men (130).

Regardless of the caloric content and macronutrient composition of the diet, obese patients with type II diabetes find the implementation of successful weight loss harder to achieve and even more difficult to maintain than does the general population (131). This was well exemplified in the recently concluded United Kingdom Prospective Diabetes Study (UKPDS). In this study, 2,597 patients with newly diagnosed type II diabetes were treated with diet alone for 3 months before being randomized to pharmacologic therapy (132). Dietary calories were restricted to an average of 1,361 kcal per day, and the average weight loss over the initial 3 months was about 5 kg, with only 16% achieving fasting plasma glucose (FPG) levels of less than or equal to 108 mg per dL. As may be expected, the rate of weight loss achieved in the initial 3 months was not sustained through the study, and, at the end of 15 years, the conventionally treated group had a weight gain of about 3 kg, and the intensively treated group showed an increase of about 6 kg. On the other hand, a few studies do document successful long-term weight loss in obese patients with type II diabetes. In the Diabetes Treatment Study (133), which was conducted in Northern Ireland, 223 obese patients with recently diagnosed type II diabetes were placed on a 1,450-kcal diet for 6 months initially and then on a 2,000-kcal diet and were followed regularly. Average weight loss at 6 months was 9 kg, and this was successfully maintained for the 6-year study period. Surprisingly, 87% of the patients at 1 year and 71% at 6 years could be managed by diet alone. However, the success of this study has been difficult to replicate in most other long-term studies.

Despite the high rate of recidivism with long-term weight loss programs, the recent availability of the oral antiobesity agents sibutramine and orlistat offers some hope that weight loss programs, in conjunction with the use of these agents, will not only enhance weight loss in obese patients with type II diabetes but, more importantly, will also help them to maintain this weight loss over the long term. What is clearly needed is the design of longer large-scale studies to investigate the optimal diet compositions for promoting weight loss in type II diabetes, the effects of such diets on metabolic control, and the role of antiobesity agents in this endeavor.

Role of Exercise Therapy in Type II Diabetes

Exercise therapy is an important component of any lifestyle regimen that is prescribed to induce weight loss in obese patients with type II diabetes. Several studies have shown a beneficial influence of physical activity on the risk of type II diabetes that is independent of age, obesity, body fat distribution, family history, and conventional cardiovascular risk factors, such as blood pressure and total cholesterol level (4). Exercise has been shown to improve insulin sensitivity and to lower blood glucose levels acutely (Fig. 10.10) (4,134). In the Nurses Health Study (135) and the Physicians' Health Study (136), those individuals who exercised at least once weekly had a one-third lower risk of developing diabetes. Similar results were reported in a recent study from Finland, where indi-

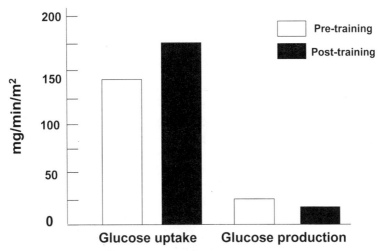

FIG. 10.10. Aerobic exercise improves insulin sensitivity. Insulin sensitivity was measured by the insulin/glucose clamp technique. *,*p* <0.05 versus pretraining.) (From DeFronzo RA, Sherman RS, Kraemer N. Effect of physical training on insulin action in obesity. *Diabetes* 1987;36: 1379–1385, with permission.)

viduals randomized to an exercise program had a dramatic decrease in the risk of developing diabetes (137).

The exact mechanism by which exercise improves insulin sensitivity remains to be determined. Both exercise and insulin are potent stimuli of glucose transport, which is the rate-limiting step for skeletal muscle glucose uptake via GLUT-4, the major glucose-transporting protein (138). However, whether insulin and exercise act through separate pathways or share the same signaling pathways is still unknown (139). In the obese Zucker rat, normal exercise-stimulated increases in glucose transport are seen, but little insulin-stimulated increases are observed (140). In human studies, patients with type II diabetes who have resistance to insulin action demonstrate increased muscle glucose uptake with exercise to the same extent as that seen in individuals without diabetes (141). Exercise increases both insulin-stimulated tyrosine phosphorylation of the insulin receptor substrate-1 (IRS-1) and phosphatidylinositol-3 kinase (PI-3K) activation (142). Wortmannin, which blocks insulin-stimulated glucose transport by inhibiting PI-3K phosphorylation, does not affect the increase in glucose transport that is seen with exercise (119,143). Several mediators that could potentially modulate the effects of exercise at the cellular level have been identified. These include calcium, nitric oxide, adenosine, bradykinin, and 5'-adenosine monophosphate (5'-AMP)–activated protein kinase. The latter enzyme is activated by high levels of AMP and creatine and is inactivated by high ATP and other mediators of energy storage. Substrates for 5'-AMP kinase include most of the enzymes of energy metabolism. Exercise has been shown to increase 5'-AMP kinase activity (144). Using 5-aminoimidazole-4-carboxamide ribonucleoside (AICAR), which activates 5'-AMP kinase, the pattern of increase in glucose uptake is the same as that seen with exercise. The action of AICAR is not blocked by wortmannin, and the greater degrees of increase in 5'-AMP kinase activity are associated with greater increases in glucose transport. Interestingly, AICAR has no additive effect on muscle contraction, but it does show an additive effect with insulin on glucose transport (144). Further research in this field is ongoing.

Overall, the effects of exercise on weight loss are generally modest, and controlled studies of exercise training have shown weight losses of about 2 to 3 kg in exercise groups compared to those of sedentary control groups (4). In patients with type II diabetes, a recent metaanalysis showed that exercise alone was associated with the poorest effects on weight loss of all the interventions evaluated (145). Even when exercise is combined with diet, the average additional weight loss is only 1.8 kg beyond that observed with diet alone. Exercise is nevertheless considered a major determinant of the long-term maintenance of weight loss, and several correlational studies have shown that individuals who exercise maintain their weight losses better than those who do not exercise (4,134). In a recent metaanalysis of 14 controlled randomized and nonrandomized trials of exercise of at least 8 weeks' duration in patients with type II diabetes, Boule et al. (146) found that patients who exercised had an average 0.66% reduction in hemoglobin A_{1C} (HbA_{1C}). This reduction is comparable in magnitude to that achieved with intensive glucose-lowering therapy in the metformin group in the UKPDS (7.4% versus 8.0%), and it may be expected to lead to a significant reduction in the risk of diabetic complications. In addition, in this metaanalysis, exercise did not have a significant impact on weight loss, thereby suggesting that the beneficial effect of exercise is not dependent on weight loss.

Despite the documented metabolic benefits of exercise, a clear indication of whether exercise therapy improved the prognosis of patients with type II diabetes or had survival benefits was not available until recently. This was addressed in a recent study by Wei et al. (147), who evaluated the prospective association of cardiorespiratory fitness and physical inactivity with mortality in 1,263 men (mean age of 50 ± 10 years) who had type II diabetes. After 12 years of follow-up, they found that patients who had a low fitness level and who were physically inactive had higher mortality rates than did men who were active and fit. The association between low fitness level or inactivity and mortality in this study was strong, and the adjusted relative risks for death were 2.1 in the low-fitness group and 1.7 in those with self-reported inactivity. These associations persisted after adjustment for age, parental history of cardiovascular disease, alcohol consumption, cigarette smoking, high cholesterol level, high blood pressure, high glucose level, overweight, and baseline cardiovascular disease. The authors of this study concluded that low cardiorespiratory fitness and physical inactivity are independent predictors of all-cause mortality in men with type II diabetes.

In another recent study, Hu et al. (148) documented that increased physical activity, including regular walking, is associated with a substantially reduced risk of cardiovascular events in diabetic women. In a prospective cohort study of 5,125 female nurses with diabetes (part of the Nurses Health Study), physical activity was assessed at baseline and after 14 years of follow-up. During 14 years of follow-up, the age-adjusted relative risks according to average hours of moderate or vigorous activity per week (less than 1, 1 to 1.9, 2 to 3.9, 4 to 6.9, and equal to or greater than 7) were 1.0, 0.93 (95% confidence interval [CI], 0.69–1.26), 0.82 (CI, 0.61–1.10), 0.54 (CI, 0.39–0.76), and 0.52 (CI, 0.25–1.09) (p <0.001 for trend) (Fig. 10.11). These figures did not change materially after adjustment for smoking, BMI, and other cardiovascular risk factors (1.0, 1.02, 0.87, 0.61, and 0.55, respectively; p =0.001 for trend). In separate analyses, the levels of physical activity were inversely associated with coronary heart disease and ischemic stroke. Among women who did not exercise vigorously, the multivariate relative risks for cardiovascular disease across quartiles of metabolic equivalent (MET) score for walking were 1.0, 0.85, 0.63, and 0.56 (p =0.03 for trend). A faster usual walking pace was also independently associated with a lower risk.

Recently, the National Institutes of Health (NIH) began the sponsorship of a large 11-year multicenter study named the "Look AHEAD (Action for Health in Diabetes)

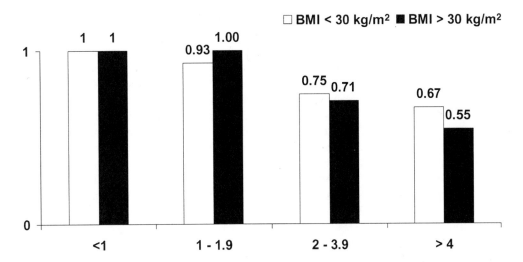

□ BMI < 30 kg/m² ■ BMI > 30 kg/m²

Average hours of moderate/vigorous activity/week

FIG. 10.11. Multivariate risks for cardiovascular events. *P* value for trend: body mass index (BMI) less than 30 kg/m² = 0.08; BMI greater than 30 kg/m² = 0.02. (Data from Hu FB, Stampfer MJ, Solomon C, et al. Physical activity and risk for cardiovascular events in diabetic women. *Ann Intern Med* 2001;134:96–105, with permission.)

study" to examine the effects of lifestyle interventions on cardiovascular events and death in patients with type II diabetes (149). In this study, 5,000 obese patients with type II diabetes will be randomized to either an intensive lifestyle program to lose at least 10% of their body weight through caloric restriction and 25 minutes of exercise daily or a conventional diabetes support and education program. This study will provide vital information on how losing weight and exercising regularly affects the cardiovascular health of those with diabetes.

Regular exercise and caloric restriction, in addition to producing metabolic benefits in established diabetes, may have an important role to play in the prevention of the disease. In recently published findings from the Nurses Health Study (150), which followed 84,941 nurses for 16 years, overweight or obesity was the single most important predictor of diabetes. In this study, lack of exercise, a poor diet, current smoking, and abstinence from alcohol use were all associated with a 91% increase in the risk of diabetes, even after adjustment for the BMI. Similar results were noted in the Male Health Professionals Follow-Up Study, in which 42,504 male health professionals were followed for 12 years. In this study, a Western dietary pattern combined with low physical activity increased the relative risk of developing type II diabetes by 96% (151). Also recently, encouraging results were published from the NIH-sponsored Diabetes Prevention Program, in which 3,234 participants were randomized to study the effect of the following three interventions on preventing diabetes in individuals at high risk of developing the disease: (a) a lifestyle intervention focusing on a 7% weight reduction in body weight through diet and increased physical activity with moderate exercise, such as brisk walking; (b) metformin administration (up to 850 mg twice a day); and (c) a placebo (152). The study was terminated 1 year early after an average follow-up of 2.8 years because of a significant reduction in the development of diabetes in the lifestyle-intervention arm. Active lifestyle intervention reduced the incidence by 58% as compared with the placebo, while the metformin group showed a 31% reduction. Thus, in this study, the lifestyle intervention was significantly more effective than metformin.

In summary, in people with type II diabetes, regular exercise has therapeutic effects on glycemic control, cardiovascular health, and psychologic well-being (4). However, caution should be advised in individuals who are treated with oral antidiabetic agents or insulin as they may require an adjustment of food intake or medication dosage (112). Also, in some patients with type II diabetes, exercise may increase the risk of cardiac events and lower extremity soft-tissue and bone injury or may exacerbate preexisting proliferative retinopathy or nephropathy (112). The ADA now recommends a graded exercise tolerance test before patients with type II diabetes embark on a moderate-intensity to high-intensity exercise program if any of the following criteria are met: age older than 35 years, type II diabetes of more than 10 years' duration, presence of any additional cardiovascular risk factors, evidence of microvascular or peripheral vascular disease, or autonomic neuropathy (112).

On the whole, all the available data suggest that obese patients with type II diabetes should be encouraged to engage in regular exercise at any level. As Dr. Joslin, a pioneer in diabetes care and research, is once reported to have stated, "It is better to discuss how far you have walked than how little you have eaten."

Role of Pharmacologic Therapy in Type II Diabetes

Although nonpharmacologic measures, including diabetes education, diet management, exercise, and weight loss, are the cornerstones of treatment in type II diabetes, maintaining weight loss and glycemic control is extremely difficult for most patients with type II diabetes. Pharmacologic treatment with one or more oral agents and/or insulin is inevitable most patients, particularly if they are to achieve and to maintain reasonable glycemic goals. In addition, pharmacotherapy may also be indicated for long-term weight control. Antiobesity agents *per se* have increasingly been shown to improve glycemic control and the adverse metabolic profile in obese patients with type II diabetes.

Four major classes of oral pharmacologic agents are available for the treatment of type II diabetes. These agents act at the major sites of defects in type II diabetes (a) by increasing insulin availability (secretagogues: SUs and meglitinides), (b) by suppressing excessive hepatic glucose output (biguanides: metformin), (c) by improving insulin sensitivity (thiazolidinediones or glitazones: rosiglitazone and pioglitazone), and (d) by delaying gastrointestinal (GI) glucose absorption (α-glucosidase inhibitors: acarbose and miglitol) (Fig. 10.8). The therapeutic objectives recommended by the ADA include a FPG level of 80 to 120 mg per dL; a bedtime plasma glucose level of 100 to 140 mg per dL; and a glycosylated HbA_{1C} level of less than 7% (Table 10.1) (112). Strong evidence from the UKPDS (114,115) shows that optimal glycemic control reduces the incidence of microvascular and possibly macrovascular complications in patients with type II diabetes. All the above-mentioned oral agents are effective as monotherapy in suitable patients, and they help maintain optimal glycemic control in the initial stages. Traditionally, SU agents—insulin secretagogues—have been used as initial agents, but, with the approval of several insulin-sensitizer agents in recent years, many physicians now use these agents as first-line therapy, particularly because insulin resistance plays an important role in hyperglycemia.

However, type II diabetes is a progressive disease, and, with time, a progressive decline in insulin secretion is seen and glycemic control inevitably deteriorates. Eventually, combination oral therapy with insulin secretagogues and insulin-sensitizer agents or, in many patients, insulin therapy will be needed to achieve optimal glycemic levels. This was clearly demonstrated in the UKPDS (114,115).

The following section reviews the clinical profile and weight gain implications of the various antidiabetic agents and the beneficial effects of the antiobesity agents on glucose control and metabolic parameters in obese patients with type II diabetes.

Antidiabetic Agents

Sulfonylurea Agents

SUs are potent insulin secretogogues whose hypoglycemic action is due to stimulation of ATP-dependent K^+ channels (K-ATP channels) in the pancreatic islet cells (153).

Clinical Profile. SUs are useful both as monotherapy agents and in combination with insulin and the other oral agents. As monotherapy, they are particularly valuable with marked hyperglycemia and evidence of impaired insulin secretion. A list of the various SUs, their dosage, and frequency of administration and dosage is provided in Table 10.5. On average, SUs reduce FPG levels by about 50 to 75 mg per dL and HbA_{1C} levels by 1.5% to 2% (154). SU antidiabetic agents are generally well tolerated, and they have a low incidence of side effects. Hypoglycemia is the most common side effect, and caution should be exercised and low doses should be used, particularly in elderly patients and in those with hepatic and renal insufficiency, to prevent hypoglycemia. The major disadvantages of SUs are weight gain and secondary failure, which may occur with all oral agents because of the progressive nature of type II diabetes.

Effects on Insulin Sensitivity, Lipids, and Other Cardiovascular Risk Factors. Whether the SUs possess insulin-sensitizing properties beyond those caused by glycemic control and the reduction of glucose toxicity *per se* is not entirely clear. *In vitro* studies show some evidence that SUs increase glucose transport and improve insulin sensitivity (155). However, in humans, one study (156) found no effect of SU treatment on insulin sensitivity, whereas another study by Pedersen et al. (157) demonstrated that SU treatment of obese patients with type II diabetes enhances insulin-stimulated peripheral glucose use in both adipose tissue and skeletal muscle, in part through a potentiation of insulin action on adipose tissue glucose transport, lipogenesis, and skeletal muscle glycogen synthase. Further studies are needed to document the insulin-sensitizing effects of the SU agents independent of their glycemic effects.

TABLE 10.5. *First-generation and second-generation sulfonyluria compounds*

Name	Initial dose (mg/d)	Daily dose range (mg/d)	Recommended maximum daily dose (mg/d)	Doses per d
First generation				
Tolbutamide	500–1,500	500–3,000	3,000	2–3
Chlorpropamide	100–250	100–500	500	1
Tolazamide	100–250	100–1,000	1,000	1–2
Acetohexamide	250–500	250–1,500	1,500	1–2
Second generation				
Glyburide	1.25–2.50	1.25–20	20	1–2
Micronized formulation	0.75–1.50	0.75–12	12	1
Glibenclamide	1.25–2.50	1.25–2.50	20	1–2
Glipizide	2.5–5	2.5–40	40	1–2
Glipizide XL	5	5–20	20	1
Gliclazide	40	40–320	320	1–2
Glimepiride	1–2	4–8	8	1

From Lebowitz HE. Insulin secretagogues: old and new. *Diabetes Rev* 1999;7:139–153, with permission.

With regard to the effects on lipid parameters, no evidence has been found that SU treatment confers any lipid-lowering benefits, other than those resulting from improved glycemic control (158).

A long-standing controversy regarding the potentially harmful cardiac effects of SUs still exists, stemming from the publication of the University Group Diabetes Group study results (159). In this study, the patients randomized to tolbutamide, an SU, had unexpected increases in cardiovascular and all-cause mortality (160). This may occur because the myocardial K-ATP channels mediate ischemic preconditioning, which is critical to myocardial protection and limitation of infarct size (161). However, the UKPDS has clearly documented that long-term SU treatment is not associated with increased cardiovascular morbidity or mortality (114,115). Some SUs (e.g., glimepiride) do not possess myocardial K-ATP channel-blocking properties (161), but the long-term cardiovascular consequences of these effects in type II diabetes remain to be determined.

Effects on Adipose Tissue and Body Weight. It is well known that insulin is one of the hormonal regulators of leptin synthesis and that it also modulates adipose tissue maintenance. Because the SU agents increase endogenous insulin secretion, the clinical use of SUs is expected to result in adipose tissue accumulation and weight gain. In a recent metaanalysis of ten randomized studies, SU treatment was associated with a mean 1.7-kg increase in body weight, compared to a mean decrease of 1.2 kg for metformin (162).

In a study from Japan, Nagasaka et al. (163) evaluated the association of endogenous insulin secretion and mode of therapy with body fat and serum leptin levels in 176 diabetic subjects treated with diet alone, with an SU, and with insulin. They observed that endogenous insulin secretion is closely associated with body fat and serum leptin in diabetic subjects treated with diet therapy and an SU. Furthermore, in insulin-treated type II diabetic subjects, both endogenous and exogenous insulin were associated with body fat and serum leptin levels, which were maintained at levels comparable to or somewhat higher than those in control subjects and diabetic patients treated without insulin.

In a recent development, Shi et al. (164) demonstrated that human adipocytes express an SU receptor (SU receptor-1 [SUR-1]) that regulates intracellular calcium and controls lipogenesis and lipolysis. They also evaluated the direct role of the human adipocyte SUR in regulating adipocyte metabolism. They used reverse transcriptase polymerase chain reaction (PCR) with primers for a highly conserved region of SUR-1 to demonstrate that human adipocytes express SUR-1. The PCR product was confirmed by sequence analysis and was used as a probe to demonstrate adipocyte SUR-1 expression by Northern blot analysis. Adipocytes exhibited dose-responsive increases in ionized calcium to glibenclamide, an SU. In addition, glibenclamide (10 μM) caused a significant 67% increase in adipocyte FA synthase activity, a 48% increase in glycerol-3-phosphate dehydrogenase activity, and a 68% inhibition in lipolysis, whereas diazoxide (10 μM) completely prevented each of these effects. These data demonstrate that human adipocytes express an SUR that regulates ionic calcium channels and consequently exerts coordinate control over lipogenesis and lipolysis.

Repaglinide and Nateglinide

Repaglinide, a carbamoyl methyl benzoic acid derivative, and nateglinide, a D-phenylalanine derivative, belong to a new class of antidiabetic agents that are structurally related to meglitinides, which were previously known as the non-SU moiety of glibenclamide. Repaglinide is available as Prandin in the United States and nateglinide, as Starlix. Like the SUs, repaglinide and nateglinide are insulin secretagogues, and their mechanism of action involves ATP-sensitive K$^+$ channels (165).

Clinical Profile. As insulin secretagogues, repaglinide and nateglinide differ from SUs in that they have a rapid onset and short duration of action, and, when taken just before meals, both agents replicate physiologic insulin profiles (165,166). In clinical studies, repaglinide has been shown to lower HbA$_{1C}$ levels by 1.6% to 1.9%, and nateglinide by 0.5% to 0.7% (161). Because repaglinide and nateglinide are quickly absorbed and have short half-lives, their use may be advantageous in subjects who are prone to delayed or missed meals (167). Like insulin secretagogues such as the SUs, hypoglycemia is the most common side effect of these agents; however, in clinical trials, hypoglycemic occurrences were lower with repaglinide and nateglinide than with SUs (168).

Effects on Insulin Sensitivity, Lipids, and Cardiovascular Risk Factors. So far, no studies have been done on the extrapancreatic effects of repaglinide or nateglinide on insulin sensitivity. These agents also do not appear to have any additional effects on lipids independent of their glucose-lowering effects. However, preliminary tissue data with nateglinide on cardiovascular effects do exist. Hu et al. (169) assessed the tissue specificity of nateglinide by examining its effect on ATP-sensitive K channels in rat tissue. Data from this study indicate that nateglinide at concentrations effective in stimulating insulin secretion is least likely, when compared to glyburide and repaglinide, to cause detrimental cardiovascular effects via the blockade of cardiovascular ATP-sensitive K channels (169). Whether these differences have clinical significance remains to be determined.

Effects on Adipose Tissue and Weight Gain. The effects of repaglinide on adipose tissue have not been studied. However, as it is an insulin secretagogue like the SUs, repaglinide use is associated with weight gain. Some data show that, compared to the SUs, repaglinide may have less weight gain properties. In one study, 576 patients with type II diabetes of at least 6 months' duration were randomized to either repaglinide or glyburide (170). At the end of the study, overall safety and changes in glycemic profile and body weight were similar with both agents. However, weight gain data for the subset of pharmacotherapy-naive patients suggested that patients on repaglinide gained less weight than those given glyburide. No similar data are available for nateglinide.

Biguanides

Metformin is an oral biguanide agent that was approved for use in the United States in 1995. Although its mechanism of action has not been clearly determined, decreased hepatic gluconeogenesis is thought to be the primary therapeutic effect of metformin in type II diabetes (171). In addition, metformin appears to improve glucose use in skeletal muscle and adipose tissue by increasing cell membrane glucose transport in the presence of insulin (171). Metformin has also been shown to decrease intestinal glucose absorption and to decrease FA oxidation (171). In a recent study, Lin et al. (172) demonstrated that, in insulin-resistant *ob/ob* mice, metformin therapy actually improved fatty liver disease and appeared to reverse hepatomegaly, steatosis, and enzyme abnormalities. The authors speculated that the likely therapeutic mechanism involved inhibition of the hepatic expression of TNF-α and TNF-inducible factors that promote hepatic lipid accumulation and ATP depletion (172).

Clinical Profile. Metformin must be taken with meals, and the starting dose (500 or 850 mg with breakfast or 500 mg with breakfast and dinner) should be increased slowly at weekly or biweekly intervals to 1,000 mg twice daily to minimize the GI side effects (171). These side effects tend to decline with continued use, and they can be minimized by initiating therapy with low doses of metformin. The risk of hypoglycemia is much less common with metformin than it is with the SUs (171). The main side effect of metformin is lactic acidosis, and the risk for this can be minimized by avoiding its use in individuals with renal insufficiency or congestive heart failure and in seriously ill patients with metabolic acidosis (171). Recently, metformin has received approval from the Food and Drug Administration (FDA) for use in adolescents with type II diabetes.

Metformin is approved for use as monotherapy and in combination with SUs, repaglinide, α-glucosidase inhibitors, glitazones, and insulin. Several controlled clinical studies of metformin monotherapy have demonstrated significant reductions in both FPG levels (60 to 70 mg per dL) and HbA$_{1C}$ levels (1% to 2%) compared to a placebo in patients poorly controlled by diet alone (173). Because of its potential to ameliorate insulin resistance, to prevent weight gain, and to improve lipid levels, metformin may be best suited as initial monotherapy in obese patients with more severe insulin resistance and dyslipidemia. In these patients, metformin does not cause weight gain, and it may even cause a modest weight loss as a result of drug-induced anorexia. Although metformin is primarily thought of as a drug for the overweight, glycemic improvement is also demonstrated in patients who are not obese, as with SUs (173).

Effects on Insulin Sensitivity, Lipids, and Cardiovascular Risk Factors. In addition to improving glycemia, evidence indicates that metformin improves insulin sensitivity; lowers triglyceride and LDL cholesterol levels; and, in some studies, improves blood pressure and HDL cholesterol levels, although these effects are not consistent (173). However, as an insulin sensitizer, metformin is less potent than the glitazones in stimulating insulin-mediated glucose uptake into muscle tissue (174). Metformin has no direct effects on insulin secretion other than those resulting from a reduction of glucose toxicity (171,173). Recently however, a direct *in vitro* effect of metformin on pancreatic beta cells has been reported (175).

In the French Biguanides and the Prevention of the Risk of Obesity-1 trial, metformin therapy reduced tissue plasminogen activator antigen and von Willebrand factor levels (176). The beneficial effects of metformin on serum lipids and other metabolic risk factors appear to have cardiovascular benefits. In the UKPDS, metformin therapy in obese patients with newly diagnosed type II diabetes was associated with a significant decrease in cardiovascular and all-cause mortality (115). Whether this benefit with metformin treatment was due to the absence of weight gain or to its other beneficial effects on the metabolic syndrome of diabetes remains to be determined. In the UKPDS, when metformin treatment was added to patients who had failed SU therapy, a significant and paradoxic increase in cardiovascular and all-cause mortality was seen. This question was analyzed in detail and was found to be due to a significant reduction in the expected number of deaths in the SU group, rather than to an increase in mortality in the SU plus metformin group (177).

Metformin's effect to prevent or delay diabetes was demonstrated in the Diabetes Prevention Program, a large randomized, placebo-controlled clinical trial being conducted by the NIH. In this study of 3,234 subjects at high risk of developing type II diabetes, after a mean of 2.8 years, metformin treatment at 850 mg twice daily significantly reduced the development of type II diabetes by 31% as compared with the placebo. In this study, metformin therapy was more effective in younger and more obese subjects. However, in the same study, intensive lifestyle intervention was more effective than metformin in reducing the development of type II diabetes (152).

Effects on Adipose Tissue and Body Weight. Unlike the insulin secretagogues and the thiazolidinediones, metformin therapy does not result in any substantial weight gain in patients with type II diabetes who receive metformin alone or in combination with other oral agents or insulin (171,178). Most studies show modest weight loss (2 to 3 kg) during the first 6 months of treatment. Metformin therapy is also associated with weight loss in nondiabetic subjects (179). The exact mechanisms by which metformin prevents weight gain or induces weight loss have not been determined. Several mechanisms have been postulated by which metformin might prevent weight gain or induce weight loss. These include a decrease in food consumption, an increase in energy expenditure, and a reduction of hyperinsulinemia (173). Some animal studies suggest an anorectic effect, but, in human studies, it has not been possible to differentiate between a central effect of metformin to decrease caloric intake versus that to increase energy expenditure (173).

The effects of metformin on body fat distribution were determined by Pasquali et al. (180), in a study of 20 obese women with polycystic ovary syndrome (PCOS) and 20 obese controls with BMIs of more than 28 kg/m^2. In both groups of women, metformin treatment for 1 month reduced body weight and BMI significantly more than the placebo. Further, in the PCOS group, as compared to the placebo, metformin therapy significantly improved hirsutism and menstrual abnormalities. Metformin treatment also decreased subcutaneous abdominal tissue (SAT) as measured by CT scan, in both the PCOS and control groups, although only in the latter group were SAT changes significantly greater than those that were observed during the placebo treatment. However, visceral adipose tissue area values significantly decreased during metformin treatment in both the PCOS and the control group, but only in the former was the effect of metformin treatment significantly higher than that of placebo. Leptin levels decreased only during metformin treatment in both groups (180).

α-Glucosidase Inhibitors

The following two α-glucosidase inhibitors are currently marketed in the United States: acarbose (Precose) and miglitol (Glyset). Both are potent inhibitors of the α-glucosidase enzymes present in the brush border of the enterocytes that are located in the proximal portion of the small intestine (181).

Clinical Profile. When used as monotherapy, both agents do not enhance insulin secretion, and, in overdose, they will not result in hypoglycemia. At recommended doses, both agents have modest effects on HbA$_{1C}$ levels (mean, 0.4% to 0.7% reductions) (181). To be maximally effective, both drugs must be administered at the start of a main meal because they are competitive inhibitors so they must be present at the site of enzymatic action at the same time that the carbohydrates are present in the small intestine. The most common adverse reactions to acarbose and miglitol are GI in nature, including abdominal discomfort, increased flatulence, and diarrhea (181). To minimize GI side effects, both acarbose and miglitol should be started at low doses and titrated upwards slowly.

Effects on Insulin Sensitivity, Lipids, and Cardiovascular Risk Factors. Studies in animal models suggest that long-term treatment with an α-glucosidase inhibitor, such as miglitol, improves insulin sensitivity and that it may have vascular protective effects in obese insulin-resistant rats (182). However, in humans, miglitol-induced improvement in postprandial hyperglycemia is not associated with improved insulin sensitivity as measured by the insulin and glucose clamp technique (183). Recently, acarbose therapy for 12 months was shown to be associated with increased insulin sensitivity in elderly patients with type II diabetes (184).

In some studies, α-glucosidase inhibitors are associated with decreases in triglyceride levels (181). In one study of 20 patients with type II diabetes from Japan (181), acarbose not only inhibited the postprandial increase of both plasma glucose and insulin but also significantly suppressed the postprandial increase of serum triglycerides and remnant-like cholesterol particles. Acarbose may also reduce triglyceride levels in nondiabetic patients, and it may be a useful adjunct to dietary therapy in nondiabetic patients affected by severe hypertriglyceridemia (181).

Currently, an international study (the Study to Prevent Noninsulin Dependent Diabetes Mellitus [STOP-NIDDM] trial) is evaluating the efficacy of an acarbose to prevent or delay the development of type II diabetes in 1,418 subjects who have been diagnosed with IGT and thus who are at increased risk of developing type II diabetes (185). The study is expected to be completed in the year 2001.

Effects on Adipose Tissue and Body Weight. In clinical practice, in contrast to animal studies, acarbose or miglitol therapy is not commonly associated with dramatic weight loss (181). This is because of polysaccharide metabolism by colonic microflora and the capacity of the large bowel to conserve calories. Thus, there is minimal calorie loss associated with acarbose and miglitol therapy. Weight loss, if it occurs, is typically mild (e.g., 0.8 to 1.4 kg over 1 year in clinical studies). The exact metabolic or pharmacologic mechanism responsible for this weight loss remains unknown. Acarbose and miglitol do appear to offset the insulinotropic effects and weight gain associated with SU treatment when they are added as combination therapy (181).

Thiazolidinediones

The thiazolidinediones or glitazones are oral antidiabetic agents that are also termed "insulin sensitizers." They act primarily by reducing insulin resistance, which is thought to be central to the development of type II diabetes and its cardiovascular complications. The two compounds in this class presently approved for use in the United States are rosiglitazone (Avandia) and pioglitazone (Actos). The first agent in this class, troglitazone (Rezulin) was marketed in the United States from March 1997 until March 2000 when it was withdrawn because the FDA determined that the risk of idiosyncratic hepatotoxicity associated with troglitazone therapy outweighed its potential benefits.

The thiazolidinediones are highly selective and potent agonists for the peroxisome PPARγ (186,187). PPARγ receptors are found in key target tissues for insulin action, such as adipose tissue, skeletal muscle, and liver, and evidence indicates that these receptors may be important regulators of lipid homeostasis, adipocyte differentiation, and insulin action (186–188). A close relationship has been shown to exist between the potency of various thiazolidinediones to stimulate PPARγ and their antidiabetic action (186–188).

Clinical Profile. Rosiglitazone is approved for use as monotherapy and in combination with metformin and SUs. Pioglitazone is approved by the FDA for use as monotherapy and in combination with SUs, metformin, and insulin (189,190). In the absence of head-to-head studies, evaluation of which glitazone is more potent in clinical use is not possible. Monotherapy with the glitazones results in significant improvements in FPG by approximately 60 to 80 mg per dL and in HbA$_{1C}$ by about 1.5% to 2.5% as compared to a placebo (189,190). Rosiglitazone and pioglitazone are also useful when they are employed in combination with SUs, metformin, and insulin (189,190). The usual dose of rosiglitazone is 4 to 8 mg daily and of pioglitazone is 15 to 45 mg daily. Unlike troglitazone, rosiglitazone and pioglitazone do not thus far appear to have hepatotoxic effects, but monitoring liver function test results periodically as advised by the FDA is still prudent.

The main side effects with glitazone use have been weight gain and edema so far, so both glitazones should be used cautiously in patients with peripheral edema or early congestive heart failure; and patients with New York Heart Association class III or IV heart failure should not receive glitazones unless the expected benefit is judged to outweigh the potential risk (189,190). Rosiglitazone and pioglitazone are both contraindicated in pregnancy and during lactation. Thiazolidinediones are active only in the presence of insulin. They should not be used to treat either diabetic ketoacidosis or type I diabetes.

Effects on Insulin Sensitivity, Lipids, and Cardiovascular Effects. Several studies have documented the insulin-sensitizing properties of the thiazolidinediones, not only in patients with type II diabetes but also in other insulin-resistant states, such as IGT, PCOS, and previous gestational diabetes (188). In addition, the glitazones have multiple beneficial effects on hepatic glucose metabolism, lipid metabolism, endothelial function, fibrinolysis, and atherogenesis (188). From the available data, differences in the lipid-modifying abilities of the various glitazones seem to exist. Pioglitazone has been shown to lower triglyceride levels by about 9% and to increase HDL levels by about 12% to 19% (190,191). Reduction in triglyceride levels appears to result from several mechanisms, including reduced FFA substrate availability, decreased hepatic triglyceride synthesis, and enhanced peripheral clearance (188). In the case of rosiglitazone, however, despite significant decreases in FFA levels by up to 22%, the initial studies demonstrated no significant lowering of triglyceride levels, although the HDL levels do increase by up to 19%. The reasons for these differences are not clear. In addition, with all the glitazones studied so far, an increase in LDL cholesterol levels, which is a matter of concern, appears to occur. In the case of troglitazone, these increases in LDL cholesterol take place without a change in atherogenic apolipoprotein B levels (188). Moreover, after troglitazone treatment, the LDL particles became larger, more buoyant, and less prone to oxidative modification (188). Data on LDL particle size and apolipoprotein B levels are still not available for rosiglitazone and pioglitazone. Long-term follow-up is needed to see if the rise in LDL has a negative impact on atherosclerosis and cardiovascular mortality.

There are limited data showing that the glitazones may have beneficial effects on blood pressure and intimal hyperplasia in type II diabetes patients both with and without coronary stent implants (192,193). These effects of the glitazones, if they are shown to persist long term, may be beneficial in terms of delaying or even preventing the development of accelerated atherosclerosis in diabetes.

Effects on Adipose Tissue and Body Weight. The effects of the glitazones on adipose tissue are complex, and they are not yet fully understood. In obese Zucker rats, treatment with the thiazolidinedione troglitazone resulted in a reduction in leptin levels and lower *ob* gene and TNF-α expression. Associated with this effect were apoptosis of large adipocytes and an increase in the number of small adipocytes with no net change in adipose tissue weight (194). The reduction in large adipocytes possibly leads to lower TNF-α and leptin levels and, consequently, to decreased insulin resistance. On the other hand, the increase in the number of small adipocytes, which are more sensitive to the antilipolytic action of insulin, might also contribute to the reduction of insulin resistance because these small adipocytes take up more glucose than do large adipocytes at submaximal insulin levels (194). This could potentially lower FFA and triglyceride levels and could improve insulin sensitivity. Although the results from this study suggest that troglitazone exerts potent effects in adipose tissue, another study (195) has demonstrated beneficial effects of troglitazone on glucose and lipid metabolism that are independent of adipose tissue in aP2/DTA mice whose white and brown fat was virtually eliminated by fat-specific expression of diphtheria toxin. In this study, despite the absence of adipose tissue, beneficial metabolic changes were seen in muscle and the liver.

In clinical practice, the use of all glitazones, even in the short term, results in varying degrees of weight gain. In the clinical studies in the United States, weight gain with rosiglitazone and pioglitazone was especially higher with monotherapy and in combination with SUs and insulin. Combination therapy with metformin appears to ameliorate or

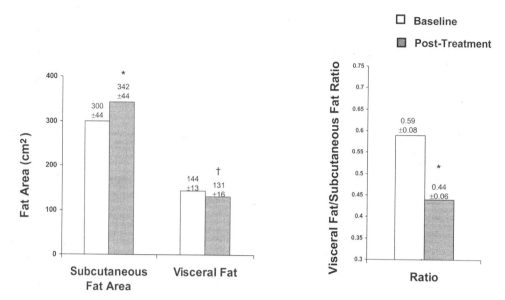

FIG. 10.12. Effects of pioglitazone (45 mg daily for 4 mo) on abdominal fat distribution in patients with type II diabetes. *,*p* <0.01; †,*p* >0.05.) (Data from Muyazaki Y, Mahankali A, Matsuda M, et al. Abstract 1245. *Diabetes* 2000;48:A299, with permission.)

to minimize this weight gain. The exact location and nature of this weight gain has been studied by numerous investigators. At the tissue level, troglitazone is known specifically to promote the differentiation of preadipocytes into adipocytes in subcutaneous, but not omental, fat (196). In one study from Japan, troglitazone at 400 mg per day for 6 months in 30 mildly obese patients with type II diabetes not only improved their glycemia and increased their BMI but also resulted in fat accumulation in the subcutaneous, rather than the visceral, adipose tissue depot. The authors speculated that this shift of energy accumulation from the visceral to the subcutaneous adipose tissue might contribute to troglitazone-mediated amelioration of insulin resistance (197). In another double-blind randomized trial, Kelly at al. (198) demonstrated that troglitazone therapy for 12 weeks significantly decreased intraabdominal fat mass as measured by MRI. In this study, no significant changes in total body fat and body weight were found compared to the placebo. In a recent study using MRI analysis, Miyazaki et al. (199) demonstrated that pioglitazone treatment at 45 mg daily for 4 months is associated with a significant increase in subcutaneous fat area. This is accompanied by a significant decrease in visceral fat area and a concomitant decrease in the visceral to subcutaneous fat ratio (Fig. 10.12). No data are yet available for rosiglitazone's effects on human adipose tissue.

Role of Antiobesity Agents in Type II Diabetes

Intensive lifestyle measures with dietary restriction and exercise therapy are associated with significant weight loss in the short term in obese patients with type II diabetes. However, maintenance of this weight loss in the long term has remained a major challenge in the field of obesity control. Moreover, in obese patients with type II diabetes, many of the pharmacologic agents used in the treatment of hyperglycemia, including SUs, thiazolidinediones, and insulin, are all associated with weight gain. Thus, a pharmacotherapeutic agent that could produce and maintain weight loss and that has a good safety profile would revolutionize the treatment of type II diabetes. Currently, two antiobesity agents—orlistat and sibutramine—have been approved for the long-term treatment of obesity. These agents have been shown to be effective in 1-year to 2-year studies in obese nondiabetic patients and in short-term studies in patients with type II diabetes. As yet, however, few studies have investigated the long-term effects of these treatments in diabetic patients. Moreover, a puzzling fact worth noting is that weight loss induced by these drugs, as well as during dietary treatment, is less pronounced in diabetic patients as compared to nondiabetic subjects. The reasons for this resistance to weight loss in diabetics remain unclear, and they could be linked to the abnormal fat metabolism (200). The effects of the two currently approved agents, sibutramine and orlistat, on body fat, glycemia, and other metabolic variables in patients with type II diabetes are discussed in the following sections.

Sibutramine

Sibutramine is a serotonin and noradrenaline reuptake inhibitor (SNRI) that induces weight loss not only by enhancing satiety but also enhancing energy expenditure through increased thermogenesis (201). The drug is generally well tolerated with mild side effects that are not treatment limiting and that are consistent with the known mechanism of action of the drug. However, mild increases in blood pressure are known to occur, and blood pressure should be carefully monitored in all patients taking this medication. Sibutramine produces statistically and clinically significant dose-related weight loss over the range of 5 to 30 mg once daily, with active weight loss occurring for 6 months. The maximum dose approved by the FDA is 15 mg every day. Weight loss with continued sibutramine therapy is maintained in long-term studies of up to 1 year. Although most studies have been performed in nondiabetic patients, a few studies have shown that in patients with type II diabetes, sibutramine-induced weight loss is associated with beneficial changes in glycemic control, serum lipids, and body fat distribution.

Effects on Glycemia. Sibutramine's effects on glycemia were documented in a 1-year study in which 139 women and 97 men with previously untreated type II diabetes (a mean BMI of 35.6 kg/m^2 and an HbA$_{1C}$ of 7.3%) were randomized to either a placebo or treatment with sibutramine, 15 mg daily. After 1 year, the sibutramine-treated patients had lost 7% of their initial body weight, whereas the placebo group had lost about 2%. Maximum weight loss was achieved by 9 months in both groups. In the sibutramine-treated group as a whole, a nonsignificant 0.3% decrease in HbA$_{1C}$ was seen, compared to a decrease of 0.2% in the placebo group. However, in those patients taking sibutramine who lost 5% of their initial body weight, a significant 0.4% drop was seen in HbA$_{1C}$, and, in those who lost 10% of their initial body weight, a 0.7% decrease in HbA$_{1C}$ was seen (202). No significant changes in blood pressure were noted in either treatment groups, although the mean pulse rate increased significantly by 5.5 beats per minute in the sibutramine group versus an increase of only 1.3 beats per minute in the placebo group. Slightly better effects on HbA$_{1C}$ were reported in another double-blind placebo-controlled study in which Finer et al. (203) combined sibutramine, 15 mg daily, with a hypocaloric diet (500 kcal per day less than individual energy needs) in 91 obese patients with type II diabetes and a mean HbA$_{1C}$ of 9.5%. After 3 months, patients in the sibutramine group had lost 2.4 kg and their HbA$_{1C}$ decreased by 0.3%, whereas the placebo group gained 0.1 kg and showed no change in their HbA$_{1C}$.

Although the maximum FDA-approved dose of sibutramine in the United States is 15 mg, studies have used sibutramine at a dose of 20 mg daily. In one international multicenter study, 175 obese patients (BMI of approximately 34 kg/m^2) with type II diabetes (HbA$_{1C}$ 8.4 ± 1.2) were randomized to either sibutramine, 20 mg daily, or placebo therapy along with a moderately hypocaloric diet (250 to 500 kcal per day below individual energy needs). After 6 months, a significant 4.3-kg weight loss in the sibutramine group was seen, compared to a 0.4-kg weight loss in the placebo group (204). Weight losses of more than 5% and of more than 10% were achieved by 33% and 8%, respectively, of the sibutramine group. Surprisingly, in the sibutramine group as a whole, the decreases in both FPG and HbA$_{1C}$ were not significant when compared to those of the placebo-treated patients. However, in the group (n = 22) who lost 5% of their body weight, the mean treatment difference in HbA$_{1C}$ was 0.53% at 24 weeks. In the group who lost 10% of body weight, the mean treatment difference in HbA$_{1C}$ was 1.65% at 24 weeks. However, there were only five patients in this group. In addition, in this study, sibutramine therapy was associated with small increases in blood pressure and pulse. In contrast to the findings of this study, in another recent study by Gockel et al. (205), 10 mg of sibutramine given twice daily for 6 months to obese female patients (BMI about 38 kg/m^2) with type II diabetes resulted not only in significant weight loss but also in improvements in glycemic control. In this study, women in the sibutramine group lost 9.6 kg and their HbA$_{1C}$ decreased by 2.7% from baseline, compared to a weight gain of 0.9 kg and a decrease of 0.5% in HbA$_{1C}$ in the placebo group. Surprisingly, in this study, the authors noted significant reductions in diastolic blood pressure and heart rate.

Effects on Insulin Sensitivity. Despite the effects of sibutramine on glycemia, no human studies as yet have documented improvements in insulin sensitivity. However, in animal studies, chronic administration of sibutramine for 6 weeks has been found to decrease hyperinsulinemia and to ameliorate insulin resistance in *ob/ob* mice, as well as to produce reduced weight gain and lower FFA concentrations (206,207).

Effects on Lipids. Concurrent with decreases in weight and blood glucose, studies have also documented favorable changes in lipids with sibutramine treatment. In the study conducted by Heath et al. (202), sibutramine treatment was associated with a significant 11.1% decrease in triglyceride levels and a 2.9% increase in HDL cholesterol, compared to the placebo group in which a detrimental 7.9% increase in triglycerides and a 3.9% decrease in HDL cholesterol levels were observed. Moreover, sibutramine-treated patients who lost 10% of their initial body weight had an impressive 10.3% increase in HDL cholesterol levels. Recently, three other multicenter studies also demonstrated similar improvements in the lipid profile of type II diabetics after treatment with sibutramine with a duration of up to 52 weeks (208).

Effects on Adipose Tissue. Visceral adiposity is well known to be strongly associated with the metabolic complications of obesity, and waist circumference and waist to hip ratio (WHR) are both secondary indicators of visceral obesity. Preliminary evidence has shown that sibutramine treatment may influence these measures of visceral obesity. In a metaanalysis of four long-term, placebo-controlled, double-blind studies, sibutramine treatment was associated with significantly greater mean decreases in waist circumference as compared to a placebo (209). Similar results were seen for the WHR. Treatment with sibutramine, 15 mg daily, produced a significant reduction in WHR compared to the placebo. In the Sibutramine Trial of Obesity Reduction and Maintenance (STORM) (210), changes in body fat distribution were examined using CT scans. In this study, a significant mean weight loss of 11.2 ± 6.3 kg from baseline occurred after 6 months of 10 mg sibutramine treatment. Importantly, decreases in total abdominal fat (18%), total subcutaneous fat (17%), and total visceral fat (22%) were all observed, in addition to a significant increase in the subcutaneous to visceral fat ratio (p =0.04). These changes in fat levels and distribution were, as may be expected, associated with improvements in FPG and insulin levels and blood pressure (209).

Orlistat

Unlike sibutramine, orlistat is a selective GI lipase inhibitor that increases fecal fat losses, enhances diet-induced weight reduction, and improves both blood glucose control and dyslipidemia in obese patients with type II diabetes. Lipase inhibition by orlistat prevents the absorption of approximately 30% of dietary fat intake. The main side effects are consistent with its fat-blocking properties, and they include oily diarrhea and fecal soiling. As with sibutramine, most studies with orlistat have been performed in nondiabetics. However, a few studies have documented beneficial effects with orlistat treatment, at the FDA-approved dose of 120 mg three times daily on glycemia, insulin sensitivity, and lipid parameters in obese patients with type II diabetes.

Effects on Glycemic Control. In a multicenter 57-week, double-blind, placebo-controlled study, Hollander et al. (211) assessed the impact of treatment with orlistat on weight loss, glycemic control, and serum lipid levels in obese patients with type II diabetes taking SU medications. They randomized 391 obese men and women with type II diabetes to 120 mg of orlistat or a placebo that was administered orally three times a day with a mildly hypocaloric diet. Study subjects had a BMI of 28 to 40 kg/m², and they were clinically stable on oral SU medication (mean HbA$_{1C}$ of approximately 8%) (211). After 1 year of treatment, the orlistat group lost 6.2% ± 0.5% of initial body weight, versus 4.3% ± 0.5% in the placebo group (p <0.001). Twice as many of the patients receiving orlistat (49% versus 23%) lost more than 5% of their initial body weight (p <0.001). Furthermore, orlistat treatment plus diet, when compared to the placebo plus diet, was associated with significant improvement in glycemic control, which was reflected in a decrease in HbA$_{1C}$ of 0.3% ± 0.1% versus an increase of 0.2% ± 0.1% in the placebo group. Those patients with an HbA$_{1C}$ level of more than 8% at the start of treatment showed a more impressive 0.5% ± 0.2% decrease in HbA$_{1C}$ levels, compared to 0.1% ± 0.3% in the placebo group. In addition, in the orlistat group, significant reductions were made in the dosage of oral SU medication. As would be expected, mild to moderate and transient GI events were reported with orlistat therapy, although their association with study withdrawal was low.

Effects on Insulin Sensitivity. As with sibutramine, no studies have specifically evaluated the effects of orlistat on insulin sensitivity in obese type II diabetic patients. However, in a large multicenter study, Davidson et al. (212) studied the long-term effects of orlistat used in combination with a hypocaloric diet in 1,187 subjects, 892 of whom were randomized to double-blind treatment. This study had a high dropout rate, and, at the end of the study, 223 placebo-treated subjects and 657 orlistat-treated subjects were evaluated in an intention-to-treat analysis. Of these, approximately 5% had diabetes (10 in the placebo group and 26 in the orlistat group). During the first year, orlistat-treated subjects lost more weight (8.8 ± 0.4 kg) than the placebo-treated subjects (5.8 ± 0.7 kg) (p <0.001). At the end of year 2, subjects who were treated with orlistat, 120 mg three times a day, had regained less weight than those who received orlistat, 60 mg, or a placebo (35.2% versus 51.3% versus 63.4% weight regain, respectively; p <0.001). Moreover, at 2 years, less of an increase in fasting serum glucose levels was observed in the orlistat group using 120 mg three times daily, compared to that of the placebo group (1 ± 0.5 mg per dL versus 5 ± 1 mg per dL; p =0.001). Along with improved glycemia, the fasting serum insulin levels also decreased significantly over 2 years in the 120-mg orlistat group, while they remained unchanged in the placebo group (84 ± 3 to 67 ± 4 pmol per L versus 86 ± 5 to 86 ± 7 pmol per L, respectively; $p=0.04$). This sustained lowering of insulin levels in the orlistat group appeared to be related to the overall greater weight loss in these subjects, rather than to an independent drug effect. Similar reductions in fasting glucose and insulin levels were obtained in another double-blind, placebo-controlled multicenter study in obese nondiabetic patients. In this study, Hauptman et al. (213) studied 796 obese patients (BMI = 30 to 44 kg/m^2) who were randomized to treatment with placebo, 60 mg of orlistat three times daily, or 120 mg of orlistat three times daily, in conjunction with a reduced-energy diet for the first year and a weight-maintenance diet during the second year. Data from these two studies, in which orlistat caused significant and sustained reductions in fasting serum insulin levels over 2 years of treatment, with concurrent decreases in fasting glucose, suggest that orlistat may improve insulin resistance.

Effects on Lipids. In obese nondiabetic subjects, orlistat treatment has been shown to have beneficial effects on glucose tolerance test status, waist circumference, blood pressure, and several lipid parameters, including total cholesterol, LDL cholesterol, triglycerides, and apolipoprotein B (214). In one study of obese patients with type II diabetes, Hollander et al. (211) demonstrated a significant 13% decrease in LDL cholesterol and an 11% decrease in triglycerides with orlistat therapy, as compared to a placebo.

Effects on Diabetes Prevention. The ultimate goal in the treatment of diabetes is the prevention of the disease itself. Well-documented studies show that weight reduction and intensive lifestyle measures might delay the progression to type II diabetes in high-risk subjects (4). Because treatment with orlistat promotes weight loss, treatment with orlistat and dietary measures may improve glucose tolerance status in subjects who have IGT and may thereby prevent progression to type II diabetes. This hypothesis has been studied by Heymsfield et al. (215). They pooled data from three randomized, double-blind, placebo-controlled multicenter clinical trials conducted at 39 United States and European research centers, involving a total of 675 obese adults (BMI = 30 to 43 kg/m^2). After a mean length of follow-up of 582 days, the subjects treated with orlistat lost significantly more weight (6.72 ± 0.41 kg) than did subjects who received a placebo (3.79 ± 0.38 kg). Concurrently, in the orlistat group, only 3.0% of subjects with IGT at baseline progressed to diabetic status versus 7.6% in the placebo group. Furthermore, among subjects with IGT at baseline, glucose levels normalized in more subjects after the orlistat treatment (71.6%) versus the placebo (49.1%; $p =0.04$). In these studies, the addition of orlistat to a conventional weight loss regimen appeared to improve oral glucose tolerance significantly and to diminish the rate of progression for the development of both IGT and type II diabetes (Fig. 10.13). No such data are available for sibutramine.

Thus, although weight management in the obese patient with type II diabetes remains a challenge for the clinician, the availability and efficacy of sibutramine and orlistat to enhance and to maintain weight loss are promising. However, further studies are required to identify responders to pharmacotherapy more effectively and to delineate further the role of antiobesity agents in the overall long-term management of obese subjects with type II diabetes. Currently, several novel pharmacologic approaches with great potential for weight loss are being tested. These include β_3-agonists, which increase energy expenditure; drugs that interfere with FFA or TNF-α release by the adipose tissue; and agents that slow gastric emptying. However, preliminary results regarding the efficacy and/or safety of some of these agents do not appear encouraging.

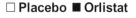

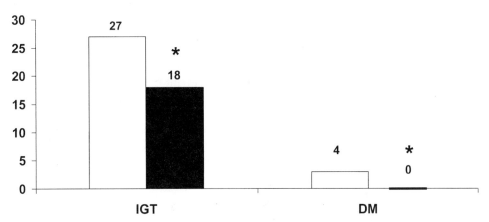

☐ Placebo ■ Orlistat

A **Subjects with Normal Glucose Tolerance at Baseline**

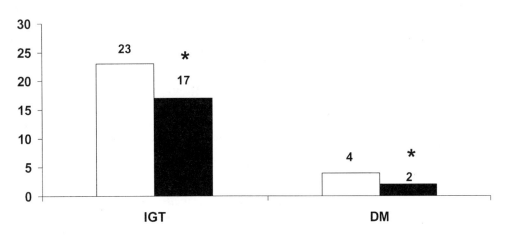

B **Subjects with Impaired Glucose Tolerance at Baseline**

FIG. 10.13. A: Effects of orlistat on progression of glucose tolerance in subjects with normal glucose tolerance at baseline. *, p =0.04. **B:** Effects of orlistat on progression of glucose tolerance in subjects with impaired glucose tolerance (IGT) at baseline. (*, p =0.04.) Abbreviation: DM, type II diabetes mellitus. (From Heymsfield SB, Segal KR, Hauptman J, et al. Effects of weight loss with orlistat on glucose tolerance and progression to type 2 diabetes in obese adults. *Arch Intern Med* 2000;160:1321–1326, with permission.)

Role of Bariatric Surgery in Type II Diabetes

When intensive lifestyle measures and pharmacologic therapy fail to produce clinically significant weight loss, bariatric surgery represents an option for well-motivated patients with morbid obesity (BMI of greater than or equal to 40 kg/m²) or for those obese patients with a BMI of more than or equal to 35 kg/m² and comorbid conditions, such as diabetes, hypertension, and dyslipidemia (216). Growing evidence points to the success of gastric banding and gastric bypass in ameliorating many of the metabolic abnormalities in type II diabetes, while maintaining an acceptable surgical risk (217). Recent reports of laparoscopic banding procedures also appear encouraging (217). Bariatric surgery allows patients with type II diabetes to reduce their antidiabetic medication substantially and to lower or even to discontinue their doses of insulin. Recently, Dixon and O'Brien (218) reported on 50 severely obese subjects with type II diabetes who underwent laparoscopic adjustable gastric banding. After 1 year, remission of diabetes occurred in 32 patients (64%), and major improvements in glucose control occurred in 13 patients (26%). In this study, remission of diabetes was predicted by greater weight loss and a shorter history of diabetes. Furthermore, in this study, early complications occurred in 6% of subjects (e.g., wound infections and respiratory support), and late complications requiring surgical intervention (e.g., gastric prolapse, band erosion, and tube leaks) were seen in 30% of subjects.

Evidence also shows that bariatric surgery may even prevent the progression from IGT to frank diabetes (219). Initial results from the Swedish Obesity Study (SOS) demonstrated that, in those individuals in the study who lost and maintained more than or equal to 12% of their body weight, none developed diabetes over 2 years (220). In the SOS, 2,000 matched patient pairs will be followed for 10 years. One pair member is surgically treated, while the other receives conventional obesity treatment. By February 2000, 1,879 patient pairs had been recruited. In a recent publication, the authors reported that, after 8 years, the weight loss in the surgical group was 28 ± 16 kg versus a gain of 0.7 ± 12 kg in the conventional nonsurgical group (221). With regard to the incidence of type II diabetes, after 2 years, the incidence of diabetes was reduced by 32-fold in the surgical group; however, after 8 years, the reduction was only 5-fold. Thus, the benefits of surgical weight reduction appear to diminish somewhat over time. Interestingly, the SOS appears to indicate the presence of discordant effects of surgical weight loss on hyperglycemia and blood pressure (221). At 2 years, the incidence of hypertension was reduced by 2.6 times, while, at 8 years, the incidence of hypertension was almost equal in both groups.

The success of bariatric surgery has even provoked a claim by both Hickey et al. (222) and Pories et al. (223) that type II diabetes may be considered a surgical disease and that surgery may represent an effective therapy for type II diabetes. However, obesity surgery still has substantial morbidity, and thus it is only an option in selected obese patients with high comorbidities.

CONCLUSION

Type II diabetes is a major worldwide problem that afflicts more than 16 million people in the United States and about 200 million people worldwide. The disease is a serious cause of morbidity and mortality, and, in 1998, the health care costs associated with diabetes were estimated to be about $98 billion in the United States alone. Unfortunately, the future appears even more bleak with the epidemic of type II diabetes continuing to grow in a genetically susceptible population that is accustomed to an increasingly sedentary and Westernized lifestyle. One of the most important risk factors for type II diabetes is obesity, and the concurrent epidemic of obesity contributes to its development by means of increased visceral fat distribution and increased insulin resistance. In predisposed individuals, this increased insulin resistance may unmask genetically determined defects in pancreatic beta-cell function, leading to glucose intolerance and hyperglycemia. However, the mechanistic links between obesity and type II diabetes remain to

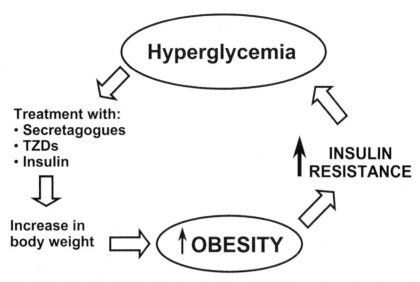

FIG. 10.14. Potential side effects of treatment with antidiabetic agents on the obese state.

be determined, and much research needs to be done to unravel the etiology of obesity and its role in the precipitation of the development of type II diabetes in predisposed individuals. In the meantime, a high priority should be assigned to the achievement of optimal glycemic goals in obese patients with type II diabetes to prevent or to delay microvascular and macrovascular complications. This may be achieved through intensive lifestyle measures and, when these fail, through pharmacologic measures. Unfortunately, many of the oral antidiabetic agents, including insulin, promote weight gain (Fig. 10.14), and, to counter this, the role of diet and exercise therapy must be emphasized. The recent availability of oral antiobesity agents that can be used long term offers hope, but well-designed long-lasting studies are needed to document their safety and efficacy with continued use. Finally, bariatric surgery offers significant benefits with acceptable risks and remains an option for selected obese patients with type II diabetes.

ACKNOWLEDGMENTS

This work was supported by the Department of Veterans Affairs and the Veteran Affairs' San Diego Healthcare System.

REFERENCES

1. Kissebah AH, Peiris AN. Biology of regional body fat distribution: relationship to non–insulin dependent diabetes mellitus. *Diabetes Metab Rev* 1989;5:83–109.
2. Harris MI, Flegal KM, Cowie CC, et al. Prevalence of diabetes, impaired fasting glucose and impaired glucose tolerance in US adults. *Diabetes Care* 1998;21:518–524.
3. National Diabetes Data Group. *Diabetes in America,* 2nd ed. NIH publication no. 95-1468. Washington, D.C.: United States Government Printing Office, 1995.
4. Pi-Sunyer FX, Maggio CA. The prevention and treatment of obesity: application to type 2 diabetes. *Diabetes Care* 1997;20:744–766.
5. DeFronzo RA, Bonadonna RC, Ferrannini E. Pathogenesis of NIDDM: a balanced overview. *Diabetologia* 1992;35:389–397.
6. West KM, Kalbfleish JM. Influence of nutritional factors on prevalence of diabetes. *Diabetes* 1971;20:99–108.

7. Resnick HE, Valsania P, Halter JB, et al. Relation of weight gain and weight loss on subsequent diabetes risk in overweight adults. *J Epidemiol Commun Health* 2000;54:596–602.
8. Everhart JE, Pettit DJ, Bennett PH, et al. Duration of obesity increases the incidence of NIDDM. *Diabetes* 1992;41:235–240.
9. Wannamethee SG, Shaper GA. Weight change and duration of overweight and obesity in the incidence of type 2 diabetes. *Diabetes Care* 1999;22:1266–1272.
10. Haffner S, Mitchell B, Hazuda H, et al. Greater influence of central distribution of adipose tissue on incidence of non–insulin-dependent diabetes in women than in men. *Am J Clin Nutr* 1991;53:1312–1317.
11. Ohlson LO, Larsson B, Svardsudd K, et al. The influence of body fat distribution on the incidence of diabetes mellitus. *Diabetes* 1985;34:1055–1058.
12. Lilloja S, Mott DM, Spraul M, et al. Insulin resistance and insulin secretory dysfunction as precursors of NIDDM. Prospective studies of Pima Indians. *N Engl J Med* 1993;329:1988–1992.
13. Ohlson LO, Larsson B, Svardsudd K, et al. The influence of body fat distribution on the incidence of diabetes mellitus. 13.5 years of follow up in the study of men born in 1913. *Diabetes* 1985;34:1055–1058.
14. Bergstrom RW, Newell-Morris LL, Leonetti DL, et al. Association of elevated C-peptide level and increased intra-abdominal fat distribution with development of NIDDM in Japanese-American men. *Diabetes* 1990;104:104–111.
15. Carey DG, Jenkins AB, Campbell LV, et al. Abdominal fat and insulin resistance in normal and overweight women: direct measurements reveal a strong relationship in subjects at both low and high risk of NIDDM. *Diabetes* 1996;45:633–638.
16. Bonora E. Relationship between regional fat distribution and insulin resistance. *Int J Obes Relat Metab Disord* 2000;24:S32–S35.
17. Wei M, Gaskill SP, Haffner SM, et al. Waist circumference as the best predictor of non–insulin-dependent diabetes mellitus (NIDDM) compared to body mass index, waist/hip ratio and other anthropometric measurements in Mexican Americans: a 7-year prospective study. *Obes Res* 1997;5:16–23.
18. Dowse GK, Zimmet PZ, Gareeboo H, et al. Abdominal obesity and physical inactivity as risk factors for NIDDM and impaired glucose tolerance in Indian, Creole, and Chinese Mauritians. *Diabetes Care* 1991;14:271–282.
19. Cassano PA, Rosner B, Vokonas PS, et al. Obesity and body fat distribution in relation to the incidence of non–insulin-dependent diabetes mellitus: a prospective cohort study of men in the normative aging study. *Am J Epidemiol* 1992;136:1474–1486.
20. Carey VJ, Walters EE, Colditz GA, et al. Body fat distribution and risk of non–insulin-dependent diabetes mellitus in women: the Nurses' Health Study. *Am J Epidemiol* 1997;145:614–619.
21. Boyko EJ, Fujimoto WY, Leonetti DL, et al. Visceral adiposity and risk of type 2 diabetes. A prospective study among Japanese-Americans. *Diabetes Care* 2000;23:465–471.
22. Colberg S, Simoneau JA, Thaete F, et al. Skeletal muscle utilization of FFA in women with visceral obesity. *J Clin Invest* 1995;95:1846–1853.
23. Lillioja S, Mott DM, Zawadzki JK, et al. Glucose storage is a major determinant of *in vivo* "insulin resistance" in subjects with normal glucose tolerance. *J Clin Endocrinol Metab* 1986;62:922–927.
24. Shulman GI, Rothman DL, Jue T, et al. Quantitation of muscle glycogen synthesis in normal subjects and subjects with non–insulin-dependent diabetes by (13)C nuclear magnetic resonance spectroscopy. *N Engl J Med* 1990;322:223–228.
25. Bogardus C, Lillioja S, Stone K, et al. Correlation between muscle glycogen synthase activity and *in vivo* insulin action in man. *J Clin Invest* 1984;73:1185–1190.
26. Damsbo P, Vaag A, Hother-Nielsen O, et al. Reduced glycogen synthase activity in skeletal muscle from obese patients with and without type 2 (non–insulin-dependent) diabetes mellitus. *Diabetologia* 1991;34:239–245.
27. Wright KS, Beck-Nielsen H, Kolterman OG, et al. Decreased activation of skeletal muscle glycogen synthase by mixed-meal ingestion in NIDDM. *Diabetes* 1988;37:436–440.
28. Kelley DE, Mintun MA, Watkins SC, et al. The effect of non–insulin-dependent diabetes mellitus and obesity on glucose transport and phosphorylation in skeletal muscle. *J Clin Invest* 1996;97:2705–2713.
29. Braithwaite SS, Palazuk B, Colca JR, et al. Reduced expression of hexokinase II in insulin-resistant diabetes. *Diabetes* 1995;44:43–48.
30. Kruszynska YT, Mulford MI, Baloga J, et al. Regulation of skeletal muscle hexokinase II by insulin in nondiabetic and NIDDM subjects. *Diabetes* 1998;47:1107–1113.
31. Rothman DL, Shulman RG, Shulman GI. ^{31}P nuclear magnetic resonance measurements of muscle glucose-6-phosphate: evidence for reduced insulin-dependent muscle glucose transport or phosphorylation activity in non–insulin-dependent diabetes mellitus. *J Clin Invest* 1992;89:1069–1075.
32. Bonadonna RC, Del Prato S, Bonora E, et al. Roles of glucose transport and glucose phosphorylation in muscle insulin resistance of NIDDM. *Diabetes* 1992;45:915–925.
33. Zierath JR, He L, Guma A, et al. Insulin action on glucose transport and plasma membrane GLUT4 content in skeletal muscle from patients with NIDDM. *Diabetologia* 1996;39:1180–1189.
34. Dohm GL, Tapscott EB, Pories WJ, et al. An *in vitro* human muscle preparation suitable for metabolic studies: decreased insulin stimulation of glucose transport in muscle from morbidly obese and diabetic subjects. *J Clin Invest* 1988;82:486–494.
35. Randle PJ, Garland PB, Hales CN, et al. The glucose fatty acid cycle: its role in insulin sensitivity and the metabolic disturbances of diabetes mellitus. *Lancet* 1963;1:785–789.

36. Kelley DE, Mandarino LJ. Fuel selection in human skeletal muscle in insulin resistance: a reexamination. *Diabetes* 2000;49:677–683.
37. Kelley DE, Goodpasteur BH. Skeletal muscle triglyceride. *Diabetes Care* 2001;24:933–941.
38. Boden G. Free fatty acids, insulin resistance, and type 2 diabetes mellitus. *Proceedings of the Association of American Physicians* 1999;111:241–248.
39. Unger RH, Zhou YT. Lipotoxicity of beta-cells in obesity and in other causes of fatty acid spillover. *Diabetes* 2001;50:S118–S121.
40. Balasse EO, Neef MA. Influence of nicotinic acid on the rates of turnover and oxidation of plasma glucose in man. *Metabolism* 1973;22:1193–1204.
41. Gomez F, Jequier E, Chabot V, et al. Carbohydrate and lipid oxidation in normal human subjects: its influence on glucose tolerance and insulin response to glucose. *Metabolism* 1972;21:381–391.
42. Kumar S, Boulton AJ, Beck-Nielsen H, et al. Troglitazone, an insulin action enhancer, improves metabolic control in NIDDM patients. Troglitazone Study Group. *Diabetologia* 1996;39:701–709
43. Brindley DN. Intracellular translocation of phosphatidate phosphohydrolase and its possible role in the control of glycerolipid synthesis. *Prog Lipid Res* 1984;23:115–133.
44. Glick BS, Rothman JE. Possible role for fatty acyl-coenzyme A in intracellular protein transport. *Nature* 1987; 326:309–312.
45. Pfanner N, Glick BS, Arden SR, et al. Fatty acylation promotes fusion of transport vesicles with Golgi cisternae. *J Cell Biol* 1991;110:955–961.
46. Pfanner N, Orci L, Glick BS, et al. Fatty acyl-co-enzyme A is required for budding of transport vesicles from Golgi cisternae. *Cell* 1989;59:95–102.
47. Rossetti L, Hawkins M, Chen W, et al. *In vivo* glucosamine infusion induces insulin resistance in normoglycemic but not in hyperglycemic conscious rats. *J Clin Invest* 1995;96:132–140.
48. Zhang Y, Proenca R, Maffei M, et al. Positional cloning of the mouse obese gene and its human homologue. *Nature* 1994;372:425–432.
49. Maffei M, Halaas J, Ravussin E, et al. Leptin levels in human and rodent: measurement of plasma leptin and *ob* RNA in obese and weight-reduced subjects. *Nat Med* 1995;1:1155–1161.
50. McNeely MJ, Boyko EJ, Weigle DS, et al. Association between baseline plasma leptin levels and subsequent development of diabetes in Japanese Americans. *Diabetes Care* 1999;22:65–70.
51. Caro JF, Sinha MK, Kolaczynski JW, et al. Leptin: the tale of an obesity gene. *Diabetes* 1996;45:1455–1462.
52. Unger RH, Zhou YT, Orci L. Regulation of fatty acid homeostasis in cells: novel role of leptin. *Proc Natl Acad Sci U S A* 1999;96:2327–2332.
53. Wan MY, Lee Y, Unger RH. Novel form of lipolysis induced by leptin. *J Biol Chem* 1999;274:17541–17544.
54. Taylor SI, Barr V, Reitman M. Does leptin contribute to diabetes caused by obesity? *Science* 1996;274:1151–1152.
55. Berti L, Cammeltoft S. Leptin stimulates glucose uptake in C2C12 muscle cells by activation of ERK2. *Mol Cell Endocrinol* 1999;157:121–130.
56. Wan Y, Kuropatwinski KK, White DW, et al. Leptin receptor action in hepatic cells. *J Biol Chem* 1997;272:16216–16223.
57. Cohen B, Novick D, Rubinstein M. Modulation of insulin activities by leptin. *Science* 1996;274:1185–1188.
58. Kulkarni RN, Wang ZL, Wang RM, et al. Leptin rapidly suppresses insulin release from insulinoma cells, rat and human islets and, *in vivo,* in mice. *J Clin Invest* 1997;100:2729–2736.
59. Kieffer TJ, Heller RS, Leech CA, et al. Leptin suppression of insulin secretion by the activation of ATP-sensitive K+ channels in pancreatic beta-cells. *Diabetes* 1997;46:1087–1093.
60. Gavrilova O, Marcu-Samuels B, Leon LR, et al. Leptin and diabetes in lipoatrophic mice. *Nature* 2000;403:850–851.
61. Shimomura I, Hammer RE, Ikemoto S, et al. Leptin reverses insulin resistance and diabetes mellitus in mice with congenital lipodystrophy. *Nature* 1999;401:850–851.
62. Ogawa Y, Masuzaki H, Hosoda K, et al. Increased glucose metabolism and insulin sensitivity in transgenic skinny mice overexpressing leptin. *Diabetes* 1999;48:1822–1829.
63. Chinookoswong N, Wang JL, Shi ZQ. Leptin restores euglycemia and normalizes glucose turnover in insulin-deficient diabetes in the rat. *Diabetes* 1999;48:1487–1492.
64. Heymsfield S, Greenberg A, Fujioka K, et al. Recombinant leptin for weight loss in obese and lean adults: a randomized, controlled, dose-escalation trial. *JAMA* 1999;282:1568–1575.
65. Hotamisligil GS, Shargill NS, Spiegelman BS, et al. Adipose expression of TNF alpha: a direct role in obesity-linked insulin resistance. *Science* 1993;259:87–91.
66. Kern PA, Saghizadeh M, Ong JM, et al. The expression of TNF alpha in human adipose tissue, regulation by obesity, weight loss and relationship to lipoprotein lipase. *J Clin Invest* 1995;95:2111–2119.
67. Stephens JM, Lee J, Pilch PF. TNF alpha induced insulin resistance in 3T3-L1 adipocytes is accompanied by a loss of IRS-1 and GLUT-4 expression without a loss of insulin receptor mediated signal transduction. *J Biol Chem* 1997;272:971–976.
68. Guo D, Donner DB. TNF alpha promotes binding of IRS-1 to PI3Kinase in 3T3L-1 adipocytes. *J Biol Chem* 1996;271:615–618.
69. Hotamisligil GS, Spiegelman BM. Tumor necrosis factor alpha: a key component of the obesity-diabetes link. *Diabetes* 1994;43:1271–1278.

70. Hurel S, Ofei F, Wells AN, et al. TNF-alpha and insulin sensitivity in humans: effects *in vivo* of antibody block-ade in obese NIDDM patients and *in vitro* upon human cultured myotubes. *Exp Clin Endocrinol Diabetes* 1996; 104:59–60.

71. Van Der Poll T, Romijn JA, Endert E, et al. Tumor necrosis factor mimics the metabolic response to acute infec-tion in healthy humans. *Am J Physiol* 1991;24:E457–E465.

72. Hotamisligil GS, Budavari A, Murray D, et al. Reduced tyrosine kinase activity of the insulin receptor in obe-sity-diabetes: central role of tumor necrosis factor-alpha. *J Clin Invest* 1994;94:1543–1549.

73. Mohamed-Ali V, Goodrick S, Bulmer K, et al. Production of soluble tumor necrosis factor receptors by human subcutaneous adipose tissue *in vivo*. *Am J Physiol* 1999;277:E971–E975.

74. Vozarova B, Weyer C, Hanson K, et al. Circulating interleukin-6 in relation to adiposity, insulin action, and insulin secretion. *Obes Res* 2001;9:414–417.

75. Tsigos C, Papanicolaou DA, Kyrou I, et al. Dose-dependent effects of recombinant human interleukin-6 on glu-cose regulation. *J Clin Endocrinol Metab* 1997;82:4167–4170.

76. Bastard JP, Jardel C, Bruckert E, et al. Elevated levels of interleukin 6 are reduced in serum and subcutaneous adipose tissue of obese women after weight loss. *J Clin Endocrinol Metab* 2000;85:3338–3342.

77. Vozarova B, Weyer C, Hanson K, et al. Circulating interleukin-6 in relation to adiposity, insulin action, and insulin secretion. *Obes Res* 2001;9:414–417.

78. Steppan CM, Bailey ST, Bhat S, et al. The hormone resistin links obesity to diabetes. *Nature* 2001;409: 307–312.

79. Hu E, Liang P, Spiegelman BM. AdipoQ is a novel adipose-specific gene dysregulated in obesity. *J Biol Chem* 1996;271:10697–10703.

80. Scherer PE, Williams S, Fogliano M, et al. A novel serum protein similar to C1q, produced exclusively in adipocytes. *J Biol Chem* 1995;270:26746–26749.

81. Weyer C, Funahashi T, Tanaka S, et al. Hypoadiponectinemia in obesity and type 2 diabetes: close association with insulin resistance and hyperinsulinemia. *J Clin Endocrinol Metab* 2001;86:1930–1935.

82. Yang WS, Lee WJ, Funahashi T, et al. Weight reduction increases plasma levels of an adipose-derived anti-inflammatory protein, adiponectin. *J Clin Endocrinol Metab* 2001;86:3815–3819.

83. Yang W, Jeng CY, Wu TJ, et al. Synthetic peroxisome proliferator-activated receptor-[gamma] agonist, rosigli-tazone, increases plasma levels of adiponectin in type 2 diabetic patients. *Diabetes Care* 2002;25:376–380.

84. Yamauchi T, Kamon J, Waki H, et al. The fat-derived hormone adiponectin reverses insulin resistance associ-ated with both lipoatrophy and obesity. *Nat Med* 2001;7:941–946.

85. Saltiel AR. You are what you secrete. *Nat Med* 2001;7:887–888.

86. Ouchi N, Kihara S, Nishida M, et al. Adipocyte derived plasma protein, adiponectin, suppresses lipid accumu-lation and class A scavenger expression in human monocyte derived macrophages. *Circulation* 2001;103: 1057–1063.

87. Lemberger T, Desvergne B, Wahli W. Peroxisome proliferator-active receptors: a nuclear receptor signaling pathway in lipid physiology. *Annu Rev Cell Dev Biol* 1996;12:335–363.

88. Saltiel AR, Olefsky JM. Thiazolidinediones in the treatment of insulin resistance in type 2 diabetes. *Diabetes* 1996;45:1661–1669.

89. Barroso I, Gurnell M, Crowley VE, et al. Dominant negative mutations in human PPAR gamma associated with severe insulin resistance, diabetes mellitus and hypertension. *Nature* 1999;402:880–883.

90. Ristow M, Muller-Wieland D, Pfeiffer A, et al. Obesity associated with a mutation in a genetic regulator of adipocyte differentiation. *N Engl J Med* 1998;339:953–959.

91. Boden G, Chen X, Rosner J, et al. Effects of 48-h fat infusion on insulin secretion and glucose utilization. *Diabetes* 1995;44:1239–1242.

92. Dobbins RL, Chester MW, Daniels MB, et al. Circulating fatty acids are essential for efficient glucose-stimu-lated insulin secretion after prolonged fasting in humans. *Diabetes* 1998;47:1613–1618.

93. Polonsky KS, Given BD, Hirsch L, et al. Quantitative study of insulin secretion and clearance in normal sub-jects. *J Clin Invest* 1988;81:435–441.

94. Grill V, Qvigstad E. Fatty acids and insulin secretion. *Br J Nutr* 2000;83:S79–S84.

95. Paolisso G, Gambardella A, Amato L, et al. Opposite effects of short and long term fatty acid infusion on insulin secretion in healthy subjects. *Diabetologia* 1995;38:1295–1299.

96. Bollheimer LC, Skelly RH, Chester MW, et al. Chronic exposure to FFAs reduces pancreatic beta cell insulin secretion that is not compensated for by a corresponding increase in proinsulin biosynthesis translation. *J Clin Invest* 1998;101:1094–1101.

97. Byrne MM, Sturis J, Cavaghan M, et al. Insulin secretion in humans. In LeRoith D, Taylor SI, Olefsky JM, eds. *Diabetes mellitus: a fundamental and clinical text.* Philadelphia: Lippincott Williams & Wilkins, 2000:105–114.

98. Liu YQ, Tornheim K, Leahy JL. Fatty acid–induced beta cell hypersensitivity to glucose: increased phospho-fructokinase activity and lowered glucose-6-phosphate content. *J Clin Invest* 1998;101:1870–1875.

99. Shimabukuro M, Ohneda N, Lee Y, et al. Role of nitric oxide in obesity-induced beta cell disease. *J Clin Invest* 1997;100:290–295.

100. Shimabukuro M, Koyama K, Lee Y, et al. Leptin or troglitazone induced lipopenia protects islets from interleukin-1 beta cytotoxicity. *J Clin Invest* 1997;100:1750–1754.

101. Shimabukuro M, Zhou YT, Levi M, et al. Fatty acid induced beta cell apoptosis: a link between obesity and dia-betes. *Proc Natl Acad Sci U S A* 1998;95:2498–2502.

102. Paul Robertson R, Harmon J, Tanaka Y, et al. Glucose toxicity of the beta cell. Cellular and molecular mechanisms. In LeRoith D, Taylor SI, Olefsy JM, eds. *Diabetes mellitus: a fundamental and clinical text.* Philadelphia: Lippincott Williams & Wilkins, 2000:125–131.

103. Kolterman OG, Gray RS, Griffin J, et al. Increase in hepatic glucose production (HGP) in patients with type 2 diabetes as compared to non-diabetic controls. *J Clin Invest* 1981;68:957–969.

104. Caro JF, Stramm LE. Biochemical defects of insulin action in humans. In LeRoith D, Taylor SI, Olefsy JM, eds. *Diabetes mellitus: a fundamental and clinical text.* Philadelphia: Lippincott Williams & Wilkins, 2000:615–626.

105. Ferrannini E, Barrett E, Bevilacqua S, et al. Effect of fatty acids on glucose production and utilization in man. *J Clin Invest* 1983;72:1737–1747.

106. Fanelli C, Calderone S, Epifano L, et al. Demonstration of a critical role for free fatty acids in mediating counterregulatory stimulation of gluconeogenesis and suppression of glucose utilization in humans. *J Clin Invest* 1993;92:1617–1622.

107. Boden G, Jadali F. Effects of lipid on basal carbohydrate metabolism in normal men. *Diabetes* 1991;40: 686–692.

108. Consoli A, Nurjhan N, Capani F, et al. Predominant role of gluconeogenesis in increasing hepatic glucose production in NIDDM. *Diabetes* 1989;38:550–557.

109. Gonzalez-Manchon C, Ayuso MS, Parrilla R. Control of hepatic gluconeogenesis: role of fatty acid oxidation. *Arch Biochem Biophys* 1989;271:1–9.

110. Williamson J, Browning E, Scholz R. Control mechanisms of gluconeogenesis and ketogenesis. *J Biol Chem* 1969;224:4607–4616.

111. Weyer C, Bogardus C, Mott DM, et al. The natural history of insulin secretory dysfunction and insulin resistance in the pathogenesis of type 2 diabetes mellitus. *J Clin Invest* 1999;104:787–794.

112. American Diabetes Association. Clinical practice recommendations 2002. *Diabetes Care* 2002;25:S1–S147.

113. Williamson DF, Thompson TJ, Thun M, et al. Intentional weight loss and mortality among overweight individuals with diabetes. *Diabetes Care* 2000;23:1499–1504.

114. United Kingdom Prospective Diabetes Study (UKPDS) Group. Intensive blood-glucose control with sulphonylureas or insulin compared with conventional treatment and risk of complications in patients with type 2 diabetes (UKPDS 33). *Lancet* 1998;352:837–853.

115. United Kingdom Prospective Diabetes Study (UKPDS) Group. Effect of intensive blood-glucose control with metformin on complications in overweight patients with type 2 diabetes (UKPDS 34). *Lancet* 1998;352: 854–865.

116. Hu FB, Manson JE, Stampfer MJ, et al. Diet, lifestyle, and the risk of type 2 diabetes mellitus in women. *N Engl J Med* 2001;345:790–797.

117. Wing RR, Koeske R, Epstein LH, et al. Long-term effects of modest weight loss in type II diabetic patients. *Arch Intern Med* 1987;147:1749–1753.

118. Lean ME, Powrie JK, Anderson AS, et al. Obesity, weight loss and prognosis in type 2 diabetes. *Diabet Med* 1990;7:228–233.

119. Wadden TA. Treatment of obesity by moderate and severe caloric restriction: results of clinical research trials. *Ann Intern Med* 1993;119:688–693.

120. Wadden TA. The treatment of obesity: an overview. In: Stunkard AJ, Wadden TA, eds. *Obesity: theory and therapy,* 2nd ed. New York: Raven Press, 1993:197–217.

121. Henry RR, Scheaffer L, Olefsky JM. Glycemic effects of intensive caloric restriction and isocaloric refeeding in non–insulin-dependent diabetes mellitus. *J Clin Endocrinol Metab* 1985;61:917–925.

122. American Diabetes Association. Nutritional recommendations and principles for individuals with diabetes mellitus. *Diabetes Care* 2002;25:S50–S60.

123. Franz MJ, Horton ES, Bantle J, et al. Nutrition principles for the management of diabetes and related complications [Technical Review]. *Diabetes Care* 1994;17:490–518.

124. National Institutes of Health. Consensus development conference on diet and exercise in non–insulin-dependent diabetes mellitus. *Diabetes Care* 1987;10:639–644.

125. Garg A. High-monounsaturated-fat diets for patients with diabetes mellitus: a meta-analysis. *Am J Clin Nutr* 1998;67:577S–582S.

126. Garg A, Bonanome A, Grundy SM, et al. Comparison of a high-carbohydrate diet with a high-monounsaturated-fat diet in patients with non–insulin-dependent diabetes mellitus. *N Engl J Med* 1988;319:829–834.

127. Garg A, Grundy S, Koffler M. Effect of high carbohydrate intake on hyperglycemia, islet function, and plasma lipoproteins in NIDDM. *Diabetes Care* 1992;15:1572–1580.

128. Vinik AI, Lauterio TJ, Wing RR. Should the bee suck honey or lard? That is the question. *Diabetes Care* 1993; 16:1045–1047.

129. Chandalia M, Garg A, Lutjohann D, et al. Beneficial effects of high dietary fiber intake in patients with type 2 diabetes mellitus. *N Engl J Med* 2000;342:1392–1398.

130. Van Dam RM, Rimm EB, Willett WC, et al. Dietary patterns and risk for type 2 diabetes mellitus in men. *Ann Intern Med* 2002;136:201–209.

131. Wing RR, Marcus MD, Epstein LH, et al. Type II diabetic subjects lose less weight than their overweight non-diabetic spouses. *Diabetes Care* 1987;10:563–566.

132. United Kingdom Prospective Diabetes Study Group. U.K. Prospective Diabetes Study 7: response of fasting plasma glucose to diet therapy in newly presenting type 2 diabetic patients. *Metabolism* 1990;39:905–912.

133. Hadden DR, Blair AL, Wilson EZ, et al. Natural history of diabetes presenting age 40–69 years: a prospective study of the influence of intensive dietary therapy. *Q J Med* 1986;59:579–598.

134. Horton ES. Role and management of exercise in diabetes mellitus. *Diabetes Care* 1988;11:201–211.

135. Manson JE, Rimm EB, Stampfer MJ, et al. Physical activity and incidence of non–insulin-dependent diabetes mellitus in women. *Lancet* 1991;338:774–778.

136. Manson JE, Nathan DM, Krolewski AS, et al. A prospective study of exercise and incidence of diabetes among US male physicians. *JAMA* 1992;268:63–67.

137. Uusitupa M, Louheranta A, Lindstrom J, et al. The Finnish Diabetes Prevention Study. *Br J Nutr* 2000;83: S137–S142.

138. Vukovich MD, Arciero PJ, Kohrt WM, et al. Changes in insulin action and GLUT-4 with 6 days of inactivity in endurance runners. *J Appl Physiol* 1996;80:240–244.

139. Cortright RN, Dohm GL. Mechanisms by which insulin and muscle contraction stimulate glucose transport. *Can J Appl Physiol* 1997;22:519–530.

140. King PA, Betts JJ, Horton ED, et al. Exercise, unlike insulin, promotes glucose transporter translocation in obese Zucker rat muscle. *Am J Physiol* 1993;265:R447–R452.

141. Usui K, Yamanouchi K, Asai K, et al. The effect of low intensity bicycle exercise on the insulin-induced glucose uptake in obese patients with type 2 diabetes. *Diabetes Res Clin Pract* 1998;41:57–61.

142. Chibalin AV, Yu M, Ryder JW, et al. Exercise-induced changes in expression and activity of proteins involved in insulin signal transduction in skeletal muscle: differential effects on insulin-receptor substrates 1 and 2. *Proc Natl Acad Sci U S A* 2000;97:38–43.

143. Smith LK, Vlahos CJ, Reddy KK, et al. Wortmannin and LY294002 inhibit the insulin-induced down-regulation of IRS-1 in 3T3-L1 adipocytes. *Mol Cell Endocrinol* 1995;113:73–81.

144. Hayashi T, Hirshman MF, Kurth EJ, et al. Evidence for 5' AMP-activated protein kinase mediation of the effect of muscle contraction on glucose transport. *Diabetes* 1998;47:1369–1373.

145. Brown SA, Upchurch S, Anding R, et al. Promoting weight loss in type II diabetes. *Diabetes Care* 1996;19: 613–624.

146. Boule NG, Haddad E, Kenny G, et al. Effects of exercise on glycemic control and body mass in type 2 diabetes mellitus: a meta-analysis of controlled clinical trials. *JAMA* 2001;286:1218–1227.

147. Wei M, Gibbons LW, Kampert JB, et al. Low cardiorespiratory fitness and physical inactivity as predictors of mortality in men with type 2 diabetes. *Ann Intern Med* 2000;132:605–611.

148. Hu FB, Stampfer MJ, Solomon C, et al. Physical activity and risk for cardiovascular events in diabetic women. *Ann Intern Med* 2001;134:96–105.

149. National Institute of Diabetes & Digestive & Kidney Diseases. The Look AHEAD project. Available at: http://www.LookAHEADstudy.org. Accessed October 18, 2002.

150. Hu FB, Manson JE, Stampfer MJ, et al. Diet, lifestyle, and the risk of type 2 diabetes mellitus in women. *N Engl J Med* 2001;345:790–797.

151. Van Dam RM, Rimm EB, Willett WC, et al. Dietary patterns and risk for type 2 diabetes mellitus in US men. *Ann Intern Med* 2001;136:201–209.

152. Diabetes Prevention Program Research Group. Reduction in the incidence of type 2 diabetes with lifestyle intervention or metformin. *N Engl J Med* 2002;346:393–403.

153. Seino S, Inagaki N, Namba N, et al. Molecular biology of the beta-cell ATP-sensitive K^+ channel. *Diabetes Rev* 1996;4:177–190.

154. Harrower AD. Comparison of efficacy, secondary failure rate, and complications of sulfonylureas. *J Diabet Complications* 1994;8:201–203.

155. Wang PH, Moller D, Flier JS, et al. Coordinate regulation of glucose transporter function, number, and gene expression by insulin and sulfonylureas in L6 rat skeletal muscle cells. *J Clin Invest* 1989;84:62–67.

156. Prigeon RL, Jacobson RK, Porte D Jr, et al. Effect of sulfonylurea withdrawal on proinsulin levels, B cell function, and glucose disposal in subjects with non insulin-dependent diabetes mellitus. *J Clin Endocrinol Metab* 1996;81:3295–3298.

157. Pedersen O, Hother-Nielsen O, Bak J, et al. Effects of sulfonylureas on adipocyte and skeletal muscle insulin action in patients with non–insulin-dependent diabetes mellitus. *Am J Med* 1991;90:22S–28S.

158. Panahloo A, Mohamed-Ali V, Andres C, et al. Effect of insulin versus sulfonylurea therapy on cardiovascular risk factors and fibrinolysis in type II diabetes. *Metabolism* 1998;47:637–643.

159. Engler RL, Yellon DM. Sulfonylurea K-ATP blockade in type II diabetes and preconditioning in cardiovascular disease: time for reconsideration. *Circulation* 1996;94:2297–2301.

160. Klimt CR, Knatterud GL, Meinert CL, et al. A study of the effects of hypoglycemic agents on vascular complications in patients with adult-onset diabetes. *Diabetes* 1970;19:747–830.

161. Lebowitz HE. Insulin secretagogues: old and new. *Diabetes Rev* 1999;7:139–153.

162. Johansen K. Efficacy of metformin in the treatment of NIDDM. *Diabetes Care* 2000;22:33–37.

163. Nagasaka S, Ishikawa S, Nakamura T, et al. Association of endogenous insulin secretion and mode of therapy with body fat and serum leptin levels in diabetic subjects. *Metabolism* 1998;47:1391–1396.

164. Shi H, Moustaid-Moussa N, Wilkison WO, et al. Role of the sulfonylurea receptor in regulating human adipocyte metabolism. *FASEB J* 1999;13:1833–1838.

165. Malaisse WJ. Mechanism of action of a new class of insulin secretagogues. *Exp Clin Endocrinol Diabetes* 1999; 107:S140–S143.

166. Keilson L, Mather S, Walter YH, et al. Synergistic effects of nateglinide and meal administration on insulin secretion in patients with type 2 diabetes mellitus. *J Clin Endocrinol Metab* 2000;85:1081–1086.

167. Damsbo P, Clauson P, Marbury TC, et al. A double-blind randomized comparison of meal-related glycemic control by repaglinide and glyburide in well-controlled type 2 diabetic patients. *Diabetes Care* 1999;22:789–794.

168. Moses R. Repaglinide in combination therapy with metformin in type 2 diabetes. *Diabetes* 1999;107: S136–S139.

169. Hu S, Wang S, Dunning BE. Tissue selectivity of antidiabetic agent nateglinide: study on cardiovascular and beta-cell K(ATP) channels. *J Pharmacol Exp Ther* 1999;291:1372–1379.

170. Marbury T, Huang WC, Strange P, et al. Repaglinide versus glyburide: a one-year comparison trial. *Diabetes Res Clin Pract* 1999;43:155–166.

171. Bailey CJ, Turner RC. Metformin. *N Engl J Med* 1996;334:574–579.

172. Lin HZ, Yang SQ, Chuckaree C, et al. Metformin reverses fatty liver disease in obese, leptin-deficient mice. *Nat Med* 2000;6:998–1003.

173. Cusi K, De Fronzo RA. Metformin: a review of its metabolic effects. *Diabetes Rev* 1998;6:89–131.

174. Inzucchi SE, Maggs DG, Spollett GR, et al. Efficacy and metabolic effects of metformin and troglitazone in type II diabetes mellitus. *N Engl J Med* 1998;338:867–872.

175. Patane G, Piro S, Agata M, et al. Metformin restores insulin secretion altered by chronic exposure to free fatty acids or high glucose: a direct metformin effect on pancreatic beta-cells. *Diabetes* 2000;49:735–740.

176. Charles MA, Morange P, Eschwege E, et al. Effect of weight change and metformin on fibrinolysis and the von Willebrand factor in obese nondiabetic subjects: the BIGPRO1 Study. Biguanides and the Prevention of the Risk of Obesity. *Diabetes Care* 1998;21:1967–1972.

177. Turner RC, Holman R, Stratton I. Correspondence. The UK Prospective Diabetes Study. *Lancet* 1999;352: 1934.

178. Lee A, Morley JE. Metformin decreases food consumption and induces weight loss in subjects with obesity and type II non–insulin dependent diabetes mellitus. *Obes Res* 1998;6:47–53.

179. Fontbonne A, Charles MA, Juhan-Vague I, et al. The BIGPRO Study Group: the effect of metformin on the metabolic abnormalities associated with upper-body fat distribution. *Diabetes Care* 1996;19:920–926.

180. Pasquali R, Gambineri A, Biscotti D, et al. Effect of long-term treatment with metformin added to hypocaloric diet on body composition, fat distribution, and androgen and insulin levels in abdominally obese women with and without the polycystic ovary syndrome. *J Clin Endocrinol Metab* 2000;85:2767–2774.

181. Lebovitz HE. Alpha-Glucosidase inhibitors as agents in the treatment of diabetes. *Diabetes Rev* 1998;6: 132–145.

182. Russell JC, Graham SE, Dolphin PJ. Glucose tolerance and insulin resistance in the JCR:LA-corpulent rat: effect of miglitol (Bay M1099). *Metabolism* 1999;48:701–706.

183. Johnson AB, Taylor R. Does suppression of postprandial blood glucose excursions by the alpha-glucosidase inhibitor miglitol improve insulin sensitivity in diet-treated type II diabetic patients? *Diabetes Care* 1996;19: 559–563.

184. Meneilly GS, Ryan EA, Radziuk J, et al. Effect of acarbose on insulin sensitivity in elderly patients with diabetes. *Diabetes Care* 2000;23:1162–1167.

185. Chiasson JL, Gomis R, Hanefeld M, et al. The STOP-NIDDM Trial: an international study on the efficacy of an alpha-glucosidase inhibitor to prevent type 2 diabetes in a population with impaired glucose tolerance: rationale, design, and preliminary screening data. Study to Prevent Non–Insulin-Dependent Diabetes Mellitus. *Diabetes Care* 1998;21:1720–1725.

186. Willson TM, Cobb JE, Cowan DJ, et al. The structure–activity relationship between peroxisome-proliferator–activated receptor & agonism and the antihyperglycemic activity of thiazolidinediones. *J Med Chem* 1996;39:665–668.

187. Desvergne B, Ijpenberg A, Devchand PR, et al. The PPAR receptors at the cross-road of diet and hormone signaling. *J Steroid Biochem Mol Biol* 1998;65:65–74.

188. Saleh YM, Mudaliar SR, Henry RR. Metabolic and vascular effects of the thiazolidinedione, troglitazone. *Diabetes Rev* 2000;7:55–76.

189. Avandia [prescribing information]. Philadelphia: SmithKline Beecham Pharmaceuticals, April 2000.

190. Actos [prescribing information]. Lincolnshire, IL: Elli Lilly Company, July 1999.

191. Shaffer S, Rubin CJ, Zhu E. Study Group—pioglitazone 001. The effects of pioglitazone on the lipid profile in patients with type 2 diabetes [Abstract]. *Diabetes* 2000;48:508P.

192. Bakris GL, Dole JF, Porter LE, et al. Rosiglitazone improves blood pressure in patients with type 2 diabetes [Abstract]. *Diabetes* 2000;48:388P.

193. Takagi T, Yoshida K, Akasaka T, et al. Troglitazone reduces intimal hyperplasia after coronary stent implantation in patients with type 2 diabetes mellitus: a serial intravascular ultrasound study [Abstract]. *J Am Coll Cardiol* 1999;33:886–882.

194. Okuno A, Tamemoto H, Tobe K, et al. Troglitazone increases the number of small adipocytes without the change of white adipose tissue mass in obese Zucker rats. *J Clin Invest* 1998;101:1354–1361.

195. Burant CF, Sreenan S, Hirano K, et al. Troglitazone action is independent of adipose tissue. *J Clin Invest* 1998; 100:2900–2908.

196. Adams M, Montague CT, Prins JB, et al. Activators of peroxisome proliferator–activated receptor-gamma have depot-specific effects on human preadipocyte differentiation. *J Clin Invest* 1997;100:3149–3153.

197. Mori Y, Murakawa Y, Okada K, et al. Effect of troglitazone on body fat distribution in type 2 diabetic patients. *Diabetes Care* 1999;22:908–912.
198. Kelly IE, Han TS, Walsh K, et al. Effects of a thiazolidinedione compound on body fat and fat distribution of patients with type 2 diabetes [published correction appears in *Diabetes Care* 1999;22:536]. *Diabetes Care* 1999;22:288–293.
199. Miyazaki Y, Mahankali A, Matsuda M, et al. Effect of pioglitazone on abdominal fat distribution and insulin sensitivity in patients with type 2 diabetes mellitus. *Diabetes* 2000;48:A299.
200. Guare JC, Wing RR, Grant A. Comparison of obese NIDDM and non diabetic women: short and long-term weight loss. *Obes Res* 1995;3:329–335.
201. Stock MJ, Macdonald IA, Astrup A. Thermogenic effects of sibutramine in humans. *Am J Clin Nutr* 1998;68: 1180–1186.
202. Heath MJ, Chong E, Weinstein SP, et al. Sibutramine enhances weight loss and improves glycemic control and plasma lipid profile in obese patients with type 2 diabetes mellitus. *Diabetes* 1999;48:A308.
203. Finer N, Bloom SR, Frost GS, et al. Sibutramine is effective for weight loss and diabetic control in obesity with type 2 diabetes: a randomized, double-blind, placebo-controlled study. *Diabetes Obes Metab* 2000;2:105–112.
204. Fujioka K, Seaton TB, Rowe E, et al. Weight loss with sibutramine improves glycemic control and other metabolic parameters in obese patients with type 2 diabetes mellitus. *Diabetes Obes Metab* 2000;2:175–187.
205. Gockel A, Karakose H, Ertorer EM, et al. Effects of sibutramine in obese female subjects with type 2 diabetes and poor blood glucose control. *Diabetes Care* 2001;24:1957–1960.
206. Day C, Bailey CJ. Effect of the antiobesity agent sibutramine in obese-diabetic *ob/ob* mice. *Int J Obes Relat Metab Disord* 1998;22:619–623.
207. Granzotto M, Pagano C, Lombardi AM, et al. Effect of sibutramine on glucose metabolism in genetically obese (fa/fa) Zucker rats. *Int J Obes Relat Metab Disord* 2000;24:S124–S126.
208. Rissanen A, Finer N, Fujioka K, et al. Sibutramine-induced weight loss improves the lipid profile in obese type 2 diabetics: results of 3 placebo-controlled trials. *Diabetes* 2000;49:A270.
209. Van Gaal LF, Wauters MA, De Leeuw IH. Anti-obesity drugs: what does sibutramine offer? An analysis of its potential contribution to obesity treatment. *Exp Clin Endocrinol Diabetes* 1998;106:35–40.
210. Van Gaal LF, Wauters MA, Peiffer FW, De Leeuw IH. Sibutramine and fat distribution: is there a role for pharmacotherapy in abdominal/visceral fat reduction? *Int J Obes Relat Metab Disord* 1998;22:S38–S42.
211. Hollander PA, Elbein SC, Hirsch IB, et al. Role of orlistat in the treatment of obese patients with type 2 diabetes. A 1-year randomized double-blind study. *Diabetes Care* 1998;21:1288–1294.
212. Davidson MH, Hauptman J, DiGirolamo M, et al. Weight control and risk factor reduction in obese subjects treated for 2 years with orlistat: a randomized controlled trial [see Comments] [published correction appears in *JAMA* 1999;281:1174]. *JAMA* 1999;281:235–242.
213. Hauptman J, Lucas C, Boldrin MN, et al. Orlistat in the long-term treatment of obesity in primary care settings. *Arch Fam Med* 2000;9:160–167.
214. Zavoral JH. Treatment with orlistat reduces cardiovascular risk in obese patients. *J Hypertens* 1998;16: 2013–2017.
215. Heymsfield SB, Segal KR, Hauptman J, et al. Effects of weight loss with orlistat on glucose tolerance and progression to type 2 diabetes in obese adults. *Arch Intern Med* 2000;160:1321–1326.
216. National Heart Lung and Blood Institute. Clinical guidelines on the identification, evaluation, and treatment of overweight and obesity in adults—the evidence report. *Obes Res* 1998;6:S51–S290.
217. Di Cosmo L, Vuolo G, Piccolomini A, et al. Bariatric surgery: early results with a multidisciplinary team. *Obes Surg* 2000;10:272–273.
218. Dixon JB, O'Brien PE. Health outcomes of severely obese type 2 diabetic subjects 1 year after laparoscopic adjustable gastric banding. *Diabetes Care* 2002;25:358–363.
219. Long SD, O'Brien K, MacDonald KG, et al. Weight loss in severely obese subjects prevents the progression of impaired glucose tolerance to type 2 diabetes. A longitudinal intervention study. *Diabetes Care* 1994;17: 372–375.
220. Sjostrom CD, Lissner L, Wedel H, et al. Reduction in incidence of diabetes, hypertension and lipid disturbances after intentional weight loss induced by bariatric surgery: the SOS Intervention Study. *Obes Res* 1999;7: 477–484.
221. Torgerson JS, Sjostrom L. The Swedish Obese Subjects (SOS) study—rationale and results. *Int J Obes Relat Metab Disord* 2001;25:S2–S4.
222. Hickey M, Pories WJ, MacDonald KG Jr, et al. A new paradigm for type 2 diabetes mellitus: could it be a disease of the foregut? *Ann Surg* 1998;227:637–644.
223. Pories WJ, Swanson MS, Macdonald KG, et al. Who would have thought it? An operation proves to be the most effective therapy for adult-onset diabetes mellitus. *Ann Surg* 1995;222:339–352.

11

Obesity, Hypertension, and Renal Disease

John E. Hall, Daniel W. Jones, Jeffrey Henegar, Terry M. Dwyer, and Jay J. Kuo

Few medical problems have generated as much interest as obesity, the most prevalent nutritional disorder in the United States and in other industrialized countries. Obesity increases the risk of cardiovascular disease through multiple mechanisms, including hypertension, diabetes, dyslipidemia, atherosclerosis, and chronic renal dysfunction, many of which are interdependent (1–3). For example, abnormal kidney function plays a central role in the etiology of obesity-related hypertension, and the increased blood pressure and metabolic abnormalities associated with obesity are important risk factors for endstage renal disease (ESRD). The constellation of cardiovascular, endocrine, renal, and metabolic disorders is often referred to as *syndrome X, the insulin-resistance syndrome, the deadly quartet,* or *the metabolic syndrome,* but obesity appears to be its root cause.

ESSENTIAL HYPERTENSION IS CLOSELY ASSOCIATED WITH OVERWEIGHT

Considerable evidence points toward excess weight as the cause of most human essential hypertension. For example, many population studies have shown that blood pressure correlates with body mass index (BMI) and other anthropometric and biochemical indexes of obesity, such as waist to hip ratio, which is an indicator of central adiposity, and plasma and leptin concentrations (4–7). Figure 11.1 shows, for example, the linear relationship between BMI and systolic and diastolic blood pressure that was observed in more than 22,000 Korean subjects, most of whom were not overweight. A similar close association between obesity and hypertension has been found in normotensive and hypertensive subjects in diverse populations throughout the world and in populations of similar origin who are living in different locations (5,8). Other cardiovascular risk factors associated with industrialization cannot fully explain this relationship because it has also been observed in multiple studies of nonindustrialized societies (8). Risk estimates from the Framingham Heart Study suggest that the causes of hypertension in approximately 78% of men and 65% of women can be attributed to obesity (6).

Clinical studies also suggest that obesity is an important cause of increased blood pressure in many patients with essential hypertension, and the therapeutic value of weight loss in reducing blood pressure has been repeatedly demonstrated (4,9–12). Even modest weight loss of 5% to 10% of baseline weight may be effective in lowering blood pressure and reducing or obviating the need for antihypertensive medication in obese hypertensive patients (10,11). Clinical trials have also demonstrated the effectiveness of weight loss in the primary prevention of hypertension (12).

Although weight loss does not always completely normalize blood pressure in obese hypertensive patients, this is perhaps not surprising in view of the many pathologic

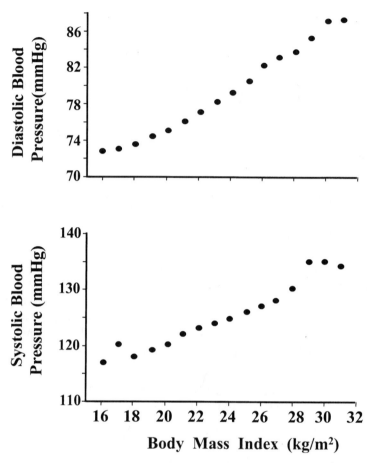

FIG. 11.1. Relationship between body mass index and systolic and diastolic blood pressures in 22,354 Korean subjects. (Data from Jones DW, Kim JS, Andrew ME, et al. Body mass index and blood pressures in Korean men and women: the Korean National Blood Pressure Survey. *J Hypertens* 1994;12:1433–1437, with permission.)

changes that occur as excess weight is maintained for long periods. For example, prolonged obesity may lead to glomerular injury, loss of functional nephrons, and resetting of the renal-pressure natriuresis to higher blood pressures (3). Effective blood pressure control under these circumstances becomes more difficult, requiring pharmacologic antihypertensive therapy. Weight loss, however, greatly enhances the effectiveness of drug therapy in controlling blood pressure in obese hypertensive patients (11).

Of importance is the observation that some obese persons are not "hypertensive" (i.e., they do not have a resting blood pressure greater than 140/90 mm Hg). However, weight loss usually lowers blood pressure in these "normotensive" obese individuals as long as marked renal disease is not present (4). This suggests that obese persons with "normal" blood pressure are hypertensive relative to their baseline pressure. Whether antihypertensive therapy, either by weight loss programs or by pharmacologic therapy, in "normotensive" obese persons provides protection against cardiovascular and renal disease remains to be tested.

TABLE 11.1. *Cardiovascular, neurohumoral, and renal changes in animal models fed a high-fat diet compared with obese humans*

Dietary model (high-fat diet)	Arterial pressure	Cardiac output	Heart rate	Renal sympathetic activity	PRA	Na$^+$ balance	GFR[a]
Human (diet and/or genetic?)	↑	↑	↑	↑	↑	↑	↑
Dog	↑	↑	↑	↑	↑	↑	↑
Rabbits	↑	↑	↑	↑	↑	↑	↑
Sprague–Dawley rat	↑	↑	↑	↑	↑	↑	↑

Abbreviations: GFR, glomerular filtration rate; Na, sodium; PRA, plasma renin activity; ↑, increased.
[a]The GFR changes indicated refer to the early phases of obesity before major loss of nephron function has occurred.

Studies in experimental animals have also shown a cause-and-effect relationship between excess weight gain and hypertension, and they have provided mechanistic insights into the molecular and physiologic events that link obesity with cardiovascular and renal disease. Weight gain induced by a chronic high-fat diet causes a reproducible rise in blood pressure in dogs, rabbits, and rats (13–16); and the cardiovascular, renal, endocrine, and metabolic changes observed in animal models of diet-induced obesity appear to mimic very closely the changes found in obese humans (3,17) (Table 11.1). Some of these changes are time dependent, occurring rapidly after excess weight gain and later becoming obscured by pathologic changes associated with prolonged obesity. For example, the glomerular hyperfiltration that is characteristic of the early phases of obesity may eventually subside as glomerular injury and nephron loss occur in association with obesity-induced hypertension.

HEMODYNAMICS AND CARDIAC FUNCTION IN OBESE SUBJECTS

Excess Weight Gain Increases Heart Rate and Cardiac Output

Rapid weight gain increases cardiac output and heart rate in experimental animals and humans. The rise in resting heart rate with chronic obesity is due primarily to the withdrawal of parasympathetic tone, rather than to increased sympathetic activity or increased intrinsic heart rate (18–20). Obesity is also associated with extracellular volume expansion and higher blood flows to many tissues (3,14,20,21). These elevated tissue blood flows summate to raise venous return and cardiac output.

Part of the increased cardiac output observed with weight gain is due to the additional blood flow required for the excess adipose tissue. However, blood flow in nonadipose tissue, including the heart, kidneys, gastrointestinal tract, and skeletal muscle, also increases with weight gain (14,21–23). The mechanisms responsible for increased regional blood flows have not been fully elucidated, but these increased regional blood flows are probably due in part to a higher metabolic rate and the local accumulation of local vasodilator metabolites, as well as to the growth of the organs and tissues in response to their increased metabolic demands.

Cardiac Hypertrophy and Remodeling and Impaired Systolic and Diastolic Function in Obesity

Obesity is associated with eccentric and concentric cardiac hypertrophy (24,25). These changes are more severe in obese subjects than they are in lean subjects with comparable hypertension (26) (Fig. 11.2). Because excess weight gain increases blood volume and venous return, the obese patient may have increased preload, cardiac dilation, and development of eccentric left ventricular hypertrophy. The rise in blood pressure in obesity also increases cardiac afterload, leading to increased left ventricular wall thickness. Thus, when obesity is combined with increased blood pressure, the cardiac workload is greatly amplified, leading to marked left ventricular hypertrophy. High sodium chloride intake, which often occurs concurrently with high caloric intake, exacerbates the obesity-induced cardiac hypertrophy (27). Moreover, the effect of high sodium chloride intake on obesity-induced cardiac hypertrophy can occur even without significant changes in arterial pressure (27).

Despite the higher cardiac output, obese subjects often develop impaired cardiac systolic and diastolic function. In animals fed a high-fat diet for 12 weeks, cardiac filling pressures were increased and diastolic dysfunction associated with decreased left ventricular compliance was evident even at this early stage of obesity (28). With more prolonged obesity, impaired systolic function may also be present. The mechanisms responsible for cardiac diastolic and systolic dysfunction in obesity are not well understood, but they probably involve structural changes in the heart, such as fibrosis, as well as functional changes, such as impaired β-adrenergic receptor signaling (29).

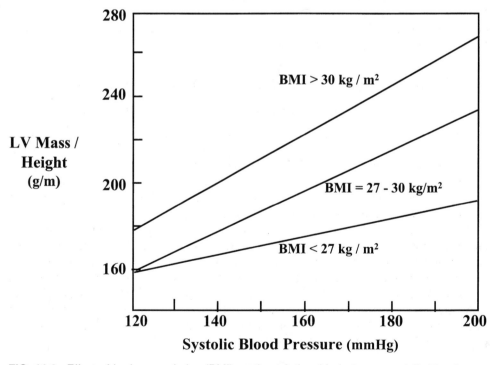

FIG. 11.2. Effect of body mass index (BMI) on the relationship between systolic blood pressure and left ventricular (LV) mass. (Data from Gottdiener JS, Reda DJ, Materson BJ, et al. Importance of obesity, race and age to the cardiac structural and functional effects of hypertension. *J Am Coll Cardiol* 1994;24:1492–1498, with permission.)

MECHANISMS OF OBESITY-RELATED HYPERTENSION: IMPAIRED RENAL PRESSURE NATRIURESIS

Excess renal sodium reabsorption appears to play a major role in initiating the rise in blood pressure associated with weight gain, and obese subjects require a higher than normal arterial pressure to maintain sodium balance, thus indicating the presence of impaired renal-pressure natriuresis (30,31). With prolonged obesity, chronic increases in arterial pressure, glomerular hyperfiltration, neurohumoral activation, and metabolic changes may cause renal injury, a further shift of pressure natriuresis, and more severe hypertension.

The following three mechanisms appear to be particularly important in mediating increased sodium reabsorption, impaired renal-pressure natriuresis, and hypertension associated with weight gain: (a) high sympathetic activity, (b) activation of the renin–angiotensin system (RAS), and (c) altered intrarenal physical forces and compression of the kidneys. Another mechanism, hyperinsulinemia, has been extensively studied, but it does not appear to be of major importance in raising blood pressure in obese subjects, although some investigators still disagree with this conclusion (32,33).

Sympathetic Activation Causes Sodium Retention and Raises Blood Pressure in Obesity

The following observations suggest that increased sympathetic activity contributes to obesity-related hypertension (3,34,35): (a) obese subjects have elevated sympathetic activity as assessed by both indirect and direct methods; (b) pharmacologic blockade of adrenergic activity reduces blood pressure to a greater extent in obese subjects than it does in lean subjects; and (c) renal denervation markedly attenuates sodium retention and the development of the obesity hypertension that is associated with a high-fat diet in experimental animals.

Obesity Increases Renal Sympathetic Activity

In comparison to lean subjects, obese people have a higher plasma norepinephrine concentration and an increased urinary excretion of norepinephrine (34,35). Norepinephrine spillover, a measure of neurotransmitter release, is also increased in the kidneys and hearts of obese hypertensive subjects compared to that in lean normotensive subjects (36–38). Muscle sympathetic activity, when measured directly with microneurographic methods, is also increased in obese humans (35). These observations suggest that obesity-related hypertension is associated with increased sympathetic activity in many tissues, although obesity *per se* appears to have a much greater effect on sympathetic activity in the kidneys than it does in some tissues, such as the heart, where sympathetic activity may actually be reduced in obese normotensive subjects (36,37,39).

Pharmacologic Blockade of Adrenergic Activity Attenuates Obesity-Related Hypertension

Studies in dogs and rabbits fed a high-fat diet indicate that the combined α-adrenergic and β-adrenergic blockade markedly attenuates the rise in blood pressure during the development of obesity (40,41). Clonidine, a drug that stimulates central α₂-receptors and reduces sympathetic activity, also markedly blunts the rise in blood pressure in dogs fed a high-fat diet (42). Finally, combining α-adrenergic and β-adrenergic blockade for 1 month reduced ambulatory blood pressure significantly more in obese essential hypertensive patients than it did in those who were lean (43). These findings suggest that increased adrenergic activity in part mediates the development and maintenance of obesity-related hypertension in experimental animals and in humans.

Renal Denervation Attenuates Sodium Retention and Increased Blood Pressure in Obesity

The renal sympathetic efferent nerves mediate much of the rise in blood pressure that is associated with sympathetic activation in obesity. In dogs fed a high-fat diet for 5 weeks, kidneys with intact renal nerves retained almost twice as much sodium as denervated kidneys (44). Also, bilateral renal denervation greatly attenuated sodium retention and hypertension in obese dogs (44) (Fig. 11.3). Thus, obesity increases renal tubular sodium reabsorption, impairs pressure natriuresis, and causes hypertension partially by increasing the renal sympathetic nerve activity.

Mechanisms of Sympathetic Activation in Obesity

Although the mechanisms that increase renal sympathetic activity in obesity have not been fully elucidated, the potential mediators include (a) hyperinsulinemia; (b) renal *afferent* nerves, which are stimulated by increased intrarenal pressures and subsequent activation of renal mechanoreceptors; (c) fatty acids; (d) angiotensin II (AngII); and (e) hyperleptinemia. Increased sympathetic activation in obesity-related hypertension has also been suggested to be caused by the potentiation of central chemoreceptor sensitivity and impaired baroreflex sensitivity (the reader is referred to other papers for discussion of these mechanisms [45,46]).

Hyperinsulinemia Does Not Mediate Obesity-Related Hypertension

Excess weight gain, particularly when associated with abdominal obesity, leads to insulin resistance, glucose intolerance, and hyperinsulinemia, which occurs as a compensation for the impaired metabolic effects of insulin. Not all tissues share in this insulin resistance, however, and the elevated insulin concentrations have been hypothesized to mediate obesity-related hypertension by stimulating sympathetic activity and by directly increasing renal tubular sodium reabsorption (35). Acute studies suggest that insulin infusion may cause modest sodium retention and increased sympathetic activity and that blood pressure is, not surprisingly, correlated with plasma insulin concentration (35).

Most of the available evidence suggests that chronic hyperinsulinemia does not mediate obesity-related hypertension. In humans and dogs, neither acute nor chronic hyperinsulinemia lasting for several weeks impairs renal-pressure natriuresis or increases arterial pressure (32). In fact, insulin infusions at rates that raise plasma concentrations to the levels found in obesity caused peripheral vasodilation and decreased arterial pressure (32) (Fig. 11.4). Insulin also did not potentiate the blood pressure or renal effects of other pressor substances, such as norepinephrine or AngII (32). Moreover, hyperinsulinemia did not increase arterial pressure in obese dogs that were resistant to the metabolic and vasodilator effects of insulin (33).

The authors also tested whether hyperinsulinemia could increase blood pressure through direct central nervous system (CNS) effects or direct renal effects by infusing

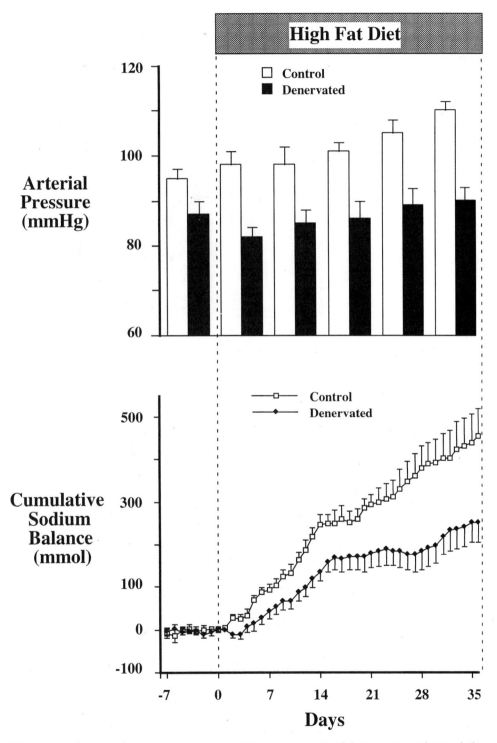

FIG. 11.3. Effects of 5 weeks of a high-fat diet on mean arterial pressure and cumulative sodium balance in dogs with innervated kidneys (control) and bilaterally denervated kidneys (denervated). (Data from Kassab S, Kato T, Wilkins C, et al. Renal denervation attenuates the sodium retention and hypertension associated with obesity. *Hypertension* 1995;25:893–897, with permission.)

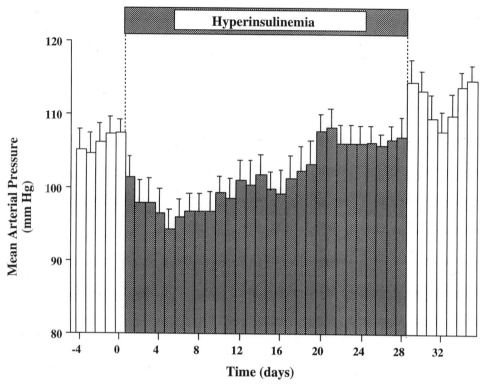

FIG. 11.4. Chronic blood pressure effects of hyperinsulinemia caused by intravenous insulin infusion in conscious, chronically instrumented dogs. Note that insulin infusion decreased arterial pressure, measured 24 hours a day. (Modified from Hall JE, Coleman TG, Mizelle HL, Smith MJ Jr. Chronic hyperinsulinemia and blood pressure regulation. *Am J Physiol* 1990;258: F722–F731, with permission.)

insulin directly into either the cerebral circulation or the renal arteries (47,48). Results from these studies have provided no evidence that selective CNS or renal hyperinsulinemia causes chronic hypertension. The observations in dogs are consistent with the finding that patients with insulinoma often have extremely high levels of insulin but no evidence of hypertension (49). Thus, multiple studies indicate that hyperinsulinemia cannot explain the sympathetic activation, increased renal tubular sodium reabsorption, impaired pressure natriuresis, or hypertension associated with obesity in humans or in dogs (32,50).

Although hyperinsulinemia can cause mild hypertension in rats, the rise in blood pressure does not appear to be mediated by sympathetic activation (51). Instead, insulin-induced hypertension in rats appears to be mediated by interactions of the RAS and thromboxane (52,53). This response may be unique for rats, in which renal thromboxane mediates most of the renal vasoconstrictor effects of AngII. This contrasts to dogs and humans, in which renal thromboxane production appears to be much less important in controlling renal function. Whether the finding that insulin raises blood pressure slightly in rats is relevant to obesity-related hypertension in humans is still unclear, but current evidence suggests that hyperinsulinemia cannot account for sympathetic activation and increased blood pressure in obese humans or obese dogs.

Renal Sensory Nerves Do Not Mediate Obesity-Related Hypertension

Intrarenal pressures are markedly elevated in obesity because of compression of the kidneys by adipose tissue and by the proliferation of the extracellular matrix in the kidney (3). The kidneys are richly endowed with mechanoreceptors that, when activated by increased intrarenal pressures, may stimulate renal afferent nerves and may potentially increase sympathetic activity (54). However, the surgical removal of renal sensory fibers by dorsal root rhizotomies between the T-10 and L-2 segments did not blunt the sodium retention or hypertension observed in dogs fed a high-fat diet (55). Thus, although the renal *efferent* sympathetic fibers contribute to sodium retention and hypertension, *afferent* pathways originating in the kidney do not appear to play a major role in stimulating sympathetic activity or raising blood pressure in obesity.

Do Elevated Fatty Acids Increase Sympathetic Activity and Blood Pressure in Obesity?

Obese hypertensive patients have high fasting plasma levels of nonesterified fatty acids (NEFAs) that are sometimes double those of normotensive subjects, and raising NEFA levels acutely increases vascular reactivity to α-adrenergic agonists (56,57). High levels of NEFA also enhance the reflex vasoconstrictor responses in the peripheral circulation (56). Both of these effects could increase the blood pressure responses to even normal levels of sympathetic stimulation.

High levels of fatty acids have also been suggested to activate the sympathetic nervous system indirectly through hepatic afferent pathways. Acute infusions of free fatty acids into the portal or systemic veins increased blood pressure and heart rate in rats; these effects were abolished by adrenergic blockade (57). Because the portal vein infusion of NEFA caused a greater increase in blood pressure than did systemic intravenous infusion, afferent pathways originating in the liver were postulated to activate the sympathetic nervous system in response to increased levels of fatty acids (57). In contrast to these observations, the authors of this chapter found no evidence in dogs to indicate that infusing a mixture of long-chain fatty acids for several days directly into the cerebral circulation or the portal vein (J.E. Hall and J. Henegar, *unpublished observations*, 1999) or intravenously either increased the arterial pressure or altered the renal function (58). Thus, the role of elevated fatty acids in linking obesity, sympathetic activation, and hypertension has not been clearly established, and it deserves further study.

Does Hyperleptinemia Link Obesity with Sympathetic Activation and Hypertension?

Another possible link between obesity and sympathetic activation is leptin, a peptide secreted by adipocytes in proportion to adiposity (59–62). Leptin from the plasma crosses the blood–brain barrier via a saturable receptor-mediated transport system, binds to its long-form receptors in the lateral and medial regions of the hypothalamus, and activates signaling pathways that regulate energy balance by reducing appetite and increasing energy expenditure through sympathetic stimulation (Fig. 11.5). Perhaps the most dramatic evidence that leptin acts as a negative feedback controller of food intake and body weight comes from the genetic studies of mice and humans. Mice that lack the ability to synthesize leptin because of a nonsense mutation of the leptin gene (e.g., *ob/ob* mice) or mice that have mutations of the leptin receptor (e.g., *db/db* mice) develop

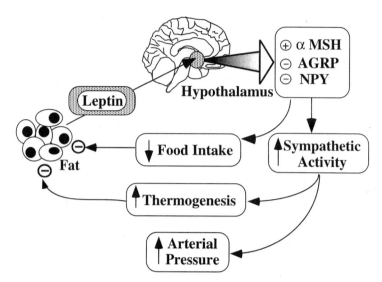

FIG. 11.5. Possible links between leptin and its effects on the hypothalamus, sympathetic activation, and hypertension. Leptin may mediate some of its effects on appetite and sympathetic activity by inhibiting (–) or stimulating (+) other neurochemical pathways, including α-melanocyte–stimulating hormone (α-MSH), agouti-related peptide (AGRP), and neuropeptide Y (NPY).

extreme obesity (59,63). Similar findings of profound early onset obesity have been reported in humans who have mutations of the leptin gene (63,64). Although the role of leptin in regulating energy balance has been extensively studied, its effects on sympathetic activity and cardiovascular function are not well understood.

Multiple studies in rats have shown that acute intravenous or intracerebroventricular infusions of leptin increase sympathetic activity in the kidneys, adrenals, and brown adipose tissue (60,62). Although leptin has very little acute effect on arterial pressure, chronic increases in leptin raise blood pressure in rodents (65–69) (Fig. 11.6). The rise in arterial pressure is slow in onset, and it occurs despite a reduction in food intake, which generally would tend to reduce arterial pressure. Transgenic mice overexpressing leptin also have increased blood pressures that are comparable to those produced by chronic leptin infusions (68,70). The chronic effects of leptin to raise arterial pressure and heart rate in rats appear to be mediated by sympathetic activation because combined α-adrenergic and β-adrenergic blockade completely abolished these responses during 14 days of leptin infusion (71).

An observation that points toward leptin as a mediator of obesity-related hypertension in rodents is the finding that obese mice that are leptin deficient and obese rats that have mutations of the leptin receptor usually have little or no increase in blood pressure compared to their lean counterparts (Table 11.2). The *ob/ob* mouse, for example, is extremely obese because it is unable to synthesize leptin, but it actually has *decreased* arterial pressure compared with its lean counterpart (72). Likewise, rat models of obesity that have mutations of the leptin receptor have normal or only slightly elevated arterial pressure compared to their lean counterparts (73). Therefore, both increased leptin synthesis and functional leptin receptors appear to be necessary for obesity to cause major increases in blood pressure in rodents. Whether this is true in other species or in humans, however, is still unclear.

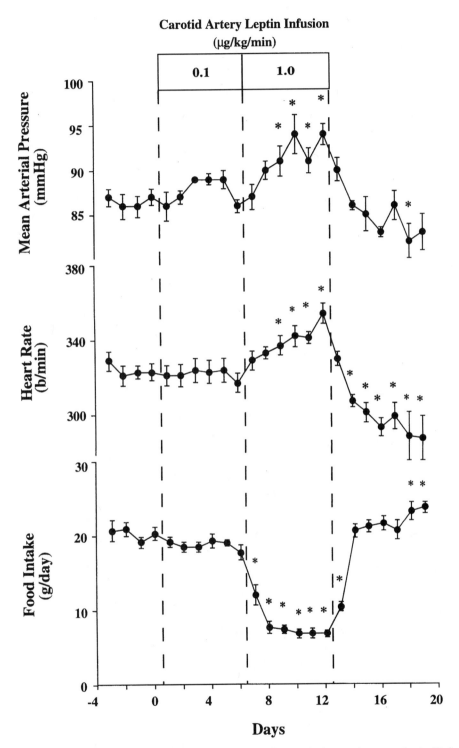

FIG. 11.6. Effect of bilateral carotid artery infusion of leptin at 0.1 g per kg per minute (5 days) and 1.0 g per kg per minute (7 days) on mean arterial pressure, heart rate, and daily food intake in conscious normal Sprague–Dawley rats. (Data from Shek EW, Brands MW, Hall JE. Chronic leptin infusion increases arterial pressure. *Hypertension* 1998;31:409–414, with permission.)

TABLE 11.2. *Genetic models of obesity with leptin abnormalities*

Model	Gene product	Hypertension
Zucker fatty rat (*fa/fa*)	Leptin receptor	Slight
Wistar fatty rat (*fa/fa*)	Leptin receptor	Slight
Diabetic mouse (*db/db*)	Leptin receptor	No
Koletsky SHR (fa^k)	Leptin receptor	No[a]
LA/N-cp/cp	Leptin receptor	No
SHR/N-cp/cp	Leptin receptor	No[b]
Dahl SS/N-cp/cp	Leptin receptor	No[b]
Osborne–Mendel	Leptin receptor	No
Obese mouse (*ob/ob*)	Leptin	No

[a]Koletsky spontaneously hypertensive rats (SHR) are hypertensive but they have lower blood pressure than their lean controls when they are fed a low sodium diet.

[b]SHR/N-cp/cp and Dahl salt-sensitive (SS)/N-cp/cp rats are hypertensive, but their blood pressures are not higher than those of their lean controls.

Is Obesity Associated with "Leptin Resistance?"

That most obese humans have high circulating leptin levels and continue to ingest excess calories has been interpreted as evidence for leptin "resistance," or a diminished responsiveness to leptin. To the extent that obesity induces resistance to the sympathoexcitatory response to leptin, the elevated leptin concentrations might cause a minimal stimulation of sympathetic activity in obese subjects (Fig. 11.7). Recently, the suggestion has

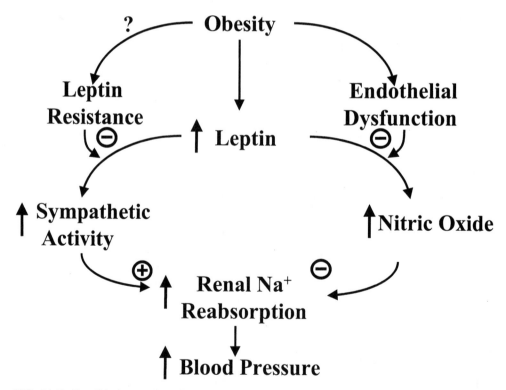

FIG. 11.7. Possible interactions between leptin, sympathetic activity, endothelial dysfunction, and leptin resistance in increasing renal tubular sodium (Na$^+$) reabsorption and mediating obesity hypertension. The net effect of leptin on blood pressure would depend on the degree of resistance to the sympathoexcitatory effects and the degree of endothelial dysfunction.

been made, however, that obesity induces "selective leptin resistance," whereby the sympathetic responses to leptin are maintained while the appetite-suppressing effects are blunted in obesity. Although some support is seen for this concept in rodents (74), no studies have assessed sympathetic responses to leptin in obese humans compared to those of lean humans.

Leptin also stimulates vasodepressor mechanisms, including nitric oxide formation, which may oppose the hypertensive effects of leptin (75,76). To the extent that obesity causes endothelial dysfunction and impaired nitric oxide release, one might expect greater blood pressure responses to hyperleptinemia in obese subjects than in lean subjects. Thus, the net effect of leptin on blood pressure in obesity depends on (a) the sensitivity of the hypothalamus to the sympathoexcitatory effects of leptin and (b) the severity of endothelial dysfunction. Currently, no studies have directly assessed the relative importance of these factors in modulating leptin's long-term effects on the control of blood pressure in obesity. Although leptin appears to contribute to increased blood pressure in obese rodents, its role in humans is less clear. At this time, no studies have evaluated the long-term cardiovascular actions of leptin in either obese or lean humans.

Activation of the Renin–Angiotensin System in Obesity

Even though excess weight gain is associated with sodium retention and the expansion of extracellular fluid volume, obese subjects usually have increases in plasma renin activity (PRA), plasma angiotensinogen, angiotensin-converting enzyme (ACE) activity, and plasma AngII levels (30,77). Possible mechanisms for increased renin secretion and activation of the RAS include (a) increased loop of Henle sodium chloride reabsorption and reduced sodium chloride delivery to the macula densa, as well as (b) activation of the renal sympathetic nerves (30,31). Increased angiotensinogen formation by adipose tissue has also been suggested to contribute to elevated AngII levels in obesity (77). Although the quantitative importance of these different pathways for forming AngII in obesity is uncertain, activation of the RAS appears to contribute to elevated blood pressure and target organ damage in obese subjects.

Blockade of the Renin–Angiotensin System Attenuates Obesity-Related Hypertension

A significant role for AngII in stimulating sodium reabsorption, impairing renal-pressure natriuresis, and causing hypertension in obesity is supported by the finding that treating dogs with an AngII antagonist or an ACE inhibitor blunts sodium retention and volume expansion and increases arterial pressure (78,79). Also, ACE inhibitors are effective in reducing blood pressure in obese humans, particularly in young patients (80).

Whether the effects of AngII to raise blood pressure in obesity are due primarily to direct actions on the kidneys or to sympathetic activation is unclear. The direct renal sodium-retaining effects of AngII are well known, and evidence also indicates that AngII has direct effects on the CNS. The physiologic role of AngII in stimulating thirst, for example, is well established, but controversy remains regarding the physiologic importance of the role of AngII in regulating sympathetic activity. Part of this controversy relates to the paucity of data on the effects of long-term physiologic increases in CNS AngII levels.

Blockade of the Renin–Angiotensin System
Attenuates Obesity-Induced Renal Injury

In addition to raising blood pressure, activation of the RAS may also contribute to the glomerular injury and nephron loss associated with obesity. Increased AngII formation constricts the efferent arterioles and exacerbates the rise in glomerular hydrostatic pressure that is caused by systemic arterial hypertension (81). Studies in patients with type II diabetes, who usually are obese, clearly indicate that ACE inhibitors slow the progression of renal disease (82). However, further studies are needed in nondiabetic obese subjects to determine the efficacy of RAS blockers compared to that of other antihypertensive agents in reducing the risk of renal injury.

Obesity May Increase Blood Pressure by Renal Compression

Adipose tissue almost completely encapsulates the kidneys, penetrates the renal hilum, and extends into the medullary sinuses of obese subjects, causing compression and increased intrarenal pressures (3,83). This may be analogous to the renal compression associated with the well-known experimental model of perinephritic hypertension, which is produced by wrapping the kidneys and by chronically increasing renal capsular pressure. The intraabdominal pressure of obese subjects also increases in proportion to the sagittal abdominal diameter, reaching levels as high as 35 to 40 mm Hg in some subjects with central obesity (84). Recent studies in dogs indicate that increasing intraabdominal pressure by 25 mm Hg for 4 weeks with an implanted inflatable balloon produced a 28-mm Hg rise in arterial pressure (85). Therefore, increases in intrarenal pressures caused by fat surrounding the kidneys and increased abdominal pressure may play a role in obesity-related hypertension (3,31).

Structural and Functional Changes in the Renal Medulla in Obesity

In addition to the external compression of the kidneys by retroperitoneal fat and fat in the abdominal cavity, changes in renal medullary histology could compress the renal medulla in obesity (31). Total glycosaminoglycan content and hyaluronan, a major component of the renal medullary extracellular matrix, are markedly elevated in the inner medulla, but not in the outer medulla or the cortex, of obese dogs and rabbits compared to their lean controls (86,87). Although the cause of increased hyaluronan in the renal medulla is unknown, its accumulation usually is associated with increased interstitial fluid pressure and tissue edema.

One possible consequence of these changes in the renal medulla is that they could further increase renal tissue pressure and compress the tubules and vasa recta. Because the kidney is surrounded by a capsule with low compliance, an increased extracellular matrix would raise interstitial fluid hydrostatic and solid tissue pressures, thus causing compression of the delicate thin loops of Henle and vasa recta. In support of this hypothesis, the authors found that renal interstitial fluid hydrostatic pressure was elevated to 19 mm Hg in obese dogs compared to a level of only 9 to 10 mm Hg in lean dogs (30). Although small increases in interstitial fluid pressure tend to inhibit renal sodium reabsorption, large increases of the magnitude found in obese dogs would tend to reduce renal medullary blood flow, slow the flow rate in the renal tubules, and raise fractional sodium reabsorption, particularly in the loop of Henle (30).

Increased loop of Henle sodium chloride reabsorption, which is caused by renal medullary compression, could also explain the elevated renal plasma flow and glomerular filtration rate (GFR), as well as the stimulation of renin secretion in obesity (Fig. 11.8). Increased sodium chloride reabsorption in the loop of Henle would decrease sodium chloride delivery to the macula densa and would cause, via tubuloglomerular feedback, reductions in the afferent arteriolar resistance and increases in the renal blood flow, GFR, and renin secretion (81). The increased GFR and elevated blood pressure resulting from sodium retention would tend to return distal sodium chloride delivery to normal in the face of increased loop reabsorption and would therefore help to restore sodium balance. Although renal compression obviously cannot explain the initial increase in blood pressure associated with rapid weight gain, it could contribute to the more sustained increases in tubular reabsorption, volume expansion, and hypertension associated with chronic obesity.

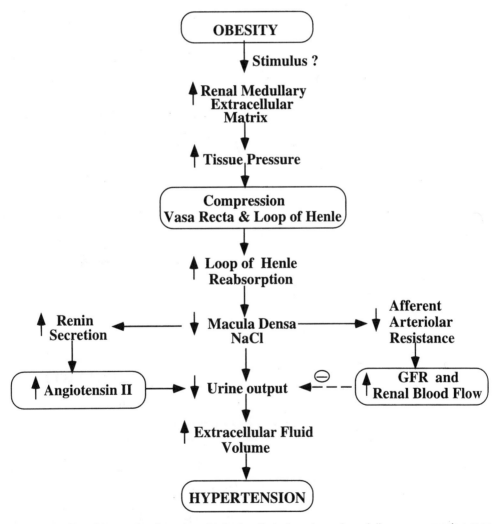

FIG. 11.8. Possible mechanisms by which obesity-induced renal medullary compression may contribute to activation of the renin–angiotensin system, increased loop of Henle sodium reabsorption, volume expansion, and hypertension. Abbreviation: GFR, glomerular filtration rate.

OBESITY AND CHRONIC RENAL DISEASE

Not only is abnormal kidney function a major cause of increased blood pressure during excessive weight gain, but chronic renal disease also appears to be an important consequence of prolonged obesity. In experimental animals, excess caloric intake causes renal disease and caloric restriction protects against glomerular injury (88). For example, more than 90% of obese Zucker rats die of ESRD (88). Restricting their food intake by only small amounts (8% to 18%) decreases renal injury and increases lifespan by about 25% to 30% (88) (Fig. 11.9). Similar observations have been made in other rodent models, indicating that food restriction can largely prevent renal pathology in obese and nonobese rats, although even "nonobese" rats fed *ad libitum* usually have large amounts of body fat (89).

No long-term studies have been done on the effects of food restriction or weight loss on renal function in humans. Although the evidence that excess weight gain *per se* causes renal disease is perhaps not as clear as it is in experimental animals, no doubt exists that

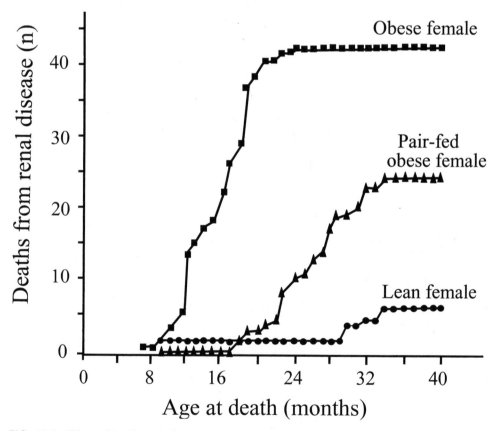

FIG. 11.9. Effect of food restriction on the cumulative death rate attributed to endstage renal disease in female obese and lean Zucker rats. Another group of obese Zucker rats was pair fed the same amount as that ingested by the lean rats. (Data from Stern JS, Gades MD, Wheeldon CM, et al. Calorie restriction in obesity: prevention of kidney disease in rodents. *J Nutr* 2001;131:913S–917S, with permission.)

obesity is closely associated with the two main causes of ESRD—diabetes and hypertension (90).

Early Glomerular Hyperfiltration May Contribute to Renal Injury in Obesity

The compensatory renal vasodilation, increased GFR, and higher blood pressure associated with obesity are important in overcoming increased sodium reabsorption. In the long term, increases in glomerular wall stress, particularly in the presence of other risk factors, such as hyperlipidemia and hyperglycemia, may eventually provoke glomerulosclerosis and the loss of functional nephrons, as has been observed in other conditions associated with glomerular hyperfiltration, such as type I diabetes.

Structural and Functional Changes in the Glomeruli in the Early Phases of Obesity

Although obesity-induced type II diabetes is recognized as a major cause of renal disease, the mechanisms that cause progressive nephron loss are unclear, and few clinical or experimental studies have examined changes in glomerular structure and function in the early stages of obesity before major disturbances of glucose metabolism occur. Obesity causes microalbuminuria, or even proteinuria, before major histologic changes occur in the glomerulus or evidence is found of glomerulosclerosis (91). In dogs with diet-induced obesity, the authors of this chapter found significant histologic changes in the glomeruli after 5 to 6 weeks of a high-fat diet (92). Substantial enlargement of the Bowman space, increased glomerular cell proliferation (i.e., increased proliferating cell nuclear antigen), increased mesangial matrix, thicker basement membranes, and increased expression of glomerular transforming growth factor β (TGF-β) were also seen (92).

In humans, an association between massive obesity and severe proteinuria was reported in 1974 by Weisinger et al. (93). In subsequent studies, obese subjects were observed to have glomerulomegaly and focal segmental glomerulosclerosis, even in the absence of diabetes (94). A review of 6,818 renal biopsies indicated that the incidence of obesity-related glomerulopathy, which was defined as combined focal segmental glomerulosclerosis and glomerulomegaly, rose tenfold from 1990 to 2000, coincident with the rapid increase in the prevalence of obesity during this period (94).

These early glomerular changes in obesity may be the precursors to the development of more severe glomerulosclerosis and the eventual loss of nephron function (Fig. 11.10). The initial renal vasodilation and glomerular hyperfiltration, in combination with increased arterial pressure, may cause marked increases in the glomerular hydrostatic pressure and stretch of glomerular capillaries and the associated mesangial cells. Thickening of glomerular basement membranes and proliferation of the mesangial matrix and fibrotic responses would initially prevent overstretching of the glomerular capillaries. However, in the long term, the structural fortification of the glomerulus would impinge on the glomerular lumen, reducing the filtration surface area, and could eventually cause glomerulosclerosis and loss of glomeruli. This would cause further impairment of the pressure natriuresis, additional sodium retention, and extra increases in arterial pressure. The increase in blood pressure would in turn serve the immediate need to maintain sodium balance, but, in the long term, it would promote further glomerular injury. Thus, glomerular hyperfiltration, particularly in the presence of hyperlipidemia and hyperglycemia, may initiate a slowly developing cycle that causes greater and greater nephron loss and higher blood pressure. In some obese persons, this cycle may progress to ESRD as diabetes and hypertension worsen. In others, the loss of renal function may occur

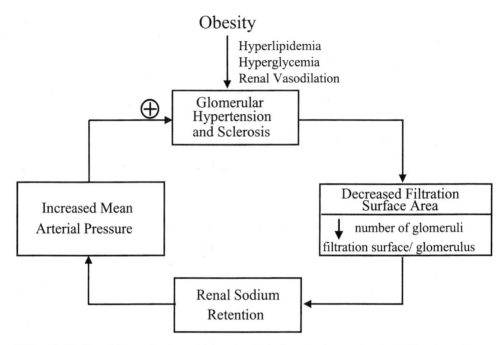

FIG. 11.10. Possible cycle by which obesity-induced glomerular hyperfiltration, hyper-glycemia, and hyperlipidemia lead to progressive renal injury. Loss of filtration surface area causes further sodium and water retention, increases in blood pressure, and more severe glomerular injury.

slowly enough that other morbidities, such as coronary artery disease, become more apparent before a serious decline of renal function occurs.

Although the mediators of the early glomerular structural changes associated with obesity are unknown, neurohumoral factors, such as AngII and sympathetic activity, and changes in intrarenal physical forces caused by high blood pressure and dilation of affer-ent arterioles probably play a significant role. The quantitative importance of these stim-uli and how they interact to cause mesangial cell proliferation and increased extracellu-lar matrix in the glomerulus are not well understood, but they probably involve a complex interplay of mechanical forces, cytokines, and growth factors. Synergistic relationships may exist among increased glomerular pressure and metabolic abnormalities such as hyperglycemia and hyperlipidemia that are similar to those that have been observed for coronary artery disease. In the Prospective Cardiovascular Munster (PROCAM) study, for example, the risk of myocardial infarction was increased about twofold by hyperten-sion and by about twofold by diabetes but by more than eightfold when hypertension and diabetes occurred together (95) (Fig. 11.11). When hypertension, diabetes, and hyper-lipidemia were present together, as occurs in many obese patients, the risk for myocardial infarction was increased by more than 20-fold (95). This suggests that hypertension, hyperglycemia, and hyperlipidemia act synergistically to cause coronary artery disease. A similar relationship may exist for renal disease, although, to the authors' knowledge, no large-scale studies have addressed this issue.

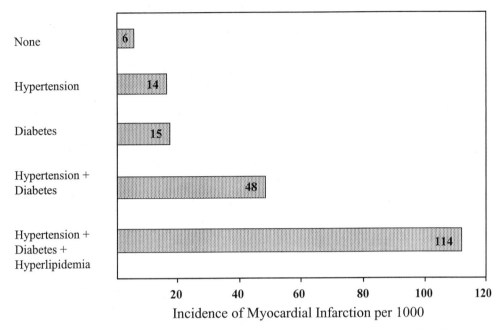

FIG. 11.11. Interaction among cardiovascular risk factors in the Prospective Cardiovascular Munster (PROCAM) study. The incidence of myocardial infarction is shown in a group of 2,574 men with no risk factors, hypertension only, diabetes only, hypertension and diabetes, or hypertension plus diabetes and hyperlipidemia. (Data from Assmann G, Schulte H. The Prospective Cardiovascular Munster Study (PROCAM): prevalence of hyperlipidemia in persons with hypertension and/or diabetes mellitus and the relationship to coronary artery disease. *Am Heart J* 1988;116:1713–1724, with permission.)

Is Obesity a Major Cause of Endstage Renal Disease?

The two leading causes of ESRD are diabetes and hypertension (90). As was discussed earlier, most essential hypertensive patients are overweight, and current evidence suggests that excess weight gain accounts for about 65% to 75% of the risk of essential hypertension. Type II diabetes, which is almost always closely linked to obesity, is responsible for at least 90% of diabetes mellitus and for most of the ESRD caused by diabetes. For example, in a study of a triethnic population in Texas, type II diabetes accounted for about 84% to 93% of diabetes-related ESRD in African Americans and Mexican Americans and for about 60% in white Americans (96). Similar results have been obtained in other populations. Thus, the two main risk factors for ESRD—hypertension and type II diabetes—are initiated mainly by obesity. In addition, the increase in the number of ESRD cases has closely paralleled the increasing prevalence of obesity in the last two decades, even though some other risk factors for vascular disease, such as smoking and hypercholesterolemia, have been decreasing (Fig. 11.12). Putting this information together suggests that excess weight gain may account for at least half of the ESRD in the United States. This conclusion, however, must be considered speculative until it has been tested with large population studies.

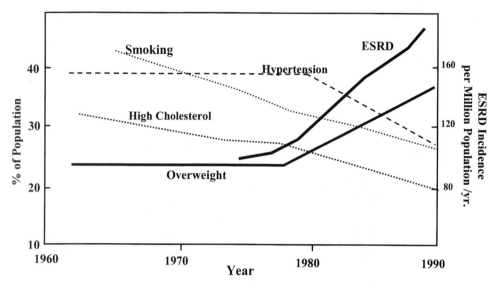

FIG. 11.12. Estimated prevalence of cardiovascular risk factors as assessed by the National Health and Nutrition Examination Surveys I, II, and III incidence of endstage renal disease (ESRD) reported by the United States Renal Data Systems Surveys.

TREATMENT OF OBESITY-RELATED HYPERTENSION AND RENAL DISEASE

As with many forms of hypertension, treatment of obesity-related hypertension and the associated renal disease is largely empiric. The kidney plays a central role in the pathophysiology of blood pressure elevation, and it is a major target for damage from elevated blood pressure. In obesity-related hypertension, the keys to breaking this cycle are reducing body weight and lowering blood pressure.

Lifestyle Modification: Weight Loss, Increased Physical Activity, and Decreased Sodium Intake

Lifestyle modifications have demonstrated their efficacy in the prevention and treatment of hypertension. Those changes that are particularly effective in the obese hypertensive patient include weight loss, increased physical activity, and decreased sodium intake (97).

Several studies have demonstrated that weight loss lowers blood pressures in normotensive or hypertensive obese subjects (98,99), and that weight loss can prevent the development of hypertension in persons with "high normal" blood pressures (98). Other studies have shown the utility of weight loss in reducing the amount of medication necessary to achieve blood pressure goals (11,100,101). Most studies on weight loss are limited by their relatively short-term duration or by the regain of weight after 6 to 12 months. The most common approach to promoting weight loss for obesity-related hypertension consists of a combination of behavior modification and education to increase energy expenditure (e.g., exercise) and/or reduce caloric intake (102). Other methods include the use of pharmacologic agents that induce satiety, increase thermogenesis, or decrease gastrointestinal fat absorption.

Surgical procedures are also options for patients with clinically severe obesity (BMI greater than or equal to 40 or BMI greater than or equal to 35 with comorbid conditions) when other methods of weight loss have failed and the patient has a high risk for obesity-associated morbidity or mortality (103). Unfortunately, the various methods that are used to promote weight loss are associated with very significant weight regain after the cessation of the intervention. Long-term maintenance of weight loss occurs in only about 20% of adults regardless of which methods are used (102).

The National Institutes of Health (NIH) recently released clinical guidelines for the treatment of obesity (102). Currently, two pharmacologic agents are approved by the Food and Drug Administration (FDA) to promote weight loss. One of these agents, sibutramine, is a sympathomimetic that induces satiety and increases thermogenesis; however, it may also cause an elevation in blood pressure even when weight loss occurs. The FDA suggests that this drug be used with caution in hypertensive patients. The current NIH guidelines on obesity suggest that sibutramine should not be used in persons with hypertension (102). The second agent, orlistat, is a gastrointestinal lipase inhibitor that reduces absorption of dietary fat by about 30% to 35%. Although clinical trials have shown that this drug can be used successfully to reduce body weight and blood pressure in some obese patients, its use is often limited by its unpleasant gastrointestinal side effects. Phentermine was used in the past in combination with fenfluramine. Fenfluramine was removed from use because of concerns about valvular heart disease and pulmonary hypertension. Few data are available regarding phentermine as monotherapy, but it is associated with elevated blood pressure in some users (102).

Increased aerobic physical activity has been demonstrated to help lower blood pressure in overweight and obese patients, partly by contributing to weight loss (102,105). Because obese patients often have exercise limitations, advice from a physician and an exercise prescription are often useful. The orthopedic problems associated with obesity sometimes limit the type of aerobic exercise that can be performed. Nonweightbearing forms of aerobic exercise, such as swimming, are often useful in obese patients (102).

Sodium restriction is beneficial in preventing and treating hypertension in some, but not all, hypertensive patients. In a metaanalysis of several studies, He et al. (106) found that obese persons had greater reductions in blood pressures than did nonobese persons when their sodium intake was restricted. However, the quantitative effect of sodium restriction on blood pressure in obese subjects depends on factors such as age, the severity of renal injury, and the presence or absence of diabetes. With progressive nephron loss in obese subjects, particularly after the onset of type II diabetes, the blood pressure becomes more and more salt sensitive, and a high sodium chloride level has a much greater effect on blood pressure. However, clinical trials addressing the factors that enhance the salt sensitivity of blood pressure in obesity have not been reported.

Pharmacotherapy of Hypertension in Obese Patients

The selection of specific drugs for management of obesity-related hypertension has been largely empiric, with little experimental evidence or guidelines as a basis for selection (97). Because most clinical trials involving patients with essential hypertension include many who are overweight or obese, some inferences can be drawn from randomized, controlled clinical trials for drug therapy of essential hypertension.

Antihypertensive agents are often chosen for their ability to lower blood pressure and to reduce other cardiovascular risk factors (e.g., hyperlipidemia and hyperglycemia), as well as with an understanding of the pathophysiology of obesity-related hypertension

(107–116). Obesity-related hypertension is often difficult to control with one drug, and it is associated with multiple factors that increase the cardiovascular risk. Therefore, combination therapy is often required for the effective management of obese hypertensive patients.

Diuretics

Diuretics are often useful for lowering blood pressure in obese hypertensive patients because of their ability to reduce renal sodium and water reabsorption and to decrease the extracellular fluid volume (109). Some clinicians prefer diuretics in obese patients because of strong evidence from randomized, controlled clinical trials that indicates that the use of diuretics to reduce blood pressure lowers cardiovascular morbidity and mortality (97). Because obese hypertensive patients often have glucose intolerance and dyslipidemia, some clinicians avoid diuretics, if possible, to avoid worsening these metabolic abnormalities (115). Although studies using high doses of diuretics have demonstrated significant adverse metabolic effects, such as worsening insulin resistance and increased plasma lipids, low-dose diuretics are less frequently associated with these effects (97), and, when used in combination with other agents, they can be quite useful in treating obesity-related hypertension.

β-Adrenergic Blockers

Like diuretics, β-adrenergic blockers have positive and negative attributes in treating the obese hypertensive patient (97). β-Blockers may be useful in countering some effects of obesity-induced sympathetic activation, such as the stimulation of renin secretion. As with diuretics, strong morbidity and mortality evidence exists for treatment of essential hypertension with β-blockers (97). Specifically, β-blockers are beneficial in patients who have had a myocardial infarction, and studies have demonstrated an effect of these drugs to decrease morbidity and mortality in diabetic patients (117). However, β-blockers clearly make losing weight more difficult for the obese patient, and, in some studies, they are associated with worsening glucose control, higher lipid levels, and an increase in body weight (117,118). Thus, although β-blockers may be indicated in obese hypertensive patients with ischemic heart disease and/or arrhythmias, other drugs may be preferable for initial therapy in obese patients who have no evidence of significant heart disease.

Angiotensin-Converting Enzyme Inhibitors

ACE inhibitors have theoretic advantages over other classes of antihypertensive agents in treating obesity-related hypertension. The activated RAS, which is manifested by elevated plasma renin levels in obese patients, suggests that these drugs should be effective in lowering blood pressure (116). The ability to attenuate glomerular hyperfiltration and urinary protein excretion presents an attractive means of managing blood pressure in this group of patients who are particularly prone to renal disease. The improved insulin sensitivity associated with ACE inhibitors is also a positive feature. One of the few randomized controlled trials in obese hypertensive patients included an ACE inhibitor. The Treatment of Obese Patients With Hypertension Study compared the blood pressure responses to the ACE inhibitor lisinopril and to the diuretic hydrochlorothiazide in obese hypertensive patients. Both agents effectively lowered systolic and diastolic blood pressure after 12 weeks of therapy. The African-American participants and the older participants were more likely to respond favorably to the diuretic, whereas the younger and white participants were more likely to respond to the ACE inhibitor (80).

Studies of hypertensive patients and patients with congestive heart failure have demonstrated that the response to ACE inhibitors depends on sodium intake and volume status. These drugs can be used with diuretics in the obese hypertensive patient for optimal blood pressure responses, even in patients who do not have elevated PRA (97).

Angiotensin II Receptor Antagonists

AngII receptor antagonists have not been studied extensively in obese hypertensive patients. In studies of patients with essential hypertension, they seem to have a blood pressure–lowering effect that is similar to that of the ACE inhibitors (97). Some differences between these two classes, including the effect of ACE inhibitors to increase kinin levels, may be responsible for subtle differences in the incidence of complications such as angioedema and cough. Obese patients would be likely to have similar blood pressure responses to ACE inhibitors and AngII antagonists. Extensive trials were recently completed in hypertensive patients, including those with diabetes, to examine the effects of AngII antagonists on cardiovascular morbidity and mortality and on the progression of renal disease. Two drugs in this class were demonstrated to prevent or to decrease proteinuria in hypertensive patients with type II diabetes mellitus (119–121).

α_1-Adrenergic Blocking Agents

Preliminary results of the Antihypertensive and Lipid-Lowering treatment to prevent Heart Attack Trial (ALLHAT) suggest that α-adrenergic blockers are not as effective as diuretics in preventing heart failure and cardiovascular disease. Therefore, these drugs will probably be used less as monotherapy for essential hypertension, including obesity hypertension. Because they have the beneficial effect of lowering plasma lipids, they may continue to play a role in combination therapy for managing obese hypertensive patients with dyslipidemia (122). They may also be useful as part of a combination of medications in many patients with resistant hypertension, which is commonly observed in obese hypertensive patients (114).

Calcium Channel Blockers

These drugs are frequently used to treat obese hypertensive patients. Their effectiveness seems to be less dependent on the status of blood volume, the RAS, and the sympathetic nervous system. Because calcium channel blockers are effective in a broad range of hypertensive patients, including obese subjects, they have gained popularity among clinicians (97). However, some studies suggest that calcium channel blockers are less effective in obese patients than they are in lean hypertensive patients (123,124).The dihydropyridine calcium antagonists have the potential disadvantage of further increasing the heart rate in obese patients. The nondihydropyridine calcium antagonists, in contrast, lower heart rate (97).

Clearly, a randomized, controlled clinical trial measuring morbidity and mortality with different treatments is needed to guide clinicians in drug selection for obese hypertensive patients. The ALLHAT study includes many overweight and obese hypertensive participants, so one may draw inferences about the relative effectiveness of the four classes tested (i.e., diuretics, ACE inhibitors, calcium antagonists, and α-blockers) in that study. In the meantime, clinicians should continue to use their best judgment, based on their understanding of the pathophysiology of obesity-related hypertension and the characteristics of the individual patient, in selecting a regimen of pharmacologic therapy that is appropriate for controlling blood pressure, attenuating the development of cardiovascular and renal disease, and avoiding the worsening of other metabolic disorders associated with obesity.

CONCLUSION

Excess weight gain is a major cause of increased blood pressure in most essential hypertensive patients, and it may be an important cause of ERSD. Obesity raises blood pressure by increasing renal tubular sodium reabsorption, impairing pressure natriuresis, and causing volume expansion. This is due in part to the activation of the sympathetic nervous system and the RAS and in part to renal compression caused by increased abdominal pressures, adhesion of adipose tissue to the renal capsule, and proliferation of the extracellular matrix in the kidneys. Although the mechanisms that cause sympathetic activation in obesity are poorly understood, current evidence suggests that increased levels of leptin acting via complex hypothalamic pathways may contribute to sympathetic activation in obese rodents. Whether this is true in obese humans is still unclear.

Renal vasodilation, glomerular hyperfiltration, and increased blood pressure initially help to compensate for increased tubular reabsorption in obesity, but the resultant increases in glomerular hydrostatic pressure and wall stress, along with the activation of neurohumoral mechanisms, hyperlipidemia, and hyperglycemia, eventually cause glomerular injury and the loss of nephron function. In experimental animals, clear evidence indicates that obesity causes a loss of glomerular function that worsens with time and that can progress to ESRD. In humans, the evidence is not as clear, although obesity is associated with proteinuria and glomerulopathy, even in the absence of diabetes. In addition, the two main causes of ESRD—diabetes and hypertension—are closely linked to obesity, suggesting that excess weight gain may account for a large component of ESRD.

Weight reduction is an essential first step in the management of obesity-related hypertension. However, currently, few specific guidelines exist for the treatment of obesity-related hypertension, other than the recommendation to reduce weight. This reflects the paucity of data available from clinical trials that compare the efficacy of different anti-hypertensive therapies in obese and lean patients. Special considerations in the obese patient with hypertension, in addition to controlling blood pressure, include correcting the metabolic abnormalities (e.g., hyperlipidemia and glucose intolerance) and protecting the kidney from injury. However, many unanswered questions about the pathophysiology and therapy of obesity linger, and these areas of research remain fruitful for further investigation, particularly in view of the current "epidemic" of obesity in most industrialized countries.

REFERENCES

1. Centers for Disease Control and Prevention, Office of Communications. *Obesity epidemic increases dramatically in the United States: CDC director calls for national prevention effort.* Rockville, MD: United States Department of Health and Human Services; October 26, 1999. Available at: www.cdc.gov/od/oc/media/pressrel/r991026.htm. Accessed September 2002.
2. Eckel RH, Krauss RM. American Heart Association call to action: obesity as a major risk factor for coronary heart disease. *Circulation* 1998;97:2099–2100.
3. Hall JE. Pathophysiology of obesity hypertension. *Curr Hypertens Rep* 2000;2:139–147.
4. Alexander J, Dustan HP, Sims EAH, et al. *Report of the Hypertension Task Force.* United States Department of Health, Education, and Welfare publication no. 70-1631. Washington, D.C.: United States Government Printing Office, 1979.
5. Jones DW, Kim JS, Andrew ME, et al. Body mass index and blood pressures in Korean men and women: the Korean National Blood Pressure Survey. *J Hypertens* 1994;12:1433–1437.

6. Garrison RJ, Kannel WB, Stokes J, et al. Incidence and precursors of hypertension in young adults: the Framingham Offspring Study. *Prev Med* 1987;16:234–251.
7. Cignolini M, Seidell JC, Targher JP, et al. Fasting serum insulin in relation to components of the metabolic syndrome in European healthy men: the European fat distribution study. *Metabolism* 1995;44:35–40.
8. Cooper, RS, Potimi CN, Ward R. The puzzle of hypertension in African-Americans. *Sci Am* 1999;280:56–63.
9. Reisen E, Abel R, Modan M, et al. Effect of weight loss without salt restriction on the reduction of blood pressure in overweight hypertensive patients. *N Engl J Med* 1978;198:1–6.
10. Blumenthal JA, Sherwood A, Gullette EC, et al. Exercise and weight loss reduce blood pressure in men and women with mild hypertension. *Arch Intern Med* 2000;160:1947–1958.
11. Jones DW, Miller ME, Wofford MR, et al. The effect of weight loss interventions on antihypertensive medication requirements in the Hypertension Optimal Treatment (HOT) study. *Am J Hypertens* 1999;12:1175–1180.
12. Stevens VJ, Obarzanek E, Cook NR, et al. Long-term weight loss and changes in blood pressure: results of the Trials of Hypertension Prevention, phase II. *Ann Intern Med* 2001;134:1–11.
13. Hall JE, Brands MW, Dixon WN, et al. Obesity-induced hypertension: renal function and systemic hemodynamics. *Hypertension* 1993;22:292–299.
14. Carrol JF, Huang M, Hester RL, et al. Hemodynamic alterations in obese rabbits. *Hypertension* 1995;26:465–470.
15. Rocchini AP, Mao HZ, Babu K, et al. Clonidine prevents insulin resistance and hypertension in obese dogs. *Hypertension* 1999;33:548–553.
16. Dobrian AD, Davies MJ, Prewitt RL et al. Development of a rat model of diet-induced obesity. *Hypertension* 2000;35:1009–1015.
17. Messerli FH, Christie B, DeCarvalho JG, et al. Obesity and essential hypertension. Hemodynamics, intravascular volume, sodium excretion and plasma renin activity. *Arch Intern Med* 1981;141:81–85.
18. Van Vliet BN, Hall JE, Mizelle HL, et al. Reduced parasympathetic control of heart rate in obese dogs. *Am J Physiol* 1995;269:H629–H637.
19. Verwaerde P, Senard JM, Galinier M, et al. Changes in short-term variability of blood pressure and heart rate during the development of obesity-associated hypertension in high-fat fed dogs. *J Hypertens* 1999;17:1135–1143.
20. Arone LJ, Mackintosh R, Rosenbaum M, et al. Autonomic nervous system activity in weight gain and weight loss. *Am J Physiol* 1995;269:R222–R225.
21. Rocchini AP. The influence of obesity in hypertension. *News Physiol Sci* 1990;5:245–249.
22. Reisin E, Messerli FH, Ventura HO, et al. Renal hemodynamics in obese and lean essential hypertensive patients. In: Messerli FH, ed. *Kidney in essential hypertension.* Boston: Martinus Nijhoff, 1984:125–129.
23. Hall JE. Renal and cardiovascular mechanisms of hypertension in obesity. *Hypertension* 1994;23:381–394.
24. Carroll JF, Braden DS, Cockrell K, et al. Obese rabbits develop concentric and eccentric hypertrophy and diastolic filling abnormalities. *Am J Hypertens* 1997;10:230–233.
25. Alpert MA. Obesity cardiomyopathy and the evolution of the clinical syndrome. *Am J Med Sci* 2001;321:225–236.
26. Gottdiener JS, Reda DJ, Materson BJ, et al. Importance of obesity, race and age to the cardiac structural and functional effects of hypertension. *J Am Coll Cardiol* 1994;24:1492–1498.
27. Carroll JF, Braden DS, Henegar JR, et al. Dietary sodium chloride (NaCl) worsens obesity-related cardiac hypertrophy [Abstract]. *FASEB J* 1998;12:A708.
28. Carroll JF, Summers RL, Dzielak DJ, et al. Diastolic compliance is reduced in obese rabbits. *Hypertension* 1999;33:811–815.
29. Carroll JF. Post–beta receptor defect in isolated hearts of obese-hypertensive rabbits. *Int J Obes Relat Metab Disord* 1999;23:863–866.
30. Hall JE, Brands MW, Henegar JR. Mechanisms of hypertension and kidney disease in obesity. *Ann N Y Acad Sci* 1999;892:91–107.
31. Hall JE. Mechanisms of abnormal renal sodium handling in obesity hypertension. *Am J Hypertens* 1997;10:S49–S55.
32. Hall JE. Hyperinsulinemia: a link between obesity and hypertension? *Kidney Int* 1993;43:1402–1417.
33. Hall JE, Brands MW, Zappe DH, et al. Hemodynamic and renal responses to chronic hyperinsulinemia in obese, insulin resistant dogs. *Hypertension* 1995;25:994–1002.
34. Tuck ML, Sowers J, Dornfield L, et al. The effect of weight reduction on blood pressure, plasma renin activity, and plasma aldosterone levels in obese patients. *N Engl J Med* 1981;304:930–933.
35. Landsberg L, Krieger DR. Obesity, metabolism, and the sympathetic nervous system. *Am J Hypertens* 1989;2:1255–1325.
36. Rumantir MS, Vaz M, Jennings GL, et al. Neural mechanisms in human obesity-related hypertension. *J Hypertens* 1999;17:1125–1133.
37. Esler M. The sympathetic system and hypertension. *Am J Hypertens* 2000;13:99S–105S.
38. Mansuo K, Mikami H, Ogihara T, et al. Weight gain–induced blood pressure elevation. *Hypertension* 2000;35:1135–1140.
39. Grassi G, Servalle G, Cattaneo BM, et al. Sympathetic activity in obese normotensive subjects. *Hypertension* 1995;25:560–563.
40. Antic V, Kiener-Belforti F, Tempini A, et al. Role of the sympathetic nervous system during the development of obesity hypertension in rabbits. *Am J Hypertens* 2000;13:556–559.

41. Zappe DH, Kassab SE, Brands MW, et al. Chronic adrenergic blockade attenuates the development of hypertension due to weight gain in dogs. *FASEB J* 1995;9:A296.
42. Rocchini AP, Mao HZ, Babu K, et al. Clonidine prevents insulin resistance and hypertension in obese dogs. *Hypertension* 1999;33:548–553.
43. Wofford MR, Anderson DC, Brown CA, et al. Antihypertensive effect of alpha and beta adrenergic blockade in obese and lean hypertensive subjects. *Am J Hypertens* 2001;14:164–168.
44. Kassab S, Kato T, Wilkins C, et al. Renal denervation attenuates the sodium retention and hypertension associated with obesity. *Hypertension* 1995;25:893–897.
45. Grassi G, Seravalle G, Columbo M, et al. Body weight reduction sympathetic nerve traffic and arterial baroreflex in obese normotensive humans. *Circulation* 1998;97:2037–2042.
46. Narkiewicz K, Kato M, Pesek CA, et al. Human obesity is characterized by selective potentiation of central chemoreflex sensitivity. *Hypertension* 1999;33:1153–1158.
47. Hildebrandt DA, Smith MJ Jr, Hall JE. Cardiovascular regulation during acute and chronic vertebral artery insulin infusion in conscious dogs. *J Hypertens* 1999;17:252–260.
48. Hall JE, Brands MW, Mizelle HL, et al. Chronic intrarenal hyperinsulinemia does not cause hypertension. *Am J Physiol* 1991;260:F663–F669.
49. Sawicki DT, Heinemann L, Starke A, et al. Hyperinsulinemia is not linked with blood pressure elevation in patients with insulinoma. *Diabetologia* 1992;35:649–652.
50. Hall JE, Summers RL, Brands MW, et al. Resistance to metabolic actions of insulin and its role in hypertension. *Am J Hypertens* 1994;7:772–788.
51. Keen HL, Brands MW, Alonso-Galicia M, et al. Chronic adrenergic receptor blockade does not prevent hyperinsulinemia-induced hypertension in rats. *Am J Hypertens* 1996;9:1192–1199.
52. Brands MW, Harrison DL, Keen HL, et al. Insulin-induced hypertension in rats is dependent on an intact renin–angiotensin system. *Hypertension* 1997;29:1014–1019.
53. Keen HL, Brands MW, Smith MS Jr, et al. Inhibition of thromboxane synthesis attenuates insulin-hypertension in rats. *Am J Hypertens* 1997;10:1125–1131.
54. DiBona GF, Kopp U. Neural control of renal function. *Physiol Rev* 1997;77:75–197.
55. Zappe DH, Capel WT, Keen HL, et al. Role of renal afferent nerves in obesity-induced hypertension [Abstract]. *Am J Hypertens* 1996;9:20A.
56. Stepniakowski KT, Goodfriend TL, Egan BM. Fatty acids enhance vascular α-adrenergic sensitivity. *Hypertension* 1995;25:774–778.
57. Grekin RJ, Dumont CJ, Vollmer AP, et al. Mechanisms in the pressor effects of hepatic portal venous fatty acid infusion. *Am J Physiol* 1997;273:R324–R330.
58. Hildebrandt DA, Kirk D, Hall JE. Renal and cardiovascular responses to chronic increases in cerebrovascular free fatty acids [Abstract]. *FASEB J* 1999;13:A780.
59. Zhjang Y, Proenca R, Maffei M, et al. Positional cloning of the mouse obese gene and its human homologue. *Nature* 1994;372:425–432.
60. Haynes WG, Sivitz WI, Morgan DA, et al. Sympathetic and cardiorenal actions of leptin. *Hypertension* 1997;30:619–623.
61. Hall JE, Shek EW, Brands MW. Is leptin a link between obesity and hypertension? *Curr Opin Endocrinol Diabetes* 1999;6:225–229.
62. Haynes WG, Morgan DA, Walsh SA, et al. Cardiovascular consequences of obesity: role of leptin. *Clin Exp Pharmacol Physiol* 1998;25:65–69.
63. Flier JS. What's in a name? In search of leptin's physiologic role. *J Clin Endocrinol Metab* 1998;83:1407–1413.
64. Flier JS, Maratos-Flier E. Obesity and the hypothalamus: novel peptides for new pathways. *Cell* 1998;92:437–440.
65. Casto RM, VanNess JM, Overton JM. Effects of central leptin administration on blood pressure in normotensive rats. *Neurosci Lett* 1998;246:29–32.
66. Mark AL, Correia M, Morgan DA, et al. Obesity-induced hypertension: new concepts from the emerging biology of obesity. *Hypertension* 1999;33:537–541.
67. Lembo G, Vecchione C, Fratta L, et al. Leptin induces direct vasodilation through distinct endothelial mechanisms. *Diabetes* 2000;49:293–297.
68. Shek EW, Brands MW, Hall JE. Chronic leptin infusion increases arterial pressure. *Hypertension* 1998;31:409–414.
69. Correia ML, Morgan DA, Sivitz WI, et al. Leptin acts in the central nervous system to produce dose-dependent changes in arterial pressure. *Hypertension* 2001;27:936–942.
70. Aizawa-Abe M, Ogawa Y, Mazuzaki H, et al. Pathophysiological role of leptin in obesity related hypertension. *J Clin Invest* 2000;105:1243–1252.
71. Carlyle M, Jones OB, Kuo JJ, et al. Chronic cardiovascular and renal actions of leptin—role of adrenergic activity. *Hypertension* 2002;39:496–501.
72. Mark AL, Shaffer RA, Correia ML, et al. Contrasting blood pressure effects of obesity in leptin-deficient *ob/ob* mice and agouti yellow mice. *J Hypertens* 1999;17:1949–1953.
73. Hall JE, Hildebrandt DA, Kuo JJ. Obesity hypertension: role of leptin and sympathetic nervous system. *Am J Hypertens* 2001;14:103S–115S.
74. Rahmouni K, Haynes WG, Morgan DA, et al. Selective resistance to central administration of leptin in agouti obese mice. *Hypertension* 2002;39:486–490.

75. Frubeck G. Pivotal role of nitric oxide in the control of blood pressure after leptin administration. *Diabetes* 1999;48:903–908.
76. Kuo J, Jones OB, Hall JE. Inhibition of NO synthesis enhances chronic cardiovascular and renal actions of leptin. *Hypertension* 2001;37:670–676.
77. Engeli S, Sharma AM. The renin angiotensin system and natriuretic peptides in obesity associated hypertension. *J Mol Med* 2001;79:21–29.
78. Hall JE, Henegar JR, Shek EW, et al. Role of renin–angiotensin system in obesity hypertension [Abstract]. *Circulation* 1997;96:I-33.
79. Robles RG, Villa E, Santirso R, et al. Effects of captopril on sympathetic activity, lipid and carbohydrate metabolism in a model of obesity-induced hypertension in dogs. *Am J Hypertens* 1993;6:1009–1019.
80. Reisen E, Weir M, Falkner B, et al. Lisinopril versus hydrochlorothiazide in obese hypertensive patients: a multicenter placebo-controlled trial. *Hypertension* 1997;30:140–145.
81. Hall JE, Brands MW, Henegar JR. Angiotensin II and long-term arterial pressure regulation: the overriding dominance of the kidney. *J Am Soc Nephrol* 1999;10:S258–S265.
82. Ravid M, Lang R, Rachmani R, et al. Long-term renoprotective effect of angiotensin-converting enzyme inhibition in non–insulin-dependent diabetes mellitus. A 7-year follow-up study. *Arch Intern Med* 1996;156: 286–289.
83. Dwyer TM, Bigler SA, Moore NA, et al. The altered structure of renal papillary outflow tracts in obesity. *Ultrastruct Pathol* 2000;24:251–257.
84. Sugarman HJ, Windsor ACJ, Bessos MK, et al. Intra-abdominal pressure, sagittal abdominal diameter and obesity co-morbidity. *J Intern Med* 1997;241:71–79.
85. Bloomfield GL, Sugarman HJ, Blocker CR, et al. Chronically increased intra-abdominal pressure produced systemic hypertension in dogs. *Int J Obes Relat Metab Disord* 2000;24:819–824.
86. Dwyer TM, Banks SA, Alonso-Galicia M, et al. Distribution of renal medullary hyaluronan in lean and obese rabbits. *Kidney Int* 2000;58:721–729.
87. Alonso-Galicia M, Brands MW, Zappe DH, et al. Hypertension in obese Zucker rats: role of angiotensin II. *Hypertension* 1996;28:1047–1054.
88. Stern JS, Gades MD, Wheeldon CM, et al. Calorie restriction in obesity: prevention of kidney disease in rodents. *J Nutr* 2001;131:913S–917S.
89. Reisin E, Azar S, DeBoisblanc BP, et al. Low calorie unrestricted protein diet attenuates renal injury in hypertensive rats. *Hypertension* 1993;21:971–974.
90. The National Institutes of Health. *United States renal data system: 1994 annual report.* Ann Arbor, MI: University of Michigan, 1994:xxi.
91. Wesson DE, Kurtzman NA, Prommer JP. Massive obesity and nephrotic proteinuria with a normal renal biopsy. *Nephron* 1985;40:235–237.
92. Henegar, JR, Bigler SA, Henegar LK, et al. Functional and structural changes in the kidney in the early stages of obesity. *J Am Soc Nephrol* 2001;12:1211–1217.
93. Weisinger JR, Kempson RL, Eldridge L, et al. The nephrotic syndrome: a complication of massive obesity. *Ann Intern Med* 1974;81:440–447.
94. Kambham N, Markowitz GS, Valeri AM, et al. Obesity related glomerulopathy: an emerging epidemic. *Kidney Int* 2001;59:1498–1509.
95. Assmann G, Schulte H. The Prospective Cardiovascular Munster Study (PROCAM): prevalence of hyperlipidemia in persons with hypertension and/or diabetes mellitus and the relationship to coronary artery disease. *Am Heart J* 1988;1116:1713–1724.
96. Pugh JA, Medina RA, Cornell JC, et al. NIDDM is the major cause of end-stage renal disease. More evidence from a tri-ethnic population. *Diabetes* 1995;44:1375–1380.
97. Joint National Committee on Prevention, Detection, Evaluation, and Treatment of High Blood Pressure. The sixth report of the Joint National Committee on Prevention, Detection, Evaluation, and Treatment of High Blood Pressure. *Arch Intern Med* 1997;157:2413–2446.
98. The Trials of Hypertension Prevention Collaborative Research Group. The effects of nonpharmacologic interventions on blood pressure of persons with high normal levels. Results of the Trials of Hypertension Prevention, phase I. *JAMA* 1992;267:1213–1220.
99. Whelton PK, Appel LJ, Espeland MA, et al. Sodium reduction and weight loss in the treatment of hypertension in older persons: a randomized controlled trial of nonpharmacologic interventions in the elderly (TONE). TONE Collaborative Research Group. *JAMA* 1998;279:839–846.
100. Davis BR, Blaufoz MD, Oberman A, et al. Reduction in long-term antihypertensive medication requirements. Effects of weight reduction by dietary intervention in overweight persons with mild hypertension. *Arch Intern Med* 1993;153:1773–1782.
101. Imai Y, Sato K, Abe K, et al. Effects of weight loss on blood pressure and drug consumption in normal weight patients. *Hypertension* 1986;8:223–228.
102. National Institutes of Health, National Heart, Lung and Blood Institutes. Clinical guidelines on the identification, evaluation, and treatment of overweight and obesity in adults: the evidence report. *Obes Res* 1998;6: 51S–209S.
103. Coelho JC, Campos AC. Surgical treatment of morbid obesity. *Curr Opin Clin Nutr Metab Care* 2001;4: 201–206.
104. Yanovski SZ, Yanovski JA. Drug therapy: obesity. *N Engl J Med* 2002;346:591–602.

105. Paffenbarger R. Physical exercise to reduce cardiovascular disease risk. *Proc Nutr Soc* 2001;59:421–422.

106. He J, Ogden LG, Vupputuri S, et al. Dietary sodium intake and subsequent risk of cardiovascular disease in overweight adults. *JAMA* 1999;282:2027–2034.

107. Fuenmayor NT, Moreira E, de los Rios V, et al. Relations between fasting serum insulin, glucose, and dihydroepiandrosterone-sulfate concentrations in obese patients with hypertension: short-term effects of antihypertensive drugs. *J Cardiovasc Pharmacol* 1997;30:523–527.

108. Edelson GW, Sowers JR. Insulin resistance in hypertension: a focused review. *Am J Med Sci* 1993;306:345–347.

109. Reisin E, Weed SG. The treatment of obese hypertensive black women: a comparative study of chlorthalidone versus clonidine. *J Hypertens* 1992;10:489–493.

110. Tuck ML. Metabolic considerations in hypertension. *Am J Hypertens* 1990;3:355S–365S.

111. Schmieder RE, Gatzka C, Schachinger H, et al. Obesity as a determinant for response to antihypertensive treatment. *BMJ* 1993;207:537–539.

112. Kuperstein R, Sasson Z. Effects of antihypertensive therapy on glucose and insulin metabolism and on left ventricular mass: a randomized, double-blind, controlled study of 21 obese hypertensives. *Circulation* 2000;102: 1802–1806.

113. Reisin E, Tuck ML. Obesity-associated hypertension: hypothesized link between etiology and selection of therapy. *Blood Press Monit* 1999;4:S23–S26.

114. Kaplan NM. Obesity in hypertension: effects on prognosis and treatment. *J Hypertens* 1998;16:S35–S37.

115. Bakris GL, Weir MR, Sowers JR. Therapeutic challenges in the obese diabetic patient with hypertension. *Am J Med* 1996;101:33S–46S.

116. Kolanowski J. Obesity and hypertension: from pathophysiology to treatment. *Int J Obes Relat Metab Disord* 1999;23:42–46.

117. United Kingdom Prospective Diabetes Study Group. Efficacy of atenolol and captopril in reducing risk of both macrovascular and microvascular complications in type 2 diabetes (UKPDS 39). *BMJ* 1998;317:713–720.

118. Zanella MT, Kohlmann O Jr, Ribeiro AB. Treatment of obesity hypertension and diabetes syndrome. *Hypertension* 2001;38:705–708.

119. Lewis EJ, Hunsicker LG, Clark WR, et al. Renoprotective effect of the angiotensive receptor antagonist irbesartan in patients with nephropathy due to type 2 diabetes. *N Engl J Med* 2001;345:851–860.

120. Brenner BM, Cooper ME, deZeeuw D, et al. Effects of losartan on renal and cardiovascular outcomes in patients with type 2 diabetes and nephropathy. *N Engl J Med* 2001;345:861–869.

121. Parving HH, Lehnert H, Brochner-Mortensen J, et al. The effect of irbesartan on the development of diabetic nephropathy inpatients with type 2 diabetes. *N Engl J Med* 2001;345:870–878.

122. Black HR. The addition of doxazosin to the therapeutic regimen of hypertensive patients inadequately controlled with other antihypertensive medications. *Am J Hypertens* 2000;13:468–474.

123. Stoa-Birketvedt G, Thom E, Aarbakke J, et al. Body fat as a prediction of the antihypertensive effect of nifedipine. *J Intern Med* 1995;237:169–173.

124. Sharma AM, Pischon T, Engeli S, et al. Choice of drug treatment for obesity-related hypertension: where is the evidence? *J Hypertens* 2001;19:667–674.

12

Hepatobiliary Complications of Obesity

Gregory T. Everson and Marcelo Kugelmas

This chapter describes a group of disorders of the liver and biliary tract that occur with increased frequency in patients with obesity. The following topics are covered: cholelithiasis, steatosis, nonalcoholic steatohepatitis (NASH), the role of steatosis and NASH in the progression of other liver diseases, and the impact of obesity on outcome after liver transplantation. The specific aims are to introduce the reader to the epidemiology and pathogenesis of these disorders, to define the key clinical syndromes, to provide methods for diagnosis, and to elucidate the natural history and impact of therapy.

BILIARY COMPLICATIONS OF OBESITY: CHOLELITHIASIS

Epidemiology and Risk Factors

Approximately 750,000 cholecystectomies are performed annually in the United States for gallstone-related disease. The estimated total cost of medical care exceeds $7 billion per year. Most gallstones are composed predominantly of cholesterol, and risk factors for gallstones include age, female gender, the use of exogenous estrogen or contraceptive steroids, pregnancy, obesity, and rapid weight loss in obese subjects (1–4). Gallstones are highly prevalent in Hispanic populations and in Native American populations of the southwestern United States (5,6). The rising prevalence of obesity in the United States population will continue to fuel gallstone risk and the rates of cholecystectomy.

The relationship of gallstone disease to obesity is particularly evident in women. In the Nurses Health Study (7), which followed nearly 90,000 women for 8 years, the annual incidence of gallstone disease was directly related to body mass index (BMI) (Table 12.1). Incidence rates in this cohort ranged from 3.7 (for BMI from 30 to 35 kilograms per meter squared [kg/m^2]) to 7.4 (for BMI greater than 45 kg/m^2) times greater than the rate of incidence of gallstone disease in women with a BMI of less than 24 kg/m^2.

The prevalence of and risk factors for gallbladder disease in adults from the ages of 20 to 74 years in the United States were recently examined in the National Health and Nutrition Examination Survey III (NHANES-III) (3). Screening ultrasonography was performed in more than 14,000 participants in NHANES-III, and gallbladder disease was defined by either the presence of cholelithiasis or prior gallbladder surgery. Based on NHANES-III results, the projected overall prevalence of gallbladder disease in the United States was estimated at 20.5 million, with 8.7 million having had a prior cholecystectomy.

The prevalence of gallbladder disease was greater in women, and it increased with age in both men and women. The difference in prevalence between men and women was greatest in the younger age-groups. In women, the risk of gallbladder disease correlated with the number of completed pregnancies, the use of cigarettes, and reduced physical

TABLE 12.1. *Incidence of cholecystectomy and symptomatic gallstones in women: direct relationship to body mass index*

Body mass index (kg/m²)	Incidence per 100,000 person-yr	Relative risk
<24	277	1 (referent)
24 to <25	389	1.43
25 to <26	482	1.74
26 to <27	582	2.11
27 to <29	685	2.53
29 to <30	729	2.67
30 to <35	1,012	3.69
35 to <40	1,287	4.72
40 to <45	1,504	5.11
>45	2,091	7.36

Data from Stampfer MJ, Maclure KM, Colditz GA, et al. Risk of symptomatic gallstones in women with severe obesity. *Am J Clin Nutr* 1992; 52:652–658, with permission.

activity. In both sexes, alcohol consumption was associated with a lower risk of gallbladder disease, and diabetes mellitus was associated with a higher risk.

In NHANES-III, gallstone risk was associated with measurements of obesity, particularly central obesity, in both men and women (8). Ultrasonography and anthropometric analysis were performed in 13,962 subjects, and fasting leptin concentration was determined in a random sample of 5,568 subjects. Multivariate analysis of risk factors in the cohort of women demonstrated independent positive correlations between gallstone risk and both BMI and waist to hip ratio (WHR) (Fig. 12.1A). Central obesity, as measured by WHR, accounted for only a proportion of the risk related to BMI. In contrast, multivariate analysis of risk factors in the cohort of men demonstrated an independent positive correlation only with the WHR (Fig. 12.1B). Central obesity did account for all of the risk related to BMI in men. The failure of BMI to correlate independently with gallstone risk is related either to the higher lean body mass and different morphology of men compared to that of women or to the uniquely dominant effect of central obesity in men. Serum leptin concentration, which correlates strongly with BMI, was only associated with gallstone disease in women after adjustment for WHR (Fig. 12.2). However, leptin concentration was not an independent predictor of gallstone risk in either women or men after adjusting for BMI. These data indicate that obesity, particularly central obesity, is a major risk factor for cholelithiasis and gallbladder disease. The magnitude of the effect of obesity on gallstone risk is greater in women than it is men.

Ethnic differences in the prevalence of cholelithiasis were also examined in NHANES-III (3). Non-Hispanic black men had the lowest prevalence of gallbladder disease (Fig. 12.3). Hispanic women had the highest prevalence of gallbladder disease, even after controlling for comorbid conditions and other risk factors. Non-Hispanic black women had a lower risk of gallbladder disease, compared to that of either Hispanic or non-Hispanic white women (Fig. 12.3). This difference among groups of women was particularly pronounced at an older age and with increasing BMI.

Weight loss in obese individuals further increases the risk of forming gallstones (9). The greatest risk occurs with rapid weight loss resulting from either following very low calorie diets (VLCDs) or undergoing weight loss operations, such as gastric bypass (10–16). The overall risk of developing gallstones within 4 to 6 months of use of a VLCD

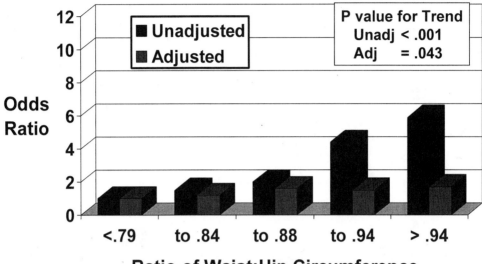

A

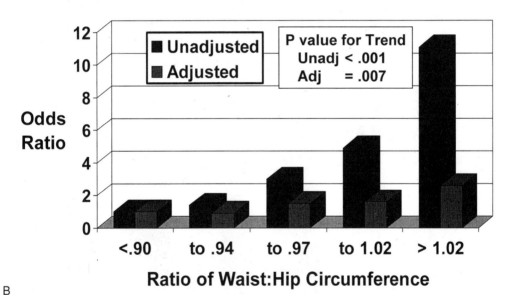

B

FIG. 12.1. **A:** Risk of gallbladder disease in women and correlation to waist to hip ratio. **B:** Risk of gallbladder disease in men and correlation to waist to hip ratio. Abbreviations: Adj, adjusted; Unadj, unadjusted.

ranges from 10% to 25%. Gallstone risk is 30% to 40% within 6 to 18 months of the performance of gastric bypass. Gallstone risk may be proportional to the rate and magnitude of weight loss. Intervention trials suggest that slower rates of weight loss, the use of aspirin or ursodeoxycholic acid, or the ingestion of as little as 10 g of fat per day may reduce the risk of formation of gallstones (9–12,14). Many surgeons perform a prophylactic cholecystectomy as part of the weight loss operation to avoid the subsequent risk of cholelithiasis and gallbladder disease.

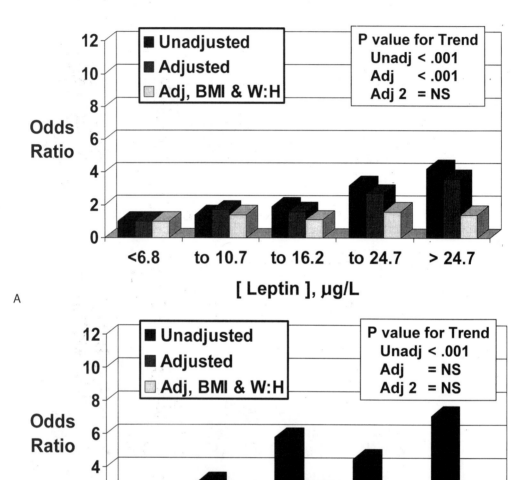

FIG. 12.2. A: Risk of gallbladder disease in women and correlation to leptin concentration. **B:** Risk of gallbladder disease in men and correlation to leptin concentration. Abbreviations: Adj, adjusted; Adj 2, adjusted for BMI and W:H; BMI, body mass index; NS, not significant; Unadj, unadjusted; W:H, waist to hip ratio.

Odds Ratio

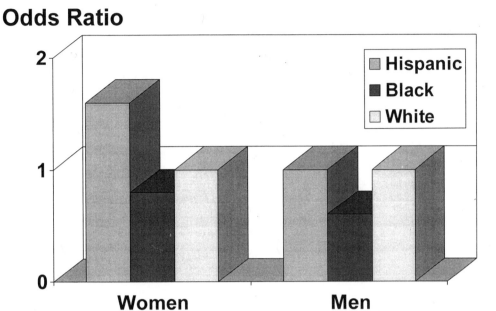

FIG. 12.3. Age-adjusted and body mass index–adjusted risk of gallbladder disease related to ethnicity.

Pathophysiologic mechanisms to explain these differences have not been completely defined, but the data indicate the presence of interactions among obesity, gender, ethnicity, and weight loss.

Types of Gallstones

Gallstones are typically classified as follows by their chemical composition: cholesterol, black pigment, and brown pigment (17,18). Cholesterol gallstones are defined as gallstones that are more than 50% cholesterol by weight. Cholesterol gallstones are not made of pure cholesterol; salts of calcium, pigments, and glycoprotein may be found in the center, in radiating spikes, or in concentric rings within the stone (Fig. 12.4).

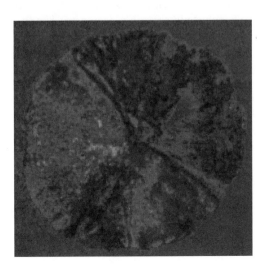

FIG. 12.4. Cross section of cholesterol gallstone.

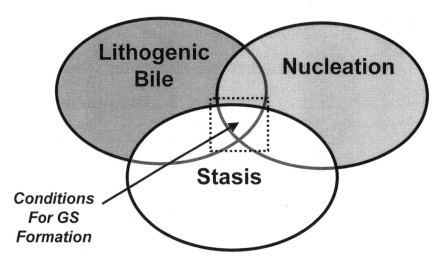

FIG. 12.5. Gallstone (GS) pathogenesis.

Pathogenesis

Current understanding of the pathogenesis of cholesterol gallstones suggests that the following three processes may be required: secretion of "lithogenic" bile by the liver, nucleation of molecules to initiate crystal formation, and stasis of bile in the gallbladder to allow crystals to elongate and agglomerate to form "sludge" and stones (Fig. 12.5) (17–20).

Secretion of Lithogenic Bile by Hepatocytes

The secretion of bile that is supersaturated with cholesterol is a prerequisite for cholesterol gallstone formation (19). Saturation of bile with cholesterol is expressed as the saturation or lithogenic index. The latter indices relate the cholesterol concentration in bile, the variable in numerator, to the concentrations of bile acid and phospholipid, both of which are variables in the denominator; and they correlate with the risk of cholesterol to precipitate from bile and to form gallstones. The lithogenic index increases when either cholesterol secretion increases or bile acid or phospholipid secretion decreases. The initial secretion of cholesterol by hepatocytes into bile is coupled tightly to phospholipid secretion in the form of unilamellar vesicles. When bile is not saturated with cholesterol, the bile acid enhances the disappearance of the vesicles in bile by promoting the transfer of cholesterol into mixed micelles of cholesterol, phospholipid, and bile acid. Changes in the composition of the bile acid pool affect the degree of micellar solubilization of cholesterol. When the bile is saturated with cholesterol, the unilamellar vesicles aggregate into large cholesterol-rich, multilamellar vesicles that favor the nucleation of cholesterol molecules, which then form crystals and ultimately gallstones.

Studies of biliary lipid composition after an overnight fast in obese subjects consistently demonstrate an increase in the lithogenic index over that of nonobese controls. The increase in lithogenic index is mainly due to the enhanced biliary secretion of cholesterol (21–23). The mechanism for the increased biliary cholesterol secretion is unclear, but some investigators have concluded that it is linked to the increased hepatic synthesis of cholesterol (18,19,24,25).

TABLE 12.2. *Lithogenic index during diet-induced weight loss*

	N	Weight loss	Lithogenic index		
			Base	8 Wk	Main
Gebhart[a]					
520 kcal	6	22%	1.25	1.40	1.00
900 kcal	7	22%	1.40	1.70	1.10
Trouillot[b]					
850 kcal	18	11%	1.10	1.42	0.92

This table depicts the results of analyses of bile samples from obese subjects at the following two phases of weight loss: early in the weight loss period after 8 wk of dieting and later, during the maintenance of weight (main).
[a]$p < 0.05$ for both base and 8 wk.
[b]$p < 0.01$ for both base and 8 wk.
Abbreviation: *N*, number of subjects.

During weight loss, the biliary cholesterol level and the lithogenic index increase (Table 12.2) (10,26,27). The exact mechanisms responsible for the augmented increase in the lithogenic index are largely undefined, but two findings may be of particular relevance. First, the biliary concentration of bile acid and the estimated biliary bile acid secretion decrease in the weight loss period. Second, one study of bile acid synthesis demonstrated a 60% reduction in bile acid synthesis during weight loss. These findings suggest that the reduced synthesis of bile acid limits the biliary bile acid secretion, resulting in a relative increase in the biliary cholesterol level and lithogenic index. Interestingly, Trouillot et al. (27) examined the hepatic and total body insulin sensitivity using the euglycemic clamp method and found a correlation between changes in bile acid synthesis and hepatic insulin sensitivity. One hypothesis is that the primary effect of weight loss is the restoration of the hepatic response to insulin, which then results in the inhibition of bile acid synthesis through the insulin-mediated inhibition of cholesterol 7α-hydroxylase (28).

Nucleation Factors

Gallbladder mucin and other glycoproteins secreted by the liver and possibly gallbladder mucosa have been proposed as pronucleation factors (20). These glycoproteins have been shown to promote the formation of cholesterol crystals from saturated biles, and they are often found in the core matrix of both cholesterol and pigment gallstones. In contrast, antinucleation factors—the apolipoproteins A-I and A-II—found in nonlithogenic bile may prevent the formation of cholesterol crystals from vesicular aggregates. Only one study has examined the time course for the concentration of selected nucleation factors in obese subjects (29). In this study, bile samples were obtained at baseline before weight loss and seven times during the first 56 days of weight loss induced by a 520-kcal diet in nine obese subjects. The cholesterol saturation index and the biliary concentrations of arachidonate, prostaglandin E_2 (PGE_2), and glycoprotein increased, and the nucleation time decreased. The nucleation time decreased before the appearance of cholesterol crystals. The increased concentration of biliary arachidonate preceded the appearance of biliary PGE_2 and the increases in biliary glycoprotein. These results suggest that two key pathogenetic mechanisms, the secretion of lithogenic bile and enhanced nucleation, are coordinately expressed during the very early phases of weight loss.

Gallbladder Motility

The healthy gallbladder prevents formation of gallstones by acidifying the bile, concentrating it, and then vigorously expelling crystals and sludge during contractions. Cholesterol nucleation takes place over days; if the gallbladder empties vigorously several times daily, removing mucus and bile from the gallbladder, crystal formation and the development of gallstones may not occur. One study evaluated gallbladder motility in obese subjects and compared the results to those of nonobese large subjects and normal-sized controls (30). The volume of the gallbladder after an overnight fast and the residual volume in response to a meal stimulus were greater in both obese and nonobese large subjects as compared to those of normal-sized individuals. Fractional emptying was similar in all three groups, but the residual volume after emptying was significantly greater in the obese and large subjects. Others have confirmed the larger gallbladder volumes in obese subjects, but they have also found impaired rates of emptying or an impaired fraction of volume emptied in response to meal stimuli (31). Thus, obesity is associated with a larger gallbladder volume but with normal or reduced fractional emptying. Even though fractional emptying may be normal, the residual volume after a meal stimulus is increased because of the greater fasting volume, indicating that the obese person retains a greater volume of bile in the gallbladder. The prolonged retention of bile in the gallbladder is thought to be a risk factor for the formation of gallstones.

A number of studies have examined the changes in gallbladder motility that occur in response to weight loss (26,27,32–37). Gallbladder contraction in response to a meal is mediated primarily by the hormone cholecystokinin (CCK). CCK is released from specialized neuroendocrine cells in the epithelium of the upper small bowel after the intraluminal digestion of dietary triglyceride to fatty acid and monoglyceride. In the case of diet-induced weight loss, the fat composition of many of the VLCDs and low-calorie diets is extremely low, ranging from 0 to 3 g of fat per day. This amount of fat is insufficient for maximal CCK release, and gallbladder contraction after these meals is typically reduced (Table 12.3). In contrast, as few as 10 g of fat may be sufficient to maintain normal gallbladder contraction and emptying and thus to reduce the risk of gallstone formation. A similar response to various amounts of fat has been observed in other studies, but not all support the notion that gallbladder motility is the final arbiter for the determination of gallstone formation. For example, Vezina et al. (38) observed a gallstone incidence rate of 11% to 18% in obese patients on weight-loss diets containing 16 and 30 g of fat. The doses of fat in these studies were demonstrated to produce maximum gallbladder contraction, yet gallstones still formed.

TABLE 12.3. *Gallbladder motility during diet-induced weight loss*

		N	Base	On diet	Gallstones
Diet	Fat/d				
520 kcal	1 g	6	68%	42%	67%
850 kcal	3 g	22	70%	53%	9%
900 kcal	10 g	7	65%	62%	0%

This table depicts the results of ultrasonographic measurements from two studies (26,27) of fractional emptying (%) of the gallbladder in response to liquid meal stimuli containing different amounts of fat, ranging from 1 to 10 g/d. The percentage of subjects who developed gallstones is given in the far right column. Meal stimuli containing 1 g and 3 g of fat do not contract the gallbladder completely. In contrast, as little as 10 g of fat may restore gallbladder emptying and may reduce the risk of gallstone formation. Abbreviation: *N*, number of subjects.

Significance of Cholelithiasis

Asymptomatic Cases

Most patients with gallstones are asymptomatic, and they will remain asymptomatic for several years. Often, gallstones are detected during performance of abdominal imaging, such as ultrasonography, that is conducted for another reason (Fig. 12.6). One study of the natural history of truly asymptomatic gallstones indicated that only 20% of the patients develop symptoms after a follow-up of up to 25 years (39).

The asymptomatic gallstone population has been suggested to be really composed of the following two populations: those who ultimately become symptomatic, usually within the first 5 years of follow-up, and those who never develop symptoms. The risk of developing symptoms is 1% to 3% per year for the first 5 to 10 years, but it then drops to 0.1% to 0.3% with prolonged observation. The risk of developing serious complications from gallstones (e.g., acute cholecystitis, cholangitis, pancreatitis, sepsis, and gangrenous gallbladder) is low at only about 0.1% per year. In the most comprehensive long-term study of the natural history, biliary colic always preceded any serious complication by several months. Given the costs associated with cholecystectomy, the relatively benign natural history, and the fact that biliary colic nearly always precedes more serious complications, prophylactic cholecystectomy is not recommended for asymptomatic patients. However, prophylactic cholecystectomy may be considered in the following circumstances: large ileal resections, patients with known gallstones who will be traveling or working in remote regions of the world, and certain populations or medical conditions that are associated with high rates of complications or can-

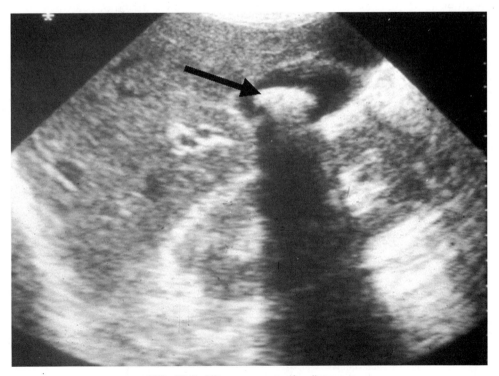

FIG. 12.6. Ultrasonogram of gallstones.

cer (e.g., Pima Indians, calcified gallbladder, porcelain gallbladder, and gallstones associated with sickle cell disease) (40). One decision analysis suggested that patients with diabetes mellitus do not benefit from the performance of a prophylactic chole-cystectomy (41).

Spontaneous Dissolution

In general, most gallstones do not spontaneously dissolve or exit the gallbladder asymptomatically. In the National Cooperative Gallstone Study, 1% of patients experienced a spontaneous clearance of gallbladder stones over a period of 2 years while taking a placebo (42). Even this low rate of clearance was questioned because the technique used to detect gallstones was oral cholecystography, which is much less sensitive than the currently recommended method of realtime ultrasonography (98% sensitivity and specificity). In contrast, two recent ultrasonographic studies suggest that one-third of the cholesterol gallstones that develop during pregnancy may dissolve (43,44). Small stones (less than 0.5 cm) that are composed predominantly of cholesterol are more likely to dissolve in the postpartum period. In general, calcified stones, pigment stones, and stones that have persisted over several years are not likely to dissolve spontaneously. Gallstones that are symptomatic are not likely to disappear of their own volition (45).

Symptomatic Cases

Biliary colic is the most specific symptom of cholelithiasis, and it is defined as pain localized to either the right upper quadrant of the abdomen or the epigastrium. It is characterized by a short crescendo period of increasing pain (5 to 15 minutes), a plateau of steady pain (15 minutes to several hours), and a decrescendo period of decreasing pain and resolution of pain (15 minutes to 2 hours). Patients are asymptomatic between the attacks of colic. Nonspecific symptoms that do not correlate well with gallstones include

TABLE 12.4. *Clinical manifestations and treatment of cholelithiasis*

Clinical manifestations
  Biliary colic (characteristic abdominal pain)
  Cholecystitis
    Murphy sign (inspiratory arrest)
    Mirrizzi syndrome (biliary obstruction from an inflamed gallbladder neck)
  Cholangitis
    Charcot triad (pain, fever, jaundice)
    Raynold pentad (pain, fever, jaundice, shock, confusion)
  Biliary obstruction
  Pancreatitis
  Gallbladder carcinoma
  Bowel obstruction (Bouveret syndrome)
Therapeutic options used to treat cholelithiasis
  "Watch and wait" for symptoms (preferred for asymptomatic gallstones)
  Cholecystectomy (typically for symptomatic patients)
    Laparoscopic (preferred surgical procedure)
    Open
  Medical treatments (rarely, if ever, used)
    Oral bile acid therapy (chenodeoxycholic or ursodeoxycholic acid)
    Extracorporeal shock-wave lithotripsy
    Methy-tert-butyl ether
  Endoscopic sphincterotomy (preferred for common bile duct stones)

nausea, vomiting, dyspepsia, diarrhea, weight loss or gain, and heartburn. Elderly, diabetic, and immunocompromised patients may present with serious complications of gallbladder disease (e.g., gangrenous gallbladder, empyema of the gallbladder, perforation of the gallbladder, and suppurative cholangitis) and may exhibit few or no localizing abdominal complaints or findings on physical examination. In these patients, gallbladder disease may present as fever, altered mental status, loss of appetite and weight loss, or sepsis. The clinical manifestations of cholelithiasis and the treatment options are given in Table 12.4.

Gallbladder Sludge

Sludge refers to gallbladder mucin with the entrapment of particulate matter nucleated from bile (Fig. 12.7). Sludge formation occurs within the gallbladder when gallbladder emptying is slow and incomplete. It is often associated with prolonged fasting or with a lack of stimulation of intestinal release of CCK. Sludge is commonly observed in ultrasonographic studies of the gallbladder in obese subjects who are undergoing rapid weight loss. Although sludge is a reversible stage in gallstone pathogenesis, gallstones may develop in a large percentage of patients and ultimately lead to symptomatic biliary tract

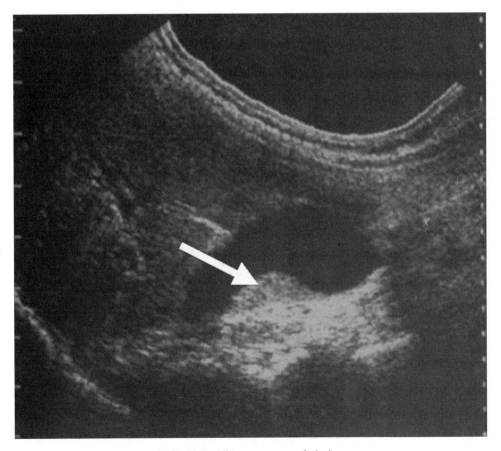

FIG. 12.7. Ultrasonogram of sludge.

disease (20,46,47). Sludge is a risk factor for gallstones, but it may be evacuated from the gallbladder, thus preventing gallstone formation.

Gallbladder Carcinoma

The incidence of carcinoma of the gallbladder is 0.1 to 0.3% in cholecystectomy specimens, and the risk increases with age and with the size of gallstones. Whether obesity further increases the risk is unknown. The highest incidence of carcinoma is seen in elderly patients with a maximum diameter of gallstones that is greater than 3 cm (48–50). Pima Indians, who have an extremely high prevalence of obesity and gallstones, have the highest rate of gallbladder cancer and mortality in the United States.

Conclusion

Cholelithiasis is highly prevalent in the United States population, affecting more than 20 million Americans. Although cholelithiasis may exhibit a benign natural history, many patients will develop symptoms and complications necessitating cholecystectomy or other medical interventions. Obesity is a major risk factor for cholelithiasis; the risk increases with increasing BMI and other measures of obesity. Mechanisms responsible for this increased risk in obesity include the increased biliary secretion of cholesterol and increased retention of bile within the gallbladder. A number of other derangements in biliary physiology, particularly during periods of rapid weight loss, may further increase the risk of formation of gallstones. These include the suppression of synthesis of bile acid, the enhanced secretion of mucin by the gallbladder mucosa, the alteration of biliary calcium concentrations and pH level, and the disordered secretion of both pronucleating and antinucleating factors. Age, gender, and ethnic differences in these pathophysiologic processes may explain the differences in the prevalence of cholelithiasis among various populations and patient groups. The increasing prevalence of obesity in the United States population is likely to continue to fuel the increased rates of cholelithiasis.

HEPATIC COMPLICATIONS OF OBESITY: NONALCOHOLIC FATTY LIVER AND STEATOHEPATITIS

Case Presentation

A nonalcoholic woman, age 50, received an orthotopic liver transplant for cryptogenic cirrhosis in 1994. Before and during the first 3 months after the transplantation, she was not obese (BMI = 27.5 kg/m^2), and she did not have either hypertension or dyslipidemia. She subsequently developed adult-onset, insulin-requiring diabetes mellitus and systolic hypertension and gained 19 kg (BMI = 35.7 kg/m^2). Her diabetes mellitus was poorly controlled; her hemoglobin A_{1C} concentration was 9%.

Her liver function test results rose threefold, and a liver biopsy, which showed changes typical of steatohepatitis, was obtained (Fig. 12.8). Five years later, her diabetes is well controlled with insulin (HbA$_{1C}$ = 6.6%), she takes antihypertensive medication, her lipid panel remains normal, she has lost weight, her BMI now is 30.6 kg/m^2, and her liver biopsy still shows typical features of NASH but without a significant progression in fibrosis.

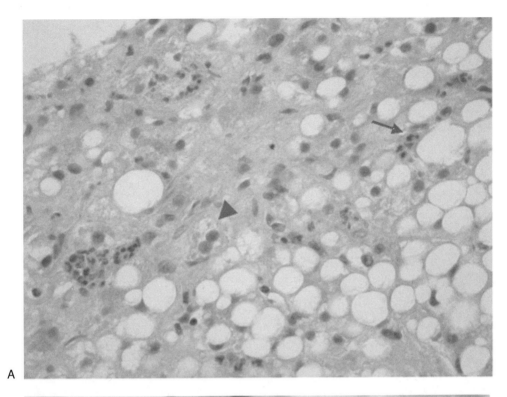

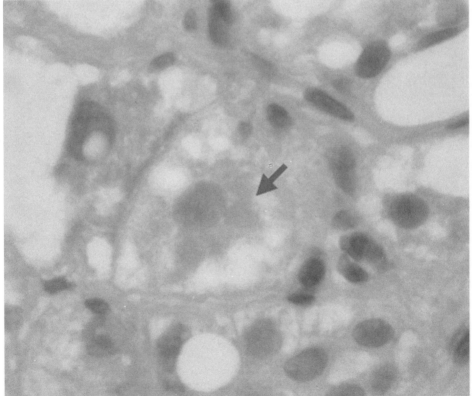

FIG. 12.8. A: Ballooning and neutrophils. **B:** Mallory hyaline. *(Figure continues on next page)*

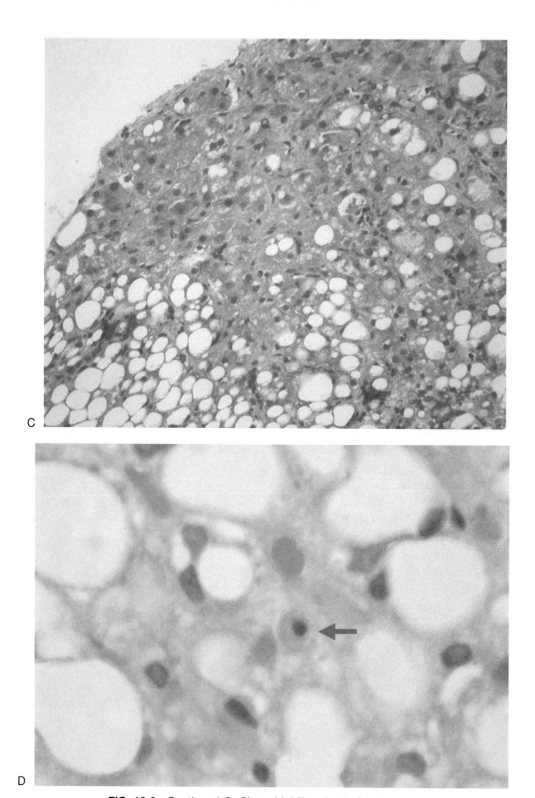

FIG. 12.8. *Continued.* **C:** Sinusoidal fibrosis. **D:** Spotty necrosis.

Definitions of Nonalcoholic Steatohepatitis and Nonalcoholic Fatty Liver Disease

Nonalcoholic Steatohepatitis

In 1980, Ludwig et al. (51) introduced the term *NASH* to the medical literature. The authors described a series of 20 patients with the typical histologic features of alcoholic steatohepatitis, who, by history, did not drink alcohol in excess. The notion that macrovesicular fat could infiltrate the liver parenchyma, causing minor elevations in the liver test results, had been well characterized before.

Nonalcoholic Fatty Liver Disease

NAFL disease without associated inflammatory or fibrotic components is a benign condition with well-defined clinical, radiologic, and biochemical characteristics and a very benign course, albeit with some minor right upper quadrant pain arising from distention of the Glisson capsule (52).

Over the past two decades, NASH has been recognized as part of the spectrum of fatty liver disease, but the key distinguishing feature is necroinflammatory damage. Hepatic injury in NASH is characterized by hepatocyte necrosis and mixed, but predominantly polymorphonuclear (PMN), inflammatory infiltrates. Unlike NAFL disease, NASH is a progressive liver disease; if it is not reversed, it may lead to cirrhosis, liver failure, and the need for liver transplantation (53). Moreover, although the pathophysiology of this condition is still not fully understood, many contributing factors are well characterized, and these merit clinical attention because intervention may affect the natural history of progression of this disease.

Initially, the typical patient at risk of developing NASH was suggested to be a middle-aged overweight woman with coexistent glucose intolerance or frank diabetes (type II) and dyslipidemia (53). Since this initial report, younger patients, men, and people who are not overweight have possibly been found to suffer from NASH. Bacon et al. (54), in their series, found that 58% of NASH patients were men and that fewer than 40% were obese. Others have reported associations of NASH with iron-overload states, gastrointestinal tract bypass surgery, and certain medications (55–57).

NASH should be considered as part of the differential diagnosis in any patient with chronically elevated liver test results. The diagnosis is confirmed by typical histologic features of steatohepatitis in a patient with a negligible alcohol intake (less than 20 g per day). The histologic features required for the diagnosis of NASH, as proposed by the NASH Pathology Working Group at the Non-Alcoholic Steatohepatitis Symposium sponsored by the National Institutes of Health in December 1998, are given in Table 12.5 and are demonstrated in the photomicrographs in Fig. 12.8. The criteria for diagnosis are rather strict, and they require the performance of liver biopsy. Although the criteria are well suited for use in clinical trials, they are not strictly followed in clinical practice or even in the NASH literature. The mere presence of steatosis with the associated lobular

TABLE 12.5. *Histology features in nonalcoholic steatohepatitis*

Steatosis **plus**
Hepatocellular injury involving acinar zone 3 (either ballooning degeneration or hepatocellular dropout) AND at least one of the following two features:
  Zone 3 mallory bodies
  Zone 3 sinusoidal fibrosis

TABLE 12.6. *Fibrosis staging in nonalcoholic steatohepatitis*

Stage 1	Zone 3 sinusoidal fibrosis
Stage 2	Stage 1 + periportal fibrosis
Stage 3	Bridging fibrosis
Stage 4	Cirrhosis

From Brunt EM. Nonalcoholic steatohepatitis: definition and pathology. *Semin Liver Dis* 2001;21:3–16, with permission.

inflammation by PMN leucocytes appears to be the minimum acceptable criteria for a diagnosis of NASH. Brunt et al. (58,59) proposed a system for the classification of histologic findings in NASH according to grade and stage, as is commonly done for other progressive liver conditions, and discussed this issue in detail (Table 12.6). Others have contributed or proposed additional modifications to these definitions (60,61).

Prevalence and Natural History of Nonalcoholic Steatohepatitis and Nonalcoholic Fatty Liver Disease

The natural history is not entirely defined. First, the exact prevalence of both NASH and NAFL is unclear because confirmation of the diagnosis requires the performance of a liver biopsy. For obvious ethical considerations, no screening surveillance studies have employed liver biopsy. A surrogate for the prevalence of NASH is the prevalence of obesity, as a reasonable correlation has been found between the risk of NASH and increasing body weight. As obesity has become an increasingly important public health problem in the United States and other developed countries, the prevalence of NASH has probably increased around the world. Second, NASH is a relatively new disorder, and a delay in the recognition and diagnosis often exists among primary care physicians and gastroenterologists. For example, undue delay may be seen in the performance of a liver biopsy in the evaluation of a patient with chronically elevated liver function test results.

Prevalence

Liver biopsy studies show that the prevalence of NAFL ranges from 15% to 39%, and that of NASH, from 1.2% to 4.8% (62–64). These studies suffer from selection bias because most patients are referred for the evaluation of elevated liver test results or right upper quadrant pain. Random autopsy studies of people who have died of miscellaneous causes may more accurately reflect the population prevalence (65,66). In these studies, the prevalence of NAFL ranges from 16% to 24%, and that of NASH, from 2.1% to 2.4%. If these estimates truly reflect the United States population prevalence, then NAFL disease is the most prevalent form of liver disease in the United States.

Natural History of Nonalcoholic Fatty Liver

That not all forms of NAFL disease are progressive must be emphasized. Teli et al. (52) identified 26 patients with histologically proven liver steatosis that was not associated with alcohol use. At a median of 11 years of follow-up, none had progressed to steatohepatitis or cirrhosis, and only one had mild fibrosis after an interval of 9.8 years from the index biopsy.

Matteoni et al. (53) investigated which clinical and pathologic characteristics of patients with NAFL were associated with the development of cirrhosis and liver death. Ninety-eight patients with NAFL who had a 10-year follow-up were identified and were divided into the following four groups: simple fatty liver (type 1), fatty liver plus inflammation (type 2), fatty liver plus ballooning degeneration (type 3), and fatty liver with ballooning degeneration and either features of alcoholic hepatitis (e.g., Mallory bodies, PMN leukocyte infiltration) or fibrosis (type 4) (see Fig. 12.8 for examples of histologic findings). Overall, mortality did not differ among the four histologic groups; however, 90% of those who developed cirrhosis or who had a liver-related death were classified as having type 3 or type 4 NAFL.

Natural History of Nonalcoholic Steatohepatitis

What factors contribute to progression in disease and the risk of fibrosis or cirrhosis (Table 12.7)? The Mayo Clinic examined 144 patients with NASH with the aim of identifying independent predictors of severe hepatic fibrosis (67). They defined severe hepatic fibrosis as bridging (stage 3) and cirrhosis (stage 4). They found that older age (older than 45 years), obesity (BMI greater than 31.1 kg/m^2 for men and greater than 32.3 kg/m^2 for women), diabetes mellitus, and, to a lesser degree, an alanine aminotransferase to aspartate aminotransferase (ALT/AST) ratio of more than 1 were significant predictors of severe liver fibrosis. In their analysis, neither iron levels nor gender was significantly associated with a worse fibrotic stage once its influence was controlled for the other variables. In contrast, George et al. (55) found iron overload to be a risk factor for worse fibrosis in 51 Australian patients with NASH. In their study, 31 of these patients were either a heterozygote or a homozygote for the C282Y mutation of the hemochromatosis gene. The presence of one or two copies of the HFE mutation was associated with an increase in all markers of increased iron stores except serum ferritin, and, for the same degree of fibrosis, these patients had less hepatic steatosis. The iron hypothesis is discussed further below (see "Pathogenesis of Hepatic Fibrosis").

Another series evaluated predictors of advanced liver fibrosis in 105 consecutive severely obese patients who underwent laparoscopic surgery for weight reduction (68). Liver biopsies obtained at the time of surgery demonstrated features of NASH in 26 cases (25%). Insulin resistance was calculated by two methods from the fasting levels of insulin, glucose, and C peptide. The best predictors of NASH were the insulin-resistance index, raised ALT levels, and hypertension. Cutoff values for the insulin-resistance index were more than 5.0, and for ALT, more than 40 IU per L. The presence of at least two of these three factors provided the best combination of sensitivity (0.8) and specificity (0.89) for predicting NASH. Eleven patients in this series had advanced fibrosis, including one case of cirrhosis. The independent predictors of fibrosis were hypertension, elevated ALT levels, and a high C-peptide level. All patients with advanced fibrosis had diabetes, hypertension, or both, and most were men. Ratziu et al. (69) also addressed the issue of predictors of advanced fibrosis in patients with NASH. In their series of 93 patients, septal fibrosis was present in 28 (30%), and cirrhosis, in 10 (11%). Age at liver biopsy of 50 years or older, a BMI of more than or equal to 28 kg/m^2, ALT level two or

TABLE 12.7. *Clinical predictors of advanced fibrosis in nonalcoholic steatohepatitis*

Angulo et al. (67)	Dixon et al. (68)	Ratziu et al. (69)
Age >45 yr	Hypertension	Age >50 yr
BMI >31.1 kg/m^2 for men and 32.3 kg/m^2 for women	Elevated C-peptide level	BMI >28 kg/m^2
Diabetes mellitus	Diabetes mellitus	ALT > twice normal
AST/ALT ratio >1	Elevated ALT	Triglycerides >1.7 mmol/L

Abbreviations: ALT, alanine aminotransferase; AST, aspartate aminotransferase; BMI, body mass index.

more times the normal level, and serum triglycerides of more than or equal to 1.7 mmol per L were significantly and independently associated with advanced fibrosis. These four independent variables were then combined in the BAAT (biopsy, age, ALT, and triglycerides) score, in which 1 point is given if the patient demonstrates the variable. BAAT scores of 0 or 1 had a sensitivity of 100%, a specificity of 47%, a positive predictive value of 45%, and a negative predictive value for septal fibrosis of 100%. At the other end of the spectrum, BAAT scores of 3 or 4 had a 100% predictive value for septal fibrosis but low sensitivity scores.

Falk-Ytter et al. (70) reviewed three series that included patients with NASH who were followed for up to 9 years with sequential liver biopsies. The combined evidence showed that 27% of those patients had a progression of the histologic stage of fibrosis and that 19% developed cirrhosis, whereas 50% showed no change and 4% had improved histology compared with the index biopsy (70). In one of these series, Powell et al. (71) followed 42 patients with NASH for a median of 4.5 years and made some very intriguing observations. First, 3 of the 42 patients had cirrhosis or bridging fibrosis on presentation, suggesting an insidious course to this disease that may be asymptomatic and undiagnosed until severe liver damage has already occurred. Second, they documented the progressive nature of this disease. One patient with cirrhosis on presentation developed hepatocellular carcinoma 4 years later and died from this complication, and four others experienced worsening of fibrosis over time. Third, they documented the reversibility of the histology in two patients—one who lost 40 kilograms and a second who had no substantial change in weight. Finally, this Australian study documented the disappearance of steatosis in two patients—one with cirrhosis at baseline and another who developed cirrhosis on subsequent biopsies over 8 years of follow-up. This latter finding led to the theory that cryptogenic cirrhosis could represent the endstage of NASH.

Nonalcoholic Steatohepatitis as the Etiology of Cryptogenic Cirrhosis

Does cryptogenic cirrhosis represent the endstage of NASH? As has been already described, the loss of fatty change in biopsies of patients with NASH who progress to fibrosis has been well documented (70). Caldwell et al. (72) compared 70 consecutive cryptogenic cirrhotic (CC) patients with 50 consecutive patients with NASH, 39 hepatitis C virus–positive patients, and 33 patients with primary biliary cirrhosis. They found that the prevalence of obesity and diabetes was no different in CC or NASH but that it was significantly higher in these two groups compared to those with either hepatitis C virus or primary biliary cirrhosis. Patients with NASH were, on average, a decade younger than the CC patients, suggesting a continuum between these two groups. Interestingly, 33% of the CC patients were heterozygotes for α1-antitrypsin genes, and 26% had abnormally high ferritin levels, suggesting a potential cofactor in the liver disease of these patients (this is called the second-hit hypothesis, see Table 12.8). A seemingly confirmatory study from Johns Hopkins University (73) compared 49 CC patients with 98 age-matched and sex-matched controls from their liver transplant waiting list. Obesity (55% vs. 24%) and type II diabetes mellitus (47% vs. 22%) were significantly more common in the CC group.

Nonalcoholic Steatohepatitis after Jejunoileal Bypass for Morbid Obesity

The natural history of NASH after jejunoileal bypass (JIB) is progressive, and it may lead to cirrhosis. Hocking et al. (74) followed 43 patients whose surgical JIB remained intact for a mean of 12.6 years. Fatty infiltration of the liver was seen in 76% of cases at the time of surgery and in 70% at follow-up. Advanced fibrosis (bridging) was present in 2 cases at the time of their JIB, whereas 16 of the 42 follow-up biopsies showed either bridging or central pericellular fibrosis. The authors calculated an actuarial 8% risk of developing cirrhosis at 15 years after the JIB (74).

Clinical Characteristics of Nonalcoholic Steatohepatitis

Most cases come to attention in the fifth and sixth decades of life, although recognition in childhood is increasing as well (52,71). Women are more likely than men to develop more severe NASH, with a prevalence ratio of close to 2 to 1 (53,54,67). NASH is extremely common in patients who suffer from obesity, type II diabetes mellitus, and dyslipidemia (51–53,67,71,72).

NASH is usually an asymptomatic condition (71). When symptoms do occur, right upper quadrant pain is most commonly seen (71). Usually the condition comes to clinical attention because of otherwise unexplained elevations in liver test results or abnormal hepatic imaging (i.e., an incidental finding when imaging for other reasons).

Liver biochemistry abnormalities are common, and, usually, modest elevations in transaminases are seen (51,52,54,71). The ALT/AST ratio is usually maintained in NASH, and an inverted ratio should raise suspicion for alcohol involvement or established cirrhosis. Derangement in albumin levels, prothrombin time, or hyperbilirubinemia is not typically seen unless liver cirrhosis and dysfunction are established.

The role of radiologic tests in NASH is mostly to rule out other liver pathology. Fatty change of the liver is well characterized by ultrasonography, computed tomographic scanning, or magnetic resonance imaging, but it does not differentiate NAFL from NASH, so it cannot replace liver histology.

Pathogenesis of Hepatic Fibrosis

The exact pathogenesis of NAFL, NASH, and the progression to hepatic fibrosis is not entirely defined. Currently, the leading theory is that an initial insult leads to fatty deposition in hepatocytes, while a second mechanism triggers the inflammation that targets lipid-laden hepatocytes (steatohepatitis). This is known as the two-hit hypothesis (75). Activation of the stellate cells by profibrotic cytokines may represent a "third hit" (Table 12.8).

Excess availability of fatty acid to the liver relative to what is required for mitochondrial oxidation, phospholipid synthesis, and cholesterol metabolism leads to steatosis in the setting of obesity, diabetes mellitus, and total parenteral nutrition (76–78). Insulin resistance is commonly found in patients with NASH, and the resulting hyperinsulinemia

TABLE 12.8. *Pathogenesis of nonalcoholic steatohepatitis*

First hit: steatosis	Second hit: steatohepatitis	Third hit: fibrosis
Obesity Diabetes mellitus Insulin resistance syndromes Dyslipidemia Miscellaneous causes (see text)	Lipid peroxidation and oxidative stress triggered by the following: Iron overload Dysregulated cytochrome P 2E1 Endotoxemia Increased tumor necrosis factor production Mitochondrial toxicity Altered hepatocyte energy homeostasis	Stellate cell activation facilitated by profibrotic cytokines

favors fatty infiltration of the liver through decreased fatty oxidation and by blocking the secretion of very low density lipoprotein triglycerides from the hepatocyte. The latter effect may involve the inhibition of the synthesis of apolipoprotein B.

The histologic features of NASH are indistinguishable from those seen in acute alcoholic hepatitis, but the clinical course is much more benign. As in alcoholic hepatitis, lipid peroxidation and oxidative stress appear to be responsible for the production of reactive oxygen species and inflammation in steatohepatitis (75). Several different factors may lead to lipid peroxidation and oxidative stress, including dysregulation of the cytochrome P450 system 2E1 (CYP 2E1); iron overload; overexpression of proinflammatory cytokines as triggered by intestinal disease; mitochondrial toxicity; and altered hepatic energy homeostasis. In turn, lipid peroxidation of organelle membranes results in cellular dysfunction, mitochondrial respiratory defects, and ultimately cellular injury and death. An elegant study from Italy (79) illustrated the point that the insulin-resistance syndrome can precede the onset of diabetes mellitus and that it can be present in nonobese patients. Nineteen nonobese nondiabetic patients with NASH were studied, and 47% were found to fulfill criteria for insulin resistance, including hypertension, central distribution of adiposity, and dyslipidemia.

Increased CYP 2E1 can generate reactive oxidative species that may trigger lipid peroxidation (80). Overexpression of CYP 2E1 has been shown in rodents and humans, and its overexpression has been associated with increased lipid peroxidation byproducts in animal models (81–83).

Controversy exists regarding the role of iron in the pathogenesis of NASH. Some investigators believe that excess iron stores play a role in the pathogenesis of NASH (54,55,84), while others do not (85). Bacon et al. (54) documented elevated serum iron test results without hemochromatosis in 18 of 31 patients with NASH, most of whom were male (58%). George et al. (55) studied 51 Australian patients with NASH and found that a significant group of men (51%) who were younger than their female counterparts had greater hepatic iron indices but less steatosis and less fibrosis. In this group of patients with NASH, those who were heterozygotes for the C282Y mutation had significantly less hepatic steatosis and the same fibrosis stage as those without the mutation. Hepatic iron overload does induce oxidative stress, lipid peroxidation, and hepatic stellate cell activation (86,87). Moreover, Mendler et al. (84) demonstrated insulin resistance, albeit by somewhat loose criteria, in 161 patients with histologically proven hepatic iron overload and elevated serum iron tests but not genetic hemochromatosis. Ninety-four percent of patients in this series fulfilled the criteria for insulin resistance, as defined by a BMI of more than 25 kg/m^2, abnormal glucose metabolism, and hyperlipidemia. As suggested in the other series already described, most patients in this large series were men (86%) (54,55). On the other hand, Younossi et al. (85) did not find an association between iron stores and the degree of fibrosis in 65 patients (48% male) with NAFL disease. These investigators did find that men had greater hepatic iron concentrations and higher hepatic iron indices than women. Overall, these data suggest that patients (more commonly men) with elevated iron stores may have steatohepatitis in the liver tissue that may represent a different pathophysiologic mechanism that is in its early stage than that which is more commonly seen in obese women with insulin resistance–induced oxidative stress and lipid peroxidation. Mendler et al. (84) suggested this could represent a distinct clinical entity that they call insulin-resistance–associated hepatic iron overload in which iron overload and steatosis are associated by the presence of insulin resistance. Whether the association among male gender, elevated hepatic iron stores, and NASH is related to greater or lesser hepatic fibrosis is still unclear.

Endotoxemia is also entertained as a possible trigger of steatohepatitis. An animal model of obese mice with fatty livers has been shown to develop NASH when it is exposed to endotoxin (88). The human "model" of this circumstance is the hepatitis that, on occasion, follows patients undergoing JIB surgery for the control of obesity (89). A broad-spectrum antibiotic metronidazole was shown to be of benefit in this condition, probably because of its intestinal decontamination features that lead to the reduction of endotoxemia (90). Endotoxemia causes the hepatocyte injury through the activation of tumor necrosis factor (TNF) by the resident macrophages in the liver (Kupffer cells). Even more interesting is the notion that TNF polymorphisms play a role in the pathogenesis of NASH (91).

Work in genetically obese mice in several laboratories has also focused attention on mitochondrial dysfunction in NASH (92,93). This work is based on the hypothesis that fatty liver cells increase the uncoupling of protein-2 in mitochondria as a means of increasing adenosine triphosphate (ATP) production. Impaired ATP homeostasis in humans with NASH has also been documented (94). Drug-induced NASH also seems to be brought on by mitochondrial dysfunction, disruption of oxidation, and decreased ATP generation from respiratory chain dysfunction (95).

The "third hit" in this disease is the activation of cytokine pathways that in turn stimulate stellate cells to differentiate and lay collagen. Stellate cell activation results in the common pathway of all chronic liver diseases, progression to cirrhosis.

Childhood and Adolescent Obesity

NAFL and NASH are increasingly being diagnosed in pediatric clinics. Franzese et al. (96) evaluated 72 consecutive obese Italian children (age of 9.5 ± 2.9 years) with serum liver tests and ultrasonography. Eighteen (25%) had transaminitis, and ultrasonographic findings for thirty-eight (53%) indicated the presence of fatty infiltration of the liver. With the loss of weight, biochemical and sonographic abnormalities resolved (96). Kinugasa et al. (97) performed a biopsy on 11 of 36 obese children with transaminitis who were seen at an obesity clinic. Five patients (45%) had fatty infiltration, another five (45%) had fibrosis changes, and one had cirrhosis (9%). The duration of obesity correlated with a worsening histology in this study.

McTigue et al. (98) studied the change in BMI of 9,179 young adults from the ages of 17 to 20 years in a survey that oversampled for minority ethnic groups from 1981 and 1998 (98). Twenty-six percent of the men and 28% of the women were obese by the age of 35 to 37 years. Significant predictors of obesity were baseline BMI and race or ethnicity. For more than 80% of the men and women who were obese in their mid-30s, the onset of obesity occurred in their early 20s. This study also demonstrated that obesity occurs earlier and develops more quickly in black and Hispanic women, compared to its occurrence in non-Hispanic white women. Many other studies implicate the early onset of obesity as a major risk factor for adult obesity (99). Some have suggested that the tendency toward obesity may develop quite early in life, perhaps even *in utero*. The increased risk of obesity in adult black women compared to that for white women is foreshadowed by differences in adipose tissue that occur as early as the age of 10 years. Other studies confirm that racial or ethnic disparities in obesity may be present in children as young as 4 to 12 years of age. These studies suggest that the groundwork for obesity, insulin resistance, and the risk of development of NAFL or NASH may be laid at an extremely early age.

Treatment

No therapy has been proven effective for NASH. Moreover, designing a study to prove a treatment's benefit to patients with NASH is quite challenging. As is true in most chronic liver conditions, an improvement in the transaminase levels has not been proven to correlate with an improved liver histology or prognosis. Extremely large series of patients should be followed for many years with serial liver biopsies to prove that therapy modifies natural history. Until better markers of fibrosis and liver function are validated, biochemical markers are the best surrogates that are available, even if they are imperfect.

Multiple series have documented an improvement in transaminase levels from diet, exercise, and weight loss (100,101). Given the multiplicity of factors leading to NASH, several interventions have been tried. Lipid-lowering agents improve biochemistries. Gemfibrozil therapy has been shown to reduce transaminase levels significantly after 4 weeks of therapy in 46 patients with NASH, compared to improvement in only 30% in the control group (102). On the other hand, clofibrate therapy has not been beneficial in patients with NASH.

Ursodeoxycholic acid (UDCA) has several mechanisms of action, and it has been shown to improve transaminase levels in different chronic liver conditions. Laurin et al. (103) conducted a pilot study in which they compared UDCA with clofibrate in patients with NASH, and the subjects in the UDCA arm of this study showed improvement in transaminitis and steatosis but no reduction in either inflammation or fibrosis (103).

Betaine is a precursor of *S*-adenosylmethionine (SAMe), a substance that may protect the liver against fatty infiltration. The Mayo Clinic reported its experience in using betaine in ten patients with NASH (104). Seven of ten patients completed 1 year of treatment and experienced a significant reduction in AST and ALT; six of these seven had paired liver biopsy results that showed a trend toward less necroinflammatory activity and an improvement in fibrosis. All patients who experienced side effects completed the 1 year of therapy. More definitive evaluation of the role of betaine in the management of NASH is being eagerly awaited.

The insulin resistance associated with NASH has been targeted with medications whose mechanism of action is sensitization to insulin. Metformin improves insulin sensitivity in patients with diabetes mellitus, and its use in obese mice was associated with a reduction in hepatomegaly and hepatic steatosis (105). Troglitazone, a thiazolidinedione that also improves insulin sensitivity, demonstrated encouraging results in humans with NASH, but it has been taken off the market because of serious hepatotoxicity (106). Both metformin and rosiglitazone are also under investigation for the treatment of NASH.

Antioxidants have also been tried in both adult and pediatric patients with NASH. Existing studies demonstrate a limited biochemical benefit, but, in the case of adults, the benefit is no greater than that which can be achieved with exercise and diet (107).

Implications for Liver Transplantation

The Mayo Clinic evaluated 1,207 patients for liver transplantation over 6 years in the mid-1990s (108). Of these patients, 2.6% were diagnosed with NASH by established criteria, pointing toward the fact that, even though this is a common disease, its progression to endstage liver disease is infrequent. Half of the patients were women, almost all were white, the mean age was 54.2 years, and the mean BMI was 35.5 kg/m^2. One of these patients developed a hepatocellular carcinoma. Of the 31 patients with NASH, 16 received a liver transplant, and the 1-year and 3-year patient survival rates were 93.7% and 81.2%, respectively. These outcomes compare very well to the other diagnostic categories for which liver transplantation is performed. Two patients died in this series, one perioperatively and another after retransplantation for allograft failure secondary to the recurrence of NASH. One year after liver transplantation in patients with NASH, 60% of patients demonstrated fatty change in their allograft biopsies, 56% had overt NASH, 33% experienced stage 2 or higher fibrosis, and two developed cirrhosis.

In another series of 51 patients who received a liver transplant for cryptogenic cirrhosis at the Cleveland Clinic Foundation (109), 25% of the patients were histologically proven to have developed NAFL disease by 6 months posttransplantation, and eight of those had NASH. Posttransplant patients with NASH were more likely to have had type II diabetes mellitus and higher fasting triglyceride levels prior to transplantation and type II diabetes mellitus after transplantation, than were those patients with benign NAFL disease. Nine patients had paired liver biopsies available for review. Patients with only steatosis or benign NAFL did not develop significant fibrosis, but 40% of patients with NASH developed cirrhosis between 37 and 80 months posttransplant.

Overall, steatosis is a common finding in posttransplant liver biopsies, and usually it is associated with a benign clinical course. *De novo* NASH has also been observed after liver transplantation, as was exemplified by the case discussed at the beginning of this section; and rapid progression to allograft cirrhosis has been described (110,111).

Conclusion

NAFL disease is very prevalent in the United States population, and it generally has a benign natural history. A small subset of patients with NAFL (5% to 10%) develop steatohepatitis (i.e., NASH), which can potentially progress to more severe liver injury ending in liver cirrhosis. Patients who are older and who have central obesity, hypertension, dyslipidemia, and diabetes mellitus are at greater risk of developing NASH. The pathophysiology of this condition is multifactorial, with several possible pathways leading to the initial insult consisting of fatty deposits in hepatocytes. Secondary or tertiary mechanisms subsequently trigger the inflammatory processes that characterize NASH. Initial reports of patients undergoing liver transplantation indicate that NASH may be an underlying cause of cryptogenic cirrhosis. Generally, outcomes after transplantation are excellent, but NASH may recur in the posttransplantation period; in these cases, the long-term consequences are uncertain. Research efforts are needed to understand this condition and its natural history better, as well as to define accurately potential medical and social interventions that may lead to the prevention of this emerging common hepatic complication.

REFERENCES

1. Kern F Jr. Epidemiology and natural history of gallstones. *Semin Liver Dis* 1983;3:87–96.
2. Diehl AK. Epidemiology and natural history of gallstone disease. *Gastroenterol Clin North Am* 1991;20:1–20.
3. Everhart J, Khare M, Hill M, et al. Prevalence and ethnic differences in gallbladder disease in the United States. *Gastroenterology* 1999;117:632–639.
4. Everhart JE. Gallstones. In: Johanson JF, ed. *Gastrointestinal diseases: risk factors and prevention.* Philadelphia Lippincott–Raven Publishers, 1998:145–172.
5. Weiss KM, Ferrell RE, Hanis CL, et al. Genetics and epidemiology of gallbladder disease in New World native peoples. *Am J Hum Genet* 1984;36:1259–1278.
6. Everhart JE, Yeh F, Elisa T, et al. Prevalence of gallbladder disease in American Indian populations: findings from the Strong Heart Study. *Hepatology* 2002;35:1507–1512.
7. Stampfer MJ, Maclure KM, Colditz GA, et al. Risk of symptomatic gallstones in women with severe obesity. *Am J Clin Nutr* 1992;55:652–658.
8. Ruhl CE, Everhart JE. Relationship of serum leptin concentration and other measures of adiposity with gallbladder disease. *Hepatology* 2001;34:877–883.

9. Everhart JE. Contributions of obesity and weight loss to gallstone disease. *Ann Intern Med* 1993;119: 1029–1035.

10. Broomfield PH, Chopra R, Sheinbaum RC, et al. Effects of ursodeoxycholic acid and aspirin on the formation of lithogenic bile and gallstones during loss of weight. *N Engl J Med* 1988;319:1567–1572.

11. Yang H, Petersen GM, Roth MP, et al. Risk factors for gallstone formation during rapid loss of weight. *Dig Dis Sci* 1992;37:912–918.

12. Liddle RA, Goldstein RB, Saxton J. Gallstone formation during weight-reduction dieting. *Arch Intern Med* 1989;149:1750–1753.

13. Festi D, Colecchia A, Larocca A, et al. Review: low caloric intake and gallbladder motor function. *Aliment Pharmacol Ther* 2000;14:51–53.

14. Festi D, Colecchia A, Orsini M, et al. Gallbladder motility and gallstone formation in obese patients following very low calorie diets. Use it (fat) to lose it (well). *Int J Obes Relat Metab Disord* 1998;22:592–600.

15. Wattchow DA, Hall JC, Whiting MJ, et al. Prevalence and treatment of gallstones after gastric bypass surgery for morbid obesity. *BMJ* 1983;286:763.

16. Shiffman ML, Sugerman HJ, Kellum JM, et al. Gallstone formation after rapid weight loss: a prospective study in patients undergoing gastric bypass surgery for treatment of morbid obesity. *Am J Gastroenterol* 1991;86: 1000–1005.

17. Trotman BW, Solway RD. Pigment gallstone disease: summary of the National Institutes of Health International Workshop. *Hepatology* 1982;2:879–884.

18. Strasberg SM, Hofmann AF, eds. Biliary cholesterol transport and precipitation: proceedings of the Workshop on Frontiers in Gallstone Formation. *Hepatology* 1990:1S–234S.

19. Cooper AD, ed. Pathogenesis and therapy of gallstone disease. *Gastroenterol Clin North Am* 1991;20:1–229.

20. Ko CW, Sekijima JH, Lee SP. Biliary sludge. *Ann Intern Med* 1999;130:301–311.

21. Bennion L, Grundy SM. Effects of obesity and caloric intake on biliary lipid metabolism in man. *J Clin Invest* 1975;56:996–1011.

22. Shaffer EA, Small DM. Biliary lipid secretion in cholesterol gallstone disease: the effect of cholecystectomy and obesity. *J Clin Invest* 1977;59:828–840.

23. Angelin B, Einarsson K, Ewerth S, et al. Biliary lipid composition in obesity. *Scand J Gastroenterol* 1981;16: 1015–1019.

24. Leijd B. Cholesterol and bile acid metabolism in obesity. *Clin Sci* 1980;59:203–206.

25. Meittinen TA, Gylling H. Cholesterol absorption efficiency and sterol metabolism in obesity. *Atherosclerosis* 2000;153:241–248.

26. Gebhard RL, Prigge WF, Ansel HJ, et al. The role of gallbladder emptying in gallstone formation during diet-induced rapid weight loss. *Hepatology* 1996;24:544–548.

27. Trouillot TE, Eckel RH, McKinley CL, et al. The link between weight loss, gallstones, and insulin action: a pathophysiologic study in humans. *Hepatology* 1997;26:399A.

28. Wang DP, Stroup D, Marrapodi M, et al. Transcriptional regulation of the human cholesterol 7 alpha-hydroxy-lase gene (CYP7A) in HepG2 cells. *J Lipid Res* 1996;37:1831–1841.

29. Marks JW, Bonorris GG, Albers G, et al. The sequence of biliary events preceding the formation of gallstones in humans. *Gastroenterology* 1992;103:566–570.

30. Vezina WC, Paradis RL, Grace DM, et al. Increased volume and decreased emptying of the gallbladder in large (morbidly obese, tall normal, and muscular normal) people. *Gastroenterology* 1990;98:1000–1007.

31. Portincasa P, De Ciaula A, Palmieri V, et al. Effects of cholestyramine on gallbladder and gastric emptying in obese and lean subjects. *Eur J Clin Invest* 1995;25:746–753.

32. Festi D, Colecchia A, Larocca A, et al. Review: low calorie intake and gallbladder motor function. *Aliment Pharmacol Ther* 2000;14:51–53.

33. Zapata R, Severin C, Manrique M, et al. Gallbladder motility and lithogenesis in obese patients during diet-induced weight loss. *Dig Dis Sci* 2000;45:421–428.

34. Wudel LJ, Wright JK, Debelak JP, et al. Prevention of gallstone formation in morbidly obese patients undergoing rapid weight loss: results of a randomized controlled pilot study. *J Surg Res* 2002;102:50–56.

35. Erlinger S. Gallstones in obesity and weight loss. *Eur J Gastroenterol Hepatol* 2000;12:1347–1352.

36. Festi D, Colecchia A, Orsini M, et al. Gallbladder motility and gallstone formation in obese patients following very low calorie diets. Use it (fat) to lose it (well). *Int J Obes Metab Disord* 1998;22:592–600.

37. Marks JW, Bonorris GG, Schoenfield LJ. Effects of ursodiol or ibuprofen on contraction of gallbladder and bile among obese patients during weight loss. *Dig Dis Sci* 1996;41:242–249.

38. Vezina WC, Grace DM, Hutton LC, et al. Similarity in gallstone formation from 900 kcal/day diets containing 16 g vs 30 g of daily fat: evidence that fat restriction is not the main culprit of cholelithiasis during rapid weight reduction. *Dig Dis Sci* 1998;43:554–561.

39. Gracie WA, Ransohoff DF. The natural history of silent gallstones, the innocent gallstone is not a myth. *N Engl J Med* 1982;307:798–800.

40. Grimaldi CH, Nelson RG, Pettitt DJ, et al. Increased mortality with gallstone disease: results of a 20 year population-based survey in Pima Indians. *Ann Intern Med* 1993;118:185–190.

41. Ransohoff DF, Miller GL, Forsyth SB, et al. Outcome of acute cholecystitis in patients with diabetes mellitus. *Ann Intern Med* 1987;106:829–832.

42. Schoenfield LJ et al. Chenodiol (chenodeoxycholic acid) for dissolution of gallstones. The National Cooperative Gallstone Study. *Ann Intern Med* 1981;95:257–282.

43. Valdivieso V, Covarrubias C, Siegel F, et al. Pregnancy and cholelithiasis: pathogenesis and natural course of gallstones diagnosed in early puerperium. *Hepatology* 1993;17:1–4.
44. Maringhini A, Ciambra M, Baccelliere P, et al. Biliary sludge and gallstones in pregnancy: incidence, risk factors, and natural history. *Ann Intern Med* 1993;119:116–120.
45. McSherry CK, Ferstenberg H, Calhoun WF, et al. The natural history of diagnosed gallstone disease in symptomatic and asymptomatic patients. *Ann Surg* 1985;202:59–63.
46. Lee SP, Maher K, Nicholls JF. Origin and fate of biliary sludge. *Gastroenterology* 1988;94:170–176.
47. Ohara N, Schaefer J. Clinical significance of biliary sludge. *J Clin Gastroenterol* 1990;12:291–294.
48. Lowenfels AB, Walker AM, Althaus DP, et al. Gallstone growth, size, and risk of gallbladder cancer: an interracial study. *Int J Epidemiol* 1989;18:50–54.
49. Polk HC Jr. Carcinoma and the calcified gallbladder. *Gastroenterology* 1966;50:582–585.
50. Weiss KM, Ferrell RE, Hanis CL, et al. Genetics and epidemiology of gallbladder disease in New World native peoples. *Am J Hum Genet* 1984;36:1259–1278.
51. Ludwig J, Viggiano TR, McGill DB, et al. Nonalcoholic steatohepatitis. Mayo Clinic experiences with a hitherto unnamed disease. *Mayo Clin Proc* 1980;55:434–438.
52. Teli MR, James OFW, Burt AD, et al. The natural history of nonalcoholic fatty liver: a follow-up study. *Hepatology* 1995;22:1714–1719.
53. Matteoni CA, Younossi ZM, Gramlich T, et al. Nonalcoholic fatty liver disease: a spectrum of clinical and pathological severity. *Gastroenterology* 1999;116:1413–1419.
54. Bacon BR, Farahvash MJ, Janney CG, et al. Nonalcoholic steatohepatitis: an expanded clinical entity. *Gastroenterology* 1994;107:1103–1109.
55. George DK, Goldwurm S, MacDonald GA, et al. Increased hepatic iron concentration in nonalcoholic steatohepatitis is associated with increased fibrosis. *Gastroenterology* 1998;114:311–318.
56. Peters RL, Gay T, Reynolds TB. Post jejunoileal bypass hepatic disease. Its similarity to alcoholic liver disease. *Am J Clin Pathol* 1975;63:318–331.
57. Poucell S, Ireton J, Valencia-Mayoral P, et al. Amiodarone-associated phospholipidosis and fibrosis of the liver. Light, immunohistochemical, and electron microscopic studies. *Gastroenterology* 1984;86:926–936.
58. Brunt EM, Janney CG, Di Bisceglie AM, et al. Nonalcoholic steatohepatitis: a proposal for grading and staging the histological lesions. *Am J Gastroenterol* 1999;94:2467–2474.
59. Brunt EM. Nonalcoholic steatohepatitis: definition and pathology. *Semin Liver Dis* 2001;21:3–16.
60. Rashid M, Roberts EA. Nonalcoholic steatohepatitis in children. *J Pediatr Gastroenterol Nutr* 2000;30:48–53.
61. Younossi ZM, Gramlich T, Chang Y, et al. Nonalcoholic fatty liver disease: assessment of variability in pathologic interpretations. *Mod Pathol* 1998;11:560–565.
62. Nonomura A, Mizukami Y, Unoura M, et al. Clinicopathologic study of alcohol-like liver disease in non-alcoholics; nonalcoholic hepatitis and fibrosis. *Gastroenterol Jpn* 1992;27:521–528.
63. Hultcrantz R, Glaumann H, Lindberg G, et al. Liver investigation in 149 asymptomatic patients with moderately elevated activities of serum aminotransferases. *Scand J Gastroenterol* 1986;21:109–113.
64. Propst A, Propst T, Judmaier G, et al. Prognosis in nonalcoholic steatohepatitis [Letter]. *Gastroenterology* 1995;108:1607.
65. Ground KE. Liver pathology in aircrew. *Aviat Space Environ Med* 1982;53:14–18.
66. Hilden M, Christoffersen P, Juhl E, et al. Liver histology in a "normal" population—examinations of 503 consecutive fatal traffic casualties. *Scand J Gastroenterol* 1977;12:593–597.
67. Angulo P, Keach JC, Batts KP, et al. Independent predictors of liver fibrosis in patients with nonalcoholic steatohepatitis. *Hepatology* 1999;30:1356–1362.
68. Dixon JB, Bhathal PS, O'Brien PE. Non-alcoholic fatty liver disease: predictors of non-alcoholic steatohepatitis and liver fibrosis in the severely obese. *Gastroenterology* 2001;121:91–100.
69. Ratziu V, Giral P, Charlotte F, et al. Liver fibrosis in overweight patients. *Gastroenterology* 2000;118:1117–1123.
70. Falk-Ytter Y, Younossi ZM, Marchesini G, et al. Clinical features and natural history of nonalcoholic steatosis syndromes. *Semin Liver Dis* 2001;21:17–26.
71. Powell EE, Cooksley WGH, Hanson R, et al. The natural history of nonalcoholic steatohepatitis: a follow-up study of forty-two patients for up to 21 years. *Hepatology* 1990;11:74–80.
72. Caldwell SH, Oelsner DH, Iezzoni JC, et al. Cryptogenic cirrhosis: clinical characterization and risk factors for underlying disease. *Hepatology* 1999;29:664–669.
73. Poonawala A, Nair SP, Thuluvath PJ. Prevalence of obesity and diabetes in patients with cryptogenic cirrhosis: a case controlled study. *Hepatology* 2000;32:689–692.
74. Hocking MP, Davis GL, Franzini DA, et al. Long-term consequences after jejunoileal bypass for morbid obesity. *Dig Dis Sci* 1998;43:2493–2499.
75. Day C, James O. Steatohepatitis: a tale of two "hits"? *Gastroenterology* 1998;114:842–845.
76. Fong D, Nehra V, Lindor K, et al. Metabolic and nutritional considerations in nonalcoholic fatty liver. *Hepatology* 2000;32:3–10.
77. Van Steenbergen W, Lanckmans S. Liver disturbances in obesity and diabetes mellitus. *Int J Obes Relat Metab Disord* 1995;19:S27–S36.
78. Fisher R. Hepatobiliary abnormalities associated with total parenteral nutrition. *Gastroenterol Clin North Am* 1989;18:645–666.
79. Pagano G, Pacini G, Musso G, et al. Nonalcoholic steatohepatitis, insulin resistance, and metabolic syndrome: further evidence for an etiologic association. *Hepatology* 2002;35:367–372.

80. Ingelman-Sundberg M, Johansson I, Yin J, et al. Lipid peroxidation dependent on ethanol-inducible cytochrome P450 from rat liver. *Adv Biophys* 1988;71:43–47.
81. Weltman M, Farrell G, Liddle C. Increased hepatocyte CYP 2E1 expression in a rat nutritional model of hepatic steatosis with inflammation. *Gastroenterology* 1996;111:1645–1653.
82. Weltman M, Farrell G, Hall P, et al. Hepatic cytochrome P450 2E1 is increased in patients with nonalcoholic hepatitis. *Hepatology* 1998;27:128–133.
83. Leclercq I, Farrell G, Field J, et al. CYP 2E1 and CYP 4A as microsomal catalysts of lipid peroxides in murine nonalcoholic steatohepatitis. *J Clin Invest* 2000;105:1067–1075.
84. Mendler MH, Turlin B, Moirand R, et al. Insulin resistance-associated hepatic iron overload. *Gastroenterology* 1999;117:1155–1163.
85. Younossi ZM, Gramlich T, Bacon BR, et al. Hepatic iron and nonalcoholic fatty liver disease. *Hepatology* 1999; 30:847–850.
86. Bonkovsky HL, Ponka P, Bacon BR, et al. An update on iron metabolism: summary of the Fifth International Conference on Disorders of Iron Metabolism. *Hepatology* 1996;24:718–729.
87. Winterbourn CC. Toxicity of iron and hydrogen peroxide: the Fenton reaction. *Toxicol Lett* 1995;82/83: 969–974.
88. Yang S, Lin H, Lane M, et al. Obesity increases sensitivity to endotoxin liver injury: implications for the pathogenesis of steatohepatitis. *Proc Natl Acad Sci U S A* 1997;94:2557–2562.
89. Haines N, Baker A, Boyer J, et al. Prognostic indicators of hepatic injury following jejunoileal bypass performed for refractory obesity: a prospective study. *Hepatology* 1981;1:161–165.
90. Drenick E, Fisler J, Johnson D. Hepatic steatosis after intestinal bypass. Prevention and reversal by metronidazole irrespective of protein-calorie malnutrition. *Gastroenterology* 1982;82:535–548.
91. Valenti L, Francazani AL, Dongiovanni P, et al. Tumor necrosis factor alpha promoter polymorphisms and insulin resistance in nonalcoholic fatty liver disease. *Gastroenterology* 2002;122:274–280.
92. Rashid A, Wu TC, Huang C, et al. Mitochondrial proteins that regulate apoptosis and necrosis are induced in mouse fatty liver. *Hepatology* 1999;29:1131–1138.
93. Chavin K, Yang S, Lin H, et al. Obesity induces expression of uncoupling protein-2 in hepatocytes and promotes liver ATP depletion. *J Biol Chem* 1999;274:5692–5700.
94. Cortez-Pinto H, Chatham J, Chacko V, et al. Alterations in liver ATP homeostasis in human non-alcoholic steatohepatitis: a pilot study. *JAMA* 1999;282:1659–1664.
95. Berson A, De Beco V, Letteron P, et al. Steatohepatitis-inducing drugs cause mitochondrial dysfunction and lipid peroxidation in rat hepatocytes. *Gastroenterology* 1998;114:764–774.
96. Franzese A, Vajro P, Argenziano A, et al. Ultrasonography and liver enzyme levels at diagnosis and during follow-up in an Italian population. *Dig Dis Sci* 1997;42:1428–1432.
97. Kinugasa A, Tsunamoto K, Furukawa N, et al. Fatty liver and its fibrous changes found in simple obesity of children. *J Pediatr Gastroenterol Nutr* 1984;3:408–414.
98. McTigue KM, Garrett JM, Popkin BM. The natural history of the development of obesity in a cohort of young US adults between 1981 and 1998. *Ann Intern Med* 2002;136:857–864.
99. Whitaker RC. Understanding the complex journey to obesity in early adulthood. *Ann Intern Med* 2002;136: 923–925.
100. Palmer M, Schaffner F. Effect of weight reduction on hepatic abnormalities in overweight patients. *Gastroenterology* 1990;99:1408–1413.
101. Kugelmas M, Vivian B, Antle A, et al. Cytokine profiles in NASH: Effects of diet, exercise, and vitamin E. *Gastroenterology* 1999;116:A1234.
102. Basaranoglu M, Acbay O, Sonsuz A. A controlled trial of gemfibrozil in the treatment of patients with nonalcoholic steatohepatitis [Letter]. *J Hepatol* 1999;31:384.
103. Laurin J, Lindor K, Crippin J, et al. Ursodeoxycholic acid or clofibrate in the treatment of nonalcoholic steatohepatitis: a pilot study. *Hepatology* 1996;23:1464–1467.
104. Abdelmalek MF, Angulo P, Jorgensen RA, et al. Betaine, a promising new agent for patients with nonalcoholic steatohepatitis: results of a pilot study. *Am J Gastrol* 2001;96:2711–2717.
105. Lin H, Yang S, Chuckaree C, et al. Metformin reverses fatty liver disease in obese, leptin-deficient mice. *Nat Med* 2000;6:998–1003.
106. Battle E, Hespenheide E, Caldwell S, et al. Pilot study of troglitazone (Rezulin) for nonalcoholic steatohepatitis. *Hepatology* 1998;28:304A.
107. Lavine J. Vitamin E treatment of nonalcoholic steatohepatitis in children: a pilot study. *J Pediatr* 2000;136: 734–738.
108. Charlton M, Kasparova P, Weston S, et al. Frequency of nonalcoholic steatohepatitis as a cause of advanced liver disease. *Liver Transpl* 2001;7:608–614.
109. Ong J, Younossi ZM, Reddy V, et al. Cryptogenic cirrhosis and post-transplantation nonalcoholic fatty liver disease. *Liver Transpl* 2001;7:797–801.
110. Carson K, Washington MK, Treem WR, et al. Recurrence of nonalcoholic steatohepatitis in a liver transplant recipient. *Liver Transpl Surg* 1997;3:174–176.
111. Molloy RM, Komorowski R, Varma RR. Recurrent nonalcoholic steatohepatitis and cirrhosis after liver transplantation. *Liver Transpl Surg* 1997;2:177–178.

13

Cancer

David Heber

A worldwide epidemic of common forms of cancer is occurring in those countries and socioeconomic groups within countries eating a so-called "Western diet," which is characterized by a dietary pattern rich in fat, sugar, and red meat but poor in fiber, fruits, and vegetables (1). Because age is the primary risk factor for cancer, all such associations are based on age-adjusted incidences, which can be up to five times higher in the so-called "high-risk countries" (e.g., the United States) than in the low-risk countries (e.g., Japan). Moreover, individuals migrating from low-risk to high-risk countries increase their risk of cancer substantially within a single generation (2). Obesity is also associated with a number of common forms of cancer (3). These data have implicated environmental and lifestyle factors, including diet, in the etiology of cancer. Evidence also suggests that obesity is associated with an increased rate of progression of cancer after initial treatment (4). With an ever-increasing population of cancer survivors and an increasing incidence of obesity, the treatment of obesity in patients with diagnosed cancer who have survived initial treatment may improve outcomes and increase the median survival. Even if these efforts had no effect on any remaining cancer cells, the treatment of obesity in cancer survivors improves their quality of life and reduces the risk of other chronic diseases, including heart disease and diabetes.

A number of plausible biologic mechanisms exist whereby obesity could promote the development and progression of cancer (5). The evidence for a connection between obesity and common forms of cancer is drawn from studies of populations, animal experiments, and limited clinical research on humans, which largely provides the biologic proof of the principle. With the exception of nonmelanoma skin cancers, in which a low-fat diet led to a reduced incidence of tumors and modest weight loss (6), no definitive large-scale clinical intervention studies have demonstrated that weight loss or dietary changes reduce cancer incidence. Nonetheless, sufficient evidence has been found to warrant advising cancer survivors to follow current dietary advice to achieve and to maintain a healthy body weight by increasing the amount of fruits, vegetables, and whole grains in the diet, while reducing fats.

INTERACTIONS OF OBESITY WITH THE ENDOCRINE, PARACRINE, AND IMMUNE SYSTEMS

Obesity, which is characterized by excess adipose tissue, has been shown to increase the risk of several common cancers. A number of biologic processes common to both obesity and cancer could lead to a causal interrelationship. Many hormones involved in obesity also play a role in the initiation and promotion of cancer at a cellular, a paracrine, and a systemic level (7). Most common forms of cancer in developed countries, including lung cancer, breast cancer, prostate cancer, colon cancer, pancreatic cancer, ovarian cancer, uterine cancer, kidney cancer, and gallbladder cancer, are epithelial cell cancers. In these cancers, interactions between epithelial and stromal components within the tissue, as well as with hormones reaching the organ via the circulation, may play a role in stimulating tumor development and growth.

At least four different mechanisms exist by which increased hormone secretion may promote cancer development (Fig. 13.1). First, obesity leads to the increased production of growth-promoting steroid hormones that can bind to the nuclear receptors in hormone-dependent tumor cells. For example, estrogens, which can promote breast cancer growth and metastasis (8), are produced in excess amounts in obese women via the aromatization of adrenal androgens by adipose stromal tissues in breast fat and the peripheral fat tissues. Second, free hormone levels can be affected by hormone–hormone interactions, such as those that occur with upper-body obesity in postmenopausal women, which is associated with reduced sex hormone–binding globulin levels, leading to increased free levels of circulating estrogens (9). Third, steroid hormone action can trigger increased oxidant stress, thus promoting cell proliferation and DNA damage (10). Androgens have been demonstrated to increase oxidant stress in prostate cancer cells, and oxidant defense mechanisms have been shown to be impaired early in the cancer process. Finally, obesity can increase the production of paracrine factors and hormones that stimulate the production of steroid hormones in cancer tissue through interactions between the stromal and epithelial compartments in tissues. Many of these paracrine factors are cytokines pro-

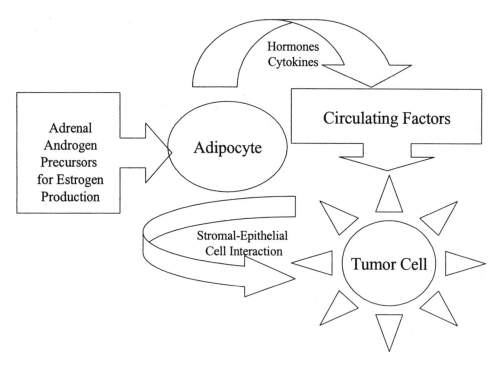

FIG. 13.1. Mechanisms of obesity-stimulated tumor growth and progression. Adrenal androgen precursors are converted to circulating estrogens by adipose tissue. Cytokines from adipose stromal tissue induce enzymatic activity in tumors and stimulate tumor growth and angiogenesis. Tumor tissue estrogens and other factors act locally through stromal–epithelial interactions and peripherally through the circulation to affect tumors with cytokine and hormone receptors.

duced by both fat cells and white blood cells. Obesity is associated with increased circulating levels of cytokines, and these levels are reduced with weight loss (11,12). These cytokines can act to increase oxidative stress in epithelial cells, which theoretically could lead to increased mutagenesis and carcinogenesis (13). The fat cell, the source of many of these so-called adipocytokines, may play a significant role in the ability of fat tissue to preserve the immune resistance to infections. Malnutrition is associated with multiple impairments of immune function, including impaired helper T-cell function, so the ability of fat to store calories provides a separate, important function for protecting the immune defenses (14). To the extent that cancer and heart disease are replacing infectious diseases as the primary cause of death as obesity becomes more common in developing countries, the increased cytokine secretion observed in obesity may have a beneficial effect on infectious disease resistance while simultaneously increasing the risk of cancer.

BREAST CANCER

More evidence exists linking obesity to breast cancer than it does to any other cancer, based on epidemiologic, clinical, and experimental studies. The effects of reproductive hormonal status on fat accumulation and mobilization are critical issues in the understanding of the pathogenesis of obesity and the common forms of cancer in women.

After the onset of puberty, women have adiposity that is increased compared to men. Obese women have higher levels of circulating estrogens than lean women because of the conversion of adrenal androgens to estrogens by an aromatase enzyme found in the adipose stromal cells (8). Premenopausal women develop gluteofemoral fat and abdominal fat, whereas men develop primarily abdominal fat (15). The gluteofemoral fat is a useful store of energy for lactation, and it increases during each pregnancy. However, in the modern society, women rarely feed their infants at the breast to the extent found in more primitive societies, so the gluteofemoral fat is not lost effectively (16). In fact, food intake can increase after pregnancy, and postpregnancy weight gain is an important factor in the epidemiology of obesity in United States women (17). Premenopausal women have two significant sources of estrogen—the ovaries and their fat tissue. After menopause, the gluteofemoral fat depots decrease in size in many women, while adiposity in the abdominal and breast fat depots increases. The use of pharmacologic amounts of estrogens by men who impersonate women leads to gynoid fat distribution, whereas the use of anabolic androgens by female weightlifters leads to male fat patterns. Although these data suggest that the gluteofemoral fat depots are estrogen dependent, estrogen receptors have not been found in cells isolated from gluteofemoral fat (18).

Age at menarche, age at menopause, parity, and the age at first full-term pregnancy are important determinants of breast cancer risk (19). Asian women living a traditional lifestyle have lower estrogen levels both before and after menopause (20), and these lower levels of estrogen have been considered important markers of the differences in breast cancer incidence observed in international epidemiologic studies (21). Increased daily alcohol intake has been associated with an increased risk of breast cancer and increased levels of endogenous estrogens in premenopausal women (22). A number of aspects of dietary intake, physical activity, and body composition affect endogenous estrogen levels. In the author's studies of more than 300 women, a decrease in fat intake was associated with a significant decrease in body fat, as measured by bioelectrical impedance (23). Bagga et al. (24) have also shown that a high-fiber, low-fat diet will reduce serum estrone and estradiol in both the follicular and the luteal phase of the cycle. Dietary fat and fiber intake have also been reported to affect the circulating concentrations of estrogens and androgens in women eating their usual diets under controlled conditions (25).

Increased estrogen production in women with excess fat compared to that of lean women (26,27) is due to the increased peripheral conversion of androstenedione to estrone by fat tissue (28,29). Obesity has been repeatedly associated with more advanced breast cancer at the time of diagnosis, higher rates of recurrence, and shorter survival times even after controlling for the tumor size and stage of disease at diagnosis (30–38). This has been explained in the past as a result of the delayed diagnosis in obese women rather than of the enhanced tumor promotion resulting from increased estrogen production. The effects of obesity on the invasiveness of breast cancers at the time of diagnosis are different in patients with estrogen receptor–positive tumors than in those with estrogen receptor–negative tumors (39). If the effects of obesity on breast tumor nodal invasion and, therefore, prognosis are simply due to delayed diagnosis, then similar associations should be seen for both the receptor–positive and the receptor–negative patients. That an effect of obesity was observed only in the receptor-positive patients strongly suggests that a hormonal mechanism accounts for the effects of obesity on breast tumor promotion.

Although obesity on a weight-for-height basis has not been associated with an increased risk of premenopausal breast cancer, adult weight gain increases the risk of postmenopausal breast cancer, and it is a predictor of breast cancer risk independent of body weight (40–49). The physiologic effects of weight gain are likely to be evident in both premenopausal and postmenopausal women, regardless of whether they are classified as obese on weight-for-height criteria.

In a case-control study of healthy premenopausal women and patients with breast cancer in Shanghai and Los Angeles, Bernstein et al. (50) found that the controls in Los Angeles had a 20.6% greater estradiol concentration than did controls in Shanghai and that adjustment for body weight accounted for only 25.7% of this difference. They concluded that the higher estrogen levels could be an important part of the twofold to threefold difference in the breast cancer incidence rates of women younger than 45 years of age in Shanghai and Los Angeles.

Therefore, obesity is related to breast cancer in a complex way that suggests that a hormonal correlate of excessive body weight might affect breast cancer growth and metastasis. The potential benefit of intentional weight loss as an adjunct to breast cancer treatment deserves further study. Many studies have suggested that drinking alcohol, even at modest levels, might also increase breast cancer risk. Because the potential benefits of modest levels of alcohol for cardiovascular disease may outweigh the risk for breast cancer, recommendations of total alcohol abstinence may be premature for women with an average risk of breast cancer. Women at an unusually high risk for breast cancer who have a lower than average risk for cardiovascular disease, however, might make an informed decision to abstain from alcohol intake. Following the current dietary advice to increase the amount of fruits, vegetables, and whole grains in the diet while reducing fats is certainly prudent for women who wish to reduce their risk of several chronic diseases.

UTERINE CANCER

The relationship between obesity and an increased risk of uterine cancer is well established. The mechanism is presumed to be the increased production of estrogens, which are also associated with menometrorrhagia in obese women. Estrogens directly stimulate the proliferation of the uterine endothelium through the direct stimulation of estrogen receptors. The relationship between body mass index (BMI) and the subsequent risk of cancer of endocrine target organs was studied in a cohort of 47,003 women examined for height and weight from 1963 to 1965 and was followed up in the Swedish Cancer Register until 1987 (51). Cancer of the ovaries and the uterine cervix were not significantly related to BMI in any age-group. In women 55 years of age or older, the relative risk of cancer of the uterine corpus when associated with BMI was higher than that for breast cancer, and this association persisted during the entire follow-up of more than 20 years. Despite the fact that endometrial cancer is less common than breast cancer, more endometrial cancer cases than breast cancer cases were attributable to obesity in this cohort because of the stronger relationship between overweight and endometrial cancer.

In a case-control study in western New York State (52), interviews were conducted with 232 incident endometrial cancer patients diagnosed between 1986 and 1991, and 631 community controls were examined to determine the effects of obesity at times before the diagnosis of uterine cancer. BMI at 16 years of age and 20, 10, and 2 years before the interview and changes in BMI between these times were considered. Although being relatively heavy at 16 years of age was associated with a slightly increased risk (adjusted odds ratio [OR] = 1.28, 95% confidence interval [CI] = 0.84–1.96), large gains over the entire period from 16 years of age to 2 years before diagnosis (OR = 3.45, CI = 2.13–5.57) and a high BMI close to the time of diagnosis (OR = 3.21, CI = 2.01–5.15) were associated with a greater risk. Differences in mean BMI between the cases and the controls increased over time.

Although obesity increases the risk of uterine cancer, it is associated with the less aggressive varieties of endometrial cancer. In a retrospective study of 492 women (53) with endometrial carcinoma, the time to recurrence was significantly increased as the BMI increased (p =0.0136). BMI was strongly related to the grade (p =0.013), the depth of myometrial invasion (p =0.031), negative cytologic findings (p =0.004), and stage (p =0.011), with obese patients having better differentiated, less invasive tumors of lower stage with negative washings. Surprisingly, morbid obesity positively affects survival in endometrial carcinoma. This effect is accounted for by the association of obesity with less aggressive disease. Despite these findings, the increased risk of uterine cancer still warrants efforts at weight reduction in women at risk.

OVARIAN CANCER

In the United States, ovarian cancer is the fourth most frequent cause of cancer death in women after lung, breast, and colorectal cancers. Each year, approximately 26,000 women are diagnosed with ovarian cancer, and 14,000 women die of it. Germline mutations in *BRCA1, BRCA2,* or other genes have been implicated in a small fraction of cases. However, for most patients, the risk of epithelial ovarian cancer could be related to the chronically repeated formation of stromal epithelial clefts and inclusion cysts after ovulation or to some type of hormonal stimulation of ovarian epithelial cells, either on the surface of the ovary or within ovarian inclusion cysts, that is possibly mediated through excessive gonadotropin secretion. From the evidence, the relative importance of these two hypotheses—ovulation and gonadotropin stimulation—cannot be distinguished. Although either or both may play a role in the development of ovarian cancer, an additional major factor may also be involved. The risk of ovarian cancer may be further increased by factors associated with excess androgenic stimulation of ovarian epithelial cells, and it may be decreased by factors related to greater progesterone stimulation.

Many features of the evidence regarding the pathophysiology of ovarian cancer appear to support a connection to androgens and progesterone.

A case-control study was conducted to assess some environmental and other risk factors for ovarian cancer from 1994 to 1996 in northern Kyushu, Japan (54). In 89 cases of epithelial ovarian cancer and 323 controls without any cancer or ovarian disorder, the ORs of ovarian cancer across increasing quartiles of the heaviest body weight were 1.00, 1.15, 1.71, and 2.29 (p =0.008, test for trend). Significantly increased risks were noted for a history of diabetes mellitus ($p < 0.05$) and for a family history of ovarian cancer ($p < 0.05$). Significantly decreased trends for risk were obtained for the number of pregnancies ($p < 0.01$) and the number of live births ($p < 0.001$). This study provides additional support for an association between obesity and the risk of ovarian cancer. As was mentioned earlier, other studies have found no association between obesity and ovarian cancer (51). Clearly, much additional research on the exact mechanisms underlying this association must be conducted.

PROSTATE CANCER

The diagnosis of prostate cancer has improved recently as a result of the development of the prostate-specific antigen (PSA) test, which detects prostate cancer before it is physically palpable as a mass on the rectal examination (55). Approximately 180,000 men were diagnosed with prostate cancer in 2000 (56). Prostate cancer develops as a result of both inherited and environmental factors. It is associated with aging, and it occurs in a latent or clinically inactive form in 30% to 40% of men by 30 to 50 years of age and in 75% of men by the age of 80 (57,58). Because latent or clinically inactive cancers had not been as effectively diagnosed before the development of the PSA test as they now are, some uncertainty about the predicted behavior of prostate cancer after diagnosis exists.

The cause of this disease is not fully understood, but a family history, the effects of androgens (e.g., testosterone) and other hormones, and environmental and dietary factors may all be involved. The international variations in the rates of prostate cancer are considerable. The county of Qidong in China has the lowest recorded incidence rate, 0.5 per 100,000 men. By comparison, Sweden has a rate of 55.3 per 100,000 men, and the United States, of 102.1 per 100,000 men (59). Diagnosing silent cancer by blood PSA tests increases the incidence because more clinically silent cancers are diagnosed. Global differences in incidence are probably not due to inheritance. If individuals with the same inherited genes are raised in two different environments, the risk of prostate cancer is associated with the country in which they are raised (60).

An American Cancer Society survey of 750,000 individuals demonstrated that obesity increased the risk of prostate cancer (61). Among the various nutritional factors examined, *per capita* total fat consumption correlates with the increased prostate cancer incidence noted in cross-national studies (62). In Japan, an increase in the risk of prostate cancer has been noted because the *per capita* intake of dietary fat has increased (63). In Hawaii, a correlation was found between saturated fat intake and prostate cancer incidence (64). In the United States, the counties with higher prostate cancer incidences have higher per capita fat intakes (65). Using questionnaires that ask how often a particular food is normally eaten, scientists have found clues to the association of dietary fat with cancer. In a retrospective study by West et al. (66) and in a prospective study by Giovannucci et al. (67), the more aggressive prostate cancers in patients were significantly correlated with high fat intake. In the study by Giovannucci et al. (67), those individuals eating the highest amount of meat had a risk of developing prostate cancer that was 2.64 times that of those eating the least. The course of prostate cancer may also be affected by fat intake. Kolonel et al. (68) found a significant relationship between dietary fat and prostate cancer mortality in men 70 years of age and older in Hawaii. In addition, several studies have demonstrated a positive association between saturated fat intake from meat and dairy products and prostate cancer (69–74). Other factors in the diet may enhance or diminish the risk of prostate cancer. The retrospective and prospective studies that have been reviewed have found an association between prostate cancer and dietary fat. Futhermore, no studies show a negative correlation.

Approximately 60% of all men have latent or clinically silent prostate cancer, and the incidence of this latent form is the same in the United States and Japan (75). These estimates are based on autopsies of men who die for reasons other than prostate cancer. At the same time, clinically significant prostate cancer occurs much more commonly in the United States than in Japan. When Japanese men migrate to the United States, their incidence of clinically detected prostate cancer rises within one generation. These facts suggest that nutrition and lifestyle practices in lower risk countries suppress the growth of prostate cancer so that it remains small and confined and thus it is never clinically diagnosed. Prostate cancer is a disease associated with aging and obesity. Some have said that, if one lives long enough, he will have prostate cancer, as more than 90% of men older than 90 years of age have detectable carcinomas in prostatic tissue. Men who die prematurely (i.e., accidental deaths) are found to have precancerous lesions, such as prostatic intraepithelial neoplasia (PIN), in their prostate glands if they are between 40 and 60 years of age. In men older than 60 years of age, not only are PIN lesions found, but foci of prostatic cancer are also found. Moreover, a shift in the prooxidant–antioxidant balance of many tissues toward a more oxidative state is commonly associated with increasing age. Recently, foci of proliferative inflammatory atrophy (PIA) have been found in prostatic cancer biopsy specimens. Although the DNA in PIN and cancerous lesions has multiple abnormalities, the PIA lesions have normal DNA. Given the common occurrence of prostatitis, both clinical and subclinical, one hypothesis is that, with aging, the prostate gland undergoes repeated inflammation leading to DNA damage, mutation, and ultimately the formation of precancerous and cancerous lesions. African-American men have a significantly higher incidence of prostate cancer compared to that of white men, and they have higher levels of insulin-like growth factor-1 (IGF-1) and androgens at puberty. Androgen exposure, which has long been associated with the development of prostate cancer, may be a means by which the prooxidant–antioxidant balance of prostate cells is altered.

In rats, prostate cancer can be induced by the prolonged administration of testosterone. The ablation of androgens has formed the basis for the first-line therapy of metastatic prostate cancer. Hormones also may play a role in the progression of prostate cancer from silent to clinically significant forms. Because diet can influence circulating sex steroid hormones, diet and androgens may alter prostate cancer biology via common pathways. The urinary levels of androgens and estrogens were decreased in a group of white and African-American men fed a diet in which the fat content was reduced from 40% to 30% of the total calories (76). A very low fat, high-fiber diet has been shown to reduce sex steroid levels in a group of normal men (77). Therefore, changes in sex hormones may mediate in part the effects of diet on prostate cancer growth.

As sedentary men age, they often experience an increase in fat mass, a decrease in lean body mass, and a change in hormone levels. These factors have been shown to increase the risk of prostate cancer. In a study of Seventh-Day Adventists, obesity was shown to increase the risk of fatal prostate cancer significantly compared to that of ideal weight (78). This association was also noted in the American Cancer Society's study of 750,000 individuals (65). With aging, the prevalence of benign prostatic hyperplasia (BPH) increases; this is an androgen-dependent chronic disorder (79). Dihydrotestosterone (DHT) formed from testosterone in the prostate and in the testes appears to promote hyperplasia in humans, dogs, and rats. Horton et al. (80) found increased levels of circulating DHT in elderly men compared to those of young men (89 ng per dL versus 49 ng per dL); in this study, nearly all the elderly men had BPH. Because the prostate can convert testosterone to DHT, some have hypothesized that the increased metabolic conversion of testosterone to DHT due to BPH may account for the increased DHT levels in elderly men.

In prostate cancer cell lines exposed to physiologic levels of 5α-dihydrotestosterone and to the synthetic androgen R1881, the proliferative responses were correlated to the changes in oxidative stress (10). Physiologic levels of androgens are capable of increasing oxidative stress in androgen-responsive LNCaP prostate carcinoma cells. The evidence suggests that this result is partially due to increased mitochondrial activity. Androgens also alter intracellular glutathione levels and the activity of certain detoxification enzymes, such as γ-glutamyl transpeptidase, that are important for maintenance of the cellular prooxidant–antioxidant balance (81).

RENAL CELL CANCER

In a population-based case-control study (82) including 449 directly interviewed cases and 707 controls, the risk increased with increasing BMI in women. A nearly fourfold risk was found in the 10% of women with the highest BMI (OR = 3.8; CI = 1.7–8.4). Among men, no clear trend was observed with usual weight or BMI, although the highest risk (30% to 50%) generally was seen in those in the upper deciles of weight or BMI. No clear indication that excess BMI early or late in life disproportionately affected risks was found. Risk also was not related to patterns of weight fluctuations or to the use of diet pills. This study supported previous observations linking renal cell cancer risk to increased BMI in women, and it suggested a weaker association in men. In a population-based case-control study conducted in Los Angeles County, California (83) to investigate the interrelationships of obesity, hypertension, and medications relative to the renal cell carcinoma risk, a total of 1,204 patients with renal cell cancer and an equal number of neighborhood controls were included. Obesity was found to be a strong risk factor for renal cancer. A fourfold increase in risk was observed for those with a BMI of more than or equal to 30 kilograms per meter squared (kg/m^2) versus that for those with a BMI of less than 22 kg/m^2. A history of hypertension was another strong independent risk factor for renal cell cancer (OR = 2.2). Little evidence that use of diuretics was directly related to renal cancer development was found. Use of diuretics for reasons other than hypertension (i.e., primarily for weight control) was unrelated to risk in self-reported normotensive subjects. Among hypertensive subjects, heavy users of diuretics experienced a risk similar to that of light users. Likewise, normotensive subjects who took nondiuretic antihypertensives regularly showed no increased risk of renal cell cancer, and intake in hypertensive subjects did not additionally increase their risk. The regular use of amphetamine-containing diet pills was associated with a twofold increase in renal cell cancer risk, and the risk increased with an increasing dose of amphetamines. However, the fraction of cases that are possibly related to this exposure is small (population-attributable risk = 5%).

Obesity and hypertension have also been implicated as risk factors for the development of renal cell cancer in a recent study from the National Cancer Institute (84). The health records of 363,992 Swedish men who underwent at least one physical examination from 1971 to 1992 were followed until death or the end of 1995. Men with cancer (renal cell cancer in 759 and renal-pelvis cancer in 136) were identified by cross-linkage of data with the nationwide Swedish Cancer Registry. Poisson regression analysis was used to estimate relative risks, with adjustments for age, smoking status, BMI, and diastolic blood pressure. Compared to men in the lowest 37.5% of BMI of the cohort, men in the middle 37.5% had a 30% to 60% greater risk of renal cell cancer, and men in the highest 25% had nearly double the risk ($p < 0.001$, for trend). A direct association was also found between higher blood pressures and a higher risk of renal cell cancer (for trend, $p < 0.001$ for diastolic pressure; $p < 0.007$ for systolic pressure). After the first 5 years of follow-up were excluded to reduce the possible effects of preclinical disease, the risk of renal cell cancer was still consistently higher in men with a higher BMI or higher blood pressure. At the 6-year follow-up, the risk rose further with increasing blood pressures and it decreased with decreasing blood pressures, after adjustment for baseline measurements. Men who were current or former smokers had a greater risk of both renal cell cancer and renal-pelvis cancer than did men who were not smokers. No relation was found between BMI or blood pressure and the risk of renal-pelvis cancer. In this study, both higher BMI and elevated blood pressure independently increased the long-term risk of renal cell cancer in men.

Many mechanisms may account for this association, including circulating hormones capable of stimulating tumor growth, increased cytokines that may increase oxidant stress in the kidney, and increased intrarenal hormone levels associated with obesity or hypertension. Given the increasing prevalence of obesity and the rising incidence of renal cell cancer in the United States, additional studies are needed to disentangle the effects of BMI from various correlates, including blood pressure, and to identify the mechanisms by which obesity affects risk.

COLON CANCER

Obesity has been reported to increase the risk of colon cancer, especially in men. The American Cancer Society's Cancer Prevention Study II (85), a nationwide mortality study of United States adults, documented 1,616 deaths from colon cancer in women and 1,792 deaths in men over 12 years of follow-up in 496,239 women and 379,167 men who were cancer free at the time of their enrollment in 1982. The authors used Cox proportional hazards analyses to control for the effects of age; race; education; smoking; exercise; alcohol; parental history of colon cancer; fat intake; vegetable and grain intake; aspirin use; and, in women, estrogen-replacement therapy. In men, death rates from colon cancer increased across the entire range of BMI. The rate ratio was highest for men with BMIs more than or equal to 32.5 kg/m^2 (relative risk [RR] = 1.90; 95% CI, 1.46–2.47) compared to that of men with BMIs between 22.00 and 23.49 kg/m^2. In women, a weaker association was seen in the three BMI categories of 27.5 to 29.9 kg/m^2 (RR = 1.26; 95% CI, 1.03–1.53), 30.0 to 32.4 kg/m^2 (RR = 1.37; 95% CI, 1.09–1.72), and more than or equal to 32.5 kg/m^2 (RR = 1.23; 95% CI, 0.96–1.59). These prospective data support the hypothesis that obesity increases the risk of colon cancer death and that the relationship of BMI to the risk of colon cancer is stronger and more linear in men than it is in women. Because BMI is a surrogate for body fat, which may be less accurate in postmenopausal women, the sex difference observed may have been due to reliance on the BMI.

Further evidence that obesity increases the risk of colon cancer and adenomas, which are precursors of cancer, and that an abdominal distribution of obesity is an independent risk factor for these events was obtained in a study of 47,723 male health professionals, 40 to 75 years of age, who responded to a questionnaire mailed in 1986 about BMI and to questionnaires in 1987 (31,055 respondents) about waist and hip circumferences (86). Between 1986 and 1992, 203 new patients were diagnosed with colon cancer, and 586 were diagnosed with adenomas. BMI was directly associated with the risk of colon cancer, independent of the level of physical activity. Waist circumference and the waist to hip ratio (WHR) were strong risk factors for colon cancer (WHR greater than or equal to 0.99 compared to a WHR less than 0.90: multivariate relative risk, 3.41; CI, 1.52–7.66; *p* for trend =0.01; waist circumference greater than or equal to 43 inches compared to waist circumference less than 35 inches: relative risk, 2.56; CI, 1.33–4.96; *p* for trend < 0.001). These associations persisted even after adjustment for BMI. Height, which can be a biomarker of prepubertal overnutrition, was also associated with a higher risk of colon cancer (height greater than or equal to 73 inches compared to height less than or equal to 68 inches: multivariate relative risk, 1.76; CI, 1.13–2.74; *p* for trend =0.02). Thus, height and obesity, particularly abdominal adiposity, were associated with an elevated risk.

A significant amount of the literature supports the concept that the direct effects of dietary fat and fiber in the colonic lumen increase the risk of colon cancer. However, because a Western dietary pattern is also associated with an increased risk of obesity, one may find that separating these two competing concepts in epidemiologic studies is difficult. The fat and fiber hypotheses, at least as originally formulated, do not adequately explain many emerging findings from recent epidemiologic studies. An alternative hypothesis stating that hyperinsulinemia promotes colon carcinogenesis was developed by Giovannucci et al. (87). Insulin is an important growth factor for colonic epithelial cells and a mitogen of tumor cell growth *in vitro*. Epidemiologic evidence supporting the insulin and colon cancer hypothesis is largely indirect, and it is based on the similarity of factors that produce elevated insulin levels with those related to colon cancer risk. Specifically, obesity—particularly central obesity, physical inactivity, and possibly a low dietary polyunsaturated fat to saturated fat ratio—is a major determinant of insulin resistance and hyperinsulinemia, and it appears to be related to the colon cancer risk. Moreover, a diet high in refined carbohydrates and low in water-soluble fiber, which is associated with an increased risk of colon cancer, causes the rapid intestinal absorption of glucose into the blood, leading to postprandial hyperinsulinemia. The combination of insulin resistance and high glycemic load produces particularly high insulin levels. Thus, hyperinsulinemia may explain why obesity, physical inactivity, and a diet low in fruits and vegetables and high in red meat and extensively processed foods—all of which are common in the West—increase the risk of colon cancer.

A number of hormonal mechanisms could account for these associations, but evidence suggests that increased circulating insulin, IGF, and leptin levels can influence colonic epithelial cell proliferation and apoptosis, and thus they may affect carcinogenesis (88). In various animal models, modulation of insulin and IGF-1 levels through various means—direct infusion; energy excess or restriction; genetically induced obesity; dietary quality, including fatty acid and sucrose content; inhibition of normal insulin secretion; and pharmacologic inhibition of IGF-1—influences colonic carcinogenesis. Human evidence also associates high levels of insulin and IGF-1 with an increased risk of colon cancer. Clinical conditions associated with high levels of insulin (e.g., non–insulin-dependent diabetes mellitus and hypertriglyceridemia) and IGF-1 (e.g., acromegaly) are related to an increased risk of colon cancer, and increased circulating concentrations of insulin and

IGF-1 are related to a higher risk of colonic neoplasia. Determinants and markers of hyperinsulinemia (e.g., physical inactivity, high BMI, and central adiposity) and high IGF-1 levels (e.g., tall stature) are also related to a higher risk. Many studies indicate that dietary patterns that stimulate insulin resistance or secretion, including high consumption of sucrose, various sources of starch, a high glycemic index, and high saturated fatty acid intake, are associated with a higher risk of colon cancer. Plasma levels of leptin increase in proportion to the level of obesity. The presence of the leptin receptor in human colon cancer cell lines has been demonstrated by the use of reverse transcriptase polymerase chain reaction (RT-PCR) and immunoblotting, and its presence in human colonic tissue has been demonstrated by immunohistochemistry. Stimulation with leptin leads to phosphorylation of the p42/44 mitogen-activated protein kinase in HT29 cells in culture, and it increases proliferation of HT29 cells *in vitro*, as well as colonic epithelial cell proliferation rates in C57BL/6 mice *in vivo*.

A number of additional nutritional factors have been implicated in colon carcinogenesis, including vitamin D and calcium and cruciferous vegetables (89,90). These may interact through additional environmental and genetic factors that affect colon cancer incidence. However, the incidence of this malignancy was invariably low before the technologic advances that rendered sedentary lifestyles and obesity common and prior to the increased availability of highly processed carbohydrates and saturated fatty acids. Therefore, obesity and the dietary constituents that make obesity more common in modern society may interact in the promotion of colon carcinogenesis, rather than being mutually exclusive hypotheses for nutritional influences on colon cancer risk.

ESOPHAGEAL CANCER

The demographics and biologic nature of esophageal cancer have changed markedly in the last few decades. Squamous cell carcinoma of the esophagus associated with smoking and alcohol ingestion that more commonly occurs in African-American men has become less common, whereas adenocarcinoma of the esophagus, which is associated with Barrett esophagus and metaplasia of the esophageal mucosa resulting from exposure to stomach acid, have become more common (91). In a Swedish nationwide case-control study, gastroesophageal reflux and obesity were identified as strong, independent risk factors for esophageal adenocarcinoma (92). A moderately strong association was found with adenocarcinoma of the gastric cardia. No significant association was found with squamous cell carcinoma of the esophagus. With increasing duration and severity of reflux symptoms and increasing BMI, the risk increased in a dose-dependent manner. When combined, reflux symptoms and obesity engender greatly increased risk estimates, with relative risks exceeding 100 compared to those of persons with neither reflux symptoms nor obesity. However, because adenocarcinoma of the esophagus and gastric cardia are rarities, the absolute risk of developing these tumors still is not high. Although more research is needed to understand the exact mechanisms involved, esophageal reflux should be aggressively treated with proton pump inhibitors during weight reduction in obese patients. This is particularly important in patients in whom esophageal reflux and obesity persist after treatment with resection of esophageal tissue for precancerous intestinal metaplasia.

PANCREATIC CANCER

Fat intake is linked with obesity and diabetes mellitus, which are risk factors for pancreatic cancer (93). Fruit and vegetable consumption appears to be protective (95). Pancreatic cancer has also been linked to reproductive hormone status. In a study designed to examine the possible role of body size and reproductive factors in pancreatic cancer, data from a population-based case-control study conducted in Shanghai, China were analyzed (95). The cases (number of subjects [n] = 451) were permanent residents of Shanghai who ranged from 30 to 74 years of age and who had been newly diagnosed with pancreatic cancer between October 1, 1990, and June 30, 1993. Deceased cases (19%) were excluded from the study. Controls (n = 1,552) were randomly selected from permanent Shanghai residents and were frequency-matched to cases by gender and age. Information on body size, reproductive status, and other possible risk factors was collected through personal interviews. After adjustments for age, income, smoking, and other confounders, a positive dose–response relation between BMI and the risk of pancreatic cancer was observed in both sexes. Among women, the risk of pancreatic cancer was significantly associated with the number of pregnancies and live births. Compared to the OR for zero to two pregnancies or live births, that for eight or more pregnancies was 1.90, whereas that for five or more births was 1.88. A modest elevation in risk, independent of parity, was associated with an early age at first birth. Risk increased by more than 40% in women with a first birth at or before the age of 19 years, relative to those in which it occurred at the age of 26 years or older. Even the use of oral contraceptives was associated with excess risk, although this was based on small numbers of users. These findings suggest that, in Shanghai, obesity, gravidity, parity, and perhaps the use of oral contraceptives are associated with moderate increases in the risk of pancreatic cancer, thus indicating that hormonal determinants deserve further investigation in the relationship between obesity and pancreatic cancer.

PEDIATRIC OBESITY, ADULT STATURE, AND CANCER

Pediatric obesity increases the lifetime risk of cancer (96). One marker of pediatric obesity is average adult height in a population. Adult height is related to both genetics and prepubertal nutrition. Overnutrition in childhood is associated with increased adult height and increased secretion of IGF-1, which may increase the risk of prostate and breast cancers later in life (97,98). Concomitant with the increased adult height in Japan, increased incidences of obesity and cancer have been noted in that country.

In a study of the relationship between adult stature and cancer incidence using data from the first United States National Health and Nutrition Examination Survey and its follow-up study of 12,554 participants, from 25 to 74 years of age, 460 cancers occurred in men and 399 in women after an average follow-up of approximately 10 years (99). The age-adjusted relative risk of cancer for the second (Q2) through the fourth (Q4) quartiles of stature compared to that for the first quartile in men were significantly increased as follows: 1.5, 1.4, and 1.4. After adjustment for race, cigarette smoking, income, and BMI, the all-sites cancer relative risk increased slightly to 1.6, 1.5, and 1.6. For most cancer sites in men, and particularly colorectal cancer (relative risk = 2.1 for Q4), the lowest incidence was observed in those in the shortest quartile of stature. A weaker positive association was detected in women and was restricted primarily to cancer of the breast and colorectum (relative risk in Q4 = 2.1 and 1.6 for the two cancers, respectively). These findings indicate that short stature is associated with a reduced risk of cancer, particularly in men; and they suggest a role for nutrition early in life in human carcinogenesis. Although reducing prepubertal nutrition to induce a reduction in adult height is not socially acceptable, treating the epidemic of obesity in the pediatric population through planned physical activities and nutritional changes is one way to reduce the lifetime risks of cancer in adulthood.

Clinical Considerations

Given the situation and the considerable evidence that nutrition and obesity may affect cancer development and progression, the clinician must develop an approach to the obese patient with cancer that is reasonable based on the available data. First, the clinician must carefully evaluate the obese patient for evidence of the development of common forms of cancer. Colonoscopy, mammography, and frequent monitoring of PSA levels in obese men are advisable. Obese women developing unusual uterine bleeding patterns should be carefully evaluated using endometrial aspiration and biopsy when necessary. Obese individuals with esophageal reflux that does not respond to usual treatment should be assessed carefully with endoscopy. Unfortunately, early diagnosis is difficult for renal cell cancer, pancreatic cancer, and ovarian cancer in all patients, including those who are obese. Second, the clinician should indicate that the final answers on the efficacy of any nutritional approach have not been proven but that a rational clinical approach attempts to reduce excess body fat based on its potential negative effects on outcome. The prevention of weight gain in men with prostate cancer undergoing androgen ablation therapies provides both aesthetic and potential medical benefits. The prevention of weight gain in the premenopausal patient with breast cancer who is undergoing an artificial early menopause as a result of chemotherapy also provides quality-of-life benefits, as well as potential medical benefits, such as reducing serum lipids. Third, the clinician must customize the approach to weight reduction so that the loss of fat, not body weight, is the outcome. Loss of lean mass may actually have untoward effects, and it can result from a weight loss approach involving simply caloric restriction. Weightlifting and other resistance exercises using equipment or free weights after proper instruction are critical elements in treating patients with breast or prostate cancer who have undergone early menopause or androgen ablation as a result of cancer therapy. With the loss of major anabolic hormones (i.e., estrogens and androgens), these patients may require instruction on building and maintaining lean muscle mass. Fourth, the clinician should address the inflammatory component of the carcinogenesis process in the course of treatment by including antiinflammatory phytonutrients from colorful fruits and vegetables in the diet plans that are designed for the patient. Diet plans that include phytochemicals, which can affect the processes of tumor growth and development, have been developed (100). These diet plans involve a marked increase in the intake of fruits and vegetables, as recommended by the American Institute of Cancer Research (101) and the National Cancer Institute (102).

Fruits and vegetables can be classified into color-coded groups that provide classes of phytonutrients (Table 13.1) and that can act in specific tissues. For example, lycopene is localized to the prostate gland, and it may have a special role in prostate cancer prevention, as the epidemiologic studies reviewed early suggested. Such diet plans may likely aid weight maintenance by reducing the caloric density while increasing nutrient density. Finally, the clinician must individualize the use of dietary supplements in these patients. Many patients with cancer will take supplements, including botanical dietary supplements. Most clinicians find discerning which ones are safe and which are dangerous difficult. This is complicated by a lack of manufacturing and labeling standards and a lack of knowledge on potential herb–drug interactions. At the very least, a complete record of all supplements being taken should be obtained, and the patient should be encouraged to stop those supplements obtained from unconventional sources. Most supplements that have been studied in animal models or in clinical settings are available over the counter in drug stores and grocery stores. Even among the accepted supplements, the possibility

TABLE 13.1. *Phytonutrient recommendations during weight loss and maintenance*

Color code	Vegetables and fruits	Phytonutrient	Benefit
Red	Tomato sauces, soups, juices	Lycopene	Antioxidant, prostate localization
Green	Broccoli, Brussels sprouts, cabbage	Isothiocyanates	Protective enzyme induction
Green/yellow	Spinach, mustard greens, collard greens, kale	Lutein	Antioxidant
Orange	Carrots, butternut squash	α-carotene and β-carotene	Antioxidant
Orange/yellow	Oranges, lemons, grapefruit	Flavonoids, ascorbate	Antioxidant enzyme induction
Red/purple	Red grapes, strawberries, raspberries, blueberries	Anthocyanidins, ellagic acid	Antioxidant, antiproliferative
White/green	Garlic, onion, chives	Allyl sulfides	Antiproliferative

From Heber D. *What color is your diet?* New York: Regan Books, 2001, with permission.

of some interactions exists. For example, some have said that, since green tea extract supplements may contain vitamin K, they should not be taken by patients on anticoagulants. While some may interpret this as just another example of a situation in which the use of a supplement has dangerous implications, one should also realize that foods such as broccoli and asparagus also contain vitamin K. Patients taking anticoagulants would normally be warned about eating these vegetables, but the vegetables would not be considered unsafe as a result. This illustrates the general bias against dietary supplements in the popular and medical literature.

Supplementation with a multivitamin and multimineral, vitamin E, vitamin C, and calcium is safe when these are given in the usual doses (Table 13.2). At the doses shown, no untoward effects have been demonstrated in clinical trials, and some benefits on immune function have been demonstrated in healthy elderly individuals (104). A full discussion of this topic is outside the scope of this chapter. Optional supplements that many patients, based on their reading of the scientific literature, often on the Internet, may wish to include are selenium and green tea extract capsules. These supplements are currently under study for their potential benefits on tumor development and progression.

The supplement prescription has several benefits. First, it enables the clinician to provide the patient with a rational supplement plan that can replace any unknown supplements the patient may have obtained from unorthodox sources. Second, it establishes the clinician's position with the patient as a physician who appreciates the nutritional orientation of many patients with cancer who often concentrate on supplements as one area of their care they can control. Finally, the supplement plan will likely enhance compliance with dietary intervention by creating a regimen that the patient can follow. In this con-

TABLE 13.2. *Vitamin supplementation recommendations*

1. Basic recommendations
   Multivitamin/multimineral providing 400 μg of folic acid
   Vitamin E at 100–400 IU/d
   Vitamin C at 250–500 mg/d
   Calcium at 1,000–1,500 mg/d from diet and supplements
2. Optional supplements resulting from patient reading
   Selenium, 50–200 μg/day
   Green-tea extract capsules containing 100–160 μg of catechins (equivalent to four cups of tea)

text, the clinician must indicate that the supplements do not substitute for the diet plan, which provides many phytonutrients not found in the vitamins and minerals that are being prescribed.

CONCLUSION

For a number of common forms of cancer, obesity is clearly associated with cancer risk, incidence, or progression. Evidence is much stronger for certain forms of cancer than for others, but no clinical trial data are available to define the benefits of weight reduction. Clearly, the endocrine and immune systems may play an important role in mediating the effects of increased adiposity on cancer risk, because of the hormones and adipocytokines produced by fat cells. Many of the changes observed in these systems in obese patients are epiphenomena of unknown significance, but others may be important in cancer development, promotion, or progression. Abnormalities in adipocytokine production and action are central to many of the observed metabolic changes in the obese patient, and they may play a role in the etiology and maintenance of the obese state, as well as in associated forms of cancer. Similarly, reproductive hormonal abnormalities appear to be closely related to obesity, and they may have special significance for understanding obesity in women throughout the various stages of development and during pregnancy. Furthermore, the development of breast cancer, uterine cancer, and ovarian cancer in women may be related to the changes in reproductive hormones during different stages of the reproductive life cycle. In designing strategies to address the problem of common forms of cancer in the United States population and around the world, the clinician must have an understanding of the roles of the endocrine and immune systems in obesity; this appreciation should be useful in both the prevention and treatment of cancer.

ACKNOWLEDGMENTS

This work was supported by the Clinical Nutrition Research Unit grant, P01 CA 42710; the Nutrition and Obesity Training Grant, T32 DK 07688; the Estradiol Metabolism in Postmenopausal Women grant, R01 CA 71052; and the Center for Dietary Supplements Research:Botanicals grant, P50 AT 000151.

REFERENCES

1. Armstrong B, Doll R. Environmental factors and cancer incidence and mortality in different countries, with special reference to dietary practices. *Int J Cancer* 1975;15:617–631.
2. Shimizu H, Ross RK, Bernstein L, et al. Cancers of the prostate and breast among Japanese and white immigrants to Los Angeles County. *Br J Cancer* 1991;63:963–966.
3. Garfinkel L. Overweight and cancer. *Ann Int Med* 1985;103:1034–1036.
4. Newman SC, Miller AB, Howe GR. A study of the effect of weight and dietary fat on breast cancer survival time. *Am J Epidemiol* 1986;123:767–774.
5. Heber D, Blackburn GL, Go VLW, eds. *Nutritional oncology* San Diego: Academic Press, 2000.
6. Jaax S, Scott LW, Wolf JE, et al. General guidelines for a low fat diet effective in the management of non-melanoma skin cancer. *Nutr Cancer* 1997;27:150–156.
7. Heber D. The role of nutrition in cancer prevention and control. *Oncology* 1992;6:9–14.
8. Nimrod A, Ryan KH. Aromatization of androgens by human abdominal and breast fat tissue. *J Clin Endocrinol Metab* 1975;40:367.
9. Kissebah AH, Evans DJ, Peiris A, et al. Endocrine characteristics in regional obesities: role of sex steroids. In: Vague J, Bjorntorp P, Guy-Grand B, et al., eds. *Metabolic complications of human obesities*. Amsterdam: Excerpta Medica, 1985:115.
10. Ripple MO, Henry WF, Rago RP, Wilding G. Prooxidant–antioxidant shift induced by androgen treatment of human prostate carcinoma cells. *J Natl Cancer Inst* 1997;89:40–48.

11. Winkler G, Lakatos P, Salamon F, et al. Elevated serum TNF-alpha level as a link between endothelial dysfunction and insulin resistance in normotensive obese patients. *Diabetes Med* 1999;16:207–211.
12. Ziccardi P, Nappo F, Giugliano G, et al. Reduction of inflammatory cytokine concentrations and improvement of endothelial functions in obese women after weight loss over one year. *Circulation* 2002;105:804–809.
13. Liebler DC, Aust AE, Wilson GL. Reactive oxidants from nitric oxide, oxidants and cellular signalling, and repair of oxidative DNA damage: a chemical pathology study section workshop. *Mol Carcinog* 1998;22: 209–220.
14. Chandra RK. The nutrition-immunity-infection nexus: the enumeration and functional assessment of lymphocyte subsets in nutritional deficiency. *Nutr Res* 1983;3:605–615.
15. Vague J. The degree of masculine differentiation of the obesities: a factor determining predisposition to diabetes, atherosclerosis, gout, and uric calculous disease. (1956). Reprinted, *Nutrition* 1999;15:89–91.
16. Rebuffe-Scrive M, Eldh J, Hafstrom LO, et al. Metabolism of mammary, abdominal, and femoral adipocytes in women before and after the menopause. *Metabolism* 1986;35:792–797.
17. Kerr MG. Significance of weight gain in pregnancy. *Lancet* 1969;1:663.
18. Rebuffe-Scrive M. Metabolic differences in fat depots. In: Bouchard C, Johnston FE, eds. *Fat distribution during growth and later health outcomes.* New York: Alan R Liss 1988:175.
19. Pike MC, Krailo MD, Henderson BE, et al. "Hormonal" risk factors, "breast tissue age," and the age-incidence of breast cancer. *Nature* 1983;303:767–770.
20. Pike MC, Spicer DV, Dahmoush L, et al. Estrogens, progestogens, normal breast cell proliferation and breast cancer risk. *Epidemiol Rev* 1993;15:17–35.
21. Kelsey JL. A review of the epidemiology of human breast cancer. *Epidemiol Rev* 1979;1:74–109.
22. Prentice R, Thompson D, Clifford C, et al. Dietary fat reduction and plasma estradiol concentration in healthy postmenopausal women. *J Natl Cancer Inst* 1990;82:129–134.
23. Heber D, Ashley JM, McCarthy WJ, et al. Assessment of adherence to a low fat diet for breast cancer prevention. *Prev Med* 1992;21:218–227.
24. Bagga D, Ashley JM, Geffrey S, et al. Effects of very low fat high fiber diet on reproductive hormones: implications for breast cancer prevention. *Cancer* 1995;22:351–355.
25. Reichman ME, Judd JT, Longcope C, et al. Effects of alcohol consumption on plasma and urinary hormone concentrations in premenopausal women. *J Natl Cancer Inst* 1993;85:722–726.
26. Grodin JM, Siiteri PK, MacDonald PC. Source of estrogen production in postmenopausal women. *J Clin Endocrinol Metab* 1973;36:207–210.
27. Siiteri PK, MacDonald PC. Role of extraglandular estrogen in human endocrinology. In: Greep RO, Astwood EB, eds. *Handbook of physiology,* Vol. 2. Washington, D.C.: American Physiological Society, 1973:15–629.
28. Schindler AE, Ebert A, Friedrich E. Conversion of androstenedione to estrone by human fat tissue. *J Clin Endocrinol Metab* 1972;35:627–630.
29. Simpson ER, Ackerman GE, Smith ME. Estrogen formation in stromal cells of adipose tissue of women: induction by glucocorticoids. *Proc Natl Acad Sci U S A* 1981;73:5690–5694.
30. Zumoff B. Relationship of obesity to blood estrogens. *Cancer Res* 1982;42:3289–3294.
31. Kalish L. Relationship of body size with breast cancer. *J Clin Oncol* 1984;2:287–293.
32. Abe R, Kumagai N, Kimura M. Biological characteristics of breast cancer in obesity. *Tohoku J Exp Med* 1976; 120:351–359.
33. Donegan WL, Hartz AJ, Rimm AA. The association of body weight with recurrent cancer of the breast. *Cancer* 1978;41:1590–1594.
34. Howson CP, Kinne D, Wynder EL. Body weight, serum cholesterol and stage of primary breast cancer. *Cancer* 1986;58:2372–2381.
35. de Waard F. Epidemiology of breast cancer: a review. *Eur J Cancer Clin Oncol* 1983;19:1671–1676.
36. Huang Z, Hankinson SE, Colditz GA, et al. Dual effects of weight and weight gain on breast cancer risk. *JAMA* 1997;278:1407–1411.
37. Coates RJ, Uhler RJ, Hall HI. Risk of breast cancer in young women in relation to body size and weight gain in adolescence and early adulthood. *Br J Cancer* 1999;81:167–174.
38. Trentham-Dietz A, Newcomb PA, Egan KM. Weight change and risk of postmenopausal breast cancer (United States). *Cancer Causes Control* 2000;116:533–542.
39. Verreault R, Brisson J, Deschenes L, et al. Body weight and prognostic indicators in breast cancer. *Am J Epidemiol* 1989;129:260–268.
40. Camoriano JK, Loprinzi CL, Ingle JN, et al. Weight change in women with adjuvant therapy or observed following mastectomy for node-positive breast cancer. *J Clin Oncol* 1990;8:1327–1334.
41. Tretli S. Height and weight in relation to breast cancer morbidity and mortality. A prospective study of 570,000 women in Norway. *Int J Cancer* 1989;44:23–30.
42. de Waard F, Poortman J, Collette BJ. Relationship of weight to promotion of breast cancer after menopause. *Nutr Cancer* 1981;2:237–240.
43. McNee RK, Mason BH, Neave LM, et al. Influence of height, weight, and obesity on breast cancer incidence and recurrence in Auckland, New Zealand. *Breast Cancer Res Treat* 1987;9:145–150.
44. Eberlein I, Simon R, Fisher S, et al. Height, weight, and risk of breast cancer relapse. *Breast Cancer Res Treat* 1985;5:81–86.
45. Hebert JR, Augustine A, Barone J, et al. Weight, height, and body mass index in the prognosis of breast cancer: early results of a prospective analysis. *Int J Cancer* 1988;42:315–318.

46. Lubin F, Ruder AM, Wax Y, et al. Overweight and changes in weight throughout adult life in breast cancer etiology. A case–control study. *Am J Epidemiol* 1985;122:579–588.
47. Le Marchand L, Kolonel LN, Earle ME, et al. Body size at different periods of life and breast cancer risk. *Am J Epidemiol* 1988;128:137–152.
48. London SJ, Colditz GA, Stampfer MJ, et al. Prospective study of relative weight, height and risk of breast cancer. *JAMA* 1989;262:2853–2858.
49. Ballard-Barbash R, Schatzkin A, Carter CL, et al. Body fat distribution and breast cancer in the Framingham study. *J Natl Cancer Inst* 1990;82:286–290.
50. Bernstein L, Yuan JM, Ross RK, et al. Serum hormone levels in pre-menopausal Chinese women in Shanghai and white women in Los Angeles: results from two breast cancer case–control studies. *Cancer Causes Control* 1990;1:51–58.
51. Tornberg SA, Carstensen JM. Relationship between Quetelet's index and cancer of the breast and female genital tract in 47,000 women followed for 25 years. *Br J Cancer* 1994;69:358–361.
52. Olson SH, Trevisan M, Marshall JR, et al. Body mass index, weight gain, and risk of endometrial cancer. *Nutr Cancer* 1995;23:141–149
53. Anderson B, Connor JP, Andrews JI, et al. Obesity and prognosis in endometrial cancer. *Am J Obstet Gynecol* 1996;174:1171–1178.
54. Mori M, Nishida T, Sugiyama T, et al. Anthropometric and other risk factors for ovarian cancer in a case–control study. *Jpn J Cancer Res* 1998;89:246–253.
55. Catalona WJ, Smith DS, Ratliff TL, et al. Detection of organ-confined prostate cancer is increased through prostate-specific antigen-based screening. *JAMA* 1993;270:948–954.
56. Landis SH, Murray T, Bolden S, et al. Cancer statistics. *CA Cancer J Clin* 1998;48:6–29.
57. Tanagho EA, McAninch JW, eds. *Smith's general urology.* Norwalk, CT: Appleton & Lange, 1995.
58. Thompson IM, Coltman CA, Brawley OW, et al. Chemoprevention of prostate cancer. *Semin Urol* 1995;13:122–129.
59. Parkin DM, Whelan SL, Ferlay J, et al, eds. *Cancer incidence in five continents,* Vol VII. Scientific Publications #143. New York: Oxford University Press, 1997.
60. Mandel JS, Schuman LM. Epidemiology of cancer of the prostate. *Rev Cancer Epidemiol* 1980;1:1–65.
61. Lew EA, Garfinkel L. Variations in mortality by weight among 750,000 men and women. *J Chronic Dis* 1979;32:563–576.
62. Whittemore AS, Kolonel LH, Wu AH, et al. Prostate cancer in relation to diet, physical activity and body size, in blacks, whites and Asians in the United States and Canada. *J Natl Cancer Inst* 1995;87:652–661.
63. Boyle P, Kevi R, Lucchuni F, et al. Trends in diet-related cancers in Japan: a conundrum? *Lancet* 1993;349:752.
64. Kolonel LN, Hankin JH, Lee J, et al. Nutrient intakes in relation to cancer incidence in Hawaii. *Br J Cancer* 1981;44:332–339.
65. Garfinkel L. Overweight and cancer. *Ann Intern Med* 1985;103:1034–1036.
66. West DW, Slattery ML, Robison LM, et al. Adult dietary intake and prostate cancer risk in Utah: a case–control study with special emphasis on aggressive tumors. *Cancer Causes Control* 1991;2:85–94.
67. Giovannucci E, Rimm EB, Colditz GA, et al. A prospective study of dietary fat and risk of prostate cancer. *J Natl Cancer Inst* 1993;85:1571–1579.
68. Kolonel LN, Yoshizawa CN, Hankin JN. Diet and prostatic cancer: a case–control study in Hawaii. *Am J Epidemiol* 1988;127:999–1012.
69. Mettlin C, Selenskas S, Natarajan N. Beta-carotene and animal fats and their relationship to prostate cancer risk. *Cancer* 1989;64:605–612.
70. Snowdon DA, Phillips RL, Choi W. Diet, obesity and risk of fatal prostate cancer. *Am J Epidemiol* 1984;120:244–250.
71. Kaul L, Heshmat MY, Kovi J, et al. The role of diet in prostate cancer. *Nutr Cancer* 1987;9:123–128.
72. Slattery ML, Schumacher MC, West DW, et al. Food consumption trends between adolescent and adult years and subsequent risk of prostate cancer. *Am J Clin Nutr* 1990;52:752–757.
73. Ross RK, Shimizu H, Paganini-Hill A, et al. Case–control studies of prostate cancer in blacks and whites in southern California. *J Natl Cancer Inst* 1987;78:869–874.
74. Talamini R, LaVecchia C, Decarli A, et al. Nutrition, social factors and prostatic cancer in a northern Italian population. *Br J Cancer* 1986;53:817–821.
75. Yatani R, Shiraishi T, Nakakuki K, et al. Trends in frequency of latent prostate carcinoma in Japan from 1965–1979 to 1982–1986. *J Natl Cancer Inst* 1988;80:683–687.
76. Hill P, Wynder EL, Garbaczewski L, et al. Diet and urinary steroids in black and white North American men and black South African men. *Cancer Res* 1987;47:2982–2985.
77. Dorgan JF, Judd JT, Longcope C, et al. Effects of dietary fat and fiber on plasma and urine estrogens in men: a controlled feeding study. *Am J Clin Nutr* 1996;64:850–855.
78. Mills PK, Beeson WL, Phillips RL, et al. Cohort study of diet, lifestyle and prostate cancer in Adventist men. *Cancer* 1989;64:598–604.
79. Geller J, Albert J. The effect of aging on the prostate. In: Korenman SG, ed. *Endocrine aspects of aging.* New York: Elsevier Science, 1982:137–161.
80. Horton R, Hsieh P, Barberia J, et al. Altered blood androgens in elderly men with prostate hyperplasia. *J Clin Endocrinol* 1975;41:793–796.
81. Lee WH, Isaacs WB, Bova GS, et al. CG Island methylation changes near the GSTP1 gene in prostatic carci-

noma cells detected using the polymerase chain reaction: a new prostatic cancer biomarker. *Cancer Epidemiol Biomarkers Prev* 1997;6:443–450.

82. Chow WH, McLaughlin JK, Mandel JS, et al. Obesity and risk of renal cell cancer. *Cancer Epidemiol Biomarkers Prev* 1996;5:17–21.

83. Yuan JM, Castelao JE, Gago-Dominguez M, et al. Hypertension, obesity, and their medications in relation to renal cell carcinoma. *Br J Cancer* 1998;77:1508–1513.

84. Chow WH, Gridley G, Fraumeni JF, et al. Obesity, hypertension, and the risk of kidney cancer in men. *N Engl J Med* 2000;343:1305–1311.

85. Murphy TK, Calle EE, Rodriguez C, et al. Body mass index and colon cancer mortality in a large prospective study. *Am J Epidemiol* 2000;152:847–854.

86. Giovannucci E, Ascherio A, Rimm EB, et al. Physical activity, obesity and risk for colon cancer and adenoma in men. *Ann Intern Med* 1995;122:327–334.

87. Giovannucci E. Insulin, insulin-like growth factors and colon cancer: a review of the evidence. *J Nutr* 2001; 131:3109S–3120S.

88. Hardwick JC, Van Den Brink GR, Offerhaus GJ, et al. Leptin is a growth factor for colonic epithelial cells. *Gastroenterology* 2001;121:79–90.

89. Richter F, Newmark HL, Richter A, et al. Inhibition of Western-diet induced hyperproliferation and hyperplasia in mouse colon by two sources of calcium. *Carcinogenesis* 1995;16:2685–2689.

90. Greenwald P, Kelloff GJ, Boone CW, et al. Genetic and cellular changes in colorectal cancer: proposed targets of chemopreventive agents. *Cancer Epidemiol Biomarkers Prev* 1995;4:691–702.

91. Li SD, Mobarhan S. Association between body mass index and adenocarcinoma of the esophagus and gastric cardia. *Nutr Rev* 2000;58:54–56

92. Lagergren J. Reflux and obesity are strong and independent risk factors according to the SECC study. *Lakartidningen* 2000;97:1950–1953.

93. Michaud DS, Giovannucci E, Willett WC, et al. Physical activity, obesity, height, and the risk of pancreatic cancer. *JAMA* 2001;286:921–929.

94. Gold EB, Goldin SB. Epidemiology of and risk factors for pancreatic cancer. *Surg Oncol Clin North Am* 1998; 7:67–91.

95. Ji BT, Hatch MC, Chow WH, et al. Anthropometric and reproductive factors and the risk of pancreatic cancer: a case-control study in Shanghai, China. *Int J Cancer* 1996;66:432–437.

96. Dietz WH. Childhood weight affects adult morbidity and mortality. *J Nutr* 1998;128:411S–414S.

97. Chan JM, Stampfer MJ, Giovannucci E, et al. Plasma insulin-like growth factor-I and prostate cancer risk: a prospective study. *Science* 1998;279:563–566.

98. Hankinson SE, Willett WC, Colditz GA, et al. Circulating concentrations of insulin-like growth factor-I and risk of breast cancer. *Lancet* 1998;351:1393–1396.

99. Albanes D, Jones DY, Schatzkin A, et al. Adult stature and risk of cancer. *Cancer Res* 1988;48:1658–1662.

100. Heber D. *What color is your diet?* New York: HarperCollins, 2001.

101. Munoz de Chavez M, Chavez A. Diet that prevents cancer: recommendations from the American Institute for Cancer Research. *Int J Cancer* 1998;11:85–89.

102. Harnack L, Block G, Subar A, et al. Association of cancer prevention-related nutrition knowledge, beliefs, and attitudes to cancer prevention dietary behavior. *J Am Diet Assoc* 1997;97:957–965.

103. High KF. Nutritional strategies to boost immunity and prevent infection in elderly individuals. *Aging Infect Dis* 2001;33:1892–1900.

14

Endocrine Disorders and Obesity

Margaret E. Wierman

The interplay between obesity and endocrine diseases is complex. Most people who have the common disorder of generalized obesity do not have an underlying endocrine disease; rather, their abnormal weight is related to an imbalance in energy intake versus energy expenditure. Rare genetic disorders that result in both endocrine disorders and abnormal body weight do exist, however. In addition, some specific endocrine disorders can cause or can contribute to obesity. Conversely, obesity from any cause may eventually result in the onset of a secondary endocrine dysfunction. This chapter reviews the data that associate obesity with endocrine disease.

GENETIC DISORDERS THAT RESULT IN ENDOCRINE DISORDERS AND OBESITY

Many genetic diseases are associated with obesity (see Chapter 2), but a subset of these present with combined endocrine disorders, which are reviewed here.

Prader–Willi Syndrome

Prader–Willi syndrome is a genetic disorder that presents in infancy with hypotonia, small hands and feet, and low birth weight, followed by massive weight gain, hyperphagia, mild mental retardation, central hypogonadotropic hypogonadism, and short stature attributable to growth hormone (GH) deficiency (1). These patients have deletions in 15q11.2 or microdeletions at 15q11-q13 in the paternal allele (2). Therapy with GH in these patients has been attempted with variable success. Carrel et al. (3) reported that 24 to 48 months of GH therapy resulted in beneficial effects on body composition with decreases in fat mass and increases in lean body mass, growth velocity, and resting energy expenditure. The long-term effects of GH or sex steroid therapy have not been reported. Very recent observations suggest that ghrelin, an enteric circulating orexigen that is important in mealtime hunger, is disordered in patients with Prader–Willi syndrome (4). Whereas other patients with obesity have low ghrelin levels, patients with Prader–Willi syndrome have been noted to have fasting plasma levels that are 4.5 times higher than those of obese controls. Efforts are underway to clone the mutated gene(s) that underlie the complex phenotype of the disorder.

Bardet–Biedl Syndrome

Bardet–Biedl syndrome is a genetically diverse, autosomal-recessive disorder with clinical manifestations of mental retardation, generalized obesity, central hypogonadism, retinal rod-cone dystrophy, polydactyly, and renal dysfunction (5,6). Genetic mutations have been mapped to five different loci, including chromosomes 11q12, 16q21, 3p13-

p12, 15q22.3-23, and 2q31 (5,6). Obesity begins after 2 years of age and retinal degeneration after the age of 8 years. It has overlapping features of the Laurence–Moon syndrome, including polydactyly, obesity kidney, and eye abnormalities (5,6). The cause of the obesity or the hypogonadism is unknown.

Mutations in Leptin or the Leptin Receptor

Mutations in leptin or the leptin receptor have been shown to be rare causes of human cases of hypogonadism and massive obesity (7–9). Because of the identification of leptin and its receptor from genetic mice models of obesity, many patients have been screened, yet, to date, only a few families have abnormalities in leptin action that account for their weight and reproductive abnormalities (7). Members of one Turkish family were shown to display leptin deficiency (9). A young girl from this family responded to exogenous leptin with weight loss and the return of reproductive axis functioning (10). Patients with leptin receptor mutations have also been identified, but these disorders are not common causes of obesity in the general population.

The role of leptin in reproduction is complex. Leptin is a peripheral hormone secreted from adipocytes that acts centrally and peripherally at all levels of the reproductive axis. In women, absence of leptin results in a lack of pubertal development, and leptin administration stimulates gonadotropin secretion in animal models (11). In girls, epidemiologic studies show that leptin levels increase across pubertal maturation (11). Leptin, however, is not the trigger for puberty, but, instead, it is a permissive protein that signals adequate body fat to allow reproductive function. In men, the role of leptin is less clear. Leptin levels in boys increase between the ages of 5 and 10 years and then decline (12). However, both animals and human males with leptin deficiency have hypogonadotropic hypogonadism. Although leptin-deficient female animals are infertile, a few *ob/ob* male mice demonstrate normal reproductive function, suggesting a larger role for leptin in signaling metabolic cues for female reproduction than for that of the male. Supporting a more prominent role of leptin in the female, leptin levels are higher in female humans than in males, and a role for leptin has been implicated in pregnancy and lactation. Cultured fat cells from women respond with increased leptin production in response to estrogen and with inhibition of leptin production in response to dihydrotestosterone (11). In contrast, fat cells from men show no leptin response to steroid hormones (11). These gender-specific differences may be the basis for the different roles of leptin in male and female reproduction and body weight regulation.

ENDOCRINE DISORDERS THAT CONTRIBUTE TO OBESITY

Hypothalamic Obesity Resulting from Tumors or Damage to the Hypothalamus

Diseases that directly involve or that have an impact on appetite centers in the hypothalamus can result in morbid obesity. Hypothalamic tumors, as well as trauma or radiation damage to the hypothalamus, disrupt the normal control of appetite and satiety mechanisms. A recent comparison of surgery outcomes in patients with suprasellar germ cell tumors versus craniopharyngiomas showed that those with craniopharyngioma tended to be more obese at presentation and that they became even heavier with therapy than those with dysgerminoma who were given the same hormonal therapy (13–15). Data from the Hospital for Sick Children in Toronto and Memorial Sloan Kettering confirm at least a 50% incidence of morbid obesity in patients with hypothalamic tumors that may or may not be improved with concomitant GH therapy (13–15). Thus, hypothalamic–

pituitary hormone insufficiency that is probably attributable to GH, thyroid hormone, and steroid hormone deficiencies, as well as to the destruction of specific appetite control centers in the hypothalamus, are implicated in the abnormal weight gain seen in patients with hypothalamic tumors or after central nervous system radiation or hypothalamic injury.

The exact neuronal connections within the ventromedial nucleus and paraventricular nucleus in the hypothalamus that mediate appetite are under active investigation (see Chapter 6). Animal models and humans with lesions in these hypothalamic areas have marked hyperphagia and disturbances in the autonomic nervous system (16,17). Investigators of these subject have observed an increase in parasympathetic nervous system and a decrease in sympathetic nervous system activity (16,17). Jung et al. (17) suggested that a dysregulation of neuropeptide Y (NPY) is present. NPY is secreted from the arcuate nucleus, and it has been shown to have diverse functions, including the activation of feeding behavior, the inhibition of reproductive function, decreases in sympathetic activity, and stimulation of parasympathetic activity. Transgenic models systems in which NPY has been deleted or overexpressed, however, do not fully replicate the disorders, thus suggesting that interaction between multiple neurotransmitters and neuropeptides is involved in the abnormal weight gain.

Cushing Syndrome

Cushing syndrome refers to the disorders of glucocorticoid excess (18–20). Exogenous Cushing syndrome refers to the clinical signs and symptoms of hypercortisolism that are related to the administration of glucocorticoids for another disorder, such as reactive airway disease, autoimmune disease, or inflammatory process (21). Endogenous Cushing syndrome results from the persistent excessive secretion of cortisol with loss of the normal diurnal variation and feedback mechanisms within the hypothalamic–pituitary–adrenal (HPA) axis (18–20). Symptoms include central weight gain with the loss of supraclavicular recession and the onset of a buffalo hump. Fatigue, weakness, and menstrual irregularities in women and a loss of libido and hypogonadism in men are common complaints. Sleep disturbance; signs of hyperandrogenism, such as acne and hirsutism; and purple striae with thinning of the skin are often present. Hypertension, glucose intolerance, and osteoporosis are frequently associated with hypercortisolism, but they are not distinguishing features. Features that are the most specific to Cushing syndrome include bruising of the thin skin and proximal muscle weakness.

Many patients with Cushing syndrome have associated mental disturbances, most commonly atypical depressive disorder (52%) and/or major affective disorder (12%) (22). A recent study suggests that, in many patients, the depressive illness remits as the hypothalamic–pituitary axis returns to normal (22). During childhood and adolescence, Cushing syndrome may present with growth retardation and delayed puberty in association with obesity. Disorders to consider that present as pseudo–Cushing syndrome include a primary mood disorder, alcoholism, and the effects of medications that alter testing for true Cushing syndrome (18–20).

The mechanisms of the abnormal weight gain and central fat redistribution with chronic excess hypercortisolism are still unknown. The distribution of weight changes is similar to that of other insulin-resistant states, such as type II diabetes mellitus, polycystic ovary syndrome (PCOS), chronic alcoholism, and android obesity. Other features of Cushing syndrome, which has already been described, distinguish patients with true Cushing syndrome from those with pseudo–Cushing syndrome. Recently, weight redistribution similar to that seen in patients with hypercortisolism has been observed in patients receiving combination antiretroviral therapy, resulting in a "protease pouch" (23,24). These patients have the buffalo hump and central weight gain, but they lack the other classic features of Cushing syndrome. Moreover, the 24-hour, urinary free-cortisol levels and dynamic testing of the HPA axis are normal in these patients. The underlying mechanism of this rapid and striking fat redistribution is also unknown, and it is now under active investigation.

Although the original descriptions of Cushing syndrome were made in the early 1900s, the diagnosis of the underlying etiology of the disorder in an individual patient remains difficult, and the appropriate evaluation is controversial. In the evaluation of the patient with hypercortisolism, the source of excess cortisol production is either dependent on or independent of adrenocorticotropic hormone (ACTH) (18–22). Approximately 70% to 80% of patients with Cushing disease have it as a result of an ACTH-secreting pituitary adenoma. Ectopic production of ACTH or corticotropin-releasing hormone from a bronchial carcinoid, pancreatic tumor, or lung cancer occurs in 10% to 15% of patients. Adrenal tumors that produce excess cortisol directly, thus causing Cushing syndrome, occur in 10% to 15% of patients.

Screening for the disorder includes the collection of 24-hour urine for free cortisol with concomitant creatinine measurement to ensure an adequate collection. Alternatively, use of a 1-mg dexamethasone-suppression test in a nonhospitalized patient can be a useful screening test. The dexamethasone is given at 11 p.m., and an 8 a.m. cortisol measurement is obtained. An 8 a.m. cortisol level of 5 or less after dexamethasone suppression and a normal 24-hour urinary free cortisol level exclude the diagnosis of Cushing syndrome. Repeated screening tests are often necessary to determine which patients should undergo continuing work-ups for the source of the abnormal cortisol secretion. Measurement of ACTH levels and high-dose dexamethasone testing with 8 mg given at 11 p.m. and measurement of an 8 a.m. cortisol level are useful to localize the source of the ACTH excess. Most patients with pituitary Cushing syndrome suppress cortisol levels by more than 50% in response to this test. Petrosal sinus catheterization is useful in patients with ACTH-dependent Cushing syndrome for confirming or refuting the pituitary localization of the tumor. Pituitary magnetic resonance imaging (MRI) is usually obtained, but it is not definitive because these ACTH-secreting adenomas are usually smaller than 1 cm and because persons without Cushing syndrome can also have abnormalities on pituitary MRI. The sensitivity and specificity of each of the tests for the diagnosis of Cushing syndrome are reviewed elsewhere (18–22).

After cure of Cushing syndrome, body fat redistribution is delayed in most patients until the glucocorticoid-replacement dosage has been tapered to physiologic levels and the reproductive axis has been reactivated. The rapid "melting" of the abnormal weight gain and the fat redistribution that is observed clinically are remarkable. Further study of the underlying mechanisms of this reversal of phenotype might shed insight into the pathophysiology of abnormal weight gain and the fat redistribution in this disorder.

Women with underlying Cushing syndrome may have features that overlap with those of women with PCOS. Kaltsas et al. (25) reviewed the presentation of female patients with Cushing syndrome and found that most had hirsutism, acne, or male pattern balding that suggested hyperandrogenism, as well as menstrual cycle disturbances. However, the gonadotropin and estradiol levels were suppressed, and the ovarian androgen levels were in the normal range in women with Cushing syndrome, in contrast to those in women with PCOS (25). Ultrasounds in some women with Cushing syndrome revealed cystic changes in the ovary which were similar to those seen in patients with PCOS, probably reflecting the chronic anovulation observed in both disorders (25).

Hypothyroidism

During infancy, hypothyroidism is manifested by mental deficiency and growth retardation (26). In the first few months of life, the symptoms include feeding problems, failure to thrive, constipation, hoarse cry, and increased somnolence. The abdomen is often protuberant, and dry skin and hair and delayed dentition are evident. Over time, the lack of thyroid hormone is manifested by significant growth retardation, with the effects on the extremities being greater than those on the trunk. Mental deficiency is severe in congenital hypothyroidism. Marked obesity is usually not a feature of the disorder.

In juvenile hypothyroidism, linear growth and sexual development are impaired (26). The children appear much younger than their chronologic age. Obesity is not a prominent feature of hypothyroidism in childhood; however, weight loss followed by weight gain associated with onset of puberty and of secretion of gonadal steroids and GH are consequences of thyroid hormone replacement.

In adulthood, hypothyroidism is associated with generalized weight gain. Myxedema coma refers to the clinical syndrome resulting from severe, long-standing thyroid hormone deficiency, and it occurs most often in the elderly (26). Clinical symptoms include a subnormal temperature, bradycardia, hypotension, severely dry skin, significant generalized weight gain with edema, and coarsening of features. The disorder is life threatening, and it requires intravenous thyroid hormone if gut motility is diminished. Management of cardiac, pulmonary, and infectious complications is often necessary. Hyperthyroidism, in contrast to hypothyroidism, is associated with weight loss. Two studies have shown that the treatment of hyperthyroidism is associated with a regain of weight (27,28). However, in the patient with hypothyroidism, physiologic replacement with thyroid hormone rarely results in significant weight loss, a result disappointing to patients and physicians alike searching for treatments that restore a lower set point for body weight regulation (27,28).

Growth Hormone Deficiency

Children with idiopathic GH deficiency and hypopituitarism have normal skeletal proportions for their age, but they tend to be overweight for their height and to have increased subcutaneous deposits of abdominal fat (29). GH-replacement therapy in both children and adults is associated with increased body weight but also with a redistribution of body fat away from a central adiposity, In addition, a significant increase in lean muscle mass is seen as a result of GH replacement (29–32). The mechanisms of the weight redistribution are unknown.

Pseudohypoparathyroidism

Patients with pseudohypoparathyroidism type Ia with a resistance to parathyroid hormone have a clinical syndrome of generalized obesity; short stature; round face; thick neck; diminished intelligence; subcutaneous calcifications; and various bone abnormalities, including shortened metacarpals and metatarsals (33). Some patients have primary hypothyroidism and hypogonadism (34). Recently, investigators have reported two children with tall stature, obesity, and pseudohypoparathyroidism (35). They have suggested the genetic mutations in the cell surface receptor $G_s\alpha$ may play a role in the underlying mechanism of obesity in this disorder of cellular resistance to hormone signaling.

Polycystic Ovary Syndrome

PCOS is a clinical disorder of patients presenting with menstrual irregularity and evidence of hyperandrogenism, either clinically (hirsutism, acne or male pattern balding) or biochemically (elevated serum androgen levels), in the absence of other diseases (36–38). Clinically, it is a disorder that begins during puberty. Girls with PCOS have irregular menses, hirsutism, and acne that begin in adolescence. The weight gain with PCOS also begins in adolescence, it is associated with an android distribution, and it occurs in 60% of patients (36–38). Insulin resistance has been postulated to contribute to the weight gain seen in women with PCOS. These women are insulin resistant in excess of the levels expected for their degree of obesity, thus suggesting the presence of a primary disorder separate from their obesity (38). An estimated 20% of women with PCOS who are obese have either impaired glucose intolerance or non–insulin-dependent diabetes mellitus by 40 years of age (37).

The underlying pathophysiology of PCOS is still controversial (37). Three major theories are prominent in the current literature. The neuroendocrine hypothesis states that an abnormal gonadotropin-releasing hormone (GnRH) pulse generator at a fixed fast frequency triggers the phenotype of hyperandrogenism and anovulation at puberty. This hypothesis is supported by data that show that many women with PCOS have high luteinizing hormone (LH) levels relative to their levels of follicle-stimulating hormone (FSH) and that use of GnRH analogs to interrupt the endogenous signaling often improves both the biochemical and clinical signs of hyperandrogenism (39). The ovarian hypothesis suggests that a primary defect of sex steroid synthesis or metabolism results in hyperresponsiveness of the ovary to normal signals from the pituitary, thereby causing hyperandrogenism. This hypothesis is supported by testing of ovarian androgen secretion *in vivo* and *in vitro* in women with PCOS in which increased 17-hydroxyprogesterone responses to GnRH agonists are demonstrated, reflecting an abnormal function of the cytochrome P450 c_{17} enzyme function in the ovaries (40).

Alternatively, the hyperinsulinism hypothesis suggests that women with PCOS are insulin resistant at all targets except the ovary, reflecting a metabolic, but not a mitogenic, defect. Hyperinsulinemia in response to insulin resistance exacerbates overproduction of ovarian androgens and triggers the phenotype. This hypothesis is supported by euglycemic clamp studies that show a 30% to 40% decrease in insulin-mediated glucose disposal in women with PCOS (38). In addition, fat cells from women with PCOS display impaired insulin sensitivity and responsiveness to glucose uptake (38). Clinically, these translate into a 15% risk of type II diabetes in postmenopausal women with prior PCOS, compared to a background rate of 2% to 3% (41,42). Recent studies suggesting that drugs, such as metformin, which improve insulin sensitivity, also improve the hyperandrogenism and rates of ovulation (43) support the importance of this system in the underlying mechanisms that result in PCOS. Because not all women who are insulin resistant and obese have features of PCOS, other factors must play a role. Whether the improvement in the function of the reproductive axis in women with PCOS treated with metformin or the thiazolidinediones, however, reflects the associated weight loss seen with the therapy or it is rather a primary effect of the insulin sensitizer on the ovary is unclear. Future studies will determine the interplay between these multiple defects seen in women with PCOS.

Treatment options in these women focus on earlier diagnosis and intervention to suppress androgens, tonic estrogens, and insulin resistance. Although no controlled studies exist, the author's clinical impression is that early suppression of ovarian and adrenal androgens with oral contraceptives and antiandrogens in adolescents with PCOS lessens the rate of weight gain and other associated abnormalities. Theoretically, inhibition of chronic changes in ovarian morphology, such as hyperthecosis, is an advantage of ovarian hormone suppression. Any approach that results in weight loss also improves the clinical features and biochemical markers of the disorder. When fertility is a goal, treatment with metformin and clomiphene citrate shows promise for higher rates of ovulation and conception than those that previously were observed with clomiphene or human menopausal gonadotropin therapy alone (43). Future research is necessary to outline the effectiveness of insulin sensitizers alone or in combination with oral contraceptives for therapy aimed at decreasing androgens and promoting weight loss in these women.

Prolactinomas

Prolactinomas have been clinically associated with a higher prevalence of weight gain. Recently, investigators compared body mass indexes (BMIs) of male patients with prolactinomas to those of male patients with glycoprotein-secreting pituitary tumors (44). They reported an overall higher BMI and a history of recent weight gain in the former group. Treatment of patients with prolactinomas with medical therapy is associated with weight loss in almost half of the patients, which correlates with the normalization of the prolactin levels. No change in body weight has been observed in patients with other types of pituitary lesions. The article does not discuss whether the weight gains and subsequent weight loss in patients with prolactinomas were associated with concomitant changes in gonadal function and sex steroid levels.

Medications that Contribute to Obesity

See Table 14.1 for a summary of these medications and their uses.

Contraceptives

The supraphysiologic doses of sex steroids used in the earlier forms of high-dose contraceptives were associated with weight gain (45). In contrast, the low-dose birth-control pills have not been associated with significant weight gain (46). In studies of patients on Norplant and Depo-Provera, weight gain was the second most common reason cited for discontinuation (the first was menstrual irregularities) (47).

TABLE 14.1. *Medications implicated in weight gain*

Contraceptives
　　Birth-control pills (dependent on estrogen dose and androgenicity of progestin)
　　Norplant (low rate <5%)
　　Depo-Provera (in women up to 20% or men treated for pulmonary disease)
　　Megace (given to patients with cancer to stimulate appetite)
　　Hormone-replacement therapy (not at physiologic doses)
Antiretroviral therapy (protease pouch)
Antiseizure medications
　　Valproic acid (hyperandrogenic anovulation and weight gain)
Antipsychotics
　　Atypicals (worse with olanzapine, can be severe)
　　Typicals (less common)

After menopause, women have been reported to gain and to redistribute weight centrally and to lose ovarian function to a more android phenotype (48,49). In contrast to the popular view, physiologic replacement doses of estrogen and progestin after menopause do not result in excess weight gain (48,49). In the Postmenopausal Estrogen/Progestin Intervention (PEPI) trial, women who were receiving hormone-replacement therapy gained less weight than did women who took a placebo (50).

High-dose progestins given to men with obstructive sleep apnea cause the suppression of the hypothalamic–pituitary–testicular axis, and their administration is accompanied by weight gain (51). High-dose progestins, such as megestrol acetate (Megace), are used in patients with cancer or in elderly patients with anorexia to stimulate appetite and weight gain (52). The effects of steroid hormone deficiency or, conversely, of supraphysiologic levels of steroid hormones on weight and body fat redistribution are poorly understood.

Antiretroviral Therapy

Recent work by many investigators has reported the appearance of a pseudo–Cushing syndrome phenotype in patients with human immunodeficiency virus infection who are taking potent antiretroviral therapy (23,24). The exact mechanism of development of the clinical features of central visceral fat redistribution, buffalo hump, and facial fullness is unknown, but the analysis of endocrine studies show that these patients have normal 24-hour urinary free cortisol levels and normal dynamic testing of the HPA axis (23,24).

Valproic Acid (Valproate)

Valproic acid, a commonly used antiseizure medication and drug used in bipolar disease, has been shown to cause a dramatic weight gain in 50% of women who take it (8 to 49 kg, mean of 21 kg) (53). The weight gain and drug administration has also been associated with anovulation and dysfunctional uterine bleeding. Many of the women display hirsutism and hyperandrogenism, with cystic ovaries appearing on ultrasound. High levels of insulin and insulin-like growth factor–binding protein-1 are observed (53). Whether the drug aggravates an underlying hyperandrogenic anovulatory disorder in these women or causes it is unclear.

Antipsychotics

Use of antipsychotic medications is associated with weight gain. However, patients with mood disorders often are inactive, they tend to have poor diets, and they may have other comorbid conditions that contribute to weight gain. Underlying mechanisms that explain the weight gain based on the neurotransmitter disorder in these patients or based on the specific actions of the medications have not been proven. Recent studies suggest that treatment with the atypical antipsychotic medications results in more significant weight gain than do the typical antipsychotics (54). Atypical antipsychotic medications are used more frequently because of their improved side-effect profile with less extrapyramidal symptoms, improved efficacy against negative symptoms and cognitive deficits, and improved quality of life (54). In the atypical class, olanzapine therapy has been associated with a greater weight gain than either clozapine or risperidone (55). Baseline BMI does not predict the amount of weight gain on therapy in this study, but others have suggested that a low pretreatment weight, a young age, and female gender predispose patients to more significant weight gain (54). Others have confirmed that adolescents are particularly sensitive to the weight-promoting effects of olanzapine and less significantly to those of risperidone (56). The potential mechanism of weight gain after antipsychotic medication administration was recently explored by Baptista et al. (57). They observed that the weight gain correlated with the levels of hyperprolactinemia associated with drug therapy. Patients with higher prolactin levels had relatively more hyperandrogenic profiles, which may contribute to the observed increased weight gain.

ENDOCRINE COMPLICATIONS OF OBESITY

Effects on the Male Reproductive Axis

Total testosterone levels are decreased in obese men, but their free testosterone levels are usually normal, unless the patient has morbid obesity (58). Sex hormone–binding globulin concentrations are decreased, resulting in low total, but normal free, testosterone levels. Concentrations of estradiol and estrone are elevated in obese men, and their estrogen-production rates are increased (59). The incidence of complications, including gynecomastia, infertility, and hypogonadism, however, is uncommon (58,59). With progressive obesity, hypogonadism occurs, perhaps as a result of the worsening obstructive sleep apnea in these patients.

Effects on the Female Reproductive Axis

Childhood obesity in girls is associated with earlier menarche. These menstrual cycles, however, are irregular and anovulatory (60–62). Menopause occurs at an earlier age in obese women. Obesity is a risk factor for early pregnancy loss after *in vitro* fertilization or intracytoplasmic sperm injection (63,64). In one study, the authors found that obese women had a decreased number of oocytes collected (65). This may be due to the number of hyperandrogenic obese women with PCOS who are attempting conception. Once pregnant, maternal fatness is associated with an increased risk for low birth weight in preterm infants and for macrosomia in full-term infants (66).

Fat distribution in women has different consequences. Most women gain fat in the gluteofemoral gynecoid distribution (i.e., the pear shape). This is associated with increased total-body estrogen action, resulting from the increased production of estrone as a result of the aromatization of androgens (67–69). This increase in total-body estrogen stores that is often unopposed by the adequate progestin effects on the uterus may be the major factor increasing the risk of endometrial cancer in obese women. In contrast, women who, like men, gain fat centrally in an android (i.e., apple) shape and who have increased visceral fat tend to have higher androgen levels. Sex hormone–binding globulin concentrations are decreased in women with central adiposity, concomitant with an increased free or bioavailable testosterone level (60,67–69). These women also have tonic levels of estrogen that put them at risk for endometrial cancer; but they also display associated hyperinsulinism, hyperlipidemia, and hypertension, with an increased risk of cardiovascular disease.

African-American women have a higher prevalence of obesity than whites, but the cause of the difference is unclear. Recent studies suggest that African-American women have a higher ACTH response to exogenous corticotropin-releasing hormone without a concomitant increase in cortisol (70). Yanovski et al. (70) compared ACTH responses to exercise in African-American and white women and found a significant increase in ACTH secretion. In the absence of subsequent increases in cortisol production, they hypothesized that ACTH may crosstalk with the hypothalamic melanocortin-4 receptors, which have been implicated in body weight control, and that this may be one of the factors underlying the greater adiposity in African-American women (70).

In many women, attainment of a specific threshold weight triggers anovulation, the onset of hirsutism, acne, and hyperandrogenic anovulation that is reversed with weight loss (68,69). Other studies have shown an increase in ovulatory rates and pregnancies in obese women with weight reduction of an average of 6.3 kg (63,64).

Effects of Obesity on Other Endocrine Axes

Prolactin

The mean levels of prolactin in obese patients are normal. Some patients have been shown to fail to have a normal prolactin response to provocative stimuli (71,72).

Growth Hormone

In obesity, GH levels and responses to provocative stimuli are reduced (73). Recent data suggest that GH clearance is increased, with a concomitant decrease in GH synthesis and secretion. Insulin-like growth factor-1 levels, the target of GH action in the liver, are normal, suggesting that, although GH levels are low, they are sufficient to maintain normal GH action (73).

Thyroid

$3,5,3'$-Triiodothyronine (T_3) levels are increased with overfeeding and suppressed after starvation. T_3 levels are stimulated by high-carbohydrate diets and are inhibited by low-carbohydrate diets, whereas thyroxine (T_4) and thyroid-stimulating hormone levels are not altered (74). In animal studies, thyroid hormone receptors were found to be low in the liver and lungs of leptin-deficient *ob/ob* mice, and this was thought to correlate with the decreased activity of Na^+K^+-adenosine triphosphatase in these tissues (75).

Vasopressin

Concentrations of vasopressin are normal in obese subjects, but they are not suppressed appropriately after a water load (71,72). The mechanism is unknown.

Adrenal

Because patients with obesity often have hypertension and glucose intolerance, they are often evaluated for Cushing syndrome. In simple obesity, the diurnal pattern of cortisol secretion is retained, and urinary free cortisol levels are usually normal or only slightly elevated. Conversely, in patients with Cushing syndrome, both are abnormal (68). In addition, dynamic testing of the adrenal axis can distinguish the two states. Overnight dexamethasone-suppression test results are abnormal in 10% of obese patients and in 98% of patients with Cushing syndrome (72). Because the evaluation for Cushing syndrome is fraught with false-positive and false-negative test results, a workup should not be performed on every obese patient; instead, the clinician should rely on his or her clinical judgment for signs and symptoms of the disorder before performing the screening tests.

Catecholamine levels in animal models of obesity have shown decreased norepinephrine turnover (17,76). In humans, however, basal norepinephrine and the response to starvation or upright posture are normal (76). Investigators reported a decrease in epinephrine response to isometric exercise in obese women but not in obese men (77). The thermogenic response to infusions of norepinephrine is somewhat blunted in obese subjects, associated with a blunted rise in oxygen uptake after a meal. Norepinephrine response to insulin is similar in obese patients to that observed in normal patients (76).

CONCLUSION

Several endocrine disorders present clinically with abnormal weight gain or fat redistribution. In addition, both supraphysiologic doses and deficiencies in sex hormone levels are associated with abnormal weight gain. Medications given to prevent seizures or psychiatric disorders often cause weight gain. Severe morbid obesity can also result in endocrine dysfunction. Surprisingly, despite careful clinical descriptions of the changes that occur in these different conditions, little is known about the basic cellular mechanisms that underlie these changes. Hopefully, the insights provided in review of basic science advances in other chapters in this book will spur investigators to study the underlying pathophysiology of abnormal weight gain and redistribution further, which in turn may lead to novel prevention or treatment strategies.

REFERENCES

1. Gunay-Aygun M, Schwartz S, Heeger S, et al. The changing purpose of Prader–Willi syndrome clinical diagnostic criteria and proposed revised criteria. *Pediatrics* 2001;108:1–5.
2. Rankinen T, Perusse L, Weisnagel SJ, et al. The human obesity gene map: the 2001 update. *Obes Res* 2002;10: 196–243.
3. Carrel AL, Myers SE, Whitman BY, et al. Benefits of long-term GH therapy in Prader–Willi syndrome: a 4-year study. *J Clin Endocrinol Metab* 2002;87:1581–1585.
4. Cummings DE, Clement K, Purnell JQ, et al. Elevated plasma ghrelin levels in Prader–Willi syndrome. *Nat Med* 2002;8:643–644.
5. Beales PL, Elcioglu N, Woolf AS, et al. New criteria for improved diagnosis of Bardet–Biedl syndrome: results of a population survey. *J Med Genet* 1999;36:437–446.
6. Leppert M, Baird I, AndersonKL, et al. Bardet–Biedl syndrome is linked to DNA markers on chromosome 11q and is genetically heterogeneous. *Nat Genet* 1994;7:108–112.
7. Campfield LA, Smith FJ, Burn P, Strategies and potential targets for obesity treatment. *Science* 1998;280: 1383–1387.
8. Tartaglia LA, Dembski M, Weng X, et al. Identification and expression cloning of a leptin receptor, OB-R. *Cell* 1995;83:1263–1271.
9. Strobel A, Issad T, Camoin L, et al. A leptin missense mutation associated with hypogonadism and morbid obesity. *Nat Genet* 1998;18:213–215.
10. Farooqi IS, Jebb SA, Langmack G, et al. Effects of recombinant leptin therapy in a child with congenital leptin deficiency. *N Engl J Med* 1999;341:879–884.
11. Casabiell X, Pineiro V, Vega F, et al. Leptin, reproduction and sex steroids. *Pituitary* 2001;4:93–99.
12. Tena-Sempere M, Barreiro ML. Leptin in male reproduction: the testis paradigm. *Mol Cell Endocrinol* 2002; 188:9–13.
13. Sklar CA Craniopharyngioma: endocrine sequelae of treatment. *Pediatr Neurosurg* 1994;21:120–123.
14. Curtis J, Daneman D, Hoffman HJ, et al. The endocrine outcome after surgical removal of craniopharyngiomas. *Pediatr Neurosurg* 1994;21:24–27.
15. Ono N, Kohga H, Zama A, et al. A comparison of children with suprasellar germ cell tumors and craniopharyngiomas: final height, weight, endocrine and visual sequelae after treatment. *Surg Neurol* 1996;46:370–377.
16. Yoshida T, Kemnitz JW, Bray GA. Lateral hypothalamic lesions and nor epinephrine turnover in rats. *J Clin Invest* 1983;72:919–927.
17. Jung RT, Shetty PS, James WPT, et al. Plasma catecholamines and autonomic responsiveness in obesity. *Int J Obes* 1982;6:131–141.
18. Nieman LK. Cushing's syndrome. *Curr Ther Endocrinol Metab* 1997;6:161–164.
19. Newell-Price J, Trainer P, Besser M, et al. The diagnosis and differential diagnosis of Cushing's syndrome. *Endocr Rev* 1998;19:647–672.
20. Meier CA, Biller BM. Clinical and biochemical evaluation of Cushing's syndrome. *Endocrinol Metab Clin North Am* 1997;26:741–762.
21. Kleerekoper M, Schiebinger R, Gutai JP. Steroid therapy for adrenal disorders—getting the dose right. *J Clin Endocrinol Metab* 1997;82:3923–3925.
22. Dorn LD, Burgess ES, Friedman TC. et. al. The longitudinal course of psychopathology in Cushing's syndrome after correction of hypercortisolism. *J Clin Endocrinol Metab* 1997;82:912–919.

23. Miller KK, Daly PA, Sentochnik K, et al. Pseudo–Cushing's syndrome in human immunodeficiency virus infected patients. *Clin Infect Dis* 1998;27:69–72.
24. Hirsch MS, Klibanski A. What price progress? Pseudo–Cushing's syndrome associated with antiretroviral therapy in patients with human immunodeficiency virus infection. *Clin Infect Dis* 1998;27:73–75.
25. Kaltsas GA, Korbonits M, Isidori AM, et al. How common are polycystic ovaries and the polycystic ovarian syndrome in women with Cushing's syndrome? *Clin Endocriol* 2000;53:493–500.
26. Larsen PR, Ingbar SH. The thyroid gland. In: Wilson J, Foster D, eds. *William's textbook of endocrinology,* 8th ed. Philadelphia: WB Saunders, 1998:445–463.
27. Hoogwerf BJ, Nuttall FQ. Long-term weight regulation in treated hyperthyroid and hypothyroid subjects. *Am J Med* 1984;76:963–970.
28. Pears J, Jung RT, Gunn A. Long-term weight changes in treated hyperthyroid and hypothyroid patients. *Scott Med J* 1990;35:180–182.
29. Baars J, Van den Broeck J, le Cessie, et al. Body mass index in growth hormone deficient children before a during growth hormone treatment. *Horm Res* 1998;49:39–45.
30. Brummer RJ. Effects of growth hormone treatment on visceral adipose tissue. *Growth Horm IGF Res* 1998;8:19–23.
31. Johannsson G, Marin P, Lonn L, et al. Growth hormone treatment of abdominally obese men reduces abdominal fat mass, improves glucose and lipoprotein metabolism and reduces diastolic blood pressure. *J Clin Endocrinol Metab* 1997;82:727–734.
32. Beshyah SA, Freemantle C, Thomas E, et al. Abnormal body composition and reduced bone mass in growth hormone deficient hypopituitary adults. *Clin Endocrinol* 1995;42:179–189.
33. Albright F, Burnett C, Smith PH, et al. Pseudohypoparathyroidism: an example of "Seabright–Bantam" syndrome. *Endocrinology* 1942;30:922–932.
34. Carter A, Bardin C, Collins R, et al. Reduced expression of multiple forms of the alpha subunit of the stimulatory GTP-binding protein in pseudohypoparathyroidism type 1a. *Proc Natl Acad Sci U S A* 1987;84:7266–7269.
35. Ong K, Dunger RA, Dunger D. Pseudohypoparathyroidism—another monogenic obesity syndrome. *Clin Endocrinol* 2000;52:389–391.
36. Taylor A. Understanding the underlying metabolic abnormalities of polycystic ovary syndrome and their implications. *Am J Obstet Gynecol* 1998;179:S94–S100.
37. Taylor AE. Polycystic ovary syndrome. *Endocrinol Metab Clin North Am* 1998;27:877–902.
38. Dunaif A. Insulin resistance and the polycystic ovary syndrome: mechanisms and implications for pathogenesis. *Endocr Rev* 1997;18:774–800.
39. Chang RJ, Laufer LR, Meldrum DR, et al. Steroid secretion in polycystic ovarian disease after ovarian suppression by a long-acting gonadotropin-releasing hormone agonist. *J Clin Endocrinol Metab* 1983;56:897–902.
40. Ehrmann DA, Rosenfield RL, Barnes R, et al. Detection of functional ovarian hyperandrogenism in women with androgen excess. *N Engl J Med* 1992;327:157–161.
41. Dahlgren E, Johansson S, Lindstedt G, et al. Women with polycystic ovary syndrome wedge resected in 1956 to 1965: a long term follow-up focusing on natural history and circulating hormones. *Fertil Steril* 1992;57:505–513.
42. Dunaif A. Selective insulin resistance in the polycystic ovary syndrome. *J Clin Endocrinol Metab* 1999;84:3110–3116.
43. Nestler JE, Jakubowicz DJ, Evans WS, et al. Effects of metformin on spontaneous and clomiphene-induced ovulation in the polycystic ovary syndrome. *N Engl J Med* 1998;338:1876–1880.
44. Greenman Y, Tordjman K, Stern N. Increased body weight associated with prolactin secreting pituitary adenomas: weight loss with normalization of prolactin levels. *Clin Endocrinol* 1998;48:547–553.
45. Oral contraceptives. *Med Lett Drugs Ther* 2000;42:42–44.
46. Rosenberg M. Weight change with oral contraceptive use and during the menstrual cycle. Results of daily measurements. *Contraception* 1998;58:345–349.
47. DeAguilar MA, Altamirano L, Leon DA, et al. Current status of injectable hormonal contraception, with special reference to the monthly method. *Adv Contracept* 1997;13:405–417.
48. Van Seumeren I. Weight gain and hormone replacement therapy: are women's fears justified? *Maturitas* 2000;34:S3–S8.
49. Chmouliovsky L, Habicht F, Lehmann T et al. Beneficial effect of hormone replacement therapy on weight loss in obese menopausal women. *Maturitas* 1999;32:147–153.
50. Simkin-Silverman LR, Wing RR. Weight gain during menopause. Is it inevitable or can it be prevented? *Postgrad Med* 2000;108:47–50,53–56.
51. Hudgel DW, Thanakitcharu S. Pharmacologic treatment of sleep-disordered breathing. *Am J Respir Crit Care Med* 1998;158:691–699.
52. Yeh SS, Wu SY, Lee TP, et al. Improvement in quality of life measures and stimulation of weight gain after treatment with megestrol acetate oral suspension in geriatric cachexia: results of a double-blind, placebo-controlled study. *J Am Geriatr Soc* 2000;48:485–492.
53. Isojarvi JI, Laatikainen TJ, Knip M, et al. Obesity and endocrine disorders in women taking valproate for epilepsy. *Ann Neurol* 1996;39:579–584.
54. Russell JM, Mackell JA. Bodyweight gain associated with atypical antipsychotics: epidemiology and therapeutic implications. *CNS Drugs* 2001;15:537–551.

55. Simpson MM, Goetz RR, Devlin MJ, et al. Weight gain and antipsychotic medication: differences between antipsychotic-free and treatment periods. *J Clin Psychiatry* 2001;62:694–700.
56. Ratzoni G, Gothelf D, Brand-Gothelf A, et al. Weight gain associated with olanzapine and risperidone in adolescent patients: a comparative prospective study. *J Am Acad Child Adolesc Psychiatry* 2002;41:337–343.
57. Baptista T, Reyes D, Hernandez L. Antipsychotic drugs and reproductive hormones: relationship to body weight regulation. *Pharmacol Biochem Behav* 1999;62:409–417.
58. Glass AR, Swerdloff RS, Bray GA, et al. Low serum testosterone and sex-hormone binding globulin in massively obese men. *J Clin Endocrinol Metab* 1977;45:1211–1219.
59. Schneider G, Kirschner MA, Berkowitz R, et al. Increased estrogen production in obese men. *J Clin Endocrinol Metab* 1981;53:828–832.
60. Kopelman PG, Pilkington TR, White N, Jeffcoate SL. Abnormal sex steroid secretion and binding in massively obese women. *Clin Endocrinol (Oxf)* 1980;12:363–369.
61. Edman CD, MacDonald PC. Effect of obesity on conversion of plasma androstenedione to estrone in ovulatory and anovulatory young women. *Am J Obstet Gynecol* 1978;130:456–461.
62. Hauner H, Ditschuneit HH, Pal SB, et. al. Fat distribution, endocrine and metabolic profile in obese women with and without hirsutism. *Metabolism* 1988;37:281–286.
63. Clark AM, Thornley B, Tomlinson L, et al. Weight loss in obese infertile women results in improvement in reproductive outcome for all forms of fertility treatment. *Hum Reprod* 1998;13:1502–1505.
64. Galletly C, Clark A, Tomlinson L, et al. Improved pregnancy rates for obese, infertile women following group treatment program. An open pilot study. *Gen Hosp Psychiatry* 1996;18:192–195.
65. Fedorcsak P, Storeng R, Dale PO, et al. Obesity is a risk factor for early pregnancy loss after IVF or IC. *Acta Obstet Gynecol Scand* 2000;79:43–48.
66. Lucas A, Morley R, Cole TJ, et al. Maternal fatness and viability of preterm infants, *BMJ* 1988;296:1495–1497.
67. Kirschner MA, Samojlik E, Drejka M, et al. Androgen-estrogen metabolism in women with upper body versus lower body obesity. *J Clin Endocrinol Metab* 1990;70:473–479.
68. Pasquali R, Antenucci D, Casimirri F, et al. Clinical and hormonal characteristics of obese amenorrheic hyperandrogenic women before and after weight loss. *J Clin Endocrinol Metab* 1989;68:173–179.
69. Guzick DS, Wing R, Smith D, et al. Endocrine consequences of weight loss in obese, hyperandrogenic anovulatory women. *Fertil Steril* 1994;61:598–604.
70. Yanovski JA, Yanovski SZ, Boyle AJ, et al. Hypothalamic–pituitary adrenal axis activity during exercise in African American and Caucasian Women. *J Clin Endocrinol Metab* 2000;85:2660–2663.
71. Foster DW. Eating disorders: obesity, anorexia nervosa, and bulimia nervosa. In: Wilson J, Foster D, eds. *William's textbook of endocrinology,* 8th ed. Philadelphia: WB Saunders, 1998:1335–1365.
72. Drenick EJ, Carlson HE, Robertson GL, et al. The role of vasopressin and prolactin in abnormal salt and water metabolism of obese patients before and after fasting and during refeeding. *Metabolism* 1977;26:309–317.
73. Cordido F, Casanueva FF, Dieguez C. Cholinergic receptor activation by pyridostigmine restores growth hormone (GH) responsiveness to GH-releasing hormone administration in obese subjects: evidence for hypothalamic somatostatinergic participation in the blunted GH release of obesity. *J Clin Endocrinol Metab* 1989;68: 290–293.
74. Danforth E Jr, Horton ES, O'Connell M, et al. Dietary-induced alterations in thyroid hormone metabolism during overnutrition. *J Clin Invest* 1979;64:1336–1347.
75. Guernsey DL, Morishige WK. Na^+ pump activity and nuclear T_3 receptors in tissues of genetically obese (*ob/ob*) mice. *Metabolism* 1979;28:629–632.
76. O'Hare JA, Minaker KL, Meneilly GS, et al. Effect of insulin on plasma norepinephrine and 3,4 dihydroxyphenylalanine in obese men. *Metabolism* 1989;38:322–329.
77. Gustafson AB, Kalkhoff RK. Influence of sex and obesity on plasma catecholamine response to isometric exercise. *J Clin Endocrinol Metab* 1982;55:703–708.

15

Psychosocial Complications of Obesity and Dieting

Suzanne Phelan and Thomas A. Wadden

This chapter explores the prevalence and nature of psychosocial complications in obese individuals. It examines the role of social factors in people's perception of and behavior toward obese individuals and reviews the psychosocial consequences of obesity in both treatment-seeking and nonclinical samples. The psychosocial complications associated with weight loss and weight regain are reviewed, and the future directions for research and treatment are outlined. Understanding the psychosocial complications of obesity will enhance practitioners' ability to assess and treat their overweight patients.

SOCIAL FACTORS

Social Pressures to Be Thin

Cultural definitions of beauty have varied over time, but they currently are thin for women and muscular and lean for men (1,2). Ironically, over the past few decades, as the Western world has become heavier, the cultural ideals of beauty have become leaner. Newspapers, magazines, videos, and television bombard people daily with images of extra lean models (3). Just as thinness is portrayed as the ideal, overweight and obesity are portrayed as unattractive and indicative of a lack of self-discipline and willpower (4,5).

The pressure to be thin is particularly strong for women. Women's magazines are replete with articles about diet foods and weight loss methods, while men's magazines are more likely to publish articles about alcoholic beverages (3). Wadden et al. (6) surveyed male and female adolescents about their level of concern regarding various issues, including weight. Results indicated that the girls worried most about their looks, figures, relationships with the opposite sex, and their weights (Table 15.1). The boys worried most about money, looks, popularity, and relationships with the opposite sex; they rated weight as 13th on their list of concerns (Table 15.2). These findings underscore the gender differences regarding the concern about weight.

Indeed, numerous studies suggest that the media's portrayal of the thin, ideal, and obese stereotype affects people's beliefs about weight and shape. In a study of adolescent girls, the frequency of reading women's magazines was significantly correlated with the prevalence of dieting, initiating an exercise program, and wanting to lose weight (7). Other research has found that women who read fashion magazines wish to weigh less and that they are less satisfied with their bodies; they also are more frustrated with their weight and are more weight preoccupied than women who do not read such magazines (8–10). Although the authors are still uncertain about whether reading such materials is a cause or a consequence of body image concerns, many people, particularly women, have internalized lean weight standards and strive for the thin ideal (11–13).

TABLE 15.1. *Degree of worry about typical concerns of female high-school students*

Variable	Mean score
Looks	7.74[a]
Figure	7.11[b]
Relationships with the opposite sex	7.03[b,c]
Weight	6.77[b,c]
Popularity with the opposite sex	6.55[c]
The future	5.92[d]
Money	5.86[d,e]
Complexion	5.82[d,e]
Grades	5.75[d,e]
Family	5.39[e,f]
Popularity with the same sex	4.95[f,g]
Parents	4.90[f,g]
Health	4.83[g]
Nuclear war	3.60[h]
Sports	3.54[h]

Means sharing a common superscript are not significantly different. Mean significance: 1, none at all; 5, moderate amount; 10, extreme amount.

Number of subjects (*N*) = 453.

From Wadden TA, Brown G, Foster GD, et al. Salience of weight-related worries in adolescent males and females. *Int J Eat Disord* 1991;10:407–414, with permission.

Negative views of obesity have also been internalized. The public has endorsed beliefs that obese individuals are ugly, sinful, psychologically impaired, and medically sick (14,15). Children as young as 3 and 6 years of age have described obese individuals as more likely to be "lazy," "stupid," and "dumb," compared to lean individuals (16,17). Other research has similarly found that both children and adults would rather have severe

TABLE 15.2. *Degree of worry about typical concerns of male high-school students*

Variable	Mean score
Money	6.57[a]
Looks	6.45[a]
Popularity with the opposite sex	6.41[a]
Relationship with the opposite sex	6.28[a]
The future	5.64[b]
Physique	5.15[b,c]
Grades	5.06[b,c,d]
Sports	4.98[c,d]
Complexion	4.82[c,d]
Family	4.74[c,d]
Health	4.60[c,d]
Parents	4.46[d,e]
Weight	3.92[e]
Popularity with the same sex	3.87[e]
Nuclear war	2.46[f]

Means sharing a common superscript are not significantly different. 1, none at all; 5, moderate amount; 10, extreme amount.

Number of subjects (*N*) = 355.

From Wadden TA, Brown G, Foster GD, et al. Salience of weight-related worries in adolescent males and females. *Int J Eat Disord* 1991;10:407–414, with permission.

handicaps, including missing hands and facial disfigurement, than be obese (18–20). College students have reported that they would rather marry embezzlers, cocaine users, shoplifters, and blind persons than obese individuals (21). Even psychologists, counselors, nurses (22–24), medical residents (25), medical students (26), and physicians (27,28) hold negative views of obesity.

Regrettably, obese individuals also endorse these negative stereotypes (16,17). For example, Rand and MacGregor (29) asked 47 formerly obese patients to evaluate their preferences for various disabilities. Unlike people with other disabilities, these formerly obese individuals almost unanimously stated that they would prefer being deaf, dyslexic, diabetic, amputated, or blind to being obese (Fig. 15.1). Moreover, all said that they would prefer to be lean and poor than severely obese and a millionaire.

The desire to be thin extends to obese patients' perceptions of treatment outcomes. Studies suggest that obese patients desire weight losses that are two to three times greater than the 10% weight loss that is recommended by professionals and is obtained by most behavioral treatment programs (30,31). For example, treatment-seeking obese women characterized a 25% weight loss as "one I would not be happy with" and a 17% weight loss as "one that I could not view as successful in any way" (Fig. 15.2) (30). Thus, the 10% weight loss achieved by most treatment programs is perceived as even less than disappointing.

African-American women may ascribe more positive qualities to overweight, such as stamina, strength, and solidity; they are also less likely to link body size to health (32). Black women, compared to white women, also report less social pressure to be slim, fewer incidences of weight-related discrimination, a lower body image dissatisfaction, a greater acceptance of overweight, and less drive to be thin (33–36). Asian women equate large body size with health, and they report less body image dissatisfaction than do other

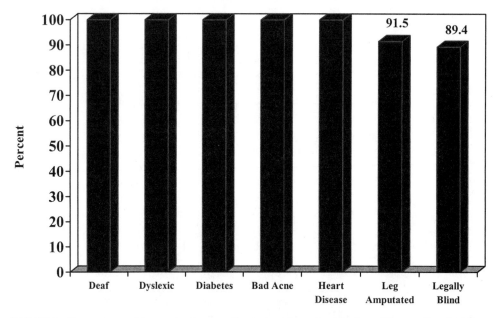

FIG. 15.1. Percentage of formerly obese patients (number of subjects = 47) reporting that they would rather have various disabilities than be obese. (Data from Rand CS, MacGregor AM. Morbidly obese patients' perceptions of social discrimination before and after surgery for obesity. *South Med J* 1990;83:1390–1395, with permission.)

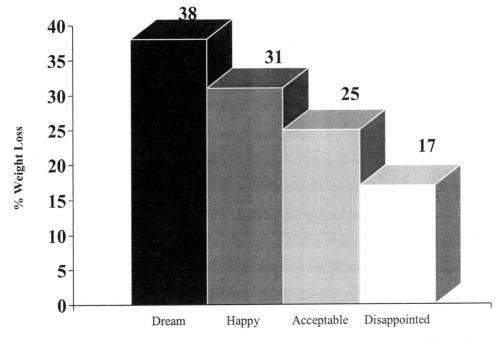

FIG. 15.2. Outcome evaluations of obese treatment seekers. (Data from Foster GD, Wadden TA, Vogt RA, et al. What is a reasonable weight loss? Patients' expectations and evaluations of obesity treatment outcomes. *J Consult Clin Psychol* 1997;65:79–85, with permission.)

ethnic groups (37,38). Data on Latino populations are needed. Thus, while the prevailing view in Western culture regards obesity as a social liability, ideals of beauty may vary across different cultures and ethnicities. Differences, however, among ethnicities may be largely attributable to differences in socioeconomic status (SES).

Social Consequences of Obesity

Unfortunately, social stigma translates into discrimination against obese individuals that may affect nearly every aspect of their lives. Socially, obese children are liked less, and they are rejected more often by their peers than are nonobese children (39). As adults, obese individuals, particularly women, have greater difficulties finding a partner, and they are less likely to marry (40,41).

Obesity also negatively affects employment, including selection, placement, compensation, promotion, discipline, and discharge (42). As early as 1976, Roe and Eickwort (43) found that 16% of employers reported that they would never hire obese individuals, and 44% said that they would hire obese individuals only under the rarest of circumstances. Similarly, other research has found that obese individuals, compared to nonobese individuals, are less likely to be employed and are more likely to earn lower salaries, to be of low SES, and to have decreases in SES over time (40,43–47). Reduced access to rental properties and housing has also been reported among obese persons (47,48).

Obesity also appears to compromise educational opportunities. Obese individuals are less likely to attain a high education level or to receive financial support from their parents for a college education (49,50). In one study, obese adolescent girls completed significantly fewer months of high school compared to their average-weight peers, despite equal intellectual functioning (40). Even in medical settings, obese individuals face limited access to health care, and they may receive biased diagnoses and treatment from both medical and mental health providers (47,51,52).

A number of possible explanations exist for the associations between obesity and these negative social outcomes. For example, decreased physical functioning—not social stigma—may be responsible for obese individuals' apparent limited access to employment and economic opportunities. However, the pervasiveness and magnitude of social stigma and the inequities experienced by obese individuals cannot be ignored. Clearly, social stigma has significant repercussions that limit an obese individual's access to many important and desirable societal and personal roles.

Less research has assessed the perception of discrimination among obese individuals themselves. However, Rand and MacGregor (29) asked 57 morbidly obese patients about their perceptions of discrimination. As Table 15.3 illustrates, 80% said that they felt that people talk behind their backs and hold a negative attitude toward them that is related to their weight. More than 65% felt that their weight had negatively affected their employment, and a similar percentage did not like to be seen in public.

In another study with a larger sample consisting of 445 members of the National Association to Advance Fat Acceptance, 98% of the respondents reported that they had experienced verbal harassment, criticism, or teasing from family or peers; 75% reported being teased at work; and 50% reported being teased or criticized by supervisors. In addition, 33% reported being called negative names by health professionals, and half of the sample felt they had been refused employment because of their size (53). The body mass index (BMI) of study participants was not reported.

Myers and Rosen (54) examined the frequency of stigmatizing situations in 112 patients with gastric bypass and in 34 less obese treatment-seeking controls. The most frequently reported situations were receiving hurtful comments from children, hearing other people make unflattering assumptions about obese persons, and encountering physical barriers (e.g., chairs that were too small). Patients reported that these occurred between "several times in my life" and "once per year."

The prevalence of discrimination has also been investigated in nonclinical samples. Falkner et al. (55) examined mistreatment because of weight in 187 men and 800 women in a population-based weight-gain–prevention program. Overall, 22% of women and 17% of men reported weight-related mistreatment. The most commonly reported sources of

TABLE 15.3. *Responses of morbidly obese patients to questions concerning their weight and psychosocial functioning*

	Always (%)	Usually (%)	Sometimes (%)	Never (%)
At work, people talk behind my back and have a negative attitude toward me related to my weight.	80.7	10.5	3.5	5.3
I feel that my weight has negatively affected whether I have been hired for a job.	67.3	20.4	10.2	2.2
I do not like to be seen in public.	66.7	17.5	14.0	1.8
I feel that I have been treated disrespectfully by the medical profession because of my weight.	45.5	32.7	16.4	2.2

From Rand CS, MacGregor AM. Successful weight loss following obesity surgery and the perceived liability of morbid obesity. *Int J Obes Relat Metab Disord* 1991;15:577–579; and Stunkard AJ, Wadden TA. Psychological aspects of severe obesity. *Am J Clin Nutr* 1992;55:524S–532S, with permission.

discrimination were from strangers (12.5% of women), from spouses (11.9% of women and 10.2% of men), and from friends (7.5% of men). Reported mistreatment was nearly ten times as prevalent among the heaviest individuals (BMI = 28.3 to 35.7 kilograms per meter squared [kg/m^2]) compared to that of the leanest individuals (BMI = 21.0 to 24.5 kg/m^2). Surprisingly, gender differences in the number of stigmatizing situations have not been consistently reported in the literature (54,55). Based on the available data, however, discrimination appears to be a fairly common experience in both treatment-seeking and non–treatment-seeking obese individuals.

PSYCHOLOGIC COMPLICATIONS

Psychologic Status of Obese Individuals in the General Population

In light of the negative social consequences of obesity, one would expect that over-weight and obese individuals experience adverse psychologic consequences as well. Population-based studies, however, in Europe and the United States prior to 1990 generally failed to find greater psychologic dysfunction in obese individuals compared to nonobese individuals (56–60). Similarly, obese individuals were not found to have a specific personality profile. However, a recent review of this literature concluded that making the assumption that obesity and psychologic distress are unrelated would be premature (61). The authors suggested that several methodologic flaws may have compromised earlier studies that found normal psychologic status in obese populations. Moreover, more recent European and United States studies, which have corrected for these shortcomings, have found slightly higher rates of depression and other complications in obese individuals (62–65). As Friedman and Brownell (61) have argued, the inconsistent effects likely reflect the heterogeneous nature of obesity. More long-term, controlled studies are needed to clarify the relationship between obesity and the risk of psychopathology in various subgroups of obese individuals within the general population.

Psychosocial Status of Obese Individuals Who Seek Treatment

Greater rates of psychologic distress, particularly depression, have been found in obese patients who seek weight loss treatment (61,66–68). For example, Berman et al. (69) reported that 50% of obese individuals presenting for treatment had a history of at least one axis I disorder (i.e., major depression and anxiety disorders) and that 55% had a history of at least one axis II disorder (i.e., personality disorders). Other research has found high rates of social avoidance, body image dissatisfaction, binge eating, and low self-esteem in obese treatment seekers (70,71).

The greater prevalence of psychologic distress in clinical populations might be expected, given that psychologic discomfort likely motivates patients to seek treatment (72). However, most obese patients in treatment settings will not have problems in psychologic functioning. As Friedman and Brownell (61) indicated, a wide range of prevalence rates of psychologic disturbance is found in obese treatment-seeking samples. Future research is needed to identify further the base rates of psychologic dysfunction among obese patients in different treatment settings.

Body Image Dissatisfaction

Body image is the perception of one's body size and appearance and the emotional response to this perception (73). An inaccurate perception of body size and/or negative emotional reactions to body size perceptions can result in varying degrees of body image dissatisfaction. Given the deviation of the average woman's weight and shape from cultural ideals, it is not surprising that dissatisfaction with weight and shape is common among women and girls, particularly those who are obese (74). In a study on the topic, Sarwer et al. (75) compared the body image of obese women to that of nonobese women and found that obese women were more likely to report moderate to extreme social embarrassment. In addition, compared to nonobese women, the obese women were more likely to camouflage their appearance with clothing, to change their posture or body movements, and to avoid looking at their body.

Body image dissatisfaction is not typically related to clinically significant anxiety or depression (75). However, a significant minority of obese patients suffer from extreme body image disparagement or disgust toward their bodies (76). These individuals are preoccupied with their physical appearance, and they often avoid social situations because of their appearance (77). Individuals with body image disparagement also tend to have comorbid emotional problems (73). Research has found a greater risk of body image disparagement in patients whose parents or peers teased them and/or in those with early onset obesity (73,74,78). As was noted earlier, African-American and Asian women tend to report less body image dissatisfaction than white women (32,38). Data on other ethnic populations are needed. In summary, many obese patients have body image dissatisfaction, but only few have severe body image disparagement.

Trauma

A few studies have reported higher rates of sexual abuse and other psychosocial trauma in obese patients compared to controls. For example, Felitti (79) reported that 25% of candidates who sought a medically supervised weight loss program reported a history of sexual abuse in childhood or adolescence, compared to a rate of 6% in average-weight controls. Greater prevalence rates of other traumatic events have also been reported. In this study (79), for example, approximately 50% of obese individuals in the sample had lost a parent in childhood or adolescence, compared to 23% for the controls; 40% had at least one alcoholic parent, compared to 17% of the controls; and 54% reported marital dysfunction compared to 16% of the controls. Physical and verbal abuse were also higher in obese individuals (29%) compared to that for controls (14%). Other correlational studies, however, have failed to find a consistent relationship between sexual abuse history and obesity (80,81). Additional research is needed to evaluate further the relationship between trauma and the development of obesity.

Level of Obesity

Most research has found significantly greater levels of distress in the severely obese individuals compared to that in less obese controls (72,82,83). For example, Wadden et al. (72) assessed depression and self-esteem in 22 severely obese (BMI = 52.4 kg/m^2) women seeking bariatric surgery and 40 less obese (BMI = 36.0 kg/m^2) women seeking pharmacologic treatment of obesity. Significantly greater levels of depression and lower self-esteem were reported in the very obese compared to the less obese individuals. Similarly, a large-scale (number of subjects [n] = 974) study of obese patients found markedly lower quality of life, as well as greater anxiety, depression, and social dysfunction, with increasing level of obesity (64). Other research has found that severely obese subjects report more stigmatizing situations than less obese patients (54). However, whether greater discrimination leads to greater psychologic burden in severely obese patients is unknown, as the next section notes.

Social Factors and Psychologic Distress

The relationship between psychologic distress and prejudice and discrimination among obese treatment seekers is an understudied topic. The authors know of only one study (54) that reported a significant relationship between the number of stigmatizing situations and mental health symptoms (correlation coefficient (r) = 0.31), negative body image (r = 0.30), and more negative self-esteem (r = −0.21), even after controlling for weight and coping style. Although this study suggested that stigmatization may lead to less optimal psychologic adjustment, the cross-sectional design of this study limits its conclusions. Additional studies are needed to examine further the relationship between stigmatization and mental health in obese patients.

QUALITY OF LIFE

The preceding review has shown that a significant minority of obese individuals who seek weight reduction may experience significant psychologic complications. More obese persons, however, are likely to experience decreased quality of life, primarily because of impairments in physical functioning. For example, a recent epidemiologic study of 5,887 men and 7,018 women from the Netherlands found that, compared to individuals with a BMI of less than or equal to 25 kg/m^2, those with a BMI of more than or equal to 30 kg/m^2 were three times more likely to have shortness of breath while walking upstairs and were twice as likely to have difficulties in performing a range of basic activities of daily living, including carrying groceries, bending, kneeling, bathing, or dressing (84). In addition, women with higher BMIs reported more problems associated with low-back pain, including more absences from work and greater limits in their activities of daily living. Similar limitations in physical functioning have been found in other studies of obese individuals (83,85–87).

Some investigators have also discovered reduced psychosocial quality of life in obese patients. Marchesini et al. (83) examined 183 obese individuals who sought standard weight loss treatment at a university setting. As might be expected, these obese individuals reported significantly greater impairments in physical functioning, compared to the population norms. However, in addition, the obese patients reported significant impairments in vitality, mental health, and social functioning. Additional analyses showed that binge eating explained most of the relationship between obesity and mental status. Thus, although most impairment in the quality of life is due to decreased physical functioning, some obese patients, particularly those with binge-eating problems, may also experience a reduced psychologic quality of life.

EATING DISORDERS

Few obese patients who seek treatment will initially have an eating disorder, which is often associated with depression or other psychologic dysfunction. The most common eating disorder in obese individuals is binge-eating disorder (BED). However, practitioners may occasionally encounter bulimia nervosa and night eating problems.

Binge-Eating Disorder

BED is characterized by the consumption of large amounts of food in a discrete period with a subjective loss of control over eating. The overeating is not followed by compensatory behaviors (e.g., vomiting, fasting, or laxative abuse). Marked distress must occur

TABLE 15.4. *Diagnostic criteria for binge-eating disorder*

A. Recurrent episodes of binge eating. An episode of binge eating is characterized by both of the following:
  1. Eating in a discrete period (e.g., within any 2-hr period) an amount of food that is definitely larger than most people would eat in a similar period under similar circumstances.
  2. A sense of lack of control over eating during the episode (e.g., a feeling that one cannot stop eating or that one cannot control what or how much one is eating).
B. The binge-eating episodes are associated with three (or more) of the following:
  1. Eating much more rapidly than normal.
  2. Eating until feeling uncomfortably full.
  3. Eating large amounts of food when not feeling physically hungry.
  4. Eating alone because of feeling embarrassed by how much one is eating.
  5. Feeling disgusted with oneself, depressed, or very guilty after overeating.
C. Marked distress regarding binge eating is present.
D. The binge eating occurs, on average, at least 2 d/wk for 6 mo.
E. The binge eating is not associated with regular performance of inappropriate compensatory behaviors (e.g., purging, fasting, excessive exercise), and it does not occur exclusively during the course of anorexia nervosa or bulimia nervosa.

From American Psychiatric Association. *Diagnostic and statistical manual of mental disorders,* 4th ed. Washington, D.C.: American Psychiatric Association, 1994, with permission.

in at least of the three areas detailed in Table 15.4 (88). Compared to nonbingers, obese individuals with BED tend to be heavier and younger, and they have increased rates of psychosocial dysfunction, including depression, low self-esteem, and body image dissatisfaction (89–92). Binge eaters are also more likely to have been teased by family members about their weight, shape, or eating (93).

Currently, BED is classified in the *Diagnostic and Statistical Manual of Mental Disorders,* 4th edition (DSM-IV) as an example of an "eating disorder not otherwise specified." Further research is needed to characterize BED before it can be considered a *bona fide* psychiatric disorder. The prevalence of BED is about 2% in community samples and is approximately 10% to 20% in obese treatment seekers (94). The wide range of prevalence estimates in treatment-seeking populations appears to be attributable to differences in assessment methods. Self-report questionnaires yield estimates of 30% to 50% (89,95). However, assessments based on structured interviews yield lower prevalence rates of approximately 10% to 15% (96,97). As identification of BED is best obtained through a clinical interview, prevalence rates of BED in treatment-seeking samples are probably less than 20% (97,98).

Other Eating Disorders

Few obese patients will have symptoms of bulimia nervosa. People with this disorder consume large amounts of food in a short period of time and report feelings of loss of control over eating, similar to symptoms found in patients with BED. However, patients with bulimia nervosa also engage in inappropriate compensatory behaviors, such as self-induced vomiting; fasting; excessive exercise; and/or use of laxatives, diuretics, or enemas (Table 15.5). Bulimia nervosa is thought to occur in 1% to 2% of women in the general population, and it is an extremely rare, but noteworthy, occurrence in obese treatment seekers.

Night Eating Syndrome

The night eating syndrome is not currently recognized by the DSM-IV. It was first described in 1955 by Stunkard et al. (99), who recently reexamined the condition (100).

TABLE 15.5. *Diagnostic criteria for bulimia nervosa*

A. Recurrent episodes of binge eating. An episode of binge eating is characterized by both of the following:
   1. Eating in a discrete period (e.g., within any 2-hr period) an amount of food that is definitely larger than most people would eat in a similar period of time under similar circumstances.
   2. A sense of lack of control over eating during the episode (e.g., a feeling that one cannot stop eating or control what or how much one is eating).
B. Recurrent inappropriate compensatory behavior to prevent weight gain, such as self-induced vomiting; misuse of laxatives, diuretics, enemas, or other medications; fasting; or excessive exercise.
C. The binge eating and inappropriate compensatory behaviors both occur, on average, at least twice a wk for 3 mo.
D. Self-evaluation is unduly influenced by body shape and weight.
E. The disturbance does not occur exclusively during episodes of anorexia nervosa.

From American Psychiatric Association. *Diagnostic and statistical manual of mental disorders,* 4th ed. Washington, D.C.: American Psychiatric Association, 1994, with permission.

Night eating is characterized by the consumption of approximately 50% of the daily total caloric intake after the evening meal. Night eaters frequently snack late into the night, and they report difficulties falling or remaining asleep. Nighttime awakenings are often accompanied by further snacking. Many patients with night eating also experience increasing depression throughout the evening and night (101). This cluster of disturbances in sleep, eating, and mood was further supported by a neuroendocrine study that found significantly lower melatonin and leptin levels and increased cortisol in night eaters compared to those of controls (100). Little research has assessed the prevalence of night eating syndrome, but estimates range from 9% to 27% of obese patients seeking weight loss treatment and 1.5% of community samples (102,103). Additional research is necessary to define and to assess further the prevalence of night eating syndrome in obese individuals.

BEHAVIORAL COMPLICATIONS OF DIETING AND WEIGHT LOSS

Dieting is the principal treatment for obesity. It involves the intentional restriction of caloric intake to induce a negative energy balance, with resulting weight loss. Some investigators have expressed concern that dieting may precipitate eating disorders, depression, and other adverse consequences. These concerns are briefly reviewed below.

Dieting and the Development of Binge Eating

The relationship between dieting and the development of eating disorders has received considerable attention in the literature. Rigid dietary restraint, coupled with a feeling of deprivation, is thought to leave the dieter emotionally vulnerable to a loss of control of eating. A minor dietary lapse, whether perceived or actual, may be interpreted by the dieter as a complete inability to maintain control and thus may lead to the total abandonment of all attempts to control food intake, with resulting binge eating. After episodes of binge eating, even stricter dieting standards are pursued and the dieting–binge eating cycle is perpetuated (104).

Aggressive dieting almost invariably precedes the development of eating disorders in normal-weight individuals (105). However, dieting alone is not considered a sufficient cause of eating disorders (106). Indeed, dieting is a common experience in the United States, with approximately 29% of men and 44% of women reporting that they are trying to lose weight at any given time (107). However, the prevalence of eating disorders is estimated at only 1% to 4% in young adult women (108). Likely, a combination of both biologic and psychosocial vulnerabilities interact with dieting to produce eating disorders in normal-weight populations.

The relationship between dieting and the development of binge eating in the obese is more complex. Wilson et al. (109) found that approximately 66% of obese binge eaters reported that the onset of binge eating occurred *before* their obesity. Similarly, Spitzer et al. (95) found that 49% of subjects with binge-eating problems reported that the onset of their binge eating preceded dieting, 14% reported that binge eating and dieting occurred at the same age, and only 37% reported that binge eating followed dieting. These are retrospective studies, however, so they must be interpreted with caution.

Prospective studies of obese adults in traditional weight loss programs have similarly found little evidence to indicate that dieting results in binge eating. In fact, most data suggest that such treatment improves binge eating in obese patients. For example, Wadden et al. (110) found that the symptoms of binge eating declined by about 40% in patients undergoing moderate caloric restriction (1,200 kcal per day) and by 27% in those who consumed a very low calorie diet (VLCD) (420 kcal per day). In addition, in a summary of data from six prospective trials evaluating binge eating in patients losing weight, the National Task Force found that most subjects were unlikely to develop binge eating and that, in fact, they experienced significant improvements in binge eating with weight loss (111). The task force concluded that "concerns that dieting induces eating disorders or other psychological dysfunction in overweight and obese adults are generally not supported by empirical studies" (111).

Thus, among normal-weight individuals with preexisting biopsychosocial vulnerabilities, dieting may trigger eating-disorder problems. However, in obese individuals, dieting does not appear to exacerbate binge eating, and it may in fact improve binge-eating symptomatology.

Psychosocial Consequences of Weight Loss And Dieting

Mood

Reports over the past 25 years suggest positive changes or, at a minimum, no change in depression and/or anxiety in obese patients undergoing various treatment modalities, including moderate calorie restriction, severe calorie restriction, the use of weight loss medications, or bariatric surgery (70,111–115). For example, Wadden et al. (110) examined the effects of a VLCD and a balanced deficit diet in 49 obese women who underwent 26 weeks of behavioral treatment and who were assessed 1 year later. As Fig. 15.3 illustrates, mood improved significantly in both groups during 26 weeks of treatment. After treatment, mood remained stable in the balanced deficit diet group, and it began to deteriorate somewhat in the VLCD group as patients began to regain weight.

Similarly, Wing et al. (116) reviewed ten studies of changes in mood during behavioral weight loss programs. The authors found no evidence of worsening of mood with weight loss. In fact, improvements in mood occurred even in subjects who lost little or no weight.

These results contrast with those of earlier studies that showed negative psychologic effects of dieting. Specifically, Stunkard and Rush (67) reviewed seven studies published between 1951 and 1973 and found that all studies showed negative psychologic effects of dieting. As others have noted, the difference between the earlier and later studies is likely a function of changes in both treatment content and study methodology (116). The more recent studies incorporated cognitive-behavioral strategies and exercise into treatment, which likely contributed to the observed improvements in mood. Additionally, the more

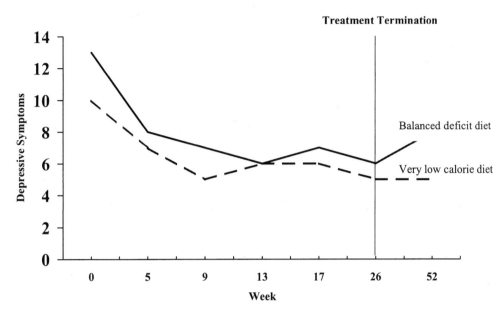

FIG. 15.3. Depressive symptoms over 52 weeks for subjects undergoing behavioral treatment with a balanced-deficit diet or very low calorie diet prescription. (Data from Wadden TA, Foster GD, Letizia KA. One-year behavioral treatment of obesity: comparison of moderate and severe caloric restrictions and the effects of weight maintenance therapy. *J Consult Clin Psychol* 1994;62:165–171, with permission.)

recent studies assessed mood prospectively, providing a more precise measure of changes during treatment. Thus, practitioners can expect obese individuals to experience, at a minimum, no adverse changes in mood as a result of participation in standard behavioral treatment programs.

Social Relationships

Surprisingly, little research has investigated the impact of weight loss on social relationships. Available data are based largely on the outcomes of patients after surgery. This literature suggests that weight loss is associated with marked improvements in social interactions, including less perceived difficulty going to restaurants and community activities, shopping for clothes, or being seen in a bathing suit, as well as increased satisfaction in personal relationships (114). Although other data have indicated that patients who have underwent surgery for their obesity may leave unsatisfactory marriages after weight loss, this may ultimately be a positive change; such patients have reported improvements in mood and psychosocial functioning (117,118). Future research is needed to assess more fully the relationship between weight loss and social functioning in patients undergoing more moderate weight loss programs.

Sexuality

For most obese individuals, sexual relationships improve with weight loss (119). Studies of patients in hospital-based weight loss programs and of those who have undergone bariatric surgery have shown increases in both the frequency of and the satisfaction with sexual relations after weight loss (120,121). However, some obese patients may experience discomfort with regard to sexuality after weight loss. Specifically, patients with a history of childhood sexual abuse appear to experience increased anxiety with weight loss; they may also lose less weight than persons without a history of sexual abuse (79,122,123).

Body Image

Significant improvements in body image have been reported in several studies of patients undergoing cognitive-behavioral treatment or surgical treatment for obesity (74,124,125). However, weight loss is not necessarily correlated with improvements in body image (124,126). In fact, improvements in body image may be obtained in the absence of weight loss. Thus, cognitive-behavioral treatment, not weight loss, may be responsible for the improvements in body image. Treatment response may vary depending on the patient's age at the onset of obesity. Specifically, patients with an early onset of obesity tend to remain dissatisfied with their body image despite achieving and maintaining a normal weight (74).

Binge Eating

As was discussed earlier, dieting and weight loss do not appear to exacerbate problem eating in obese binge eaters. In fact, weight loss may decrease binge-eating episodes and the associated psychologic complication (127). Although some research has found higher attrition rates, lower weight loss, and a greater risk of weight regain among binge eaters, most studies have found weak effects or no effects of binge eating on weight loss and attendance (72,89,127–130).

Quality of Life

Available data indicate that patients experience significant improvements in quality of life after weight loss. In particular, improvements in physical functioning have been observed (114,131). Enhanced psychosocial quality of life has also been reported. Specifically, improvements in well-being, pain, and fatigue after weight loss have been observed, which may contribute to the overall improved psychosocial status observed in patients who lose weight (72,114,115).

Magnitude of Weight Loss and Psychosocial Improvement

Whether greater weight loss leads to a greater improvement in psychosocial status remains unclear. In patients who have had surgery for their obesity, Karlsson et al. (114) reported significant correlations ($r = 0.11$ to 0.30) between 1-year weight losses and improvements in perceived health, degree of comfort in social settings, and mental well-being (e.g., overall mood, anxiety, and depression). In addition, quality of life continued to be significantly more positive in patients with greater (i.e., ≥20 kg) weight losses at 2 years.

However, research in patients undergoing behavioral interventions has shown that greater weight losses are not clearly related to greater improvements in mood or other psychosocial variables. For example, Jeffery et al. (132) found no relationship between improvements in psychologic well-being and weight losses in participants undergoing 18 months of behavior therapy and a 30-month follow-up visit. Similarly, research in patients undergoing 17 weeks of behavioral treatment with a VLCD found that improved psychologic status was not significantly correlated with weight loss over the course of the 2-year study (133).

In randomized trials, greater psychosocial improvements are often observed in interventions producing greater magnitudes of weight loss (110,114,134). For example, Karlsson et al. (114) reported that improvements in patients who underwent surgery for their obesity (average weight loss of 28 kg) were significantly greater than those observed in conventionally treated controls (average weight loss of 1 kg) 2 years after treatment. However, such data do not explain whether the greater improvements in psychosocial functioning are due to greater weight losses or to other variables, such as treatment modality (e.g., exercise versus VLCD). In addition, heavier patients (i.e., those who underwent surgery) may experience greater psychosocial burdens related to obesity and may thus have a higher probability of improvement, compared to leaner patients who lose weight.

The mixed findings in the literature may also be a function of differences in assessment method. Psychosocial functioning is a complex construct that includes several variables, such as mood, body image, intimate relationships, and work functioning. Different measurement tools or aspects of the construct could yield different findings in relation to weight loss. Clearly, additional empiric studies are needed to provide further understanding of the relationship between the degree of weight loss and the corresponding psychosocial improvements. Nonetheless, significant improvements in psychosocial status occur with only modest weight losses (i.e., 5% to 10%), which may be more sustainable than larger weight losses.

Psychosocial Consequences of Weight Regain

Most obese patients who lose weight will regain it within 5 years. The psychologic ramifications of this have been investigated in a number of studies. Most research suggests that the initial improvements in mood and body image that occur with weight loss deteriorate as patients regain the lost weight. Patients, however, do not become more depressed than they were at baseline, even with full weight regain (111,114,115,135). In addition, some research has found that psychosocial improvements can be maintained despite subsequent weight regain (136). Thus, individuals who regain lost weight apparently will experience improvements or, at a minimum, will be no worse psychologically than they were before they lost weight. However, most patients are frustrated and disappointed when they regain lost weight, even if they do not display clinically significant distress.

Psychosocial Consequences of Weight Cycling

The psychosocial effects of repeated weight loss and regain (i.e., weight cycling) have also been investigated. Two recent reviews concluded that weight cycling does not appear to be associated with clinically significant increases in psychosocial dysfunction (111,137). Both reviews cite several studies that found no relationship between weight cycling and increased psychopathology, depression, or psychologic distress. However, decreases in general mental and physical well-being, as well as body image, were noted in a few studies (111). In addition, binge eating is consistently related to cycles of weight loss and regain. Whether binge eating is a cause or a consequence of these repeated weight loss attempts is unclear, however. Additional prospective studies are needed to delineate further the relationship among weight cycling, reduced quality of life, and binge-eating severity.

FUTURE DIRECTIONS

Stigmatization of obesity is pervasive in Western society, and it appears to limit significantly an obese individual's access to a wide variety of social and vocational opportunities. Although most obese individuals in the general population do not have psychologic complications, a significant minority of those who seek weight reduction will suffer from depression, binge eating, and related problems. These adverse psychologic effects may be due, in part, to internalized stigmatization.

A significant challenge facing practitioners, researchers, and the public at large is the identification of methods to decrease stigmatization of the obese. The law offers an important avenue, as it did in ameliorating racial discrimination in this country. Some states and municipalities have passed laws against weight-based discrimination (e.g., Michigan; Washington, D.C.; Santa Cruz, California; and San Francisco), an example that the authors wish would be followed by the federal government. Very little discrimination against the obese appears to violate federal law (42). The 1990 Americans with Disabilities Act may protect some individuals from discrimination, but this approach has been successfully used in only a few instances (40).

Another approach to reducing stigmatization is increased understanding of its causes. As has been noted previously, many people believe that obesity is attributable to moral shortcomings. Education may help the public realize that obesity has a strong genetic component in some individuals and that all Americans are at risk of becoming overweight because of the nation's fat-inducing lifestyle. On a promising note, research in medical students has found that stigmatization can be decreased through education that increases knowledge, sensitivity, and empathy (138). Research in methods to facilitate this in other populations is needed.

Another approach is to find ways to help obese individuals cope with stigmatization. Generally, people believe that the best way to reduce unwanted negative attention is to lose weight. However, weight loss is rarely maintained. In light of this dilemma, several educational and psychotherapeutic approaches have been designed specifically to help obese individuals cope with stigmatization (47). These include education in identifying and reacting to stigmas in ways that minimize the negative effect (22,139). In addition, antidieting and size acceptance movements that reject the societal emphasis on thinness and that promote healthy eating habits without a focus on weight have emerged (22). The limited research available on antidieting approaches suggests that they improve self-esteem, mood, and eating behavior at a rate similar to that found in standard weight loss programs, but they fail to induce clinically significant short- or long-term weight losses (111). Thus, although appealing from the standpoint of improving self-esteem, nondieting approaches are unlikely to provide improvements in medical complications associated with obesity.

Finally, efforts to design weight control interventions will benefit from assessing the fit between weight loss programs and the various subtypes of obese patients. For instance, patients with clinically significant antifat attitudes may benefit most from treatments aimed at ameliorating such internalized stigmas. Similarly, patients with body image disparagement may benefit from treatment specifically targeting body image problems. A detailed review of psychosocial measures can be found in other com-

TABLE 15.6. *Instruments to assess psychosocial factors of obesity*

Instrument	Source
Social factors	
Attitudes toward obese persons scale	Allison et al., 1991 (148)
Beliefs about obese persons scale	Allison et al., 1991 (148)
Fat phobia scale	Robinson et al., 1993 (139)
Anti-fat attitudes scale	Crandall and Biernat, 1990 (149)
Quality of life	
Short-form general health survey (SF-36)	Ware and Sherbourne, 1992 (142)
Eating behavior	
Eating disorders inventory	Stunkard and Messick, 1985 (143)
Mood	
Beck depression inventory-II	Beck et al., 1996 (144)
Binge eating	
Questionnaire on eating and weight patterns-R	Spitzer et al., 1992 (94)
Body image	
Overweight preoccupation scale (four items selected from the Body self-relations questionnaire of Brown et al., 1990 [146])	Cash et al., 1991 (145)

prehensive texts, but a sample of easily administered instruments is provided in Table 15.6 (140).

Practitioners should continue to evaluate overweight individuals' need for weight reduction. Extending the range of possible treatment goals to include psychosocial outcomes may further enhance practitioners' care of their overweight and obese patients.

REFERENCES

1. Massara EB, Stunkard AJ. A method of quantifying cultural ideals of beauty and the obese. *Int J Obes* 1979;3:149–152.
2. Brown PJ. Cultural perspectives on the etiology and treatment of obesity. In: Stunkard AJ, Wadden TA, eds. *Obesity: theory and therapy.* New York: Raven Press, 1993:73–77.
3. Silverstein B, Peterson B, Perdue L. Some correlates of the thin standard of bodily attractiveness for women. *Int J Eat Disord* 1986;5:895–905.
4. Harris MB, Harris RJ. Fat, four-eyed and female: stereotypes of obesity, glasses, and gender. *J Appl Soc Psychol* 1982;12:503–516.
5. Brownell KD. Personal responsibility and control over our bodies: when expectation exceeds reality. *Health Psychol* 1991;10:303–310.
6. Wadden TA, Brown G, Foster GD, et al. Salience of weight-related worries in adolescent males and females. *Int J Eat Disord* 1991;10:407–414.
7. Field AE, Cheung L, Wolf AM, et al. Exposure to mass media and weight concerns among girls. *Pediatrics* 1999;103:E36.
8. Turner SL, Hamilton H, Jacobs M, et al. The influence of fashion magazines on the body image satisfaction of college women: an exploratory analysis. *Adolescence* 1997;32:603–614.
9. Stice E, Schupak-Neuberg E, Shaw HE, et al. Relation of media exposure to eating disorder symptomatology: an examination of mediating mechanisms. *J Abnorm Psychol* 1994;103:836–840.
10. Pinhas L, Toner BB, Garfinkel PE, et al. The effects of the ideal of female beauty on mood and body satisfaction. *Int J Eat Disord* 1999;25:223–226.
11. Crocker J, Cornwall B, Major B. The stigma of overweight: affective consequences of attributional ambiguity. *J Pers Soc Psychol* 1993;64:60–70.
12. Rodin J, Silberstein LR, Striegel-Moore R. Women and weight: a normative discontent. *Nebr Symp Motiv* 1984;32:267–307.
13. Pliner P, Chaikern S, Flett GL. Gender differences in concern with body weight and physical appearance over the lifespan. *Pers Soc Psychol Bull* 1990;16:262–273.
14. Allon N. The stigma of overweight in everyday life. In: Bray GA, ed. *Obesity in perspective.* Washington, D.C.: United States Government Printing Office, 1973:83–102.
15. Crandall CS. Prejudice against fat people: ideology and self-interest. *J Pers Soc Psychol* 1994;66:882–894.
16. Cramer P, Steinwert T. Thin is good, fat is bad: how early does it begin? *J Appl Dev Psychol* 1998;19:429–451.

17. Staffieri JR. A study of social stereotype of body image in children. *J Pers Soc Psychol* 1967;7:101–104.
18. Goodman N, Dornbusch SM, Richradson SA, et al. Variant reactions to physical disabilities. *Am Sociol Rev* 1963;28:429–435.
19. Maddox GL, Back K, Liederman V. Overweight as social deviance and disability. *J Health Soc Behav* 1968;9: 287–298.
20. Richardson SA, Goodman N, Hastorf AH, et al. Cultural uniformity in reaction to physical disabilities. *Am Sociol Rev* 1961;26:241–247.
21. Venes AM, Krupka LR, Gerard RJ. Overweight/obese patients: an overview. *Practitioner* 1982;226:1102–1109.
22. Sobal J, Devine CM. Social aspects of obesity: influences, consequences, assessments, and interventions. In: Dalton S, ed. *Overweight and weight management: the health professional's guide to understanding and practice.* Gaithersburg, MD: Aspen, 1997:313–331.
23. Hoppe R, Ogden J. Practice nurses' beliefs about obesity and weight related interventions in primary care. *Int J Obes Relat Metab Disord* 1997;21:141–146.
24. Maroney D, Golub S. Nurses' attitudes toward obese persons and certain ethnic groups. *Percept Mot Skills* 1992;75:387–391.
25. Brotman AW, Stern TA, Herzog DB. Emotional reactions of house officers to patients with anorexia nervosa, diabetes, and obesity. *Int J Eat Disord* 1984;3:71–77.
26. Blumberg P, Mellis LP. Medical students' attitudes toward the obese and the morbidly obese. *Int J Eat Disord* 1985;4:169–175.
27. Maisman LA, Wang VL, Becker MH, et al. Attitudes toward obesity and the obese among professionals. *J Am Diet Assoc* 1979;74:331–336.
28. Price JH, Desmond SM, Krol RA, et al. Family practice physicians' beliefs, attitudes and practices regarding obesity. *Am J Prev Med* 1987;3:215–220.
29. Rand CS, MacGregor AM. Successful weight loss following obesity surgery and the perceived liability of morbid obesity. *Int J Obes* 1991;15:577–579.
30. Foster GD, Wadden TA, Vogt RA, et al. What is a reasonable weight loss? Patients' expectations and evaluations of obesity treatment outcomes. *J Consult Clin Psychol* 1997;65:79–85.
31. Foster G, Wadden TA, Phelan S, et al. Obese patients' perceptions of treatment outcomes and the factors that influence them. *Arch Intern Med* 2001;161:2133–2139.
32. Rosen J, Gross J. Prevalence of weight reducing and weight gaining in adolescent girls and boys. *Health Psychol* 1987;6:131–147.
33. Kumanyika S, Wilson JF, Guilford-Davenport M. Weight-related attitudes and behaviors of black women. *J Am Diet Assoc* 1993;93:416–422.
34. Striegel-Moore R, Schreiber G, Pike KM, et al. Drive for thinness in black and white preadolescent girls. *Int J Eat Disord* 1995;18:59–69.
35. Stevens J, Kumanyika SK, Keil JE. Attitudes toward body size and dieting: differences between black and white clinic patients with NIDDM. *Am J Public Health* 1994;84:1322–1325.
36. Rucker CE, Cash TF. Body image, body-size perceptions, and eating behaviors among African-American and white college women. *Int J Eat Disord* 1992;12:291–299.
37. Bush HM, Williams RG, Lean ME, et al. Body image and weight consciousness among South Asian, Italian and general population women in Britain. *Appetite* 2001;37:207–215.
38. Cachelin FM, Rebeck RM, Chung GH, et al. Does ethnicity influence body-size preference? A comparison of body image and body size. *Obes Res* 2002;10:158–166.
39. Strauss CC, Smith K, Frame C, et al. Personal and interpersonal characteristics associated with childhood obesity. *J Pediatr Psychol* 1985;10:337–343.
40. Gortmaker SL, Must A, Perrin JM, et al. Social and economic consequences of overweight in adolescence and young adulthood. *N Engl J Med* 1993;329:1008–1012.
41. Sobal J, Nicolopoulos V, Lee J. Attitudes about overweight and dating among secondary school students. *Int J Obes* 1995;19:376–381.
42. Roehling MV. Weight-based discrimination in employment. Psychological and legal aspects. *Personnel Psychology* 1999;52:969–1016.
43. Roe DA, Eickwort K. Relationships between obesity and associated health factors with unemployment among low income women. *J Am Med Womens Assoc* 1976;31:193–204.
44. Sobal J, Rauschenbach B, Frongillo E. Marital status, fatness, and obesity. *Soc Sci Med* 1992;35:915–923.
45. Puhl R, Brownell KD. Bias, discrimination, and obesity. *Obes Res* 2001;9:788–805.
46. Sobal J, Stunkard AJ. Socioeconomic status and obesity: a review of the literature. *Psychol Bull* 1989;105: 260–275.
47. Sobal J. Obesity and nutritional sociology: A model for coping with the stigma of obesity. *Clin Sociol Rev* 1991; 9:125–141.
48. Karris L. Prejudice against obese renters. *J Soc Psychol* 1977;1:159–160.
49. Canning H, Mayer J. Obesity: its possible effects on college admissions. *N Engl J Med* 1966;275:1172–1174.
50. Crandall CS. Do parents discriminate against their heavy-weight daughters? *Pers Soc Psychol Bull* 1995;21: 724–735.
51. Adams CH, Smith NJ, Wilbur DC, et al. The relationship of obesity to the frequency of pelvic examinations: do physician and patient attitudes make a difference? *Women Health* 1993;20:45–57.

52. Young LM, Powell B. The effects of obesity on the clinical judgments of mental health professionals. *J Health Soc Behav* 1985;26:233–246.
53. Rothblum ED, Brand PA, Miller C, et al. Results of the NAAFA survey on employment discrimination: part II. *NAAFA Newsletter* 1989;17:4–6.
54. Myers A, Rosen JC. Obesity stigmatization and coping: relation to mental health symptoms, body image, and self-esteem. *Int J Obes Relat Metab Disord* 1999;23:221–230.
55. Falkner NH, French SA, Jeffery RW, et al. Mistreatment due to weight: prevalence and sources of perceived mistreatment in women and men. *Obes Res* 1999;7:572–576.
56. Crisp AH. Jolly fat: relation between obesity and psychoneurosis in the general population. *BMJ* 1976;3:7–9.
57. Silverstone JT. Psychosocial aspects of obesity. *Proc R Soc Med* 1968;61:371–375.
58. Hallstrom T, Noppa H. Obesity in women in relation to mental illness, social factors, and personality traits. *J Psychosom Res* 1981;25:75–82.
59. Wadden TA, Stunkard AJ. Psychosocial consequences of obesity and dieting: research and clinical findings. In: Stunkard AJ, Wadden TA, eds. *Obesity: theory and therapy.* New York: Raven Press, 1993:163–179.
60. Wadden TA, Stunkard AJ. Psychopathology and obesity. *Ann N Y Acad Sci* 1987;499:55–65.
61. Friedman MA, Brownell KD. Psychological correlates of obesity: moving to the next research generation. *Psychol Bull* 1995;117:3–20.
62. Lapidus L, Bengtsson C, Hallstrom T, et al. Obesity, adipose tissue distribution and health in women: results from a population study in Gothenburg, Sweden. *Appetite* 1989;12:25–35.
63. Carpenter KM, Hasin DS, Allison DB, et al. Relationships between obesity and *DSM-IV* major depressive disorder, suicide ideation, and suicide attempts: results from a general population study. *Am J Public Health* 2000; 90:251–257.
64. Sullivan M, Karlsson J, Sjostrom L, et al. Swedish Obese Subjects (SOS)—an intervention study of obesity. Baseline evaluation of health and psychosocial functioning in the first 1743 subjects examined. *Int J Obes Relat Metab Disord* 1993;17:503–512.
65. Lissau I, Sorensen TI. Parental neglect during childhood and increased risk of obesity in young adulthood. *Lancet* 1994;343:324–327.
66. Fitzgibbon ML, Stolley MR, Kirschenbaum DS. Obese people who seek treatment have different characteristics than those who do not seek treatment. *Health Psychol* 1993;12:342–345.
67. Stunkard AJ, Rush A. Dieting and depression reexamined: a critical review of untoward responses during weight reduction for obesity. *Ann Intern Med* 1974;81:526–533.
68. Prather RC, Williamson DA. Psychopathology associated with bulimia, binge eating, and obesity. *Int J Eat Disord* 1988;7:177–184.
69. Berman WH, Berman ER, Heymsfield S, et al. The incidence and comorbidity of psychiatric disorders in obesity. *J Pers Disord* 1992;6:168–175.
70. Solow C, Silberfarb PM, Swift K. Psychological effects of intestinal bypass surgery for severe obesity. *N Engl J Med* 1974;290:300–303.
71. Kolotkin RL, Head S, Hamilton M, et al. Assessing the impact of weight on quality of life. *Obes Res* 1995;3:49–56.
72. Wadden TA, Sarwer DB, Arnold MA, et al. Psychosocial status of severely obese patients before and after bariatric surgery. *Probl Gen Surg* 2000;17:13–22.
73. Cash TF, Hicks KL. Being fat versus thinking fat: relationships with body image, eating behaviors, and well-being. *Cogn Ther Res* 1990;14:327–341.
74. Adami GF, Gandolfo P, Campostano A, et al. Body image and body weight in obese patients. *Int J Eat Disord* 1998;24:299–306.
75. Sarwer DB, Wadden TA, Foster GD. Assessment of body image dissatisfaction in obese women: specificity, severity, and clinical significance. *J Consult Clin Psychol* 1998;66:651–654.
76. Stunkard AJ, Mendelson M. Obesity and the body image: characteristics of disturbances in the body image of some obese persons. *Am J Psychiatry* 1967;123:1296–1300.
77. Tiggermann M, Rothblum ED. Gender differences in social consequences of perceived overweight in the United States and Australia. *Sex Roles* 1988;18:75–86.
78. Grilo CM, Wilfley D, Brownell KD, et al. Teasing, body image, and self-esteem in a clinical sample of obese women. *Addict Behav* 1994;19:443–450.
79. Felitti VJ. Childhood sexual abuse, depression, and family dysfunction in obese persons. *South Med J* 1993;86: 732–736.
80. Sansone RA, Sansone LA, Fine MA. The relationship of obesity to borderline personality symptomatology, self-harm behaviors, and sexual abuse in female subjects in a primary-care medical setting. *J Pers Disord* 1995; 9:254–265.
81. Wiederman MW, Sansone RA, Sansone LA. Obesity among sexually abused women: an adaptive function for some? *Women Health* 1999;29:29–100.
82. Black DW, Goldstein RB, Mason EE. Prevalence of mental disorder in 88 morbidly obese bariatric clinic patients. *Am J Psychiatry* 1992;149:227–234.
83. Marchesini G, Solaroli E, Baraldi L, et al. Health-related quality of life in obesity: the role of eating behavior. *Diabetes Nutr Metab* 2000;13:156–164.
84. Lean ME, Han TS, Seidell JC. Impairment of health and quality of life using new US federal guidelines for the identification of obesity. *Arch Intern Med* 1999;159:837–843.

85. Stewart AL, Brook RH. Effects of being overweight. *Am J Public Health* 1983;73:171–178.
86. Han TS, Tijhuis MA, Lean ME, et al. Quality of life in relation to overweight and body fat distribution. *Am J Public Health* 1998;88:1814–1820.
87. Launer LJ, Harris T, Rumpel C, et al. Body mass index, weight change, and risk of mobility disability in middle-aged and older women: the epidemiologic follow-up study of NHANES I. *JAMA* 1994;27:1093–1098.
88. American Psychiatric Association. *Diagnostic and statistical manual of mental disorders,* 4th ed. Washington, D.C.: American Psychiatric Association, 1994.
89. Marcus MD, Wing RR, Hopkins J. Obese binge eaters: affect, cognitions, and response to behavioral weight control. *J Consult Clin Psychol* 1988;56:433–439.
90. Marcus MD, Wing RR, Lamparski DM. Binge eating and dietary restraint in obese patients. *Addict Behav* 1985; 10:163–168.
91. Grilo CM, Wilfley DW, Brownell KD, et al. The social self, body dissatisfaction, and binge eating in obese females. *Obes Res* 1994;2:24–27.
92. Cargill BR, Clark MM, Pera V, et al. Binge eating, body image, depression, and self-efficacy in an obese clinical population. *Obes Res* 1999;7:379–386.
93. Fairburn CG, Doll HA, Welch SL, et al. Risk factors for binge eating disorder: a community-based, case-control study. *Arch Gen Psychiatry* 1998;55:425–432.
94. Spitzer RL, Devlin M, Walsh TB, et al. Binge eating disorder: a multisite field trial of the diagnostic criteria. *Int J Eat Disord* 1992;11:191–203.
95. Spitzer RL, Yanovski SZ, Wadden TA, et al. Binge eating disorder: its further validation in a multisite study. *Int J Eat Disord* 1993;13:137–153.
96. Brody ML, Walsh TB, Devlin M. Binge eating disorder: reliability and validity of a new diagnostic category. *J Consult Clin Psychol* 1994;62:381–386.
97. Varnado PJ, Williamson DA, Bentz BG, et al. Prevalence of binge eating disorder in obese adults seeking weight loss treatment. *Eat Weight Disord* 1997;2:112–117.
98. Greeno CG, Marcus MD, Wing RR. Diagnosis of binge eating disorder: discrepancies between a questionnaire and clinical interview. *Int J Eat Disord* 1995;17:153–160.
99. Stunkard AJ, Grace WJ, Wolff HG. The night-eating syndrome. *Am J Med* 1955;19:78–86.
100. Birketvedt G, Florholmen J, Sundsfjord J, et al. Behavioral and neuroendocrine characteristics of the night-eating syndrome. *JAMA* 1999;282:657–663.
101. Stunkard AJ, Grace WJ, Wolff HG. The night-eating syndrome. A pattern of food intake among certain obese patients. *Am J Med* 1955;19:78–86.
102. Stunkard AJ. Eating patterns and obesity. *Psychiatr Q* 1959;33:284–294.
103. Rand CS, Macgregor MD, Stunkard AJ. The night eating syndrome in the general population and among postoperative obesity surgery patients. *Int J Eat Disord* 1997;22:65–69.
104. Herman CP, Polivy J. From dietary restraint to binge eating: attaching causes to effects. *Appetite* 1990;14:123–125.
105. Ruderman AJ. Restraint, obesity, and bulimia. *Behav Res Ther* 1985;23:151–156.
106. Wilson GT. Relation of dieting and voluntary weight loss to psychological functioning and binge eating. *Ann Intern Med* 1993;119:727–730.
107. Serdula MK, Mokdad AH, Williamson DF, et al. Prevalence of attempting weight loss and strategies for controlling weight. *JAMA* 1999;282:1353–1358.
108. American Psychiatric Association. Practice guidelines for eating disorders. *Am J Psychiatry* 1993;150:212–228.
109. Wilson GT, Nonas CA, Rosenblum GD. Assessment of binge eating in obese patients. *Int J Eat Disord* 1993; 150:1472–1479.
110. Wadden TA, Foster GD, Letizia KA. One-year behavioral treatment of obesity: comparison of moderate and severe caloric restrictions and the effects of weight maintenance therapy. *J Consult Clin Psychol* 1994;62:165–171.
111. National Task Force on the Prevention and Treatment of Obesity. Dieting and the development of eating disorders in overweight and obese adults. *Arch Intern Med* 2000;160:2581–2589.
112. Wadden TA, Stunkard AJ, Smoller JW. Dieting and depression: a methodological study. *J Consult Clin Psychol* 1986;54:869–871.
113. Stunkard AJ, Stinnet JL, Smoller JW. Psychological and social aspects of the surgical treatment of obesity. *Am J Psychiatry* 1986;143:417–429.
114. Karlsson J, Sjostrom L, Sullivan M. Swedish Obese Subjects (SOS)—an intervention study of obesity. Two-year-follow-up of health-related quality of life (HRQL) and eating behavior after gastric surgery for severe obesity. *Int J Obes Relat Metab Disord* 1998;22:113–126.
115. Waters GS, Pories WJ, Swanson MS, et al. Long-term studies of mental health after the Greenville gastric bypass operation for morbid obesity. *Am J Surg* 1991;161:154–158.
116. Wing RR, Epstein LH, Marcus MD, et al. Mood changes in behavioral weight loss programs. *J Psychosom Res* 1984;28:345–346.
117. Rand CS, Kowalski K, Kuldau JM. Characteristics of marital improvement following obesity surgery. *Psychosomatics* 1984;25:221–226.

118. Wadden TA, Steen SN, Wingate BJ, et al. Psychosocial consequences of weight reduction: how much is enough? *Am J Clin Nutr* 1996;63:461–465.
119. Peace K, Dyne J, Russell G, et al. Psychobiological effects of gastric restriction surgery for morbid obesity. *N Z Med J* 1989;102:76–78.
120. Werlinger K, King TK, Clark MM, et al. Perceived changes in sexual functioning and body image following weight loss in an obese female population: a pilot study. *J Sex Marital Ther* 1997;23:74–78.
121. Stunkard AJ, Wadden TA. Psychological aspects of severe obesity. *Am J Clin Nutr* 1992;55:524S–532S.
122. King TK, Clark MM, Pera V. History of sexual abuse and obesity treatment outcome. *Addict Behav* 1996;21: 283–290.
123. Felitti VJ. Long-term medical consequences of incest, rape, and molestation. *South Med J* 1991;84:328–331.
124. Foster GD, Wadden TA, Vogt RA. Body image before, during and after weight loss treatment. *Health Psychol* 1997;16:226–229.
125. Cash TF. Body image and weight changes in a multisite comprehensive very-low-calorie diet program. *Behav Ther* 1994;25:239–254.
126. Rosen JC, Orosan P, Reiter J. Cognitive behavioral therapy for negative body image in obese women. *Behav Ther* 1995;26:25–42.
127. Keefe PH, Wyshogrod D, Weinberger E, et al. Binge eating and outcome of behavioral treatment of obesity: a preliminary report. *Behav Res Ther* 1984;22:319–321.
128. Yanovski SZ, Gormally JF, Lesser MS, et al. Binge eating disorder affects outcome of comprehensive very-low-calorie diet treatment. *Obes Res* 1994;2:205–212.
129. Wadden TA, Foster GD, Letizia KA. Response of obese binge eaters to treatment by behavior therapy combined with very low calorie diet. *J Consult Clin Psychol* 1992;60:808–811.
130. Kalarchian MA, Wilson GT, Brolin RE, et al. Effects of bariatric surgery on binge eating and related psychopathology. *Eat Weight Disord* 1999;4:15–23.
131. Fontaine KR, Cheskin LJ, Barofsky I. Health-related quality of life in obese persons seeking treatment. *J Fam Pract* 1996;43:265–270.
132. Jeffery RW, Wing RR, Mayer RR. Are smaller weight losses or more achievable weight loss goals better in the long term for obese patients? *J Consult Clin Psychol* 1998;66:641–645.
133. Pekkarinen T, Takala I, Mustajoki P. Two year maintenance of weight loss after VLCD and behavioural therapy for obesity: correlation to the scores of questionnaires measuring eating behaviour. *Int J Obes* 1996;20: 332–337.
134. Wadden TA, Vogt RA, Foster GD, et al. Exercise and the maintenance of weight loss: 1-year follow-up of a controlled clinical trial. *J Consult Clin Psychol* 1998;66:429–433.
135. Wadden TA, Stunkard AJ, Liebschutz J. Three year follow-up of the treatment of obesity by very-low-calorie diet, behavior therapy, and their combination. *J Consult Clin Psychol* 1988;56:925–928.
136. Foster GD, Wadden TA, Kendall PC, et al. Psychological effects of weight loss and regain: a prospective evaluation. *J Consult Clin Psychol* 1996;64:752–757.
137. Foster GD, Sarwer DB, Wadden TA. Psychological effects of weight cycling in obese persons: a review and research agenda. *Obes Res* 1997;5:474–488.
138. Wiese JC, Wilson JF, Jones RA, et al. Obesity stigma reduction in medical students. *Int J Obes Relat Metab Disord* 1992;16:859–868.
139. Robinson BE, Bacon JG, O'Reilly J. Fat phobia: measuring, understanding, and changing anti-fat attitudes. *Int J Eat Disord* 1993;14:467–480.
140. St. Jeor ST, ed. *Obesity assessment: tools, methods, interpretations*. New York: Chapman & Hall, 1997.
141. Garner DM, Garfinkel PE, Schwartz D. Cultural expectation of thinness in women. *Psychol Rep* 1980;47: 483–491.
142. Ware JE, Sherbourne CD. The MOS 36-item short-form health survey (SF-36), I. Conceptual framework and item selection. *Med Care* 1992;30:473–483.
143. Stunkard AJ, Messick S. The Three-Factor Eating Questionnaire to measure dietary restraint, disinhibition and hunger. *J Psychosom Res* 1985;29:71–83.
144. Beck AT, Steer RA, Brown GK. *Manual for Beck Depression Inventory-II*. San Antonio: Psychological Corporation, 1996.
145. Cash TF, Wood KC, Phelps KD, et al. New assessment of weight-related body image derived from extant instruments. *Percept Mot Skills* 1991;73:235–241.
146. Brown TA, Cash TF, Mikulka PJ. Attitudinal body image assessment: factor analysis of the Body-Self Relations Questionnaire. *J Pers Assess* 1990;55:135–144.
147. Rand CS, MacGregor AM. Morbidly obese patients' perceptions of social discrimination before and after surgery for obesity. *South Med J* 1990;83:1390–1395.
148. Allison DB, Basile VC, Yuker HE. The measurement of attitudes toward and beliefs about obese persons. *Int J Eat Disord* 1991;10:599–807.
149. Crandall CS, Biernat M. The idealogy of anti-fat attitudes. *J Appl Soc Psy* 1990;20:227–243.

16

Dyslipidemia of the Metabolic Syndrome

John D. Brunzell

HISTORY

To understand the dyslipidemia associated with obesity better, one needs to consider the interaction of a common population trait—visceral obesity and insulin resistance—with the oligogenic disorders in which this dyslipidemia occurs and by which it is modified. In 1988, Gerald Reaven coined the term "syndrome X" for a Banting Lecture at the American Diabetes Association and popularized the concept that a cluster of findings occur that are related to diabetes and atherosclerosis. Syndrome X included insulin resistance at the level of glucose and of free fatty acid (FFA) metabolism, hyperinsulinemia, hypertension, increased plasma triglyceride (TG) levels, and decreased high-density lipoprotein cholesterol (HDL-C) levels (1). A search of the National Library of Medicine's PubMed of the terms "obesity and lipids" in the summer of 2001 produced 10,000 articles. Several excellent reviews have recently been published (2–5).

An association among obesity, hyperinsulinemia, insulin resistance, impaired glucose tolerance, hypertension, hypertriglyceridemia, and atherosclerosis had been appreciated since the early 1960s. Albrink et al. (6–9) had recognized an association among truncal skinfold thickness, hyperinsulinism, serum TG levels, and blood sugar levels in normal individuals and in those with coronary disease. The relation between hyperinsulinism and TG levels (10), including in cases of obesity (11–13), was confirmed by others. The early reports of hypertriglyceridemia and decreased HDL-C seem to be due to associations of this dyslipidemia specifically with the central distribution of body fat and insulin resistance.

Vague (14) had described differences in body fat distribution in obese men and women. He noted that men with central obesity were at higher risk of diabetes, hypertension, and atherosclerosis than were men with generalized obesity or obese women, who accumulated fat in the hips and thighs. Many years later, Kissebah et al. (15), Krotkiewski et al. (16), Fujioka et al. (17), and Despres et al. (18) substantiated these findings. Albrink et al. (19) demonstrated a relationship between central obesity and HDL$_2$, and Peeples et al. (20) described the association between obesity with small dense low-density lipoprotein (LDL) particles.

Many terms have been used to describe the various components of the association of central obesity and insulin resistance with hypertension, diabetes, dyslipidemia, and premature atherosclerosis. These include android obesity (14), the metabolic syndrome (11), syndrome X (1), the central obesity syndrome (5), the insulin-resistance syndrome (21), the deadly quartet (22), visceral adiposity syndrome (23), and the atherogenic lipoprotein phenotype (24). The terminology has been driven by the particular component of the syndrome of interest to the authors. Recently, the National Cholesterol Education Program (NCEP) (25) suggested the use of the term *metabolic syndrome,* which appears to be sufficiently specific without being too generalized.

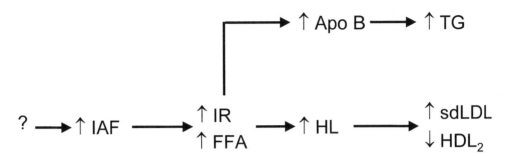

FIG. 16.1. Proposed order of events. Unknown factors lead to maldistribution of body fat with an increase in intraabdominal fat (IAF). This leads to insulin resistance (IR) and an increase in plasma free fatty acid (FFA) levels. The following two effects result at the level of the liver: (1) the increased FFAs lead apolipoprotein B (Apo B) away from degradation toward secretion as triglyceride (TG)-containing very low density lipoprotein (VLDL), and (2) increased hepatic lipase (HL) activity leads to the conversion of large buoyant low-density lipoprotein (LDL) to small dense LDL and to a decrease in high-density lipoprotein-2 (HDL$_2$).

VISCERAL OBESITY AND INSULIN RESISTANCE ARE PRECURSORS OF METABOLIC SYNDROME

With the advent of computed tomography (CT) an increase of visceral fat, rather than subcutaneous fat (SCF), accumulation has been documented in individuals with central body fat distribution. Fujioka et al. (17) reported that glucose and TG levels are increased with increased visceral fat, while Shuman et al. (26) demonstrated that type II diabetes is associated with increased visceral fat, but not SCF. Despres et al. (27) found that the extent of visceral obesity is associated with variations in the TG and HDL-C levels in obese women. Men have been found to have more visceral fat than do women, even when matched for body mass index (BMI) (28–30). These differences in visceral fat and the resultant changes in lipoproteins and blood pressure have been suggested to account for the difference in risk of premature coronary disease between men and premenopausal women (29,30). Although adipose tissue characteristically accumulates in the hips and thighs in women, those women who have increased visceral fat have a dyslipidemia similar to that of centrally obese men (15,16,27). In all of these studies, adverse changes in glucose or lipid parameters have been associated with increased visceral fat and not with other body fat or lean tissue compartments.

Increased visceral fat is associated with insulin resistance and elevated plasma FFA levels. Visceral obesity has been associated with hyperinsulinism (31,32) and insulin resistance as measured by the frequently sampled intravenous glucose-tolerance test (23). The accumulation of visceral fat has been suggested to precede and to cause insulin resistance because the insulin-sensitivity index increases and FFAs levels fall when visceral fat is decreased after caloric restriction (Fig. 16.1) (33).

COMPONENTS OF METABOLIC SYNDROME

The metabolic syndrome consists of central or visceral obesity, insulin resistance, elevated plasma FFA levels, impaired glucose tolerance, hypertension, predisposition to thrombosis, and dyslipidemia (Table 16.1). Multiple features of this syndrome are candidates that might predispose men and women to premature coronary artery disease (CAD) (34).

TABLE 16.1. *Components of
metabolic syndrome*

Visceral obesity
Insulin resistance
Elevated free fatty acids
Impaired glucose tolerance
Hypertension
Elevated plasminogen activator inhibitor-1
Dyslipidemia

Abnormalities in body fat distribution and insulin resistance were discussed in the section titled "Visceral Obesity and Insulin Resistance Are Precursors of Metabolic Syndrome." The levels of insulin, glucose, plasminogen activator inhibitor-1 (PAI-1), TG, HDL-C, and blood pressure are increased when compared with nonaffected individuals, but not all individuals have abnormal levels of these parameters. A continuum of values exists for each variable that is at a higher level than normal but that does overlap with normal. Multiple genetic and environmental factors seem to affect the distribution of these variables both in normal individuals and in those with the metabolic syndrome. Type II diabetes, familial combined hyperlipidemia (FCHL), and polycystic ovary syndrome (PCOS), specific syndromes in which the metabolic syndrome is a component, are discussed in the following section.

Age is an important variable in the metabolic syndrome. The metabolic syndrome begins in early adult life after the completion of adolescent growth. Although the LDL-C level does not appear to predict the primary onset of atherosclerosis in the elderly, central obesity, hypertension, and insulin resistance might continue to be risk factors for atherosclerosis in the elderly (35–39). This would be consistent with the increased risk of atherosclerosis seen with low HDL levels in the elderly (40).

Susceptibility to thrombosis has been suggested to occur with insulin resistance, diabetes, and dyslipidemia. An increase in PAI-1 has been consistently associated with hyperinsulinemia, insulin resistance, central obesity, and hypertriglyceridemia (41–46). The finding that PAI-1 is expressed in visceral adipose tissue but not in SCF in humans may explain the elevation in PAI-1 in the metabolic syndrome (47).

Albuminuria has also been associated with CAD (48,49). Although the metabolic syndrome has been suggested to be associated with albuminuria, careful studies of albuminuria in the metabolic syndrome have not uncovered a relationship with albuminuria (50–53). In addition, elevated plasma uric acid levels and inflammatory markers have also suggested to be part of the metabolic syndrome. The increase in inflammatory markers is probably the result of inflammatory processes in the arterial wall resulting from the complications of atherosclerosis (54).

The NCEP Adult Treatment Panel III (NCEP ATPIII) (25) has suggested a paradigm for the diagnosis of the metabolic syndrome that involves five easily measured clinical features. These include an increased waist circumference ($\geq$102 cm for men, $\geq$88 cm for women), a TG level of more than or equal to 150 mg per dL, a decreased HDL-C level (<40 mg per dL for men, <50 mg per dL for women), blood pressure of 135/88 mm Hg or higher, and a fasting plasma glucose level of 110 mg per dL or more. A diagnosis of the metabolic syndrome would be made with the presence of at least three of these clinical variables. The National Health and Nutrition Examination Survey III (NHANES-III) measured these variables in 8,814 adult men and women and found that about 24% of United States adults meet the criteria for the metabolic syndrome (55). The dyslipidemia of the metabolic syndrome in either the presence or absence of other oligogenic syndromes is discussed in the following section.

METABOLIC SYNDROME IN OLIGOGENIC DISORDERS

Common Oligogenic Disorders Associated with Visceral Obesity and Insulin Resistance

Visceral obesity and insulin resistance form an important component of a number of clinical syndromes (Table 16.2). In some instances, the visceral obesity interacts with other traits as two independent "hits" to manifest these clinical syndromes, such as that which occurs in FCHL, in type II diabetes mellitus, and perhaps in some forms of essential hypertension. Visceral obesity may play a similar role in PCOS; the combination of visceral obesity and insulin resistance may interact with hyperandrogenemia, leading to the full syndrome of PCOS.

Other syndromes, such as type I diabetes, not covered here may exhibit major changes in their clinical manifestations when they occur in the setting of a familial predisposition for visceral obesity, (56). Moreover, some forms of familial partial lipodystrophy seem to be associated with visceral fat accumulation and severe insulin resistance (57). A predisposition for visceral obesity may contribute to the lipodystrophy seen in patients infected with human immunodeficiency virus, particularly those on antiviral therapy.

Familial Combined Hyperlipidemia

FCHL was first described in the families of survivors of myocardial infarctions when elevations in TG, total cholesterol, or both were found in affected relatives (58). Subsequent reports confirmed these findings and their association with premature CAD (59–61). Subjects with FCHL characteristically have elevations in apolipoprotein B (apoB) levels and an increased amount of small dense LDL particles compared with normal controls (62–64) that persist even after the reduction of TG levels with gemfibrozil (65). One mechanism thought to play a major role in the elevation of apoB levels comes from kinetic studies, which have shown an increase in production rates of apoB-containing lipoprotein particles in subjects with FCHL compared with normal controls and other genetic forms of hypertriglyceridemia (66–68).

Although initially described as a monogenic disorder (58), inheritance of the lipid phenotype has been shown to be more complex than that (Fig. 16.2). Segregation and linkage analyses have provided evidence for major gene effects that influence the elevation

TABLE 16.2. *Metabolic syndrome in oligogenic disorders*

Major component
    Familial combined hyperlipidemia
    Type II diabetes mellitus
    Possibly essential hypertension
    Possibly polycystic ovary syndrome
Population trait effects
    Adult men
    Postmenopausal women
    Type I diabetes mellitus
Acquired
    Cushing syndrome
    Acquired immune deficiency syndrome

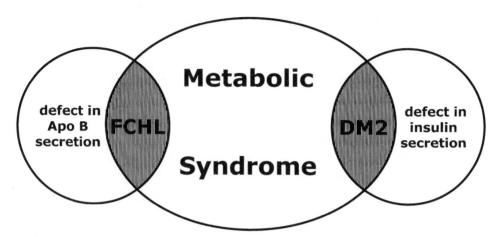

FIG. 16.2. The metabolic syndrome is a common population trait, which includes central obesity, insulin resistance, and mild dyslipidemia. The metabolic syndrome interacts with defects in insulin secretion to cause type II diabetes (DM2) and with defects in hepatic apolipoprotein B (Apo B) secretion to cause familial combined hyperlipidemia (FCHL).

in apoB levels (69), as well as the presence of small dense LDL particles in families with a history of FCHL (70,71). Further evidence for genetic heterogeneity comes from studies showing that 36% of subjects with FCHL have reduced postheparin lipoprotein lipase (LPL) activity (72). Patients with FCHL with this diminished LPL activity have slightly higher TG levels than do patients with FCHL with normal LPL activity (72). Several mutations of the apoA-IV gene (73); regulatory elements of the LPL gene (74); and variants in the apoA-I, apoC-III, apoA-IV cluster have been described that could contribute to the diminished LPL activity and variable hyperlipidemia in this group. In addition, several groups have shown that polymorphisms of the LPL gene are associated with higher lipid levels, specifically TG levels, in subjects with FCHL who carry these mutations than they are in noncarriers (75).

In the general population, small, dense LDL particles are common, with an estimated prevalence rate of 25% (76,77). Subjects with small, dense LDL have a number of other lipid abnormalities in common with subjects with FCHL, including elevated TG levels, apoB production rates, and apoB levels (78–80). Insulin resistance has also been reported in subjects with small, dense LDL particles (23,32), and recent studies have shown that subjects with FCHL are also insulin resistant (81–87).

Given the similarities in metabolic phenotype (e.g., insulin resistance and dyslipidemia), some authors have hypothesized that insulin resistance is a major determinant of the hyperlipidemia phenotype in FCHL, including elevated apoB levels (82,86,88). The question remains, however, of whether the increased apoB levels in FCHL can be entirely accounted for by the finding of the insulin-resistance syndrome in this population. In a study of families with a history of FCHL, Jarvik et al. (89) suggested that mechanisms that result in the small, dense LDL phenotype (e.g., insulin resistance) may contribute to the lipid phenotype of FCHL but that they do not fully explain the elevated apoB levels in this disorder. In physiologic studies, the apoB levels were higher in patients with FCHL than in those with isolated obesity when individuals with FCHL were matched to individuals of similar BMI, visceral fat, and insulin sensitivity who did not have FCHL (90). This indicates that the elevation in apoB is not related entirely to insulin resistance. Both the family data and the physiologic data indicate that FCHL is an oligogenic disorder with an apoB-raising locus, which interacts with hypertriglyceridemic factors, such as visceral obesity or modest reductions in LPL.

Type II Diabetes Mellitus

Type II diabetes is associated with visceral obesity and insulin resistance (91,92). A defect in insulin secretion is present in those insulin-resistant individuals who develop hyperglycemia. First-degree relatives of individuals with type II diabetes may be centrally obese and insulin resistant, they may display decreased insulin secretion in response to glucose, or they may have both in addition to type II diabetes. Although the genes contributing to central obesity, insulin resistance, and defective insulin secretion are unknown, type II diabetes is a classic example of an oligogenic disorder. To determine the genes involved will require the careful phenotypic characterization of subsets of individuals with type II diabetes.

Essential Hypertension

Essential hypertension is a heterogeneous group of disorders. One subset of individuals demonstrates a common familial form of essential hypertension that has been characterized as nonmodulating, salt-sensitive hypertension (93). Phenotypic characterization of these individuals is complex, and it includes normal or high renin levels. These individuals alter neither the renal blood flow during an angiotensin II infusion while on a high-salt diet nor the aldosterone response to angiotensin II while on a low-salt diet. Nonmodulating salt-sensitive hypertension is seen in about 25% of hypertensive men, but it is uncommon in women until after menopause (93). A single nucleotide polymorphism at codon 235 in the angiotensinogen gene has been associated with this form of hypertension, which is in linkage disequilibrium with a promoter variant of the gene (94).

Central obesity and insulin resistance are common in those who manifest nonmodulating, salt-sensitive hypertension. The interaction of the common population trait–central obesity–with genetic defects in the renin–angiotensin system may be another example of an oligogenic disorder. This may explain the frequent inclusion of dyslipidemia in reports of essential hypertension (24).

Polycystic Ovary Syndrome as an Oligogenic Disorder

PCOS has been suggested to be a complex genetic disease and perhaps an oligogenic disorder (95–97). Hyperandrogenism has been suggested to be inherited independently from visceral obesity and insulin resistance (95,96). In family studies of women with PCOS, sisters with PCOS, some with hyperandrogenism without amenorrhea, some with obesity alone, and others who are normal all appear (97). This is compatible with the independent segregation of obesity and hyperandrogenism in these families. The hyperandrogenism and polycystic ovary component appears to be an autosomal dominant trait in families with PCOS (98).

When women with PCOS undergo ovarian cautery, the hyperandrogenism improves without a change in insulin resistance as measured by clamp studies (99). Treatment with flutamide, an androgen-receptor blocker, improves hyperandrogenism without a change in clamp-determined insulin resistance (100). These studies suggest that the hyperandrogenism is, in part, separate from the insulin resistance. When women are treated with troglitazone, a decrease in testosterone and a concomitant improvement in insulin resistance and hypertriglyceridemia are seen (101–103). This is compatible with the idea of insulin resistance contributing to hyperandrogenism. Alternatively, insulin resistance may aggravate an underlying primary androgen defect (104).

To determine whether PCOS is an oligogenic disorder in which visceral obesity and insulin resistance segregate independently in families, the determination of whether visceral obesity segregates independently from hyperandrogenism should be made in family studies.

Menopause

When women become postmenopausal, some develop central obesity with increased visceral fat (105–111), some become insulin resistant with an increased incidence of diabetes, some become hypertensive, and some develop dyslipidemia characterized by hypertriglyceridemia with small, dense LDL particles (112). Postmenopausal women treated with estrogen-replacement therapy have been reported to have decreased intraabdominal fat (113–116), insulin resistance, diabetes (117), and hypertension. Although menopause in some women is associated with the development of hypertriglyceridemia and small, dense LDL, treatment with *oral* estrogen causes an increase in TG-rich very low density lipoproteins (VLDL), an increase in HDL, and the development of small dense LDL (118). In this circumstance, the effect of estrogen to decrease visceral fat and to increase plasma TG may have competing effects with LDL size and density. Less of an increase in TG is seen with transdermal estrogen replacement (119–122).

The subset of women who develop visceral obesity, insulin resistance, and the other components of the metabolic syndrome may have a genetic predisposition to the syndrome that is expressed only after the loss of endogenous estrogen. Austin et al. (24) have suggested that the presence of small, dense LDL is a marker for the presence of the metabolic syndrome. They also note that the prevalence of small, dense LDL particles increases across menopause from 10% to almost 25%, a level that may be seen in men. The prevalence of metabolic syndrome X in the general population is 25% (1). A similar prevalence in the United States population has been reported by the NHANES studies (55).

Common Modifiers of Dyslipidemia in Central Obesity

Untreated Diabetes

Defects in insulin secretion in *untreated* non–insulin-dependent type II diabetes mellitus affect dyslipidemia, in addition to the effects associated with central obesity and insulin resistance (123). The hypertriglyceridemia seen in untreated diabetes can result from increased FFA levels, leading to increased hepatic TG synthesis or to decreased LPL-mediated TG removal (123). These VLDL particles are often bigger and more TG-enriched than are those seen in obesity, and the may lead to further small, dense LDL via the cholesteryl ester transfer protein (CETP). HDL-C also is often lower in untreated diabetes (123). After therapy for hyperglycemia, much of the remaining dyslipidemia in type II diabetes is a reflection of the underlying central obesity and insulin resistance.

Hepatic Lipase Promoter Polymorphism

Four common polymorphisms, which are in linkage disequilibrium, have been reported in the hepatic lipase promoter (124,125). The less common variant in whites is associated with increased HDL-C levels, which are caused by increased HDL_2-C levels (124–126). This less common variant is also related to more buoyant LDL particles (126). This genetic variant has been shown to modify the relation among central obesity, insulin resistance, and the dyslipidemia present. In whites, these promoter variants may account for 20% to 30% of the variance in hepatic lipase activity (124–126). In African

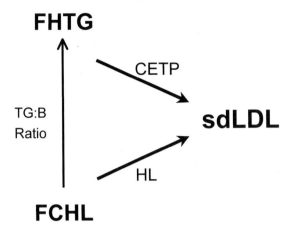

FIG. 16.3. The role of cholesteryl ester transfer protein (CETP) and hepatic lipase (HL) in determining the size and density (sd) of low-density lipoprotein (LDL) and high-density lipoprotein (HDL) is dependent on other factors that influence the size and triglyceride-to-apolipoprotein B (TG:B) ratio in very low density lipoprotein over a wide spectrum of triglyceride levels. Abbreviations: FCHL, familial combined hyperlipidemia; FHTG, familial hypertriglyceridemia. (From Brunzell JD, Hokanson JE. Dyslipidemia of central obesity and insulin resistance. *Diabetes Care* 1999;22:C10–C13, with permission.)

Americans, Hispanic Americans, Japanese Americans, and Chinese, the "rare" allele occurs with a frequency of up to 50% (127). This may account for increased HDL₂-C levels in these ethnic groups compared with Europeans.

Primary Increase in Hepatic Triglyceride Synthesis

Increased TG synthesis with TG-enriched VLDL can lead to LDL and HDL heterogeneity independent of visceral obesity. TG-enriched VLDLs exchange TG for cholesteryl ester in LDL in a process mediated by CETP (128). This process probably is exaggerated in conditions with very TG-enriched VLDL, such as familial hypertriglyceridemia, estrogen-replacement therapy, and high-carbohydrate diets (63,129,130). Each of these conditions can be associated with low levels of small, dense LDL particles (131). This effect appears to occur at one end of a spectrum of VLDL particle size, with the small VLDL of the central obesity–insulin resistance syndrome at the other end (Fig. 16.3). With large VLDLs, the effect on LDL size and density is predominantly determined by CETP. With small VLDLs and insulin resistance, hepatic lipase is the major determinant of LDL size and density. HDL-C levels and composition also reflect the effects of both CETP and hepatic lipase.

Cushing Syndrome: An Acquired Form of Central Obesity

Cushing syndrome is associated with redistribution of body fat from the periphery to the trunk. Patients with Cushing syndrome have been shown by CT scan to have an increase in visceral fat (132). This increase in visceral fat is associated with the insulin resistance, hypertension, and dyslipidemia seen in Cushing syndrome. This dyslipidemia differs in some ways from isolated visceral obesity in that HDL-C levels often are elevated (133).

MECHANISM OF DYSLIPIDEMIA OF THE METABOLIC SYNDROME
Lipoprotein Physiology (134)

ApoB is constitutively secreted into the lumen of the hepatocyte endoplasmic reticulum. This apoB is destined for degradation if it is not incorporated into VLDL particles. In an independent process, TG is synthesized in the hepatocyte and is added to the apoB-containing particle. This process is completed in the Golgi complex, and the VLDL, with apoB and TG, is secreted into the plasma. The VLDL delivers TG fatty acids to the muscle for energy or to adipose tissue for storage. LPL, which is bound to adipose and muscle capillary proteoglycans, hydrolyzes the TG to FFAs for energy or storage. The lipoproteins remaining after the removal of much of the TG are recognized by the hepatocyte in a complex process that leads to the conversion of the remnant particles to LDL particles.

These LDL particles, which normally contain most of the plasma cholesterol, can experience several fates. LDL provides cholesterol to extrahepatic tissues via the LDL cell surface receptor. Although this mechanism provides cholesterol to cells for cell membranes and to steroid-producing tissues for hormone synthesis, most of the LDL-C is recycled back to the liver via hepatic LDL receptors.

LDL also can permeate the arterial wall and, if modified (e.g., through oxidation of lipids or proteins), can be taken up by arterial wall macrophages to form foam cells. Hepatic lipase can accelerate this proatherogenic process by converting large LDL particles into smaller LDL particles. The smaller LDL particles are more proatherogenic than the large LDL particles because they enter the arterial wall more easily, they are bound to and are retained more easily in the arterial wall, they bind to the proteoglycan matrix, and they are more easily oxidized. All of these steps promote uptake of these particles by macrophages, and they enhance atherogenesis.

Cholesterol can be removed from peripheral tissues and returned to the liver through processes termed *reverse cholesterol transport*. ApoA-I and other HDL proteins promote the removal of cholesterol from tissues via the ABC-A1 cell surface receptors. ApoA-I causes the translocation of cholesterol to the cell surface via the ABC-A1 receptor, with the AI–cholesterol complex forming nascent HDL particles. Cholesterol also can be added to plasma apoA-I particles by phospholipid transfer protein from the surface of the VLDL as the VLDL core is processed by LPL. This cholesterol in nascent HDL particles is then esterified to cholesteryl ester, leading to a larger HDL particle. The cholesteryl ester can be returned to the liver directly by HDL or by transfer via CETP to LDL in exchange for TG, with subsequent hepatic uptake of the LDL particle.

Mechanism of Dyslipidemia in Metabolic Syndrome

Visceral obesity and insulin resistance are major contributors to the dyslipidemia associated with the metabolic syndrome. The lipid abnormalities seen include an increase in TG, a decrease in HDL$_2$-C levels, and an increase in small, dense LDL particle number (Table 16.3) (5). However, in normal randomly selected populations, isolated visceral obesity and insulin resistance raise TG levels only slightly (increase by 36%), and they decrease HDL-C levels (135). In populations that are selected by measuring large, buoyant versus small, dense LDL particles, the TG level separating these populations is around 150 mg per dL. In contrast, visceral obesity and insulin resistance contribute to a

---

TABLE 16.3. *Dyslipidemia of metabolic syndrome*

Elevated triglyceride level (in small very low density lipoprotein)
Increased intermediate-density lipoprotein level
Increased small, dense low-density lipoprotein particles
Increased apolipoprotein B levels
Decreased high density lipoprotein 2 cholesterol level

more severe dyslipidemia, such as that seen with type II diabetes and FCHL, as well as with other oligogenic syndromes.

The hypertriglyceridemia associated with visceral obesity and insulin resistance formerly was thought to be secondary to the effects of elevated plasma insulin levels, which cause increased hepatic fatty acid esterification of glycerol and hepatic TG synthesis (136,137). This concept required that the liver was uniquely insulin sensitive, which appears to be unlikely when measured directly (138). Insulin resistance also may lead to elevated TG levels in obesity through decreased adipose tissue LPL. However, kinetic studies suggest plasma TG removal is saturable, but not defective, in obesity and that adipose tissue LPL activity per cell is elevated in obesity (139,140). Hirsch and Knittle (141) and Imbeault et al. (142) suggested that increased fat cell size in adult-onset obesity is the form of obesity that is related to insulin resistance, particularly intraabdominal obesity. The sequential relation of increased adipose tissue LPL per cell leading to obesity with increased fat cell size with subsequent insulin resistance has been suggested to occur (Fig. 16.1).

A unique explanation for the association of central obesity and insulin resistance with hypertriglyceridemia is that it takes place via an increase in portal vein long-chain FFAs, resulting in increased apoB-100 secretion by the liver (143,144). The long-chain fatty acids would divert apoB away from degradation in the endoplasmic reticulum and toward secretion. This would easily explain the presence of increased numbers of smaller VLDL particles in insulin-resistant states with a decreased VLDL TG-to-apoB ratio compared with normal (145). This would result in increases in LDL apoB levels as well. Alternative explanations for the insulin resistance include the role of increased hepatic fat or intramyocellular fat (146,147).

Increases in insulin resistance and FFA levels appear to have two divergent effects at the level of the liver. The first is to cause an increase in the number of apoB-containing particles secreted from the liver, leading to the increase in VLDL TG and the number of LDL particles. The second outcome is to increase the enzyme hepatic lipase on hepatic cell surface proteoglycans. This enzyme contributes in a minor way to plasma remnant lipoprotein recognition by the liver via a noncatalytic action. More importantly, hepatic lipase activity hydrolyzes TG and phospholipid in LDL and HDL particles to convert big, buoyant LDL particles to small, dense LDL particles and HDL$_2$ particles to HDL$_3$ particles (Fig. 16.4) (5). Hepatic lipase acts in concert with CETP in this process. Which of these proteins is predominant depends on the TG content of VLDL and the secretion rate of VLDL (5).

Despres et al. (148) and Pouliot et al. (149) noted an association between visceral fat by CT scan and increased hepatic lipase activity in women and in men, respectively. This increase in hepatic lipase was related to visceral fat and not to SCF or total body fat (29,148). This increase in hepatic lipase was associated with the presence of small, dense LDL particles (150), decreased HDL$_2$-C levels (151), and possibly decreased remnant lipoprotein particles (152). The gender differences in LDL particle size and HDL$_2$ levels between men and premenopausal women could largely be accounted for by gender differences in visceral fat (29,153). An increase in visceral fat as the cause of the insulin resistance, the increase in hepatic lipase, and the dyslipidemia are supported by studies of before and after 10% loss of weight by caloric restriction. After weight loss resulting in decreased visceral fat content, insulin resistance, hepatic lipase, and the dyslipidemia all improved (33).

Visceral obesity and insulin resistance contribute to the dyslipidemia seen in FCHL, but they cannot account for the elevation in apoB levels characteristic of FCHL (90).

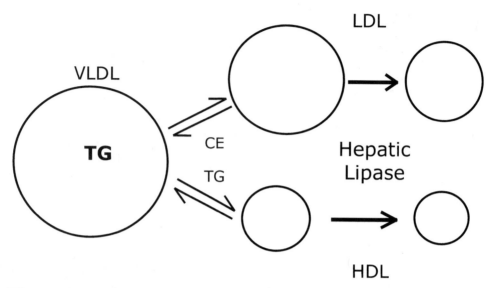

FIG. 16.4. Exchange of cholesteryl ester (CE) and triglyceride (TG) between TG-rich very low density lipoprotein (VLDL) and low-density lipoprotein (LDL) and high-density lipoprotein (HDL) is mediated by cholesteryl ester transfer protein. Hepatic lipase hydrolyzes TG and phospholipid in LDL and HDL to generate smaller particles.

Intensive lipid-lowering therapy in the Familial Atherosclerosis Treatment Study (FATS) led to decreased hepatic lipase activity; decreased small, dense LDL particles; and elevated HDL_2-C, with subsequent regression of CAD by angiography (151). The benefit of clearing small, dense LDL particles in FATS and the subsequent regression of atherosclerosis was seen in those individuals who had FCHL with small, dense LDL particles or elevated lipoprotein (a) with small, dense LDL particles at baseline (154).

Several single-nucleotide polymorphisms (SNPs), which are in nearly complete linkage disequilibrium, have been identified in the promoter of the hepatic lipase gene by Jansen and by Cohen (127). The C-514 T allele has a frequency of 20% to 25% in whites and of about 50% in African Americans and Asians. The C-514 T allele is associated with decreased hepatic lipase activity; big, buoyant LDLs; and increased HDL_2 levels. Although accumulation of visceral fat raises hepatic lipase activity and leads to smaller LDL and HDL particles, the C-514 T variant attenuates this effect (155). The C-514 T SNP also attenuates the effect of intensive lipid-lowering therapy to decrease hepatic lipase activity to correct the small, dense LDL and to decrease HDL_2 (156). Thus, this SNP in hepatic lipase can be antiatherogenic by decreasing the hepatic lipase activity leading to big, buoyant LDL particles and higher HDL_2 levels. In contrast, it is proatherogenic by blocking the effect of lipid-lowering drugs to decrease hepatic lipase activity.

Small, dense LDL particles and decreased HDL, predominantly HDL_3, have been seen in situations in which VLDL are secreted as very TG-rich VLDL. In these circumstances, an exchange of TG in VLDL for cholesteryl ester in LDL and HDL can lead to accumulation of small amounts of small, dense LDL and decreased HDL_3 levels. The decrease is mediated by excess TG transfer via CETP, followed by lipid hydrolysis by low levels of hepatic lipase. These changes are different from those seen with the metabolic syndrome, in which VLDLs are less TG rich, greater amounts of small dense LDL particles are present, and HDL_2 is decreased rather than HDL_3. Increased CETP-mediated TG levels for cholesteryl ester exchange can occur with oral hormone-replacement therapy, high car-bohydrate feeding, and with certain drugs, such as Accutane and retroviral protease inhibitors.

The dyslipidemia of the metabolic syndrome can be diagnosed by demonstrating increased apoB levels in the presence of mild to moderate increases in plasma TG and decreased HDL-C levels. Ascertaining LDL peak size by gradient gel electrophoresis or LDL peak density by density gradient ultracentrifugation is not necessary. Total HDL levels reflect changes in the HDL_2 levels, indicating that HDL subfractions do not need to be measured (157). Nuclear magnetic resonance imaging is a good method for detect-ing HDL subspecies, but it has not been validated for apoB-containing lipoproteins (158).

COMPLICATIONS OF METABOLIC SYNDROME

Premature Coronary Artery Disease

Complications of atherosclerosis are the most common cause of death in the central obesity associated with FCHL and type II diabetes. This may be related to dyslipidemia, hypertension, or other components of the metabolic syndrome or to hyperglycemia in dia-betes. Often cardiovascular death can occur in generalized obesity because of the effect on the cardiorespiratory systems (see Chapter 9) .

An increase in plasma LDL-C and a decrease in HDL-C have independently been shown to lead to atherosclerosis, particularly to premature CAD. Plasma TG levels often have been shown to be associated with an increased risk of atherogenesis, but they usu-ally are not independent of the effects of LDL-C or HDL-C. Elevated plasma TG levels, however, are a marker for the dyslipidemia seen in the metabolic syndrome, consisting of increased amounts of small, dense LDL and decreased HDL_2-C levels.

Austin et al. (24) demonstrated that small, dense LDL particles are more common than big, buoyant LDL in patients with CAD. Small, dense LDL particles have been shown prospectively to predict cardiovascular events and to predict response to therapy (159–161). Intensive lipid-lowering therapy, which selectively decreases small, dense LDL particles, predicted regression of CAD by repeated angiography (151). These changes in LDL particle physical characteristics were at least as important as changes in LDL levels or levels of HDL_2-C and were determined by the drug-induced decrease in hepatic lipase activity.

The differences in the risk of premature coronary disease between men and pre-menopausal women and between men and centrally obese men can be accounted for, in large part, by the dyslipidemia resulting from increased hepatic lipase activity in the pres-ence of visceral obesity and insulin resistance. Therapy ideally is directed toward visceral obesity, but it can be directed toward any of the steps in the cascade leading to early atherogenesis.

Nonalcoholic Fatty Liver Disease

Fatty liver has been associated with the metabolic syndrome, and it is related to cen-tral obesity, insulin resistance, and hypertriglyceridemia (162–164). Indeed, fatty liver seems to occur in both genetic and acquired hypertriglyceridemia, and it may represent excess synthesis of hepatic TG as compared with hepatic apoB, leading to hepatic accu-mulation of TG instead of VLDL TG transport (156–167). Fatty liver also may occur in heterozygous familial hypobetalipoproteinemia, in which decreased synthesis of hepatic apoB occurs (168).

On the other hand, any severe hypertriglyceridemia with defective VLDL catabolism can be associated with fatty liver and hepatosplenomegaly (169). In fact, familial LPL deficiency, a form of hypertriglyceridemia due entirely to an extrahepatic defect in TG hydrolysis, is commonly associated with fatty liver, which regresses rapidly with the restriction of dietary fat intake. In one report, 29 of 34 individuals with LPL deficiency had severe hypertriglyceridemia with hepatosplenomegaly (170).

Central obesity and insulin resistance with hypertriglyceridemia, particularly when aggravated by other prohypertriglyceridemia medications, can cause fatty liver. Treatment to lower TG is associated with a decrease in liver size. Some individuals who develop fatty liver progress on to steatohepatitis with fibrosis and necrosis for reasons that are not clear. Perhaps these individuals have the second "hit" required to develop nonalcoholic steatohepatitis.

Chylomicronemia Syndrome

Severe hypertriglyceridemia can lead to pancreatitis and the development of eruptive xanthomata (169). These do not occur in the common forms of the metabolic syndrome with mild hypertriglyceridemia. However, the metabolic syndrome might contribute to severe hypertriglyceridemia when other forms of TG elevation are present (169).

DIAGNOSIS AND ASSESSMENT OF DYSLIPIDEMIA

Generally, the initial assessment of dyslipidemia is the measurement of plasma TG, total cholesterol, and HDL-C, with calculation of the LDL-C level. Mild elevations in TG with a reduction in HDL-C are seen in the metabolic syndrome; LDL-C levels are often normal. In spite of the normal LDL-C level, the number of LDL particles is often increased in the form of small, dense LDL particles, which are cholesterol poor. The presence of small, dense LDL can be determined by direct measurement of LDL size or density by gradient gel electrophoreses or density gradient ultracentrifugation, respectively (171). LDL particle number can be assessed by measurement of apoB, where one molecule of apoB is present in each LDL particle (172).

The NCEP ATPIII panel suggests indirect assessment of small, dense LDL by the determination of the pressure of the metabolic syndrome and discourages the use of measures of LDL particle heterogeneity. However, many lipid clinics add the measurement of apoB to the routine lipid profile in the assessment of the patient at risk of premature CAD.

TREATMENT OF DYSLIPIDEMIA

The NCEP ATPIII suggests lifestyle modification for the treatment of most people with the metabolic syndrome (25). Loss of weight by caloric restriction has been demonstrated to decrease plasma TG levels in many studies by decreasing hepatic TG production and secretion (173). An increase in HDL-C also occurs after weight loss. Confusion about lipoprotein responses to weight loss is present because studies performed during weight loss in a hypocaloric state provided more extreme results than those performed after weight stabilization at the lower weight (174). The studies of significance are those performed at a stable weight. Maintenance of weight loss is difficult, and it has high degrees of recidivism (175). However, low-fat dietary intake and aerobic exercise have been demonstrated to maintain weight loss better than caloric restriction, as well as to

TABLE 16.4. *Drug therapy for dyslipidemia[a]*

	Triglyceride	LDL-C	Selective small dense LDL	HDL-C	Selective HDL$_2$ C	Reference
Monotherapy						
Statin (variable dose)	±↓	↓↓	—	±↑	—	175
Niacin (0.5 g three times a day)	↓	↓	↓	↑	↑	188
TZD (variable dose)	↓	↑	↓	↑	↑	189
Combination therapy						
Statin + resin	±↓	↓↓	↓	↑	↑	148
Niacin + resin	↓	↓	↓	↑	↑	148
TZD + statin	↓	↓	↓	↑	↑	189

Abbreviations: HDL-C, high-density lipoprotein cholesterol; LDL-C, low-density lipoprotein cholesterol; TZD, thiazolidinedione.

[a]↓, decreased; ↓↓, greatly decreased ↑, increased; ±, small change; statin, HMG-CoA reductase inhibitor.

lead to decreases in TG and small, dense LDL particles and to raise HDL-C levels, in particular, HDL$_2$-C (33,176–180). These changes in dyslipidemia are related in part to the decrease in dietary saturated fat content and in part to the decrease in body fat with changes in hepatic lipase and LPL (33,181). Aerobic exercise has been suggested to reduce visceral fat selectively (182–184). Low-dose aspirin therapy for increased susceptibility to thrombosis and aggressive treatment of hypertension also are recommended (25,185).

Drug therapy might be used to treat the central obesity of the metabolic syndrome, but effective drugs are limited. However, drug therapy aimed at the dyslipidemia, combined with diet and exercise, is recommended when more severe dyslipidemia occurs, as is seen in type II diabetes or FCHL (Table 16.4). Several studies have demonstrated that statin therapy in type II diabetes lowers LDL-C levels and decreases cardiovascular events (186). Statins combined with bile acid–binding resins are effective. The use of insulin sensitizers, such as thiazolidinediones, will selectively decrease small, dense LDL particle levels and will raise HDL$_2$-C levels, and thus they might be considered complementary drugs to statin therapy (187). Therapy with niacin acid, with or without a bile acid sequestrant, is highly effective in treating the dyslipidemia seen in the metabolic syndrome.

Patients with the metabolic syndrome, such as those as seen in type II diabetes or in FCHL, should be treated for hypertension and hyperglycemia with low-dose aspirin therapy and dietary and lipid-lowering therapy. A multifaceted approach seems to be indicated in metabolic syndrome until the cause of the visceral obesity and insulin resistance can be directly treated; this helps prevent the other features of the syndrome, including cardiovascular disease.

ACKNOWLEDGMENTS

Portions of this work were supported by National Institutes of Health grants DK02456, HL30086, and HL64322; the University of Washington Clinical Research Center, RR37; the Diabetes Endocrine Research Center, DK17047; and the Clinical Nutrition Research Unit, DK35816.

REFERENCES

1. Reaven GM. Role of insulin resistance in human disease. *Diabetes* 1988;37:1595–1607.
2. Despres JP, Krauss RM. Obesity and lipoprotein metabolism. In: Bray GA, Bouchard C, James WPT, eds. *Handbook of obesity.* New York: Marcel Dekker Inc, 1998:651–676.
3. Wajchenberg BL. Subcutaneous and visceral adipose tissue: their relation to the metabolic syndrome. *Endocr Rev* 2000;21:697–738.
4. Lamarche B, Lemieux I, Despres JP. The small, dense LDL phenotype and the risk of coronary heart disease: epidemiology, pathophysiology and therapeutic aspects. *Diabetes Metab* 1999;25:199–211.
5. Brunzell JD, Hokanson JE. Dyslipidemia of central obesity and insulin resistance. *Diabetes Care* 1999;22:C10–C13.
6. Albrink MJ, Meigs JW. Interrelationship between skinfold thickness, serum lipids and blood sugar in normal men. *Am J Clin Nutr* 1964;15:255–261.
7. Albrink MJ, Meigs JW, Granoff MA. Weight gain and serum triglycerides in normal men. *N Engl J Med* 1962;266:484–489.
8. Davidson P, Albrink MJ. Abnormal plasma insulin response with high plasma triglycerides independent of clinical diabetes or obesity. *J Clin Invest* 1966;45:1000.
9. Albrink MK, Mann EB. Serum triglycerides in coronary artery disease. *Arch Intern Med* 1959;103:4–8.
10. Reaven GM, Lerner RL, Stern MP, et al. Role of insulin in endogenous hypertriglyceridaemia. *J Clin Invest* 1967;46:1756–1767.
11. Avogaro P, Crepaldi G, Enzi G, et al. Association of hyperlipaemia, diabetes mellitus and mild obesity. *Acta Diabetol Lat* 1967;4:572.
12. Bagdade JD, Bierman EL, Porte D Jr. The significance of basal insulin levels in the evaluation of the insulin response to glucose in diabetic and non-diabetic subjects. *J Clin Invest* 1967;46:1549–1557.
13. Bierman EL, Bagdade JD, Porte D Jr. Obesity and diabetes: the odd couple. *Am J Clin Nutr* 1968;21:1434–1437.
14. Vague J. La differenciation sexuelle, facteur determinant des formes de l'obesite. *Presse Med* 1947;30:339–340.
15. Kissebah AH, Vydelingum N, Murray RW, et al. Relation of body fat distribution to metabolic complications of obesity. *J Clin Endocrinol Metab* 1982;54:254–260.
16. Krotkiewski M, Björntorp P, Sjöström L, et al. Impact of obesity on metabolism in men and women. Importance of regional adipose tissue distribution. *J Clin Invest* 1983;72:1150–1162.
17. Fujioka S, Matsuzawa Y, Tokunaga K, et al. Contribution of intra-abdominal fat accumulation to the impairment of glucose and lipid metabolism in human obesity. *Metabolism* 1987;36:54–59.
18. Despres JP, Moorjani S, Lupien PJ, et al. Regional distribution of body fat, plasma lipoproteins, and cardiovascular disease. *Arteriosclerosis* 1990;10:497–511.
19. Albrink MJ, Krauss RM, Lindgrem FT, et al. Intercorrelations among plasma high density lipoprotein, obesity and triglycerides in normal population. *Lipids* 1980;15:668–676.
20. Peeples LH, Carpenter JW, Israel RG, et al. Alterations in low-density lipoproteins in subjects with abdominal adiposity. *Metabolism* 1989;38:1029–1036.
21. Haffner SM, Valdez RA, Hazuda HP, et al. Prospective analysis of the insulin-resistance syndrome (syndrome X). *Diabetes* 1992;41:715–722.
22. Kaplan NM. The deadly quartet, upper-body obesity, glucose intolerance, hypertriglyceridemia, and hypertension. *Arch Intern Med* 1989;149:1514–1520.
23. Fujimoto WY, Abbate SL, Kahn SE, et al. The visceral adiposity syndrome in Japanese-American men. *Obes Res* 1994;2:364–371.
24. Austin MA, King MC, Vranizan KM, et al. Atherogenic lipoprotein phenotype. A proposed genetic marker for coronary heart disease risk. *Circulation* 1990;82:495–506.
25. Executive summary of the third report of the National Cholesterol Education Program (NCEP) Expert Panel on Detection, evaluation and treatment of high blood cholesterol in adults (Adult Treatment Panel III). *JAMA* 2001;285:2486–2497.
26. Shuman W, Newell-Morris L, Leonetti D, et al. Abnormal body fat distribution detected by computed tomography in diabetic men. *Invest Radiol* 1986;21:483–487.
27. Despres JP, Moorjani S, Ferland M, et al. Adipose tissue distribution and plasma lipoprotein levels in obese women, importance of intra-abdominal fat. *Arteriosclerosis* 1989;9:203–210.
28. Enzi G, Gasparo M, Biodetti PR, et al. Subcutaneous and visceral fat distribution according to sex, age, and overweight, evaluated by computed tomography. *Am J Clin Nutr* 1986;44:739–746.
29. Carr MC, Hokanson JE, Zambon A, et al. The contribution of intra-abdominal fat to gender differences in hepatic lipase activity and LDL/HDL heterogeneity. *J Clin Endocrinol Metab* 2001;86:2831–2837.
30. Lemieux S, Despres JP, Moorjani S, et al. Are gender differences in cardiovascular disease risk factors explained by the level of visceral adipose tissue? *Diabetologia* 1994;37:757–764.
31. Sparrow D, Borkan GA, Gerzof SG, et al. Relationship of fat distribution to glucose tolerance. Results of computed tomography in male participants of the normative aging study. *Diabetes* 1986;35:411–415.
32. Tchernof A, Lamarche B, Prudhomme D, et al. The dense LDL phenotype. Association with plasma lipoprotein levels, visceral obesity, and hyperinsulinemia in men. *Diabetes Care* 1996;19:629–637.

33. Purnell JQ, Kahn SE, Albers JJ, et al. Effect of weight loss with reduction of intra-abdominal fat on lipid metabolism in older men. *J Clin Endocrinol Metab* 2000;85:977–982.
34. Brunzell JD, Hokanson JE. LDL and HDL subspecies and risk for premature coronary artery disease. *Am J Med* 1999;107:16S–18S.
35. Bermudez OI, Tucker KL. Total and central obesity among elderly Hispanics and the association with type 2 diabetes. *Obes Res* 2001;9:443–451.
36. Lempiainen P, Mykkanen L, Pyorala K, et al. Insulin resistance syndrome predicts coronary heart disease events in elderly nondiabetic men. *Circulation* 1999;100:123–128.
37. Mykkanen L, Kuusisto J, Haffner SM, et al. Hyperinsulinemia predicts multiple atherogenic changes in lipoproteins in elderly subjects. *Arterioscler Thromb* 1994;14:518–526.
38. Cefalu WT, Wang ZQ, Werbel S, et al. Contribution of visceral fat mass to the insulin resistance of aging. *Metabolism* 1995;44:954–959.
39. Cefalu WT, Werbel S, Bell-Farrow AD, et al. Insulin resistance and fat patterning with aging: relationship to metabolic risk factors for cardiovascular disease. *Metabolism* 1998;47:401–408.
40. Brown CD, Higgins M, Donato KA, et al. Body mass index and the prevalence of hypertension and dyslipidemia. *Obes Res* 2000;8:605–619.
41. Mansfield MW, Stickland MH, Grant PJ. PAI-1 concentrations in first-degree relatives of patients with non–insulin-dependent diabetes: metabolic and genetic associations. *Thromb Hemost* 1997;77:357–361.
42. Asplund-Carlson A, Hamsten A, Wiman B, et al. Relationship between plasma plasminogen activator inhibitor-1 activity and VLDL triglyceride concentration, insulin levels and insulin sensitivity: studies in randomly selected normo- and hypertriglyceridaemic men. *Diabetologia* 1993;36:817–825.
43. Sakkinen PA, Wahl P, Cushman M, et al. Clustering of procoagulation, inflammation, and fibrinolysis variables with metabolic factors in insulin resistance syndrome. *Am J Epidemiol* 2000;152:897–907.
44. De Mitrio V, De Pergola G, Vettor R, et al. Plasma plasminogen activator inhibitor-I is associated with plasma leptin irrespective of body mass index, body fat mass, and plasma insulin and metabolic parameters in premenopausal women. *Metabolism* 1999;48:960–964.
45. Schneider DJ, Sobel BE. Synergistic augmentation of expression of plasminogen activator inhibitor type-1 induced by insulin, very-low-density lipoproteins, and fatty acids. *Coronary Artery Dis* 1996;7:813–817.
46. Meigs JB, Mittleman MA, Nathan DM, et al. Hyperinsulinemia, hyperglycemia and impaired hemostasis. *JAMA* 2000;283:221–228.
47. Shimomura I, Funahashi T, Takahashi M, et al. Enhanced expression of PAI-1 in visceral fat: possible contributor to vascular disease in obesity. *Nat Med* 1996;2:800–803.
48. Kuusisto J, Mykkanen L, Pyorala K, et al. Hyperinsulinemic microalbuminuria: a new risk indicator for coronary heart disease. *Circulation* 1995;91:831–837.
49. Bianchi S, Bigazzi R, Valtriani C, et al. Elevated serum insulin levels in patients with essential hypertension and microalbuminuria. *Hypertension* 1994;23:681–687.
50. Nielsen S, Jensen MD. Relationship between urinary albumin excretion, body composition, and hyperinsulinemia in normotensive glucose-tolerant adults. *Diabetes Care* 1999;22:1728–1733.
51. Jensen JS, Borch-Johnsen K, Jensen G, et al. Insulin sensitivity in clinically healthy individuals with microalbuminuria. *Atherosclerosis* 1996;119:69–76.
52. Jager A, Kostense PJ, Nijpels G, et al. Microalbuminuria is strongly associated with NIDDM and hypertension, but not with the insulin resistance syndrome: the Hoorn Study. *Diabetologia* 1998;41:694–700.
53. Pedrinelli R, Di Bello V, Catapano G, et al. Microalbuminuria is a marker of left ventricular hypertrophy but not hyperinsulinemia in nondiabetic atherosclerotic patients. *Arterioscler Thromb* 1993;13:900–906.
54. Festa A, D'Agostino R, Howard G, et al. Chronic subclinical inflammation as part of the insulin resistance syndrome: the insulin resistance atherosclerosis study (IRAS). *Circulation* 2000;102:42–47.
55. Ford E, Giles W, Dietz W. Prevalence of the metabolic syndrome among US adults; findings from the third National Health and Nutrition Examination Survey. *JAMA* 2002;287:356–359.
56. Purnell JQ, Hokanson JE, Marcovina SM, et al. Effect of excessive weight gain with intensive therapy of type 1 diabetes on lipid levels and blood pressure: results from the DCCT. Diabetes Control and Complications Trial. *JAMA* 1998;280:140–146.
57. Garg A, Peshock RM, Fleckenstein JL. Adipose tissue distribution pattern in patients with familial partial lipodystrophy (Dunnigan variety). *J Clin Endocrinol Metab* 1999;84:170–174.
58. Goldstein JL, Schrott HG, Hazzard WR, et al. Hyperlipidemia in coronary heart disease, II. Genetic analysis of lipid levels in 176 families and delineation of a new inherited disorder, combined hyperlipidemia. *J Clin Invest* 1973;52:1544–1568.
59. Rose H, Kranz P, Weinstock M, et al. Inheritance of combined hyperlipoproteinemia: evidence for a new lipoprotein phenotype. *Am J Med* 1973;54:148–160.
60. Nikkila E, Aro A. Family study of serum lipids and lipoproteins in coronary heart-disease. *Lancet* 1973;1:954–959.
61. Brunzell JD, Schrott HG, Motulsky AG, et al. Myocardial infarction in the familial forms of hypertriglyceridemia. *Metabolism* 1976;25:313–320.
62. Sniderman AD, Shapiro S, Marpole D, et al. Association of coronary atherosclerosis with hyperapobetalipoproteinemia (increased protein but normal cholesterol levels in human plasma low density lipoproteins). *Proc Natl Acad Sci U S A* 1980;77:604–608.

63. Brunzell JD, Albers JJ, Chait A, et al. Plasma lipoproteins in familial combined hyperlipidemia and monogenic familial hypertriglyceridemia. *J Lipid Res* 1983;24:147–155.

64. Hokanson JE, Austin MA, Zambon A, et al. Plasma triglyceride and LDL heterogeneity in familial combined hyperlipidemia. *Arterioscler Thromb* 1993;13:427–434.

65. Hokanson JE, Krauss RM, Albers JJ, et al. LDL physical and chemical properties in familial combined hyperlipidemia. *Arterioscler Thromb Vasc Biol* 1995;15:452–459.

66. Chait A, Albers JJ, Brunzell JD. Very low density lipoprotein overproduction in genetic forms of hypertriglyceridemia. *Eur J Clin Invest* 1980;10:17–22.

67. Janus ED, Nicoll AM, Turner PR, et al. Kinetic bases of the primary hyperlipidemias: studies of apolipoprotein B turnover in genetically defined subjects. *Eur J Clin Invest* 1980;10:161–172.

68. Kissebah AH, Alfarsi S, Adams PW. Integrated regulation of very low density lipoprotein triglyceride and apolipoprotein B kinetics in man: normolipemic subjects, familial hypertriglyceridemia and familial combined hyperlipidemia. *Metabolism* 1981;30:856–868.

69. Pairitz G, Davignon J, Mailloux H, et al. Sources of interindividual variation in the quantitative levels of apolipoprotein B in pedigrees ascertained through a lipid clinic. *Am J Hum Genet* 1988;43:311–321.

70. Austin MA, Wijsman E, Guo S, et al. Lack of evidence for linkage between low density lipoprotein subclass patterns and the apolipoprotein B locus in familial combined hyperlipidemia. *Genet Epidemiol* 1991;8:287–297.

71. Austin MA, Horowitz H, Wijsman E, et al. Bimodality of apolipoprotein B levels in familial combined hyperlipidemia. *Atherosclerosis* 1992;92:67–77.

72. Babirak S, Brown BG, Brunzell JD. Familial combined hyperlipidemia and abnormal lipoprotein lipase. *Arterioscler Thromb* 1992;12:1176–1183.

73. Deeb SS, Nevin DN, Iwasaki L, et al. Two novel apolipoprotein A-IV variants in individuals with familial combined hyperlipidemia and diminished levels of lipoprotein lipase activity. *Hum Mutat* 1996;8:319–325.

74. Yang WS, Nevin DN, Iwasaki L, et al. Regulatory mutations in the human lipoprotein lipase gene in patients with familial combined hyperlipidemia and coronary artery disease. *J Lipid Res* 1996;37:2627–2637.

75. Aouizerat B, Allayee H, Cantor R, et al. Linkage of a candidate gene locus to familial combined hyperlipidemia: lecithin:cholesterol acyltransferase on 16q. *Arterioscler Thromb Vasc Biol* 1999;19:2730–2736.

76. Austin MA, King MC, Vranizan KM, et al. Inheritance of low-density lipoprotein subclass patterns: results of complex segregation analysis. *Am J Hum Genet* 1988;43:838–846.

77. Campos H, Blijlevens E, McNamara J, et al. LDL particle size distribution: results from the Framingham Offspring Study. *Arterioscler Thromb* 1992;12:1410–1419.

78. McNamara JR, Campos H, Ordovas JM, et al. Effect of gender, age, and lipid status on low density lipoprotein subfraction distribution. Results from the Framingham Offspring study. *Arteriosclerosis* 1987;7:483–490.

79. Austin MA, Breslow JA, Hennekens CH, et al. Low density lipoprotein subclass pattern and risk of myocardial infarction. *JAMA* 1988;260:1917–1921.

80. Packard C, Demant T, Stewart J, et al. Apolipoprotein B metabolism and the distribution of VLDL and LDL subfractions. *J Lipid Res* 2000;41:305–318.

81. Hunt SC, Wu LL, Hopkins PN, et al. Apolipoprotein, LDL subfraction, and insulin associations with familial combined hyperlipidemia in Utah patients with familial dyslipidemic hypertension. *Arteriosclerosis* 1989;9:335–344.

82. Aitman T, Godsland I, Farren B, et al. Defects of insulin action on fatty acid and carbohydrate metabolism in familial combined hyperlipidemia. *Arterioscler Thromb Vasc Biol* 1997;17:748–754.

83. Bredie S, Tack C, Smits P, et al. Nonobese patients with familial combined hyperlipidemia are insulin resistant compared with their nonaffected relatives. *Arterioscler Thromb Vasc Biol* 1997;17:1465–1471.

84. Ascaso J, Lorente R, Merchante A, et al. Insulin resistance in patients with familial combined hyperlipidemia and coronary artery disease. *Am J Cardiol* 1997;80:1481–1487.

85. Ascaso J, Merchante A, Lorente R, et al. A study of insulin resistance using the minimal model in nondiabetic familial combined hyperlipidemic patients. *Metabolism* 1998;47:508–513.

86. Karjalainen L, Pihlajamaki J, Karhapaa P, et al. Impaired insulin-stimulated glucose oxidation and free fatty acid suppression in patients with familial combined hyperlipidemia: a precursor defect for dyslipidemia? *Arterioscler Thromb Vasc Biol* 1998;18:1548–1553.

87. Pihlajamaki J, Karjalainen L, Karhapaa P, et al. Impaired free fatty acid suppression during hyperinsulinemia is a characteristic finding in familial combined hyperlipidemia, but insulin resistance is observed only in hypertriglyceridemic patients. *Arterioscler Thromb Vasc Biol* 2000;20:164–170.

88. Castro Cabezas M, de Bruin T, de Valk H, et al. Impaired fatty acid metabolism in familial combined hyperlipidemia: a mechanism associating hepatic apolipoprotein B overproduction and insulin resistance. *J Clin Invest* 1993;92:160–168.

89. Jarvik GP, Brunzell JD, Austin MA, et al. Genetic predictors of FCHL in four large pedigrees. Influence of apolipoprotein B level major locus predicted genotype and LDL subclass phenotype. *Arterioscler Thromb Vasc Biol* 1994;14:1687–1694.

90. Purnell JQ, Kahn SE, Schwartz RS, et al. Relationship of insulin sensitivity and apoB levels to intra-abdominal fat in subjects with familial combined hyperlipidemia. *Arterioscler Thromb Vasc Biol* 2001;21:567–572.

91. Kahn S, Prigeon R, Schwartz R, et al. Obesity, body fat distribution, insulin sensitivity and islet beta-cell function as explanations for metabolic diversity. *J Nutr* 2001;131:354S–360S.

92. Carey D, Jenkins A, Campbell L, et al. Abdominal fat and insulin resistance in normal and overweight women: direct measurements reveal a strong relationship in subjects at both low and high risk of NIDDM. *Diabetes* 1996;45:633–638.
93. Williams GH, Fisher ND, Hunt SC, et al. Effects of gender and genotype on the phenotypic expression of non-modulating essential hypertension. *Kidney Int* 2000;57:1404–1407.
94. Hopkins PN, Lifton RP, Hollenberg NK, et al. Blunted renal vascular response to angiotensin II is associated with a common variant of the angiotensinogen gene and obesity. *J Hypertens* 1996;14:199–207.
95. Poretsky L, Piper B. Insulin resistance, hypersecretion of LH, and a dual-defect hypothesis for the pathogenesis of polycystic ovary syndrome. *Obstet Gynecol* 1994;84:613–621.
96. Franks S, Gharani N, Waterworth D, et al. The genetic basis of polycystic ovary syndrome. *Hum Reprod* 1997;12:2641–2648.
97. Legro RS, Spielman R, Urbanek M, et al. Phenotype and genotype in polycystic ovary syndrome. *Recent Prog Horm Res* 1998;53:217–256.
98. Govind A, Obhrai MS, Clayton RN. Polycystic ovaries are inherited as an autosomal dominant trait: analysis of 29 polycystic ovary syndrome and 10 control families. *J Clin Endocrinol Metab* 1999;84:38–43.
99. Lemieux S, Lewis GF, Ben-Chetrit A, et al. Correction of hyperandrogenemia by laparoscopic ovarian cautery in women with polycystic ovarian syndrome is not accompanied by improved insulin sensitivity or lipid-lipoprotein levels. *J Clin Endocrinol Metab* 1999;84:4278–4282.
100. Diamanti-Kandarakis E, Mitrakou A, Raptis S, et al. The effect of a pure antiandrogen receptor blocker, flutamide, on the lipid profile in the polycystic ovary syndrome. *J Clin Endocrinol Metab* 1998;83:2699–2705.
101. Ehrmann DA, Schneider DJ, Sobel BE, et al. Troglitazone improves defects in insulin action, insulin secretion, ovarian steroidogenesis, and fibrinolysis in women with polycystic ovary syndrome. *J Clin Endocrinol Metab* 1997;82:2108–2116.
102. Hasegawa I, Murakawa H, Suzuki M, et al. Effect of troglitazone on endocrine and ovulatory performance in women with insulin resistance–related polycystic ovary syndrome. *Fertil Steril* 1999;71:323–327.
103. Dunaif A, Scott D, Finegood D, et al. The insulin-sensitizing agent troglitazone improves metabolic and reproductive abnormalities in the polycystic ovary syndrome. *J Clin Endocrinol Metab* 1996;81:3299–3306.
104. Ciampelli M, Fulghesu AM, Cucinelli F, et al. Impact of insulin and body mass index on metabolic and endocrine variables in polycystic ovary syndrome. *Metabolism* 1999;48:167–172.
105. Ley CJ, Lees B, Stevenson JC. Sex- and menopause-associated changes in body-fat distribution. *Am J Clin Nutr* 1992;55:950–954.
106. Poehlman E, Toth M, Gardner A. Changes in energy balance and body composition at menopause: a controlled longitudinal study. *Ann Intern Med* 1995;123:673–675.
107. Zamboni M, Armellini F, Milani M, et al. Body fat distribution in pre- and post-menopausal women: metabolic and anthropometric variables and their inter-relationships. *Int J Obes Relat Metab Disord* 1992;16:495–504.
108. Svendsen O, Hassager C, Christiansen C. Age- and menopause-associated variations in body composition and fat distribution in healthy women as measured by dual-energy X-ray absorptiometry. *Metabolism* 1995;44:369–373.
109. Tremollieres F, Pouilles J, Ribot C. Relative influence of age and menopause on total and regional body composition changes in postmenopausal women. *Am J Obstet Gynecol* 1996;175:1594–1600.
110. Kotani K, Tokunaga K, Fujioka S, et al. Sexual dimorphism of age-related changes in whole-body fat distribution in the obese. *Int J Obes Relat Metab Disord* 1994;18:207–212.
111. Bjorkelund C, Lissner L, Andersson S, et al. Reproductive history in relation to relative weight and fat distribution. *Int J Obes Relat Metab Disord* 1996;20:213–219.
112. Carr MC, Kim KH, Zambon A, et al. Changes in LDL density across the menopausal transition. *J Investig Med* 2000;48:245–250.
113. Haarbo J, Marslew U, Gotfredsen A, et al. Postmenopausal hormone replacement therapy prevents central distribution of body fat after menopause. *Metabolism* 1991;40:1323–1326.
114. Reubinoff B, Wurtman J, Rojansky N, et al. Effects of hormone replacement therapy on weight, body composition, fat distribution, and food intake in early postmenopausal women: a prospective study. *Fertil Steril* 1995;64:963–968.
115. Gambacciani M, Ciaponi M, Cappagli B, et al. Body weight, body fat distribution, and hormonal replacement therapy in early postmenopausal women. *J Clin Endocrinol Metab* 1997;82:414–417.
116. Espeland M, Stefanick M, Kritz-Silverstein D, et al. Effect of postmenopausal hormone therapy on body weight and waist and hip girths. Postmenopausal Estrogen-Progestin Interventions Study Investigators. *J Clin Endocrinol Metab* 1997;82:1549–1556.
117. Manning P, Allum A, Jones S, et al. The effect of hormone replacement therapy on cardiovascular risk factors in type 2 diabetes. *Arch Intern Med* 2001;161:1772–1776.
118. Campos H, Sacks FM, Walsh BW, et al. Differential effects of estrogen on low-density lipoprotein subclasses in healthy postmenopausal women. *Metabolism* 1993;42:1153–1158.
119. Chetkowski R, Meldrum D, Steingold K, et al. Biologic effects of transdermal estradiol. *N Engl J Med* 1986;314:1615–1620.
120. Fahraeus L, Larsson-Cohn U, Wallentin L. Lipoproteins during oral and cutaneous administration of oestradiol-17 beta to menopausal women. *Acta Endocrinol* 1982;101:597–602.
121. Basdevant A, De Lignieres B, Guy-Grand B. Differential lipemic and hormonal responses to oral and parenteral 17 beta-estradiol in postmenopausal women. *Am J Obstet Gynecol* 1983;147:77–81.

122. Walsh B, Li H, Sacks F. Effects of postmenopausal hormone replacement with oral and transdermal estrogen on high density lipoprotein metabolism. *J Lipid Res* 1994;35:2083–2093.

123. Brunzell JD, Chait A. Diabetic dyslipidemia-pathology and treatment. In: Porte D Jr, Sherwin J, eds. *Ellenberg and Rifkin's diabetes mellitus.* Norwalk: Appleton & Lange, 1996:1077–1096.

124. Guerra R, Wang S, Grundy S, et al. A hepatic lipase (LIPC) allele associated with high plasma concentrations of high density lipoprotein cholesterol. *Proc Natl Acad Sci U S A* 1997;94:4532–4537.

125. Murtomaki S, Tahvanianen E, Antikainen M, et al. Hepatic lipase gene polymorphism influence plasma HDL levels: results from Finnish EARS participants. *Arterioscler Thromb Vasc Biol* 1997;17:1879–1884.

126. Zambon A, Deeb S, Hokanson J, et al. Common variants in the promoter of the hepatic lipase gene are associated with lower levels of hepatic lipase activity, buoyant LDL and higher HDL₂ cholesterol. *Arterioscler Thromb Vasc Biol* 1998;18:1723–1729.

127. Zambon A, Brown BG, Deeb SS, et al. Hepatic lipase as a focal point for the development and treatment of coronary artery disease. *J Investig Med* 2001;49:112–118.

128. Deckelbaum R, Granot E, Oschry Y, et al. Plasma triglyceride determines structure-composition in low and high density lipoproteins. *Arteriosclerosis* 1984;4:225–231.

129. Walsh BW, Schiff I, Rosner B, et al. Effects of postmenopausal estrogen replacement on the concentrations and metabolism of plasma lipoproteins. *N Engl J Med* 1991;325:1196–1204.

130. Melish J, Le N, Ginsberg H, et al. Dissociation of apoprotein B and triglyceride production in very-low-density lipoproteins. *Am J Physiol* 1980;239:E354–E362.

131. Purnell JQ, Brunzell JD. The central role of dietary fat, not carbohydrate, in the insulin resistance syndrome. *Curr Opin Lipidol* 1997;8:17–22.

132. Wajchenberg BL, Bosco A, Marone MM, et al. Estimation of body fat and lean tissue distribution by dual energy X-ray absorptiometry and abdominal body fat evaluation by computed tomography in Cushing's disease. *J Clin Endocrinol Metab* 1995;80:2791–2794.

133. Kissebah A, Krakower G. Endocrine disorders. In: Betteridge D, Illingworth D, Shepherd J, eds. *Lipoproteins in health and disease.* New York: Oxford University Press, 1999:931–941.

134. Scriver C, Beaudet A, Sly W, et al. *The metabolic & molecular bases of inherited disease.* New York: McGraw-Hill, 2001:2705–2988.

135. Nieves D, Cnop M, Retzlaff B, et al. The atherogenic lipoprotein profile associated with obesity and insulin resistance is largely attributable to intra-abdominal fat. *Diabetes* (*in press*).

136. Grundy SM, Mok HY, Zech L, et al. Transport of very low density lipoprotein triglycerides in varying degrees of obesity and hypertriglyceridemia. *J Clin Invest* 1979;63:1274–1283.

137. Olefsky J, Farquhar J, Reaven G. Reappraisal of the role of insulin in hypertriglyceridemia. *Am J Med* 1974;57:551–560.

138. Sparks JD, Sparks CE. Insulin regulation of triacylglycerol-rich lipoprotein synthesis and secretion. *Biochim Biophys Acta* 1994;1215:9–32.

139. Pykalisto OJ, Smith PH, Brunzell JD. Determinants of human adipose tissue LPL. *J Clin Invest* 1975;56:1108–1117.

140. Brunzell JD, Schwartz RS, Eckel RH, et al. Insulin and adipose tissue lipoprotein lipase in humans. *Int J Obes* 1981;5:685–694.

141. Hirsch J, Knittle J. Cellularity of obese and nonobese human adipose tissue. *Fed Proc* 1970;29:1516–1521.

142. Imbeault P, Lemieux S, Prud'homme D, et al. Relationship of visceral adipose tissue to metabolic risk factors for coronary heart disease: is there a contribution of subcutaneous fat cell hypertrophy? *Metabolism* 1999;48:355–362.

143. Homan R, Grossman JE, Pownall HJ. Differential effects of eicosapentaenoic acid and oleic acid on lipid synthesis and secretion by HepG2 cells. *J Lipid Res* 1991;32:231–241.

144. Xu X, Shang A, Jiang H, et al. Demonstration of biphasic effects of docosahexaenoic acid on apolipoprotein B secretion in HepG2 cells. *Arterioscler Thromb Vasc Biol* 1997;17:3347–3355.

145. Packard CJ, Shepherd J. Lipoprotein heterogeneity and apolipoprotein B metabolism. *Arterioscler Thromb Vasc Biol* 1997;17:3542–3556.

146. Kim J, Fillmore J, Chen Y, et al. Tissue-specific overexpression of lipoprotein lipase causes tissue-specific insulin resistance. *Proc Natl Acad Sci U S A* 2001;98:7522–7527.

147. Kelley D, Williams K, Price J, et al. Plasma fatty acids, adiposity, and variance of skeletal muscle insulin resistance in type 2 diabetes mellitus. *J Clin Endocrinol Metab* 2001;86:5412–5419.

148. Despres JP, Ferland M, Moorjani S, et al. Role of hepatic-triglyceride lipase activity in the association between intra-abdominal fat and plasma HDL cholesterol in obese women. *Arteriosclerosis* 1989;9:485–492.

149. Pouliot MC, Despres JP, Nadeau A, et al. Visceral obesity in men: associations with glucose tolerance, plasma insulin, and lipoprotein levels. *Diabetes* 1992;41:826–834.

150. Zambon A, Austin MA, Brown BG, et al. Effect of hepatic lipase on LDL in normal men and those with coronary heart disease. *Arterioscler Thromb* 1993;13:147–153.

151. Zambon A, Hokanson JE, Brown BG, et al. Evidence for a new pathophysiological mechanism for coronary artery disease regression: hepatic lipase mediated changes in LDL density. *Circulation* 1999;99:1959–1964.

152. Zambon A, Deeb SS, Bensadoun A, et al. *In vivo* evidence of a role for hepatic lipase in human apoB-containing lipoprotein metabolism, independent of its lipolytic activity. *J Lipid Res* 2000;41:2094–2099.

153. Lemieux S, Prud'homme D, Bouchard C, et al. Sex differences in the relation of visceral adipose tissue accumulation to total body fatness. *Am J Clin Nutr* 1993;58:463–467.

154. Zambon A, Brown B, Hokanson J, et al. Genetic variants of dyslipidemia differ in their angiographic response to intensive lipid-lowering therapy in premature coronary artery disease. *Circulation* 2002 (*in press*).

155. Carr MC, Hokanson JE, Deeb SS, et al. A hepatic lipase gene promoter polymorphism attenuates the increase in hepatic lipase activity with increasing intra-abdominal fat in women. *Arterioscler Thromb Vasc Biol* 1999;19:2701–2707.

156. Zambon A, Deeb SS, Brown BG, et al. Common hepatic lipase gene promoter variant determines clinical response to intensive lipid-lowering treatment. *Circulation* 2001;103:792–798.

157. Lamarche B, Moorjani S, Cantin B, et al. Associations of HDL_2 and HDL_3 subfractions with ischemic heart disease in men. *Arterioscler Thromb Vasc Biol* 1997;17:1098–1105.

158. Otvos J, Jeyarajah E, Bennett D, et al. Development of a proton nuclear magnetic resonance spectroscopic method for determining plasma lipoprotein concentrations and subspecies distributions from a single, rapid measurement. *Clin Chem* 1992;38:1632–1638.

159. Lamarche B, Tchernof A, Moorjani S, et al. Small, dense low-density lipoprotein particles as a predictor of the risk of ischemic heart disease in men. Prospective results from the Quebec Cardiovascular Study. *Circulation* 1997;95:69–75.

160. Stampfer MJ, Krauss RM, Ma J, et al. A prospective study of triglyceride level, low-density lipoprotein particle diameter, and risk of myocardial infarction. *JAMA* 1996;276:882–888.

161. Gardner CD, Fortmann SP, Krauss RM. Association of small low-density lipoprotein particles with the incidence of coronary artery disease in men and women. *JAMA* 1996;276:875–881.

162. Marchesini G, Brizi M, Bianchi G, et al. Nonalcoholic fatty liver disease: a feature of the metabolic syndrome. *Diabetes* 2001;50:1844–1850.

163. Marchesini G, Brizi M, Morselli-Labate AM, et al. Association of nonalcoholic fatty liver disease with insulin resistance. *Am J Med* 1999;107:450–455.

164. Assy N, Kaita K, Mymin D, et al. Fatty infiltration of liver in hyperlipidemic patients. *Dig Dis Sci* 2000; 45:1929–1934.

165. Maruhama Y, Ohneda A, Tadaki H, et al. Hepatic steatosis and the elevated plasma insulin level in patients with endogenous hypertriglyceridemia. *Metabolism* 1975;24:653–664.

166. Luyckx FH, Lefebvre PJ, Scheen AJ. Non-alcoholic steatohepatitis: association with obesity and insulin resistance, and influence of weight loss. *Diabetes Metab* 2000;26:98–106.

167. Marceau P, Biron S, Hould FS, et al. Liver pathology and the metabolic syndrome X in severe obesity. *J Clin Endocrinol Metab* 1999;84:1513–1517.

168. Mars H, Lewis L, Robertson A, et al. Familial hypobetalipoproteinemia: a genetic disorder of lipid metabolism with nervous system involvement. *Am J Med* 1969;46:886.

169. Brunzell J, Deeb S. Familial lipoprotein lipase deficiency, apo CII deficiency, and hepatic lipase deficiency. In: Scriver C, Beaudet A, Sly W, et al, eds. *The metabolic and molecular basis of inherited disease.* New York: McGraw-Hill, 2001:2789–2816.

170. Fredrickson DS, Lees RS. Familial hyperlipoproteinemia. In: Stanbury JB, Wyngaarden JB, Fredrickson DS, eds. *The metabolic basis of inherited disease.* New York: McGraw-Hill, 1966:429–485.

171. Hokanson JE, Austin MA, Brunzell JD. Measurement and clinical significance of low-density lipoprotein subclasses. In: Rifai N, Warnick GR, Dominiczak MH, eds. *Handbook of lipoprotein testing.* Washington, D.C.: American Association of Clinical Chemistry Press, 1997:267–282.

172. Brunzell JD, Sniderman AD, Albers JJ, et al. Apoproteins B and A-1 and coronary artery disease in humans. *Arteriosclerosis* 1984;4:79–83.

173. Olefsky JM, Reaven GM, Farquhar JW. Effects of weight reduction on obesity: studies of carbohydrate and lipid metabolism. *J Clin Invest* 1974;53:64–76.

174. Schwartz RS, Brunzell JD. Increase of adipose tissue lipoprotein lipase activity with weight loss. *J Clin Invest* 1981;67:1425–1430.

175. Pronk NP, Wing RP. Physical activity and long-term maintenance of weight loss. *Obesity Res* 1994;2:587–599.

176. Williams PT, Krauss RM, Stefanick ML, et al. Effects of low-fat diet, calorie restriction, and running on lipoprotein subfraction concentrations in moderately overweight men. *Metabolism* 1994;43:655–663.

177. Halle M, Berg A, Garwers U, et al. Influence of 4 weeks' intervention by exercise and diet on low-density lipoprotein subfractions in obese men with type 2 diabetes. *Metabolism* 1999;48:641–644.

178. Tuomilehto J, Lindstrom J, Eriksson J, et al. Prevention of type 2 diabetes mellitus by changes in lifestyle among subjects with impaired glucose tolerance. *N Engl J Med* 2001;344:1342–1350.

179. Knowler WC, Barrett-Connor E, Fowler SE, et al. Reduction in the incidence of type 2 diabetes with lifestyle intervention or metformin. *N Engl J Med* 2002;346:393–403.

180. Franz M, Bantle J, Beebe C, et al. Evidence-based nutrition principles and recommendations for the treatment and prevention of diabetes and related complications. *Diabetes Care* 2002;25:148–198.

181. Eckel R, Yost T. HDL subfractions and adipose tissue metabolism in the reduced-obese state. *Am J Physiol* 1989;256:E740–E746.

182. Heim DL, Holcomb CA, Loughin TM. Exercise mitigates the association of abdominal obesity with high-density lipoprotein cholesterol in premenopausal women: results from the third National Health and Nutrition Examination Survey. *J Am Diet Assoc* 2000;100:1347–1353.

183. Goodpaster BH, Kelley DE, Wing RR, et al. Effects of weight loss on regional fat distribution and insulin sensitivity in obesity. *Diabetes* 1999;48:839–847.
184. Pratley RE, Hagberg JM, Dengel DR, et al. Aerobic exercise training-induced reductions in abdominal fat and glucose-stimulated insulin responses in middle-aged and older men. *J Am Geriatr Soc* 2000;48:1055–1061.
185. Aspirin for the primary prevention of cardiovascular events: recommendation and rationale. *Ann Intern Med* 2002;136:157–160.
186. Pyörälä K, Pedersen TR, Kjekshus J, et al. Cholesterol lowering with simvastatin improves prognosis of diabetic patients with coronary heart disease. A subgroup analysis of the Scandinavian Simvastatin Survival Study (4S) [published erratum appears in *Diabetes Care* 1997;20:1048]. *Diabetes Care* 1997;20:614–620.
187. Cohen BR, Kreider M, Biswas N, et al. Rosiglitazone in combination with an HMG CoA reductase inhibitor: safety and effects on lipid profile in patients with type 2 diabetes. *Diabetes* 2001;50:A451.
188. Knopp R. Evaluating niacin in its various forms. *Am J Cardiol* 2000;86:51–56.
189. Freed M, Ratner R, Marcovina S, et al. Rosiglitazone alone and in combination with atorvastatin on the metabolic abnormalities in type 2 diabetes mellitus. *Am J Cardiol* 2002;90:947–952.

17

Orthopedic Complications

David T. Felson and Susan L. Edmond

Obesity increases the force across weight-bearing joints. In some persons, this is well tolerated, but in others, it may lead to joint or musculoskeletal injury. Moreover, it may not produce the same effect in all weight-bearing joints. This chapter reviews the effect of obesity on the most common form of arthritis, osteoarthritis (OA), and on low back pain.

MUSCULOSKELETAL PAIN AND OSTEOARTHRITIS

Musculoskeletal pain is remarkably common, with knee pain the most frequent daily health complaint among women 65 years of age and older and the second most widespread health complaint among middle-aged men and women (1). The other site at which musculoskeletal pain is extraordinarily prevalent is in the lower back. Acute low back pain afflicts most of the adult population at some point in their life, and 20% to 30% of middle-aged and elderly adults report experiencing back pain on most days of the most recent month (2). Although hip pain is less frequent than knee pain, hip pain on most days affects up to 10% of middle-aged and elderly persons.

Knee, hip, and back pain can be caused by multiple diseases. Knee pain can be due to bursitis or tendinitis or even to referred pain from the hip, but if the pain is chronic and if it affects a middle-aged or elderly person, the knee pain is most often due to OA. Hip pain is usually localized to the groin or anterior thigh and, when it is chronically present with weight-bearing activities, it reflects the presence of OA more often than any other cause. OA of the knee affects 11% to 13% of persons aged 65 years and older (3), and it affects roughly 6% of the adult population aged 30 years and older. Hip OA is less than half as prevalent as knee OA, affecting perhaps 2% of the adult population aged 30 and older (3).

OA is a disease in which all elements of the joint are affected pathologically, from the hyaline articular cartilage, which serves to buttress the force between two apposing bones; to the synovium, which is often modestly inflamed; to ligaments that become lax; to bridging muscles that are weak; to the underlying bone itself, which remodels and becomes sclerotic. Although many persons whose knees show pathologic evidence of disease do not have pain, when pain does occur, it is generally brought on by activities. Typically, for example, persons with knee OA will not have pain in the morning on awakening but will experience discomfort or pain going up and down stairs, walking long distances, or getting up out of a chair. Symptomatic OA has a predilection for weight-bearing joints in the body, particularly the knees and hips, and it frequently occurs in hand joints. Other joints, such as ankles and wrists, are rarely affected by this disease. The high frequency of OA in the knee and hip may be because of the weight-bearing stresses, although this does not explain the absence of ankle involvement. Hands may often be affected because they evolved at a time when humans were still brachiating apes;

since then, the pincer grip has become the dominant hand activity, which puts excess stresses on hand joints ill designed for these stresses.

OA can be defined in different ways. Structural pathology may be visualized on x-ray film, and OA on radiographs may reflect biologic changes of disease (Fig. 17.1). However, many persons with such structural disease may have few, if any, symptoms. Symptomatic and clinical disease consists of frequent joint pain and coexistent evidence of structural joint disease (e.g., an x-ray film showing OA).

The etiology of OA is multifaceted, but the earliest lesions appear to be related to episodes of articular cartilage injury and, occasionally, of injury to the bone underlying it. Repeated insults ultimately induce a wearing away of cartilage, changes in the underlying bone, and angulation deformities with ligamentous stretching or even rupture. With increasing inflammation and loss of cartilage, the increase in synovial fluid stretches the joint capsule. Capsular stretching and disuse, perhaps along with other factors, induces muscle weakness. With muscle weakness, a vicious cycle ensues because muscle conditioning and strength play an important role in stabilizing the joint and in protecting it from further joint injury (4,5). With muscle weakness already present, the joint becomes less able to protect itself, and the cycle of arthritic destruction progresses more rapidly.

The course of OA is variable. Although remission is distinctively unusual, episodic symptoms are common, and persons with disease often have severe pain one month and then feel much better the next for no obvious reason. Symptoms can stabilize, can gradually improve, or can slowly worsen. When the disease is advanced, the pain becomes less episodic and more continuous.

OA treatment is multifaceted, consisting of antiinflammatory drugs; injectables; physical therapy and muscle strengthening; the use of canes or crutches; and perhaps nutriceuticals, such as glucosamine and chondroitin (6). When a person with OA of the knee or hip has reached the point at which he or she is experiencing pain at night or when his or her function is limited because of pain, a total joint replacement, an operation that is highly cost-effective and that leads to major improvements in pain and function, is indicated (7).

Back pain is most often episodic, with bouts lasting up to several weeks. Pain can be localized to the lower back, or it can radiate down the back of one or both thighs.

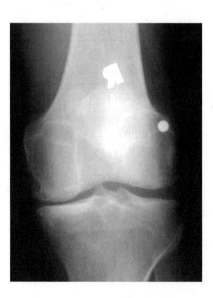

FIGURE 17.1. Knee osteoarthritis as seen on radiograph.

Although uncommon treatable disorders, such as vertebral fractures, cancer, infections, and certain forms of arthritis, may cause back pain, it is most often idiopathic (8). Because the understanding of the pathogenesis of back pain is poor, back pain is generally evaluated without ascribing causation. Current treatments include analgesic treatments and early mobilization with avoidance of triggering activities.

The effect of obesity on these musculoskeletal conditions varies by site and condition, but obesity is one of the best studied risk factors for musculoskeletal conditions, including low back pain and knee and hip OA. Studies evaluating the effect of being overweight or obese on musculoskeletal disorders have used widely varying definitions of these entities.

EXCESS WEIGHT AND THE RISK OF OSTEOARTHRITIS

Knee Osteoarthritis

Cross-sectional studies have consistently shown that obese persons have a higher prevalence of OA of the knee than do nonobese controls (9,10). Estimates of risk vary and depend on both the criteria for obesity and how OA is defined. In one United States nationwide survey in which radiographs were included, obese women (body mass index [BMI] less than 30 kilograms per meter squared [kg/m^2] and up to 35 kg/m^2) had almost four times the risk of knee OA by radiograph as women whose BMI was less than 25 kg/m^2 (10). For men in the same category, the risk was increased 4.8-fold.

Any cross-sectional association could be explained by a tendency for persons with OA to become sedentary and secondarily obese. However, recent longitudinal data disprove this notion and suggest that obesity precedes the development of disease. In the first such study, Felson et al. (11) found that Framingham Heart Study subjects who were overweight during middle age (mean age of 37 years) were at much higher risk of knee OA in their elderly years (mean age of 73 years). Subsequent longitudinal studies from the United States and Europe have proven beyond question that obesity is an important risk factor for the development of OA of the knee (12–14). When followed over time, those who were obese at baseline had a substantially higher risk of developing disease than those who were not. The relationship between weight and the development of OA appears fairly linear, particularly in women, such that, for every increment in increased weight, the risk of knee OA increases. Women in the United States of average weight have a higher risk than thin women.

The knee consists of three connected, but somewhat separate, joints, the medial and lateral tibiofemoral joints and the patellofemoral joint. Disease in at least two of these three compartments (medial and patellofemoral) appears to be increased in prevalence in those who are obese (15,16). The exception to this may be lateral tibiofemoral disease. Obesity increases the risk of bilateral disease in the knees more often than it does that of unilateral disease (17), which is more often associated with an identified knee injury. Moreover, the strong association between obesity and knee OA persists regardless of how the disease is defined. Strong associations have been seen in studies of radiographic disease, of knee symptoms only, and of symptomatic OA. For example, in a recent case-control study of persons seeking care for the first time for their knee OA (18), those with weights of more than 80 kg were at 10.3 times the risk of presenting with symptomatic knee OA as those with weights of less than 63.6 kg.

Although some studies suggest that men who are obese have a similarly high risk of knee OA to women who are obese, many studies report a weaker relationship between obesity and knee OA in men. For example, in the Framingham Study, men who were overweight had no increased risk of incident radiographic disease, whereas women had a substantial risk evaluation (10). Although gender differences are not consistently found, their explanation is unclear.

The timing of obesity's effect on knee OA is unclear. If obesity in childhood were associated with OA in later life, this might suggest effects on the hormonal milieu or on skeletal joint development. It could also speak to early joint injury as a critical precursor to later joint failure. If obesity's effect were strongest in later life before the development of disease, than this might suggest that mechanical factors at a time when the joint was beginning to experience the vulnerabilities of aging would be most likely to cause disease. The latter finding might also offer opportunities for disease prevention. In the Framingham Study, results suggest that weight in middle age and older years is a stronger predictor of disease than is weight earlier in life (11). In contrast, a recent report from the John Hopkins precursor study, a study of male physicians, suggests that BMI between ages 20 and 39 years is more strongly associated with self-reported OA in men than is an increased BMI later in life (19).

Not only are obese people at high risk for developing knee OA, longitudinal studies suggest that, for those who already have knee OA, obesity predisposes them to a higher risk of progression (20). Women who are overweight and who have unilateral OA of the knee may be at much higher risk of developing bilateral disease than are their nonobese counterparts (21).

Hip Osteoarthritis

Like the knee, the hip is a weight-bearing joint in which obesity leads to increased loading. Not surprisingly therefore, most studies suggest that people who are overweight have a higher-than-expected risk of hip OA. Whereas the relationship of obesity with knee OA is strong and consistent across studies, the same cannot be said for studies of obesity and hip OA (3).

Studies evaluating the relationship between obesity and *radiographic* hip OA have been particularly inconsistent, especially for unilateral disease (Table 17.1). Based on the results of at least three studies, bilateral hip OA disease is clearly related to obesity (22–24). Among 5,000 women who had undergone hip radiographs as part of the Study of Osteoporotic Fractures, obesity was associated with an 80% increase in odds of bilateral hip OA (odds ratio [OR] = 1.8) but only a 40% increase in unilateral OA (OR = 1.4).

TABLE 17.1. *Obesity and the prevalence of bilateral and unilateral hip osteoarthritis*

Author (yr)	Reference	Disease definition	Odds ratio (95% CI) for association of obesity with bilateral OA	Odds ratio (95% CI) for association of obesity with unilateral OA
Tepper and Hochberg (1993) (NHANES)	23	Radiographic	2.0 (0.97, 4.2)	0.5 (0.3, 1.2)
Heliovaara et al. (1993)	22	Clinical	For BMI more than 30–35 kg/m^2: 2.3 (1.5, 3.5)	1.6 (1.0, 2.5)
			For BMI more than 35 kg/m^2: 2.8 (1.4, 5.7)	1.0 (0.5, 3.0)
Nevitt et al. (1993)	24	Radiographic	For heaviest quintile: 1.8 (1.1, 2.9)	1.4 (0.9, 2.1)

Abbreviations: BMI, body mass index; CI, confidence interval; NHANES, National Health and Nutrition Examination Survey; OA, osteoarthritis.

TABLE 17.2. *Studies of weight and prevalent clinical hip osteoarthritis*

Reference	Total number (number of cases)	Disease definition	General findings
Saville and Dickson (1968)	121 (121)	Clinical	Negative (no internal controls)
Kraus et al. (1978)	200 (100)	Severe clinical	Obese, RR = 2.7, $p < .0005$
Vingard (1991)	569 (247)	THR patients (clinical)	Overweight age 40 yr, OR = 3.5 (1.4, 4.5)
Heliovaara et al. (1993) (reference 22)	7217 (369)	Clinical	Obese, OR = 2.0
Vingard et al. (1997)	540 (242)	THR patients (clinical)	BMI ≥25 vs. BMI <20 kg/m^2: OR = 2.9 (1.3, 6.5)
Karlson et al. (2000)	121,700 (567)	THR patients (clinical)	Highest vs. lowest quintile of weight; OR = 2.6 (1.7, 3.9)

Abbreviations: BMI, body mass index; OR, odds ratio; RR, relative risk; THR, total hip replacement.

Obese persons have a high risk of developing *symptomatic* hip OA (Table 17.2). Persons with symptomatic hip OA consistently tend to be heavier than those without it, and, compared with persons of normal weight, those who are obese have a twofold to three-fold increased risk of developing the symptomatic form of the disease, a risk, however, that is not as high as that seen for knee OA.

Why does the relationship of obesity and hip OA differ depending on how *disease* is defined? The association of obesity with symptomatic disease could be explained by the idea that obesity induces hip symptoms in those with structural disease. Alternatively, the failure to detect an association of obesity with unilateral radiographic hip OA could reflect the inexactitude of the definition. That the association is stronger with bilateral as opposed to unilateral radiographic disease suggests that when radiographic disease is clear-cut in both hips, the association with obesity emerges. The most likely explanation for these differences is that the more precisely defined or severe the hip OA is, then the greater the likelihood is that it is associated with obesity.

Why obese persons do not have as high a risk of hip OA as they do of getting the disease in the knee is still unclear. The force across the hip joint during weight bearing is distributed broadly across a large weight-bearing surface, whereas in the knee, 60% to 70% of the force is concentrated in the medial compartment and it may not be distributed evenly throughout that compartment. Thus, the multiplier effect of obesity in the knee may increase local cartilage stresses to the point of injury, whereas the stress or force per square inch that bears on hip joint cartilage may be less. In addition, some of the adiposity in obese persons may be located below the hip joint, which does not increase loading on that joint. Lastly, factors other than loading, such as developmental abnormalities, may play a prominent role in causing hip OA; because of this, many cases of hip OA may not be related to obesity.

Explaining Why Obesity Causes Osteoarthritis

Weight could, in theory, act in three ways to cause OA. First and most logically, being overweight increases the loading across weight-bearing joints, thereby inducing cartilage breakdown. Second, adipose tissue could affect the concentrations of metabolic products, which themselves act on articular cartilage or on other joint structures to produce joint degradation. Third, obesity could be a confounder associated, but not casually, with another factor that itself produces OA. Some have suggested, for example, that a genetic mutation or abnormality may be responsible for both obesity and OA. The last explanation—that obesity itself is a confounder—is unlikely. Relationships found between obesity and knee OA are very strong, and, as noted by Walker (25), to qualify as an explanatory factor, a factor such as inheritance must be a stronger risk factor for disease than the associated factor (obesity) is, and it must be highly correlated with the associated factor (i.e., it must be strongly correlated with obesity). Based on the strength of association of obesity with knee OA and the inconsistently reported heritability of knee OA, that genetic or even other confounding factors could cause both knee OA and obesity appears highly unlikely. Thus, the third explanation listed previously is probably incorrect. Thus, the medical community is left with weighing the persuasiveness of mechanical versus metabolic explanations.

Complex Mechanical Effects of Excess Weight

In terms of joint mechanics, the overall force across the knee and hip are approximately two to three times the body weight during walking (26). Every pound of excess weight can be multiplied by this factor to determine its effect on knee and hip forces. During certain activities, such as climbing stairs and getting up out of a chair, knee and hip forces reach levels that are even higher, and every pound of excess weight exerts its force according to this even higher multiplier. Thus, although the tolerable limits of stress (force per unit area) inside the knee and hip are unknown, obesity in the face of ongoing daily activity substantially increases mechanical stress across the joint.

In the face of this loading assault, the body brings to bear several joint-protective mechanisms that ideally prevent any joint damage and later OA. These mechanisms include joint surfaces with excellent lubrication that are frictionless; ligaments and tendons, which assume the proper tension and position to minimize joint loading; and particularly muscles that, when they contract, serve as shock absorbers, cushioning sudden impulse loads, such as those that occur when the heel hits the floor during gait or going down stairs. The cushioning impact of footwear could also be viewed as another way of absorbing the shock of the impulse that occurs during gait. With faster walking, this impulse becomes greater and, with running, even greater. These counterbalancing forces are depicted in Fig. 17.2, in which body weight and speed of walking are potential magnifiers of force on the left side while shock absorption on the right side of the figure serves as a likely protector. Shock absorption is a function of the joint-protective mechanisms noted earlier, particularly muscle contraction. High cartilage stresses result when body weight and/or speed of gait overcome the intrinsic protective mechanisms.

If this pathophysiologic explanation for joint injury is correct, then logically, obese persons who are weak are at a high risk of OA, and, moreover, when weak obese persons perform activities that load weight-bearing joints, they are at exceedingly high risk. Indeed, recent work in a population study looking at the prevalence of knee OA suggests that, among women who are overweight with knee OA, quadriceps weakness may be a centrally important factor distinguishing obese women with knee OA from those without it (27). Quadriceps generally become stronger with increased weight, because quadriceps and other weight-bearing muscles have to cope with the increased loading conferred by obesity. Paradoxically, in women with knee OA, lower quadriceps strength is present. Interestingly, quadriceps weakness is not necessarily a feature of knee OA in men. This may explain why obesity is such a potent risk factor for knee OA in women and why it is less so in men; in women, knee OA is often coupled with quadriceps weakness, whereas in men, it is not.

Injurious activities may include going up and down stairs and participating in active leisure time activities. In the Framingham Study, both of these types of activities were

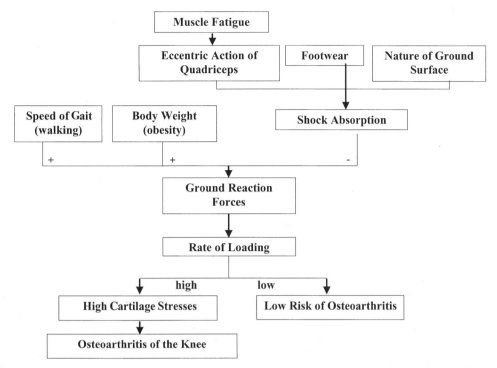

FIGURE 17.2. The effect of counterbalancing forces of body weight, gait, and joint shock absorption on joint loading and osteoarthritis risk. (From Syed Y, Davis BL. Obesity and osteoarthritis of the knee: hypotheses concerning the relationship between ground reaction forces and quadriceps fatigue in long-duration walking. *Med Hypotheses* 2000;54:182–185, with permission.)

associated with high rates of subsequent development of symptomatic knee OA (28), but these activities were especially likely to induce disease if the subjects at baseline were above average body weight. Thus, any explanation of the effect of obesity on OA must incorporate an understanding of other injurious activities, such as joint injuries, and must account for joint-protective mechanisms, such as muscle strength. With these complex data, insight into how obesity works to cause knee and hip OA can be achieved. Further, an understanding of these other protective and injurious factors can provide guidance about how individuals may lower their risk of disease. In theory, those with quadriceps weakness and obesity are at particularly high risk of OA when participating in weight-bearing exercise programs. To optimize joint protection in these vulnerable persons, the clinician may recommend quadriceps strengthening and gradual gentle entry into weight-bearing exercise activities.

Certain persons may be at higher risk of obesity-related knee OA than are others. Specifically, most loading in the knee occurs across the medial or inner aspect of the joint. This is particularly true of persons whose knees are aligned in a varus (or bow-legged) fashion. Such persons bear even more loading across the inner aspect of their knee than do persons whose knees are oriented or aligned in a valgus (knock-kneed) manner. Those with varus alignment may be more vulnerable to the OA effects of obesity than are those with valgus alignment, in which forces may be more equitably distributed across both compartments of the knee (29).

Metabolic Concomitants of Adiposity

Explaining the effect of obesity on the risk of OA by invoking mechanical explanations fails to explain one intriguing observation that has been inconsistently reported. Women who are overweight in some, but not all, studies have an increased risk of developing hand OA (30). This increased risk may be mediated mechanically because overweight women and men are stronger and they exert more force across even non–weight-bearing joints, and this could lead to hand OA. Nonetheless, a possible association of obesity with hand OA begs for other explanations. These other explanations consist of metabolic features of adiposity, which may in turn have direct effects on intraarticular structures, such as cartilage. By metabolic features, the authors mean that persons with excess adipose tissue may have abnormal levels of certain hormones or growth factors that affect cartilage or underlying bone in such a way that predisposes them to the development of OA.

Because the location of adipose tissue has been linked to specific metabolic abnormalities, evaluating fat distribution and its relationship to OA might provide clues about whether metabolic factors explain some of this relationship. However, studies evaluating waist to hip ratio, waist circumference, and other anthropometric measurements of adiposity have reported that these do not explain the relationship of body weight with OA. Once body weight is incorporated as a risk factor, these measures of localized tissue distribution of adipose tissue yield no additional information (31–33).

Another factor might be diabetes, which is obviously increased in prevalence in obese people. Furthermore, insulin is a potent growth factor for bone and cartilage, and levels of insulin are usually elevated early in diabetes. However, the obesity–knee OA association is not attenuated by adjusting for the presence of diabetes in general, and evidence suggests that, at best, a weak correlation exists between the occurrence of diabetes and knee OA (34–36).

OA is often conceived of as a disorder in which cartilage matrix repair is overwhelmed by degradative process. Factors that increase cartilage matrix synthesis would protect against OA. One such factor may be insulin-like growth factor-1 (IGF-1), which increases cartilage matrix synthesis, and high circulating levels might, in theory, protect against OA. Epidemiologic studies, unfortunately, have not confirmed that high serum levels of IGF-1 are associated with the reduced risk in OA. In fact, two such studies have been conducted: One of them has shown no relationship between IGF-1 levels and the development or progression of OA, and the other study paradoxically has shown that high IGF-1 levels actually increase the risk of developing progressive disease in the knee (37,38). IGF-1 levels may be decreased in those with abdominal adiposity, but without additional evidence to suggest that these lower than normal levels predispose these individuals to OA, supporting the notion that this accounts for the effect of obesity on OA may be difficult.

Obese postmenopausal women not only have a higher risk of OA than nonobese women, but they also have higher circulating estrogen levels. Little evidence exists to suggest that these high estrogen levels predispose to OA. First, women with hand OA appear to have no different levels of estradiol than women without it (39). Second, a series of epidemiologic studies evaluating the rate of OA in postmenopausal estrogen users versus nonusers reports in general that estrogen-replacement therapy, if anything, lowers the risk of OA, rather than increasing it (40).

One clear-cut intermediary by which obesity may cause OA is its effect on increasing bone mineral density. Overweight and obese women have substantially higher bone mineral density at all body sites than do thin women. Furthermore, women with high bone density are at high risk of getting OA (41,42). In studies in which the relationship between obesity and knee OA is tested, however, adjusting additionally for bone mineral density does not attenuate the strong associations seen between obesity and knee OA much. These analyses would suggest that, although high bone density may be one mechanism by which obesity acts to cause knee OA, this is not the main explanation.

While a specific metabolic explanation accounting for the relationship between obesity and OA is as yet not forthcoming, an unidentified metabolic factor may play an important role. In a study in which monozygotic twins who differed in their weight were evaluated, the heavier twin was much more likely to develop knee OA than was the lighter one but he or she was not more likely to develop hand OA in most hand joints (43). The one exception to this was the base of the thumb where the overweight twin was indeed more likely to get OA, although the risk in that obese twin was not nearly the same as the heightened risk of disease in the knee. If one uses the knee OA increase in the heavier monozygotic twin as evidence of a mechanical effect and the absence of hand OA in that same twin as lack of evidence of a metabolic effect, then one can conclude that mechanical effects probably account for more of the association between obesity and OA than do metabolic ones.

WEIGHT LOSS TO PREVENT OR TREAT OSTEOARTHRITIS

Prevention

Persons who are overweight or those who are overweight with incipient knee or hip symptoms might wish to lower their risk of getting OA (or a worse disease) by losing weight. No clinical trials have been performed to test whether weight loss has an effect on the risk of developing OA in those considered at high risk. In the Framingham Osteoarthritis Study, in subjects tracked longitudinally, weight change over time affected the risk of developing OA; those who gained weight were at increased risk and those who lost weight lowered their risk. For example, the odds of developing radiographically evidenced OA decreased by 40% for every 10-lb loss in weight over 8 years (44). This effect of weight change was seen in women but not in men.

Treatment

Many clinicians recommend weight loss to their patients with knee and hip OA, but a remarkable paucity of information supports this recommendation. In a study of morbidly obese subjects who were more than 40 kg above ideal weight and who were subjected to gastroplasty operations leading to a loss of an average 44 kg, the percentage of subjects with frequent knee pain decreased from 57% to 14% (45). Although drastic weight loss may certainly affect the prevalence and severity of knee symptoms, the effects of more modest weight losses are unclear. In a clinical trial evaluating the efficacy of an appetite suppressant in patients with knee and hip OA, Williams and Foulsham (46) found no significant effect of the appetite suppressant compared with the placebo, but they did report that, in their subjects with knee OA, the amount of weight loss correlated well (correlation coefficient $[r] = 0.45$, $p < 0.05$) with clinical improvement. They found no such correlation in persons with hip OA, in whom, as was noted earlier, the relationship with obesity is somewhat weaker. A randomized pilot trial comparing exercise with exercise and weight loss did not have enough subjects to evaluate the effect of weight loss on knee OA symptoms definitively, but it did show that those in the weight loss and exercise group lost more weight and that they experienced a normalization of their gait with a willingness to walk faster with a longer stride length and cadence. Furthermore, although the effect was nonsignificantly different from the control group, those in the weight loss group experienced a significant and absolute improvement in their ability to ambulate without assistance or difficulty (47). Thus, although no definitive evidence is available, studies suggest that weight loss is likely to be efficacious in persons with knee OA, but the amount of weight loss necessary to trigger substantial improvement may be difficult to achieve readily.

Exercise is a central element in the treatment of OA in obese and nonobese patients. First, muscle weakness is a consequence of disease, and stronger muscles may provide better shock absorption for weight-bearing impulse loads. Further, in OA, the degree of muscle weakness correlates directly with the severity of disability. Exercise has been shown to lessen pain and disability in knee OA (48).

OBESITY AND THE OUTCOMES OF TOTAL KNEE AND HIP REPLACEMENT

As was noted earlier, overweight persons are at high risk of developing knee and hip OA, and the optimal treatment for advanced disease in these joints is total joint replacement, which is also known as *total joint arthroplasty*. The sites at which this operation is most often conducted are the knees and hips. Total joint arthroplasty is extremely effective in alleviating pain and improving function. Most patients undergoing these operations experience dramatic improvements in disabling pain and an enhanced ability to walk. Arthroplasties last from 10 to 20 years. A cost-effectiveness analysis suggests that, because arthroplasty usually eliminates most of the ongoing costs of care for persons with OA, these operations may actually be cost saving (49). Because obese persons are at higher risk of both diseases for which total joint arthroplasty is usually performed, their experience with total joint arthroplasty in terms of effectiveness and of complication rates is of great importance.

Orthopedists were initially reluctant to perform these operations on obese persons because of the theoretical concerns that obesity would impart destructive stresses on the synthetic components of the arthroplasty, thus wearing it out quickly. Therefore, any increased weight would be magnified in its effect on an artificial joint by the multiplier effect of body weight on joint loading as described earlier. As predicted, initial case series of obese patients undergoing hip arthroplasty showed frequent operative complications, such as a high rate of wound infections; and natural history studies have suggested high rates of failure of total hip arthroplasty in overweight persons with loosening of both femoral and acetabular components at a rate that is much higher than that among those who are not obese (50,51). Although orthopedists do perform hip replacements on obese patients, the long-term survival of these implants may be abbreviated.

In contrast to these results regarding hip arthroplasty, long-term follow-up data of persons with total knee arthroplasty from different centers suggest that obese persons (defined as weights of more than 80 kg or as BMI > 30 kg/m^2) have similar functional outcomes as those of nonobese persons (52–54). In a large series from an orthopedic hospital in New York, in which patients were followed for more than 10 years, functional improvements in obese patients (BMI > 30 kg/m^2) were similar to or perhaps even greater than improvements in nonobese persons (53). In a large hospital series from the Midwest, obese persons did as well after total knee replacement (TKR) as those who were not obese (54). Even so, complications of obesity in total knee arthroplasty do occur. First, obese persons appear to have an increased frequency of lucent lines around the prosthetic components, especially on the tibial side, although these often do not progress and their meaning is unknown (53). They can be a harbinger of loosening of the component. Second, obese persons have a higher rate of patellofemoral symptoms after TKR. These symptoms include pain on arising from a chair and when going up and down stairs, and they are thought to be due to the increased stress across the patella during these activities. Finally, despite some reassuring follow-up data, given the multiplier effect of weight on knees and the concentration of stresses on the medial compartment of the knee during weight bearing, loosening rates among obese persons undergoing TKR are still likely to be higher than those among nonobese persons.

Despite these cautionary concerns, orthopedic surgeons are increasingly performing total joint replacements in obese persons with knee and hip OA.

OBESITY AND BACK PAIN

Back pain is widely considered a major health problem. The lifetime prevalence of low back pain in industrialized countries has been estimated to be as high as 84%, and as high as 33% of individuals have suffered from low back pain in the past month (55,56). In industrialized countries, back pain prevalence is two to four times greater than it is in rural low-income countries (57). Back pain is also less prevalent in children and adolescents. For children aged 12 years, the point prevalence of low back pain has been estimated at 1%. This prevalence increases to 10% by the age of 20 years for women and by the age of 25 years for men (58).

Back pain is seldom considered life threatening. Nevertheless, disability secondary to back pain can be severe, and it frequently includes occupational, psychologic, behavioral, and avocational components. In older adults, disability from back pain often includes difficulty performing basic activities of daily living. In the United States, low back pain has been estimated to cost up to $50 billion dollars yearly in health care expenditures alone (59).

Numerous studies have explored the association between obesity and back pain. The premise behind these studies is that an increase in mechanical loading on the spine from greater weight is a contributing factor to the onset of back pain. Leboeuf-Yde (60) conducted a review of 65 studies published between 1965 and 1997 on obesity and low back pain. Approximately half of these studies reported a positive, albeit often weak, association between obesity and low back pain. The author concluded that not enough evidence was available to make the determination of whether a causal relation between body weight and low back pain exists. The author also concluded that no meaningful differences in study results were found when considering gender, the definition of body weight, the population studied, or the type of analysis conducted (60). Work published since this review has not necessarily been more revealing. A twin study showed no relation between BMI differences of monozygotic twins and their likelihood of having low back pain (61).

Most studies on obesity and back pain have analyzed cross-sectional data. This study design does not address the issue of whether obesity precedes and causes the back symptoms or whether back pain precedes the obesity. This latter possibility is a reasonable concern because obesity can be caused by the decrease in activity that commonly results from back pain. Lake et al. (62) performed a longitudinal study assessing the association between obesity and back pain in a population of more than 8,000 men and women. The investigators concluded that obese women had an increased risk of subsequent back pain that could not be explained by an effect of back pain on obesity. This association was absent among men (62).

The question of whether weight change is associated with a reduction in back symptoms has also been investigated. In one study, 105 subjects who underwent vertical banded gastroplasty for obesity were followed for an average of 22.5 months. Before surgery, all of the subjects were at least 45 kg overweight. On average, subjects lost 44 kg during the follow-up. At follow-up, the number of subjects with low back pain had decreased from 62 to 11 individuals (46). However, in another study with less dramatic weight change, no association was found between either weight at baseline or a change in weight by follow-up 10 years later and the onset of low back pain (63).

Thus, the causal association between obesity and back pain is most likely either weak or absent. Although obesity has been shown to have a strong effect on other aspects of health, it does not appear to have a large impact on back pain.

CONCLUSION

Obesity increases the risk of knee and to a lesser extent hip OA, which combined affect a large percentage of middle-aged and elderly adults and which are a major source of disability. Increased loading of weight-bearing joints probably explains this increase in risk, although metabolic concomitants of obesity may also play a role in joint injury. Weight loss, perhaps even a modest amount, prevents disease from developing and structural progression from occurring when it is already present. Although an absence of large-scale trials exists, weight loss appears to ameliorate knee, but not necessarily hip, symptoms. Obese patients with knee OA are good candidates for TKR, with prosthesis survival rates that are comparable to those of nonobese persons. Hip replacements, however, loosen more quickly in obese than in nonobese patients, leading to prosthesis failure.

Despite a widespread perception that obese persons are at increased risk of back pain, evidence suggests a tenuous association at best.

ACKNOWLEDGMENTS

The authors would like to thank Kitty Bentzler for expert technical assistance and Dr. Thomas Einhorn for advice regarding the advisability of joint replacement in obese subjects. Dr. Felson's work is supported by National Institutes of Health grant AR47785.

REFERENCES

1. Verbrugge LM. From sneezes to adieux: stages of health for American men and women. *Soc Sci Med* 1986;22: 1195–1212.
2. Edmond S, Felson DT. Prevalence of back symptoms in elders. *J Rheumatol* 2000;27:220–225.
3. Felson DT, Zhang Y. An update on the epidemiology of knee and hip osteoarthritis with a view to prevention. *Arthritis Rheum* 1998;41:1343–1355.
4. Brandt KD. Putting some muscle into osteoarthritis. *Ann Intern Med* 1997;127:154–156.
5. O'Reilly S, Jones A, Doherty M. Muscle weakness in osteoarthritis. *Curr Opin Rheum* 1997;9:259–262.
6. Hochberg MC, McAlindon T, Felson DT. Systemic and topical treatments. Osteoarthritis, new insights part 2: treatment approaches. *Ann Intern Med* 2000;133:726–737.
7. Chang RW, Pellisier JM, Hazen GB. A cost-effectiveness analysis of total hip arthroplasty for osteoarthritis of the hip. *JAMA* 1996;275:858–865.
8. Engstrom JW. Back and neck pain. In: Braunwald E, Fauci AS, Kasper DL, et al., eds. *Harrison's principles of internal medicine,* 15th ed. New York: McGraw-Hill, 2001:79–90.
9. Felson DT, Chaisson CE. Understanding the relationship between body weight and osteoarthritis. *Billieres Clin Epidemiol* 1997;11:671–681.
10. Anderson JJ, Felson DT. Factors associated with osteoarthritis of the knee in the first National Health and Nutrition Examination Survey (NHANES I). *Am J Epidemiol* 1988;128:179–189.

11. Felson DT, Anderson JJ, Naimark A, et al. Obesity and knee osteoarthritis: the Framingham Study. *Ann Intern Med* 1988;109:18–24.
12. Felson DT, Zhang Y, Hannan MT, et al. Risk factors for incident radiographic knee osteoarthritis in the elderly: the Framingham Study. *Arthritis Rheum* 1997;40:728–733.
13. Manninen P, Riihimaki H, Heliovaara M, et al. Overweight, gender and knee osteoarthritis. *Int J Obes* 1996;20: 595–597.
14. Cooper C, Snow S, McAlindon TE, et al. Risk factors for the incidence and progression of radiographic knee osteoarthritis. *Arthritis Rheum* 2000;43:995–1000.
15. McAlindon T, Zhang Y, Hannan M, et al. Are risk factors for patellofemoral and tibiofemoral knee osteoarthritis different? *J Rheumatol* 1996;23:332–337.
16. Cicuttini FM, Baker JR, Spector TD. The association of obesity with osteoarthritis of the hand and knee in women: a twin study. *J Rheumatol* 1996;23:1221–1226.
17. Davis MA, Ettinger WH, Neuhaus JM. The role of metabolic factors and blood pressure in the association of obesity with osteoarthritis of the knee. *J Rheum* 1988;15:1827–1832.
18. Oliveria SA, Felson DT, Cirillo PA, et al. Body weight, body mass index, and incident symptomatic osteoarthritis of the hand, hip and knee. *Epidemiology* 1999;10:161–166.
19. Gelber AC, Hochberg MC, Mead LA, et al. Body mass index in young men and the risk of subsequent knee and hip osteoarthritis. *Am J Med* 1999;107:542–548.
20. Dougados M, Gueguen A, Nguyen M, et al. Longitudinal radiologic evaluation of osteoarthritis of the knee. *J Rheumatol* 1992;19:378–383.
21. Spector TD, Hart DJ, Doyle DV. Incidence and progression of osteoarthritis in women with unilateral knee disease in the general population: the effect of obesity. *Ann Rheum Dis* 1994;53:565–568.
22. Heliovaara M, Mkel M, Impivaara O, et al. Association of overweight, trauma and workload with coxarthrosis: a health survey of 7,217 persons. *Acta Orthop Scand* 1993;64:513–518.
23. Tepper S, Hochberg MC. Factors associated with hip osteoarthritis: data from the First National Health and Nutrition Examination Survey (NHANES-I). *Am J Epidemiol* 1993;137:1081–1088.
24. Nevitt MC, Lane NE, Scott JC, et al. Relationship of hip osteoarthritis to obesity and bone mineral density in older American women: preliminary results from the Study of Osteoporotic Fractures. *Acta Orthop Scand* 1993; 64:2–5.
25. Walker AM. *Observation and Inference. An introduction to the methods of epidemiology.* Chestnut Hill, MA: Epidemiology Resources, 1991.
26. Schipplein OD, Andriacchi TP. Interaction between active and passive knee stabilizers during level walking. *J Orthop Res* 1991;9:113–119.
27. Slemenda C, Brandt KD, Heilman DK, et al. Quadriceps weakness and osteoarthritis of the knee. *Ann Intern Med* 1997;127:97–104.
28. McAlindon TE, Wilson PW, Aliabadi P, et al. Level of physical activity and the risk of radiographic and symptomatic knee osteoarthritis in the elderly: the Framingham study. *Am J Med* 1999;106:151–157.
29. Sharma L, Lou C, Cahue S, et al. The mechanism of the effect of obesity in knee osteoarthritis. *Arthritis Rheum* 2000;43:568–575.
30. Carman WJ, Sowers M, Hawthorne VM, et al. Obesity as a risk factor for osteoarthritis of the hand and wrist: a prospective study. *Am J Epidemiol* 1994;139:119–129.
31. Davis MA, Neuhaus JM, Ettinger WH, et al. Body fat distribution and osteoarthritis. *Am J Epidemiol* 1990;132:710–707.
32. Hart DJ, Spector TD. The relationship of obesity, fat distribution and osteoarthritis in women in the general population: the Chingford Study. *J Rheumatol* 1993;20:331–335.
33. Hochberg MC, Lethbridge-Cejku M, Scott WW Jr, et al. The association of body weight, body fatness and body fat distribution with osteoarthritis of the knee: data from the Baltimore Longitudinal Study of aging. *J Rheumatol* 1995;22:488–493.
34. Davis M, Ettinger WH, Neuhaus JM. The role of metabolic factors and blood pressure in the association of obesity with osteoarthritis of the knee. *J Rheumatol* 1988;15:1827–1832.
35. Felson DT, Anderson JJ, Naimark A, et al. Obesity and knee osteoarthritis. *Ann Intern Med* 1988;109:18–24.
36. Frey MI, Barrett-Connor E, Sledge PA, et al. The effect of non–insulin-dependent diabetes mellitus on the prevalence of clinical osteoarthritis. A population based study. *J Rheumatol* 1996;23:716–722.
37. Fraenkel L, Zhang Y, Trippel SB, et al. Longitudinal analysis of the relationship between serum insulin-like growth factor-I and radiographic knee osteoarthritis. *Osteoarthritis Cartilage* 1998;6:362–367.
38. Schouten JS, Van den Ouweland FA, Valkenburg HA, et al. Insulin-like growth factor-1: a prognostic factor of knee osteoarthritis. *Br J Rheumatol* 1993;32:274–280.
39. Cauley JA, Kwoh CK, Egeland G, et al. Serum sex hormones and severity of osteoarthritis of the hand. *J Rheumatol* 1993;20:1170–1175.
40. Nevitt MC, Felson DT. Sex hormones and the risk of osteoarthritis in women: epidemiological evidence. *Ann Rheum Dis* 1996;55:673–676.
41. Hannan MT, Anderson JJ, Zhang Y, et al. Bone mineral density and knee osteoarthritis in elderly men and women. *J Bone Miner Res* 1992;7:547–553.
42. Dequeker J, Boonen S, Aerssens J, et al. Inverse relationship osteoarthritis-osteoporosis: what is the evidence? What are the consequences? *Br J Rheumatol* 1996;35:813–818.

43. Cicuttini FM, Baker JR, Spector TD. The association of obesity with osteoarthritis of the hand and knee in women: a twin study. *J Rheumatol* 1996;23:1221–1226.

44. Felson DT, Zhang Y, Hannan MT, et al. Risk factors for incident radiographic knee osteoarthritis in the elderly: the Framingham Study. *Arthritis Rheum* 1997;40:728–733.

45. McGoey BV, Deitel M, Saplys RJ, et al. Effect of weight loss on musculoskeletal pain in the morbidly obese. *J Bone Joint Surg Br* 1990;72:322–323.

46. Williams RA, Foulsham BM. Weight reduction in osteoarthritis using phentermine. *Practitioner* 1981;225: 231–232.

47. Messier SP, Loeser RF, Mitchell MN, et al. Exercise and weight loss in obese older adults with knee osteoarthritis: a preliminary study. *J Am Geriatr Soc* 2000;48:1062–1072.

48. Baker K, McAlindon TE. Exercise for knee osteoarthritis. *Curr Opin Rheum* 2000;12:456–463.

49. Chang RW, Pellisier JM, Hazen GB. A cost-effectiveness analysis of total hip arthroplasty for osteoarthritis of the hip. *JAMA* 1996;275:858–865.

50. Surin VV, Sundholm K. Survival of patients and prostheses after total hip arthroplasty. *Clin Orthop* 1983;177: 148–153.

51. Olsson SS, Jernberger A, Tryggo D. Clinical and radiological long-term results after Charnley–Müller total hip replacement. *Acta Orthop Scand* 1981;52:531–542.

52. Stern SH, Insall JN. Total knee arthroplasty in obese patients. *J Bone Joint Surg Am* 1990;72:1400–1404.

53. Griffin FM, Scuderi GR, Insall JN, et al. Total knee arthroplasty in patients who were obese with 10 years follow-up. *Clin Orthop* 1998;356:28–33.

54. Smith BE, Askew MJ, Gradisar IA, et al. The effect of patient weight on the functional outcome of total knee arthroplasty. *Clin Orthop* 1992;276:237–243.

55. Cassidy JD, Carroll LJ, Cote P. The Saskatchewan health and back pain survey. *Spine* 1998;23:1860–1867.

56. Skovron ML, Szpalski M, Nordin M, et al. Sociocultural factors and back pain: a population-based study in Belgian adults. *Spine* 1994;19:129–137.

57. Volinn E. The epidemiology of low back pain in the rest of the world: a review of surveys in low- and middle-income countries. *Spine* 1997;22:1747–1754.

58. Leboeuf-Yde C, Kyvik KO. At what age does low back pain become a common problem? A study of 29,424 individuals aged 12–41 years. *Spine* 1998;23:228–234.

59. Frymoyer JW, Cats-Baril WL. An overview of the incidence and costs of low back pain. *Orthop Clin North Am* 1991;22:263–271.

60. Leboeuf-Yde C. Body weight and low back pain: a systematic literature review of 56 articles reporting on 65 epidemiologic studies. *Spine* 2000;25:226–237.

61. Leboeuf-Yde C, Kyvik KO, Bruun NH. Low back pain and lifestyle. Part II: obesity information from a population-based sample of 29,424 twin subjects. *Spine* 1999;24:779–784.

62. Lake JK, Power C, Cole TJ. Back pain and obesity in the 1958 British birth cohort: cause or effect? *J Clin Epidemiol* 2000;53:245–250.

63. Aro S, Leino P. Overweight and musculoskeletal morbidity: a ten-year follow-up. *Int J Obes* 1985;9:267–275.

64. Syed Y, Davis BL. Obesity and osteoarthritis of the knee: hypotheses concerning the relationship between ground reaction forces and quadriceps fatigue in long-duration walking. *Med Hypotheses* 2000;54:182–185.

PART III

Therapeutics

18

Behavioral Treatment of Obesity: Strategies to Improve Outcome and Predictors of Success

Rena R. Wing and Suzanne Phelan

Behavioral approaches to the treatment of obesity are designed to help participants learn new behaviors related to energy balance. Simply put, this involves teaching participants to reduce caloric intake and to increase energy expenditure. This chapter reviews the history of behavioral approaches, describes the results that are currently achieved, and then discusses new strategies that are being used to improve the efficacy of behavioral programs. Predictors of outcome in behavioral treatment programs are then reviewed.

HISTORY OF BEHAVIORAL TREATMENT FOR OBESITY

Behavioral techniques were first applied to the problem of obesity in 1960 to 1970 (1). These approaches grew out of learning theory, and they emphasized the importance of focusing on eating and exercise behaviors and of changing the antecedents and consequences (reinforcers) that controlled these behaviors (2). The goal in these early programs was to make patients aware of their behaviors and to change their behavioral patterns (e.g., where and when food was eaten), rather than changing the actual caloric intake or energy balance. Key strategies included self-monitoring (participants were taught to write down what they ate and the circumstances associated with eating), stimulus control (which emphasized removing cues for inappropriate eating, increasing cues for appropriate eating, eating in only one place, and slowing the act of eating), and self-reinforcement (participants were taught to identify alternative sources of reinforcement) (3). Patients were encouraged to increase lifestyle activity, but the focus again was on behavioral patterns rather than on the calories used in the activity.

Although the earliest behavioral program was conducted individually with the client (1), the field rapidly moved to group interventions. Initially, these programs involved weekly meetings for 8 to 10 weeks (4). On average, participants lost 3.8 to 4.2 kg over this interval. When followed up 15 weeks later, the average weight loss was 4.0 kg (2,5). Weight losses achieved in these early behavioral programs were shown to be greater than those achieved with nutrition therapy or psychotherapy.

Behavioral treatment programs evolved from 1970 to 1990 to include heavier patients at entry, longer treatment intervals, and longer duration of follow-up. In addition, the treatment program began to focus more explicitly on energy balance. Patients were given specific goals for caloric intake and for energy expenditure from exercise. Stimulus-control approaches were expanded not only to deal with physical cues related to eating and exercising but also to address the psychologic and social cues. The results of these interventions gradually improved to an average weight loss of 8.5 kg at 21 weeks (2,4). At 1-

415

year follow-up, patients maintained a weight loss of 5.6 kg (i.e., 66% of their initial weight loss).

Since 1990, there has been further strengthening of behavioral approaches aimed at improving both initial weight loss and long-term maintenance. The current state of the art for behavioral treatment of obesity is described below.

CURRENT BEHAVIORAL TREATMENT PROGRAMS

Currently, most behavioral programs are offered in a group format with 6 months of weekly meetings followed by 6 months of biweekly meetings and 6 months of monthly meetings. A closed group format, in which 10 to 20 participants begin the group program together and remain together as they proceed through the program, is typically used. The program is led by a multidisciplinary team of therapists, including individuals trained in nutrition, exercise physiology, and clinical psychology.

Behavioral programs provide a structured series of lessons that are designed to teach participants to modify their diet and exercise behaviors. An example of a 26-lesson series and an overview of the principles being taught in these lessons are found in Table 18.1.

A key component of behavioral programs is *self-monitoring* (6). Participants are given a calorie and fat goal for intake and are taught to write down everything they eat, to figure out calories and fat in those foods using a resource book, and to keep a running total of their intake to ensure they stay within their calorie and fat goal. Dietary intake is recorded every week for the first 6 months and periodically thereafter. These records are often reviewed by a therapist, who provides specific guidance on food choices and supportive feedback to the participant. Similarly, participants self-monitor their physical activity using either calories per bout of activity or minutes of activity. Again, this infor-

TABLE 18.1. *Lessons covered during first 6 months of a behavioral treatment program*

Behavioral approach to changing your eating and exercise habits
Increasing your physical activity: programmed exercise
Developing a healthy low-fat eating plan
Cues in your physical environment for eating and exercise
Building social support
Increasing physical activity through lifestyle changes
Eating in social situations
Modifying eating patterns
Overcoming common barriers to exercise
Problem solving
Changing the quality of your diet
Eating out in restaurants
Thoughts and weight control
Exercising for aerobic fitness
High-fiber low-fat eating
Strength training
Recipe modification
High-risk situations
Assertion and eating
Motivation
Getting back on track—dealing effectively with lapses
Maintenance of behavior change and weight loss

From Jeffery RW, Wing RR, Thorson C, et al. Strengthening behavioral interventions for weight loss: a randomized trial of food provision and monetary incentives. *J Consult Clin Psychol* 1993;61:1038–1045; and Wing RR, Jeffery RW, Burton LR, et al. Food provision vs. structured meal plans in the behavioral treatment of obesity. *Int J Obes Relat Metab Disord* 1996;20:56–62, with permission.

mation is recorded daily for the first 6 months of the program; subsequently, the activity is recorded either periodically or daily throughout the remainder of the program.

Self-monitoring is often considered the single most important component of a behavioral program (7). This information allows participants to identify behaviors that need to be changed and to monitor their progress in making these changes. Self-monitoring is often not totally accurate; in fact, estimates of dietary intake obtained from such recording underestimate actual intake by an average of 30% (8,9). Therefore, this technique should be viewed more as a tool for behavior change rather than as an assessment technique.

To help patients change their eating and exercise behaviors, it is important to help them change the environment in which they live. Often, unhealthy eating and lack of exercise are responses to cues in the environment (e.g., the serving of large portion sizes, friends going out for a meal, television ads). Therefore, behavioral programs teach *stimulus-control* techniques to reduce the cues for inappropriate behaviors and to strengthen the cues for appropriate eating and activity. For example, participants are taught to remove high-calorie foods from their shelves and to keep a variety of low-calorie snack foods readily available.

Problem-solving approaches become increasingly important in the later weeks of a behavioral program. Participants are taught to identify problem situations, to brainstorm solutions to these problems, and then to implement and evaluate the effectiveness of one solution (10). The problem situations that occur most commonly (e.g., eating out in restaurants, lack of time for exercise, and dealing with nonsupportive family members) are each presented during weekly lessons, and strategies are proposed for overcoming these obstacles.

Based on the theory of *relapse prevention* by Marlatt and Gordon (11,12), programs now include discussion of the fact that lapses are to be expected. Participants are taught to anticipate and to plan for such occurrences to prevent them from escalating into relapses.

Recent behavioral programs have evaluated the impact of stronger behavioral strategies, such as food provision (13), structured meal plans (14–16), supervised exercise (17–20), or home exercise equipment (21). These studies have all included some ongoing treatment contact through 12 to 18 months. With these approaches, the weight losses achieved in the *most* successful group has averaged 10.5 kg at 6 months, 11.5 kg at 12 months, and 8.3 kg at 18 months. These results probably reflect the very best that can be achieved with current behavioral approaches. These stronger behavioral techniques are discussed in detail later in this chapter.

SPECIFIC STRATEGIES TO IMPROVE OUTCOME

Increasing Physical Activity

A large number of randomized clinical trials have compared diet only, exercise only, and the combination of diet plus exercise in the treatment of obesity. These studies have recently been reviewed by the Expert Panel on the Identification, Evaluation, and Treatment of Overweight and Obesity in Adults (22) and by Wing (23) as part of the American College of Sports and Medicine Consensus Conference. Findings from the latter are summarized in Table 18.2. Based on approximately 10 to 12 studies, it appears that exercise alone (i.e., without caloric restriction) produces modest weight losses of approximately 2 kg. Whether these weight losses are due to the physical activity *per se* or to changes in dietary intake in these exercising individuals is difficult to determine. Similarly, the combination of diet plus exercise, compared with diet only, produces a small (1-

TABLE 18.2. *Effect of exercise on weight loss and maintenance*

Type of comparison	Number of studies[a]	Number with significant difference between groups	Weight loss (kg)		
			Exercise	No exercise	Difference
Exercise alone vs. no treatment	10	6	−2.58	+0.75	3.3
Exercise plus diet vs. diet only (short)	13	2	−8.43	−7.79	0.65
Exercise plus diet vs. diet only (long)	6	2	−6.88	−2.61	4.27

[a]Mean weight loss based on 7 out of 10 studies; 12 out of 13 studies; and 6 out of 6 studies, respectively.

From Wing R. Physical activity in the treatment of adulthood overweight and obesity: current evidence and research issues. *Med Sci Sports Exerc* 1999;31:S547–S552, with permission.

to 2-kg) increase in weight loss. Although significant differences in weight loss for diet plus exercise versus diet only were observed in only 2 of the 13 studies on this topic, almost all of the 13 studies pointed in this direction.

The strongest impact of exercise is considered to occur in the area of maintenance of weight loss (24). As this chapter discusses later, exercise has consistently been associated with long-term weight loss maintenance in correlational analyses (24). However, results from randomized, controlled trials are weaker than is often assumed. Wing (23) identified six studies comparing diet only to diet plus exercise that included at least a 1-year follow-up. Although all six of the studies favored the combination, with a mean difference of 4.7 kg in weight loss between conditions, only two of the six showed statistically significant long-term differences in weight loss between the two conditions. The failure to observe statistically significant differences between conditions, in spite of the strong correlations between activity level and weight loss in *post hoc* analyses, may be due to the fact that many participants assigned to diet plus exercise stop exercising over time and that participants in the diet condition begin to exercise. Moreover, those individuals who maintain their exercise long term may also maintain other behavior changes (e.g., low-calorie, low-fat eating) and thereby maintain their weight losses.

These studies suggest that weight loss is increased, albeit modestly, by adding exercise to a weight loss program. Thus, almost all current behavioral weight loss programs include exercise as a key component of treatment. The goal now is to determine how best to increase the proportion of participants who adopt and maintain their exercise behaviors long term.

Lifestyle and Structured Exercise

To improve adoption and maintenance of physical activity, behavioral programs encourage participants to use a combination of lifestyle and programmed (structured) exercise. Lifestyle exercises include activities such as using stairs rather than elevators, parking at the far end of the lot and walking from store to store, and getting off the bus one stop earlier. Such lifestyle activities are important because they can easily become part of the daily routine; however, most individuals are unable to achieve marked increases in overall energy expenditure through lifestyle activity alone. Therefore, lifestyle activity is recommended in combination with structured exercise. Structured exercise involves setting aside times specifically for the purpose of activity, such as participating in an aerobic class 3 days per week or walking a 2-mile route 5 days a week.

Choosing a Type of Structured Exercise

The most important factor in selecting the type of physical activity to recommend is participant preference. Enjoying a type of physical activity helps increase the likelihood of adherence to that activity long term. Because most participants in behavioral weight-control programs choose walking as their primary mode of physical activity, programs stress walking but do allow patients to choose other activities as well. Recently, research has focused on the question of whether resistance training should be recommended either alone or in combination with aerobic training (14,23). The advantage of resistance training is that it can preserve or increase lean body mass and can thereby increase energy expenditure. A recent controlled trial compared the weight losses achieved with a diet-only program to those obtained through a diet program with either aerobic exercise, resistance exercise, or the combination of aerobic plus resistance training (14). The three activity programs were initially offered onsite to ensure adherence and to match the programs for caloric expenditure. No differences in weight loss were seen among any of the treatment conditions. Several other studies have likewise found no differences in weight loss from aerobic versus resistance activity (23).

Interestingly, no research has compared different types of structured exercises. As was noted earlier, walking is typically recommended. Whether adding some other type of activity to this routine would improve long-term adherence is not clear. Aerobic dance was used in the study by Wadden et al. (14), but no comparisons have been made between walking and other activities, such as bicycling, swimming, or golf.

How Much Exercise Should Be Recommended?

Typically, behavioral programs encourage participants to increase gradually the amount of activity they are doing until they reach a level of 1,000 kcal per week. This level would be achieved by walking 2 miles on 5 days each week. The caloric equivalents of various activities are listed in Table 18.3.

Recently, researchers have begun to question whether this recommendation is high enough. For example, participants in the National Weight Control Registry who have been successful at long-term maintenance of weight loss (on average, they have lost more than 60 lb and have kept it off for longer than 6 years) report that they expend an average of 2,800 kcal per week (25). They typically achieve this level through a combination of different activities, including walking, bicycling, strength training, or aerobic dance. Approximately 500 kcal per week are expended in medium-intensity activities and 800 kcal per week are used in heavy-intensity activities (Table 18.4).

TABLE 18.3. *Caloric values for 10 minutes of physical activity*

Activity	Calories
Walking (4 mi/hr)	72
Running (7 mi/hr)	164
Swimming	56
Tennis	80
Dancing	48
Cycling (13 mi/hr)	124
Light gardening	42
Shoveling snow	89

Values based on 175-lb person.

TABLE 18.4. *Calories expended per week in different types of activity by successful weight loss maintainers*

Type of activity	Subjects in top quartile of energy expenditure in TRIM study (19)	Energy expenditure of successful weight maintainers in the NWCR (25)
Walking	1,125	1,093
Stairs	259	188
Other activities:		
Light (5 kcal/min)	167	211
Medium (7.5 kcal/min)	390	526
Heavy (10 kcal/min)	608	798
Total calories/wk	**2,549**	**2,829**

Abbreviations: NWCR, National Weight Control Registry.

As shown in Table 18.4, the activity profile reported by the registry participants is quite similar to that reported by individuals who were in the top quartile of exercise after 18 months of participation in a weight loss program (19). Again, these participants reported expending 2,600 kcal per week in exercise, with approximately 1,000 kcal of that in walking. These participants in the highest quartile of exercise were also most successful in maintaining their weight loss long term, whereas no differences in long-term maintenance of weight loss was observed for participants in the three lower quartiles of activity.

Based on these data, several studies are now comparing weight loss programs that prescribe 1,000 kcal per week of physical activity to programs with 2,000- to 2,500-kcal-per-week goals and varying levels of intensity of these activities.

Supervised Versus Home-Based

Two recent weight loss studies compared weight losses achieved in behavioral programs that included either supervised exercise with ones in which exercise was completed by the participant on his or her own (17,18). Both found that initial weight losses were not affected by the exercise recommendation but that the maintenance of weight loss was better in the unsupervised condition. Andersen et al. (18) found that the supervised condition regained 1.6 kg from 6 to 18 months, whereas the unsupervised group regained only 0.8 kg ($p = 0.06$). Perri et al. (17) reported that the weight losses were comparable at 6 months but that, at 15 months, the supervised group had an average weight loss of 7.01 kg and the unsupervised condition maintained a weight loss of 11.65 kg. The increased flexibility of being able to schedule activities at times of day and locations that are best suited to the individual may be a factor in the long-term effectiveness of unsupervised activity prescription.

Strategies to Increase Exercise Adherence

In addition to defining the appropriate amount and type of activity to recommend for weight loss, one should identify strategies that will promote long-term adherence to exercise. Participants note that lack of time is the primary barrier to increase exercise. One approach to dealing with this issue has been to recommend that exercise be divided into multiple short sessions each day, rather than trying to find one extended period for exercise. Jakicic et al. (26) randomly assigned overweight women to behavioral weight loss programs that differed only in the way in which exercise was prescribed. One group was instructed to exercise in one 40-minute bout each day (long bout group), whereas the other condition was asked to complete the activity in four 10-minute bouts (short bout group). The short bout prescription led to better adherence to exercise and to somewhat better weight losses at 6 months. Both groups experienced a comparable improvement in fitness.

Recently, Jakicic et al. (21) replicated this study and extended the treatment to 18 months. The study also included a third treatment condition, in which participants were instructed to exercise in short bouts and were given a home treadmill for their use. This study again found that prescribing exercise in short bouts, rather than long bouts, improved initial exercise participation; however, from months 6 to 18 of the program, the short and long bout groups had comparable exercise adherence. Moreover, weight losses from 0 to 18 months were comparable (3.7 kg for the short bout group and 5.8 kg for a long bout group), as were the long-term improvements in fitness. Thus, prescribing exercise in short bouts may be a particularly helpful strategy for initiating exercise.

The short bout group that was given the home exercise equipment demonstrated the best overall outcome in this study. This group had the best maintenance of physical activity from 13 to 18 months of the program and the largest overall weight losses (7.4 kg). Making the exercise equipment easily accessible to participants thus appeared to influence the long-term outcome.

Decreasing Sedentary Behavior

Epidemiologic studies have shown a strong correlation between the number of hours of television viewing and body weight. Based on these data, Epstein et al. (27) have studied the effectiveness of decreasing sedentary activity in overweight children. Overweight children from the ages of 8 to 12 years were given a standard behavioral weight-control program that included diet, behavioral strategies, and the involvement of the parents. In addition to these components, one group of children was randomly assigned to work on increasing aerobic activity; the second group focused on decreasing sedentary activity; and the third group combined the two. Group 2, which focused on decreasing sedentary activity, displayed the largest decreases in percent overweight at 1 year (18.7% vs. 8.7% in group 1 and 10.3% in group 3). The improvements in fitness were equivalent across the three groups. These data suggest that children in group 2 probably substituted physical activity for their reduced sedentary activities; the fact that they made this substitution by choice, without having an increase in activity mandated by this study, may have increased their preference for physical activity. To date, these findings have not been applied to overweight adults.

Modifying Dietary Intake

Behavioral researchers have also devoted a great deal of attention to defining the type of diet that is most effective for short-term and long-term weight loss. Again, the issues are related to the magnitude of caloric restriction, the composition of the diet, and strategies that may promote adherence to new eating patterns.

Choosing a Calorie Goal

Caloric restriction is a key element of a weight loss program, but the optimal degree of restriction remains unclear. Typically, behavioral weight loss programs recommend diets of approximately 1,200 to 1,500 kcal per day. In some programs, more individualized calorie goals are prescribed. Baseline caloric intake is estimated (sometimes by multiplying weight in pounds by 12 to 15, depending on the person's physical activity level) and then 1,000 kcal per day is subtracted from this estimate to produce a weight loss of 2 lb per week.

Low-Calorie Versus Very Low Calorie Diets

Several studies have compared the results of weight loss programs with low-calorie diets (1,000 to 1,500 kcal per day) to those with very low calorie diets (VLCDs) (28–31). VLCDs are diets of 400 to 800 kcal per day that include high levels of protein, typically consumed as liquid formula or lean meat, fish, and fowl. VLCDs have been shown to produce excellent initial weight loss, which averages 20 kg at 12 weeks. Maintenance, however, has been problematic. Patients have typically returned to their baseline weights once the VLCD is terminated (Fig. 18.1).

Behavioral researchers have conducted several studies in which they have attempted to use VLCDs to promote initial weight loss, combined with behavior modification to help sustain the effect (29,30). However, even with this combination, weight losses at a 1-year follow-up were not significantly different for behavioral programs with VLCDs versus behavioral programs with low-calorie diets. Thus, there does not appear to be long-term data to justify the use of VLCDs.

Recently, Williams et al. (32) experimented with the possibility of using VLCDs intermittently. Subjects in this study had type II diabetes treated with diet only or oral medication, which was stopped at the initiation of the weight loss program. Participants were randomly assigned to one of three weight loss programs. All groups met weekly for 20 weeks and each was given the same behavioral program and exercise prescription. Group 1 was prescribed a diet of 1,500 to 1,800 kcal per day throughout the 20 weeks. Group 2 started the program with 5 days of a VLCD and then followed the VLCD on 1 day of each week for the remainder of the 20 weeks. Group 3 consumed the VLCD for 5 days during the initial week of the program and then used the VLCD for 5 consecutive days every 5 weeks during the remainder of the program. Weight losses for the standard behavioral

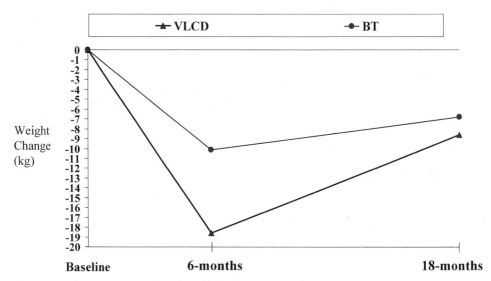

FIG. 18.1. Weight loss using behavioral therapy (BT) versus very low calorie diet (VLCD). (Adapted from Wing RR, Marcus MD, Salata R, et al. Effects of a very-low-calorie diet on long-term glycemic control in obese type 2 diabetic subjects. *Arch Intern Med* 1991;151:1334–1340, with permission.)

program (group 1) over the 20-week program averaged 5.4 kg. Both group 2 and group 3 achieved almost double the weight losses (9.6 and 10.4 kg, respectively). Moreover, 93% of subjects in group 3 lost more than 5 kg, compared with 69% of the subjects in group 2 and 50% of the subjects in group 1, the standard behavioral group. The number of patients who needed to restart diabetes medication and the fasting glucose levels was similar across the three treatment groups, but more subjects in group 3 attained a normal hemoglobin A_{IC}. This benefit appeared to be independent of the effects of weight loss. Thus, these results suggest that using a VLCD periodically may be helpful to patients, but further research evaluating the long-term impact of this approach is clearly needed.

Structured Meal Plans

The benefits of VLCDs may derive not only from their low calorie levels but also from the fact that they simplify food selection and shopping for participants. In many cases, the participant is given the food or the liquid formula they are to consume. Several studies have suggested that this structure may be very helpful for improving dietary adherence.

Jeffery et al. (13) investigated food provision as a strong behavioral approach to modifying the environmental cues for eating. They reasoned that participants in a behavioral weight loss program would find it easier to remain on their diet if they were given the food they should eat in the appropriate portion sizes. Thus, they randomly assigned some participants to self-select their diet within a prescribed calorie goal (1,000 or 1,500 kcal per day) and others to the same program with the same calorie goal but with food provided to the participant. Subjects in the food provision group were given a box of food each week for 18 months; the box contained exactly what they should eat for five breakfasts and five dinners each week. Suggested meal plans and shopping lists were provided for the other meals. Food provision was found to improve weight loss markedly. Whereas the standard group lost 7.7, 4.5, and 4.1 kg at 6, 12, and 18 months, respectively, the group given the food had weight losses of 10.1, 9.1, and 6.4 kg at these same time points.

The food provision intervention included several components that could have been related to its effectiveness. Food provision involved receiving food, which was given free, and a structured meal plan indicating exactly what should be eaten at each of the meals. To try to identify which components of food provision were necessary, these investigators recruited 163 overweight women and randomly assigned them to one of four groups (15). Group 1 received a standard behavioral weight loss program with a prescribed calorie goal. Group 2 received the same program, but participants were also given meal plans for five breakfasts and five dinners each week and a grocery list to help them purchase the required foods. Group 3 received a box of food with these meals provided and shared the cost of the food with the study. Group 4 received the food free. Weight losses at the end of 6 months averaged 8.0, 12.0, 11.7, and 11.4 kg for groups 1 to 4, respectively (Fig. 18.2).

These results suggest that providing the meal plan and grocery list was the essential component. No further benefit was obtained by giving the food. However, all groups given meal plans or food lost significantly more weight than the standard behavioral group.

Several other recent studies have documented the benefits of food provision approaches. A multicenter study of 202 type II diabetic patients compared the effects of a self-selected low-calorie diet with those of a comprehensive prepackaged meal plan (33). Both diets were designed to provide 55% to 60% carbohydrate, 20% to 30% fat, and 15% to 20% protein and to produce a weight loss of 1 kg per week. Average weight losses were 3.4 kg in the group that received a comprehensive meal plan and 2.9 kg in the self-

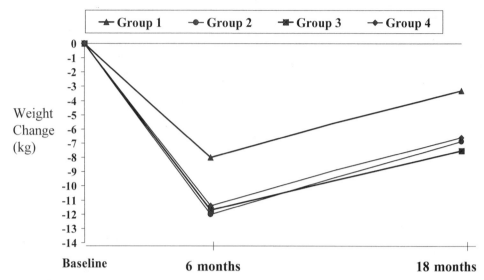

FIG. 18.2. Weight loss for group 1 (standard behavior therapy [SBT]), group 2 (SBT plus meal plans), group 3 (SBT plus food with cost sharing), and group 4 (SBT plus food provided free). (Adapted from Wing RR, Jeffery RW, Burton LR, et al. Food provision vs. structured meal plans in the behavioral treatment of obesity. *Int J Obes Relat Metab Disord* 1996;20:56–62, with permission.)

selected diet group. Improvements in glycemic control, lipids, and blood pressure were comparable in the two diet conditions.

Wadden et al. (14) used a diet of 900 to 925 kcal that consisted of four servings of a liquid diet formula (Sandoz Nutrition; 150 kcal per day per serving) and a shelf-stable entree (Healthy Recipes, Sandoz Nutrition; 280 to 300 kcal per serving) and 2 cups of salad for dinner. This diet was prescribed for 18 weeks; after that time, the liquid diet was gradually reduced and the consumption of conventional foods was increased until the patient was consuming 1,500 kcal per day with 15% to 30% fat and 55% to 60% carbohydrate. Weight losses averaged 10 kg during the first 8 weeks and 14.3 kg by week 17, which was the end of the 925-kcal diet. Average weight loss was 16.5 kg at week 24. These outstanding weight losses suggest this type of diet regimen deserves further study.

Two recent reports likewise document benefits of using Slim-Fast as part of a weight loss regimen (34,35). One hundred participants were instructed to follow a diet of 1,200 to 1,500 kcal per day for 3 months, with group 1 consuming a self-selected diet of conventional foods and group 2 using two Slim-Fast meal replacements per day and two Slim-Fast nutrition bars. Participants in group 1 lost 1.3 kg (1.5%) over 3 months, whereas participants in group 2 lost 7.1 kg (7.8%). Following this 3-month randomized trial, all participants were instructed to consume a reduced-calorie diet with one meal and one snack of Slim-Fast each day for the next 24 months. At the 27-month follow-up, which was completed on 63% of the original 100 participants, the mean weight loss was 5.9% for group 1 and 11.3% for group 2.

The results for 75 of the 100 patients at 4 years were recently reported (35). After 4 years, group 1 has maintained a total mean weight loss of 3.2%, and group 2 has maintained a weight loss of 8.4%. Moreover, both groups attained significant long-term improvements in glucose and insulin, and group 2 also had long-term improvements in triglycerides and blood pressure.

Macronutrient Composition of the Diet

Behaviorists have conducted several studies examining the impact of limiting fat intake on weight loss and maintenance. These studies have stemmed from the recognition that fat has more calories per gram than carbohydrate or protein and from findings in the breast cancer literature that a low-fat diet with no caloric restriction produces weight loss.

Jeffery et al. (36) compared the effectiveness for weight loss of limiting calories with no restriction on fat to the effectiveness of limiting fat intake with no restriction on calories. No differences in weight loss were observed at 6 or 18 months. However, weight losses in both groups were quite modest. Better results were obtained by Schlundt et al. (37) and Pascale et al. (38), who examined the combination of dietary fat restriction plus calorie restriction. Schlundt et al. (37) found that the combination intervention improved weight loss compared with restricting fat only, and Pascale et al. (38) found that the combination improved weight loss compared with reducing calories only. Based on these suggestive findings, the field has started to recommend routinely that participants monitor both calories and fat and that they aim to keep fat intake at less than 20% of calories.

Recently, there has been renewed interest in diets that severely restrict carbohydrate intake. Such diets have not been formally evaluated in weight loss trials. However, an analysis of participants in the National Weight Control Registry who have successfully maintained their weight loss long term reveals that very few (less than 1%) of these successful weight losers report consuming a diet that is as severely limited in carbohydrates (39). Rather, on average, registry participants consume a low-calorie, low-fat diet with less than 24% of kcal from fat (25).

Increasing Support and Motivation for Weight Loss Maintenance

Almost all studies in the weight loss literature show that patients achieve their maximum weight loss at approximately 6 months, followed by weight regain (40). A tremendous amount of attention has consequently been directed at reducing this weight regain. Several of the techniques described earlier in this chapter (e.g., providing home exercise equipment) have been modestly effective in this regard. However, maintenance of weight loss remains difficult for several reasons. First, physiologic changes may occur with weight loss (e.g., lower metabolic rate and lower leptin levels) that serve to promote weight regain (41–43). Second, the reinforcement associated with weight loss (e.g., attention from others, fitting into smaller size clothes, and improvements in risk factors) is far greater than that for weight loss maintenance (5). Third, many people never really achieve their desired weight loss during a treatment program, and thus they may be disappointed with the outcome (44). Finally, "boredom" is the single most commonly reported explanation for the failure to maintain behavior changes and weight loss long term (45).

Ongoing continued contact between the participants and therapist appears to be the most effective approach to the prevention of weight regain. Perri et al. (46), in an elegant series of maintenance studies, have systematically examined the benefit of continued contact. In one study, a 20-week treatment program was compared with a 40-week program (47). Although the educational content of the two programs was identical, the 40-week program produced better weight loss effects. Weight losses in the two conditions were comparable at 20 weeks, but from weeks 20 to 40, the 20-week group started to regain and the 40-week group continued to lose weight. At week 40, the weight losses averaged 6.4 kg in the 20-week program and 13.6 kg in the extended program. Both groups regained weight between weeks 40 and 72, but the 40-week group achieved a greater overall weight loss (9.8 vs. 4.6 kg). These results suggest that lengthening the program served to delay, but not to prevent, weight regain.

Maintaining weekly contact for 40 weeks or a full year has been difficult in other studies, with attendance at meetings decreasing markedly over time (48). Therefore, many programs begin with weekly meetings for 6 months and then taper to biweekly meetings for the next 6 to 12 months. Perri et al. (49) compared the effects of offering no contact from 6 to 18 months to offering biweekly contact with various types of content (e.g., aerobic exercise and social support). The nature of contact had no significant impact, but continuing to see the participants did improve the outcome.

Spouses have also been used as a source of ongoing support for patients. In some cases, the spouse has been asked to change his or her behavior along with the participant, whereas, in other studies, the spouse is taught only to support the participants' effort. A metaanalysis of this literature suggests a small positive effect of involving the spouses (50). Wing et al. (51) found no overall benefit of including the spouse in the treatment program, but they did observe a significant interaction with gender; including the spouse in the program increased weight losses of the women in the program, but it decreased weight losses of the men.

More recently, Wing and Jeffery (52) examined the effect of recruiting participants with a "team" of three other friends or family members. This approach to promoting natural social support was crossed with an experimental manipulation of social support—most notably, financial rewards given to teams who were most successful at weight loss maintenance—in a 2-by-2 treatment design. Those participants who were recruited with friends and who were given the social support intervention had the best long-term results; 75% of these individuals completed the 10-month study, and 66% maintained their weight loss in full from months 4 to 10. This contrasted sharply with the standard behavioral group, which was recruited without friends and not given the social support manipulation, in which only 76% of participants completed the 10 months and only 24% maintained their weight loss in full from months 4 to 10.

PATIENT AND TREATMENT PREDICTORS OF OUTCOME

The emphasis in behavioral treatment research is typically on the average weight losses achieved. Far less attention has been directed to the variability in outcome. Unfortunately, the variability in results achieved in behavioral programs is extremely large. At 6 months, the standard deviation of weight loss is typically about 5 to 7 kg, and 1 year after treatment, the standard deviation increases to about 7 to 9 kg (16,21). Thus, some individuals do quite well in behavioral programs and others are far less successful. Knowing the variables that predict who will succeed or fail in behavioral treatment could help practitioners identify appropriate candidates.

However, it is important to recognize the limitations of studies of predictors that examine the correlation between pretreatment factors or treatment process variables and weight change. The homogeneity among participants may make identifying pretreatment predictors of outcome difficult. Moreover, in studies of treatment variables, the directionality of relationships cannot be determined. For example, a positive correlation between decreased fat intake and weight loss could mean (a) that a reduction in fat intake causes weight loss, (b) that reduction in fat intake is a consequence of weight loss, or (c) that the correlation is due to other unmeasured variables. The randomized controlled trials described earlier are far more conclusive than predictor studies for this reason. A further limitation to "predictor" and other research is that outcomes are likely biased because of selective dropout. In other words, the ability to generalize findings is limited because those who complete the study may be different from those who drop out.

With these caveats in mind, this section reviews the patient characteristics (e.g., demographic and psychologic) and process measures (e.g., attendance and adherence to diet and exercise) that have been examined in relation to short-term and long-term outcomes in behavioral weight loss programs and selected weight gain prevention studies. Although biologic markers, such as resting metabolic rate and fat cell number, have been shown to correlate positively with weight loss, such measures are not accessible to most practitioners and are therefore not discussed (53).

Patient Characteristics

Demographics

The average patient in a behavioral weight-control study is white, middle-aged, middle income, 100 kg, and female. Thus, the likelihood of detecting differential outcomes based on demographic variables is minimized in many studies. Nonetheless, research has examined several demographic variables. Gender has generally failed to predict outcomes in behavioral treatment. In some studies, men have achieved larger weight losses than women, but these differences typically disappear after adjusting for initial body weight. French et al. (54) evaluated the predictive value of gender in 186 men and women participating in a behavioral weight-control program. Although at 6 months men had lost significantly more weight than women (19.3 vs. 13.3 kg, respectively), no differences in weight loss were obtained at 12 (12.9 vs. 10.2 kg) or 18 months (9.0 vs. 5.9 kg) after adjusting for baseline differences in weight and other variables. One study found greater weight losses, adjusted for baseline weight, in men compared with women at 8 weeks; however, the correlation was modest ($r = 0.23, p < 0.001$), and the differences disappeared at 13 months (55). Several other studies have found no long-term predictive value for gender in behavioral treatment (56).

Similarly, behavioral treatment studies suggest no relationship between age and treatment outcomes, although one study found that attrition was higher in younger individuals (55–58). Marital status, education, and employment similarly do not appear to predict behavioral treatment outcomes (56,59).

Ethnicity

Ethnic differences in weight loss in behavioral treatment programs have been reported with marked consistency. Reviewing weight losses in two hypertension prevention trials, Kumanyika et al. (60) noted that in both trials blacks lost less weight than whites. This difference was observed in both studies for men (a 1.4-kg to 2.0-kg difference in weight loss of black and white men) and for women (a 2.2-kg to 2.7-kg difference in weight loss for black and white women). Similarly, two studies with VLCDs have observed smaller weight losses in blacks than in whites (61,62). Anglin and Wing (62) reported a marked difference in weight loss (7.1 kg in blacks and 13.9 kg in whites), which was due primarily to poor attendance and greater weight regain during the latter 6 months of the program in the black participants. Whether these differences are due to physiologic differences between ethnic groups or to the culture relevance of the treatment program remains unclear.

Initial Body Weight

Initial body weight is the most consistent pretreatment predictor of behavioral treatment outcome. Specifically, heavier individuals achieve larger short-term and long-term weight losses (63). This finding is of interest because behavioral programs are typically recommended primarily for less overweight patients, whereas more stringent diets, such as VLCDs or drug treatments, are recommended for heavier individuals. Interestingly, greater initial waist circumference has also been found to predict greater sustained weight loss, independent of initial body weight and BMI (57). This suggests that patients with greater waist circumference may attain not only greater health benefits but also greater weight losses. Some studies show greater attrition in heavier patients, but other studies contradict these findings (64,65). Overall, there appears to be little basis for discouraging heavier patients from joining behavioral treatment programs.

Medical Status

Preliminary research indicates that poor medical status in addition to the diagnosis of obesity may negatively affect outcomes in behavioral treatment. Clark et al. (58) examined the relationship between physician-assessed health status and attendance during 26 weeks of a VLCD and behavioral therapy program in 143 obese individuals. Although hyperlipidemia and total number of medical diagnoses were unrelated to outcome, higher baseline systolic blood pressure was related to lower attendance ($r = -0.27$). Furthermore, patients with untreated hypertension were less likely to attend sessions, compared to those with treated hypertension. In another study, Karlsson et al. (66) examined the relationship between health status, as assessed by the Sickness Impact profile, and weight change in 66 moderately obese women following two 1,300-kcal diets over 2 years. Results indicated that baseline functional status was significantly related to weight regain. Other studies have found that weight loss may be poorer in diabetic compared with nondiabetic individuals (67,68). Certain medications (e.g., psychotropics) may make losing weight more difficult for patients. Although these findings suggest that medical illnesses will lessen success at weight loss, certain medical events (e.g., myocardial infarction) may trigger enhanced motivation for weight control, leading to better weight losses.

Psychologic Variables

Numerous studies of psychopathology and behavioral treatment outcome have yielded inconsistent and contradictory findings. Most research suggests that pretreatment levels of depression, anxiety, and personality fail to differentiate success or failure in short-term and long-term behavioral treatment outcomes (56,63,66,69,70). However, notable exceptions to all of these findings exist (59,71–73).

Binge eaters, who tend to have greater psychopathology, are commonly thought to fare worse in treatment compared with non–binge eaters (74). However, the empiric evidence regarding the prognostic value of binge eating is mixed. Sherwood et al. (75) assessed binge eating as a predictor of short-term and long-term weight loss in a large (n = 444) sample of women undergoing behavioral treatment. Results indicate that baseline binge status was not associated with 6-month weight loss and that it was only a weak predictor of diminished weight loss at 18 months. Interestingly, the weak relationship between binge status and weight change was lessened when depressive symptomatology scores were added to the analyses, suggesting that depression may moderate the relationship between binge eating and weight loss. The directionality of the relationships between depression, binge eating, and weight loss could not be determined in this study.

Individuals with high levels of depression and binge eaters may be at greater risk of dropping out of treatment, which might explain the inconsistent findings reviewed earlier (58,69,75). However, at present, there is no evidence to suggest that psychologic variables are useful in predicting weight loss.

Stress and Coping

Although few studies have evaluated differential treatment response according to pretreatment level of stress, some reports indicate that major life stress, financial difficulties, job changes, and/or major family illness are related to early dropout (76). Coping style may also moderate treatment outcome. Drapkin et al. (77) examined 93 patients after 6 months of behavioral treatment and found that the ability to generate coping responses to a variety of situations was positively related to weight loss, explaining about 8% of the variance.

Dieting History

Although a history of weight cycling is often considered a risk factor for poor performance in weight loss programs, the literature on this topic is quite inconsistent. Some studies found that greater dieting history is related to diminished weight loss and weight maintenance, as well as to greater attrition (78–80). However, other studies contradict these findings (55,56).

Social Factors

Social factors also have a powerful influence on obese individuals' treatment response (52). Patients with greater social support have more positive short-term and long-term weight losses, and they are more likely to complete treatment (80,81). The social support provided by other group members in behavioral treatment programs may be helpful to those who lack other sources of support.

Summary

In summary, the only demographic characteristics that consistently predict outcome are initial body weight and race. Specifically, patients who are heavier lose more weight than those who are lighter, and whites lose more weight than blacks. Patients with binge eating, depression, major stress, and major medical problems may be at a greater risk of attrition, and they could require greater patient–provider contact and/or referral for adjunct psychiatric care. Table 18.5 summarizes the patient predictors of treatment outcomes.

TABLE 18.5. *Patient predictors of treatment outcomes*

Variables associated with outcomes	Variables with mixed or scant evidence	Variables not associated
Ethnicity Initial body weight	Waist circumference Health status Social support Stress Psychopathology Weight cycling	Gender Age Marital status Education Employment

Treatment Variables

Surprisingly, little research has examined the relationship between adherence to specific behavioral strategies taught during treatment (e.g., stimulus control and cognitive restructuring) and subsequent outcome. The variables that have been examined include the magnitude of initial weight loss, the consumption of low-fat and/or low-calorie foods, the performance of regular exercise, attendance, and self-monitoring. Although predictor studies of treatment components are weaker methodologically than the randomized trials described earlier, these studies are reviewed here to show the consistency of results across the two types of literature.

Initial Weight Loss

Several studies indicate that weight loss during the first few weeks of treatment is positively correlated with weight loss at the end of treatment. For example, Wadden et al. (16) reported that weight loss at as early as 8 weeks correlated significantly ($r = 0.45$) with weight loss at 1-year follow-up. In addition, patients who lost more weight at the end of treatment have larger weight losses at follow-up (16,82). Jeffery et al. (83) examined weight loss maintenance at 30 months and found that the individuals who lost the most weight initially (i.e., at approximately 6 months) had the best long-term weight losses. These data suggest that individuals who fail to lose weight during the first few weeks of treatment do not "catch up" and that they may benefit from additional provider contact and monitoring during treatment. Moreover, weight losses at 6 months predict overall weight loss, indicating the importance of maximizing initial weight losses.

Food Intake

A reduction in caloric consumption is clearly integral to successful short-term and long-term weight control (20,84). Surprisingly, however, reduction in caloric intake has accounted for only 9% of the variance in weight loss in behavioral programs (16,20). This modest effect may reflect difficulties in assessing intake (85). Alternatively, the findings may suggest that changes in the percentage of total energy from fat and level of activity are stronger determinants of weight loss than is total caloric intake.

Fat Intake

Several studies suggest that greater decreases in the percentage of calories from fat intake are significantly related to greater short-term and sustained weight losses (13,57). Harris et al. (86) reported that fat intake was the most important caloric contributor to weight change among 157 men and women participating in a behavioral weight loss program over 18 months. Similarly, Jeffery et al. (13) reported that the change in percentage of calories from fat over 6 months accounted for 7% of the variance in weight change over the same period, as well as from 12 to 18 months. Larger effects (i.e., 20% of variance) have been reported in other studies (57). Research has also begun to identify the consumption of specific foods as markers for weight loss (86,87). For example, French et al. (88) found that the decreased consumption of French fries, dairy products, sweets, and meats was positively associated with change in BMI over time. Decreased consumption of fast food has also been associated with weight loss (87).

Physical Activity

Similar to the findings from randomized controlled trials reviewed earlier, physical activity appears to be only weakly related to short-term weight loss in correlational studies. By contrast, consistent and strong relationships have been reported between physical activity and long-term outcomes (17,20,57,87). Perri et al. (17) found that exercise participation in 49 obese women undergoing long-term behavioral treatment was not associated with initial weight loss from baseline to 6 months ($r = 0.12$) but that it was associated with weight maintenance during months 7 through 12 ($r = 0.33$, $p < 0.05$). Similarly, Leermakers et al. (20) reported that weight gain after 6 months of behavioral treatment correlated significantly with the amount of weekly exercise during months 6 though 12 ($r = -0.42$, $p < 0.005$) and months 6 through 18 ($r = -0.34$, $p < 0.005$). Whether different types of structured activity (e.g., vigorous vs. lifestyle) predict differential treatment outcomes awaits further investigation. Clearly, however, correlational data support the conclusion that physical activity is the single best predictor of long-term weight loss maintenance (24). In addition, higher levels of physical activity before treatment may predict better weight loss 1 year after treatment and may guard against attrition (56,58).

Eating Control

The degree of restraint, or conscious control over one's eating, has been shown to increase during behavioral treatment and to be positively related to weight loss outcome. For example, Foster et al. (89) reported a significant inverse relationship ($r = -0.29$) between increases in cognitive restraint and decreases in weight during 5 to 6 months of comprehensive behavioral treatment. Similar findings have been reported in both short-term and long-term outcomes (56,58,89,90). Disinhibition scores, which reflect the propensity to lose control over one's eating, tend to decrease during treatment. However, most studies report only modest correlations between decreases in disinhibition and weight loss or regain (56,79,89–91).

Treatment Attendance

Attendance at treatment sessions is clearly related to initial success in behavioral treatment, accounting for about 15% to 25% of the variance in short-term weight loss (13,19,76,92). However, the relationship between attendance and the maintenance of weight loss is less consistent. Wadden et al. (14) reported that treatment attendance was the only variable among several behavioral and physiologic measures that significantly correlated with the maintenance of weight loss during 48 weeks of treatment. Other research has found no relationship between the attendance of weight-maintenance sessions and outcome (63). Similarly, findings are mixed about whether past attendance protects against subsequent weight regain. Some studies suggest that attendance continues to be associated with success 1 year later, but other studies contradict these findings (76,93).

Self-Monitoring and Other Behaviors

Research has shown that self-monitoring is one of the most important predictors of weight loss in behavioral treatment programs (7). In fact, it has been deemed "the cornerstone of behavioral treatment" (94). A number of clinical studies have found self-monitoring to be significantly correlated with both short-term and long-term weight loss, accounting for approximately 30% of the variance in weight loss (13,76). For instance, Baker and Kirschenbaum (7) examined the relationship between self-monitoring and weight control in 56 subjects over 18 weeks. Participants who self-monitored consistently lost more weight than those who monitored less consistently or not at all. In addition, individuals lost more weight during their "best" weeks of monitoring than they did in their "worst" monitoring periods.

Few studies have examined the prognostic significance of adhering to other weight-control behaviors. In one of the few studies to examine specific behaviors in relation to outcome, slow eating was positively correlated ($r = .67$) with weight loss after 28 weeks of behavioral treatment, but 14 weeks later a faster eating rate returned (95). Perri et al. (47) reported a significant positive relation between a composite rating of adherence (e.g., to self-monitoring, eating in one place, and slowed eating) and long-term weight loss ($r = 0.43$, $p < 0.05$), and similar findings have been reported elsewhere (87). In addition, a decrease in the number of barriers to adherence has also been related to improved long-term (i.e., 30-month) weight loss outcomes (93). Little research has examined the impact of cognitive factors in weight loss. However, Smith et al. (96) found that cognitive appraisals (e.g., "all or nothing," "rationalization," and "matter of degree" thinking) were not associated with weight loss during 20 weeks of treatment with a low-calorie diet. Clearly, additional research is needed to replicate these findings and to determine the relationship between adherence to other behaviors and subsequent treatment outcome.

Summary

As patients begin treatment, their early weight loss, consistent attendance, increased levels of restraint, and compliance to weight-control behaviors (e.g., self-monitoring, a reduced-fat diet, and exercise) are signs that they will succeed in treatment. Failure to implement these strategies early in treatment should be interpreted as a warning to reexamine patients' motivation and commitment to treatment and the need to consider providing additional care.

CONCLUSION

Both randomized controlled trials and predictor studies show the importance of behavioral strategies specifically related to decreasing intake, especially dietary fat intake, and increasing physical activity. New stronger approaches for producing long-term changes in both of these aspects of energy balance are clearly needed.

Clinicians should recognize that most patients will be able to achieve modest weight losses in behavioral treatment programs, so referrals to such programs are typically appropriate. Helping patients get off to a good start in such programs and maximizing motivation through strategies such as social support may promote long-term successful weight loss and maintenance.

ACKNOWLEDGMENTS

This research was supported in part by a grant (DK 29757) awarded to Dr. Wing from the National Institutes of Health.

REFERENCES

1. Stuart RB. Behavioral control of overeating. *Behav Res Ther* 1967;5:357–365.
2. Wing RR. Behavioral approaches to the treatment of obesity. In: James P, ed. *Handbook of obesity.* New York: Marcel Dekker Inc, 1993:855–873.
3. Wing RR. Behavioral strategies for weight reduction in obese type II diabetic patients. *Diabetes Care* 1989;12: 139–144.
4. Jeffery RW, Wing RR, Stunkard AJ. Behavioral treatment of obesity: the state of the art. *Behav Ther* 1978;9: 189–199.
5. Wadden TA. The treatment of obesity: an overview. In: Wadden TA, ed. *Obesity theory and therapy.* New York: Raven Press, 1993:197–218.

6. Kazdin AE. Self-monitoring and behavior change. In: Thoresen CF, ed. *Self-control: power to the person.* Monterey: Brooks/Cole, 1974.
7. Baker RC, Kirschenbaum DS. Self-monitoring may be necessary for successful weight control. *Behav Ther* 1993;24:377–394.
8. Goris AH, Westerterp-Plantega MS, Westerterp KR. Undereating and underrecording of habitual food intake in obese men: selective underreporting of fat intake. *Am J Clin Nutr* 2000;71:130–134.
9. Lichtman SW, Pisarska K, Berman ER, et al. Discrepancy between self-reported and actual caloric intake and exercise in obese subjects. *N Engl J Med* 1992;327:1893–1898.
10. D'Zurilla TJ, Goldfried MR. Problem solving and behavior modification. *J Abnorm Psychol* 1971;78:107–126.
11. Marlatt GA, Gordon JR. *Relapse prevention: maintenance strategies in addictive behavior change.* New York: Guilford, 1985.
12. Marlatt GA, Gordon JR. Determinants of relapse: implications for the maintenance of behavior change. In: Davidson SM, ed. *Behavioral medicine: changing health lifestyles.* New York: Brunner/Mazel, 1979:410–452.
13. Jeffery RW, Wing RR, Thorson C, et al. Strengthening behavioral interventions for weight loss: a randomized trial of food provision and monetary incentives. *J Consult Clin Psychol* 1993;61:1038–1045.
14. Wadden TA, Vogt RA, Andersen RE, et al. Exercise in the treatment of obesity: effects of four interventions on body composition, resting energy expenditure, appetite, and mood. *J Consult Clin Psychol* 1997;65:269–277.
15. Wing RR, Jeffery RW, Burton LR, et al. Food provision vs. structured meal plans in the behavioral treatment of obesity. *Int J Obes Relat Metab Disord* 1996;20:56–62.
16. Wadden TA, Vogt RA, Foster GD, et al. Exercise and maintenance of weight loss: 1-year follow-up of a controlled clinic trial. *J Consult Clin Psychol* 1998;66:429–433.
17. Perri MG, Martin AD, Leermakers EA, et al. Effects of group- versus home-based exercise in the treatment of obesity. *J Consult Clin Psychol* 1997;65:278–285.
18. Andersen R, Frankowiak S, Snyder J, et al. Effects of lifestyle activity vs. structured aerobic exercise in obese women: a randomized trial. *JAMA* 1998;281:335–340.
19. Jeffery RW, Wing RR, Thorson C, et al. Use of personal trainers and financial incentives to increase exercise in a behavioral weight-loss program. *J Consult Clin Psychol* 1998;66:777–783.
20. Leermakers EA, Perri MG, Shigaki CL, et al. Effects of exercise-focused versus weight focused maintenance programs on the management of obesity. *Addict Behav* 1999;24:219–227.
21. Jakicic J, Wing R, Winters C. Effects of intermittent exercise and use of home exercise equipment on adherence, weight loss, and fitness in overweight women. *JAMA* 1999;282:1554–1560.
22. National Heart, Lung, and Blood Institute. Clinical guidelines on the identification, evaluation, and treatment of overweight and obesity in adults—the evidence report. *Obes Res* 1998;6:51S–210S.
23. Wing R. Physical activity in the treatment of the adulthood overweight and obesity: current evidence and research issues. *Med Sci Sports Exerc* 1999;31:S547–S552.
24. Pronk NP, Wing RR. Physical activity and long-term maintenance of weight loss. *Obes Res* 1994;2:587–599.
25. Klem ML, Wing RR, McGuire MT, et al. A descriptive study of individuals successful at long-term maintenance of substantial weight loss. *Am J Clin Nutr* 1997;66:239–246.
26. Jakicic JM, Wing RR, Butler BA, et al. Prescribing exercise in multiple short bouts versus one continuous bout: effects on adherence, cardiorespiratory fitness, and weight loss in overweight women. *Int J Obes Relat Metab Disord* 1995;19:893–901.
27. Epstein LH, Valoski AM, Vara LS, et al. Effects of decreasing sedentary behavior and increasing activity on weight change in obese children. *Health Psychol* 1995;14:109–115.
28. Wadden TA, Stunkard AJ. Controlled trial of very low calorie diet, behavior therapy, and their combination in the treatment of obesity. *J Consult Clin Psychol* 1986;54:482–488.
29. Wadden TA, Foster GD, Letizia KA. One-year behavioral treatment of obesity: comparison of moderate and severe caloric restriction and the effects of weight maintenance therapy. *J Consult Clin Psychol* 1994;62:165–171.
30. Wing RR, Blair E, Marcus M, et al. Year-long weight loss treatment for obese patients with type II diabetes: does inclusion of an intermittent very low calorie diet improve outcome? *Am J Med* 1994;97:354–362.
31. Wing RR, Marcus MD, Salata R, et al. Effects of a very-low-calorie diet on long-term glycemic control in obese type 2 diabetic subjects. *Arch Intern Med* 1991;151:1334–1340.
32. Williams KV, Mullen ML, Kelley DE, et al. The effect of short periods of caloric restriction on weight loss and glycemic control in type 2 diabetes. *Diabetes Care* 1998;21:2–8.
33. Pi-Sunyer F, Maggio C, McCarron D, et al. Multicenter randomized trial of a comprehensive prepared meal program in type 2 diabetes. *Diabetes Care* 1999;22:191–197.
34. Ditschuneit HH, Flechtner-Mors M, Johnson TD, et al. Metabolic and weight-loss effects of a long-term dietary intervention in obese patients. *Am J Clin Nutr* 1999;69:198–204.
35. Flechtner-Mors M, Ditschuneit HH, Johnson TD, et al. Metabolic and weight loss effects of long-term dietary intervention in obese patients: four-year results. *Obes Res* 2000;8:399–402.
36. Jeffery RW, Hellerstedt WL, French SA, et al. A randomized trial of counseling for fat restriction versus calorie restriction in the treatment of obesity. *Int J Obes* 1995;19:132–137.
37. Schlundt DG, Hill JO, Pope-Cordle J, et al. Randomized evaluation of a low fat ad libitum carbohydrate diet for weight reduction. *Int J Obes Relat Metab Disord* 1993;17:623–629.
38. Pascale RW, Wing RR, Butler BA, et al. Effects of a behavioral weight loss program stressing calorie restriction versus calorie plus fat restriction in obese individuals with NIDDM or a family history of diabetes. *Diabetes Care* 1995;18:1241–1248.

39. Wyatt HR, Seagle HM, Grunwald GK, et al. Long-term weight and very low carbohydrate diets in the National Weight Control Registry. *Obes Res* 2000;8:875.
40. Jeffery R, Drewnowski A, Epstein L, et al. Long-term maintenance of weight loss: current status. *Health Psychol* 2000;19:37–41.
41. Yost TJ, Jensen DR, Eckel RH. Weight regain following sustained weight reduction is predicted by relative insulin sensitivity. *Obes Res* 1995;3:583–587.
42. Leibel RL, Rosenbaum M, Hirsch J. Changes in energy expenditure resulting from altered body weight. *N Engl J Med* 1995;332:621–628.
43. Yost TJ, Eckel RH. Fat calories may be preferentially stored in reduced-obese women: a permissive pathway for resumption of obese state. *J Clin Endocrinol Metab* 1988;67:259–264.
44. Foster GD, Wadden TA, Vogt RA, et al. What is a reasonable weight loss? Patients' expectations and evaluations of obesity treatment outcomes. *J Consult Clin Psychol* 1997;65:79–85.
45. Smith C, Wing R, Burke L. Vegetarian and weight loss diets among young adults. *Obes Res* 2000;8:123–129.
46. Perri MG, Nezu AM, Viegener BJ. *Improving the long-term management of obesity.* New York: John Wiley and Sons, 1992.
47. Perri MG, Nezu AM, Patti ET, et al. Effect of length of treatment on weight loss. *J Consult Clin Psychol* 1989; 57:450–452.
48. Wing RR, Venditti EM, Jakicic JM, et al. Lifestyle intervention in overweight individuals with a family history of diabetes. *Diabetes Care* 1998;21:350–359.
49. Perri MG, McAllister DA, Gange JJ, et al. Effects of four maintenance programs on the long-term management of obesity. *J Clin Psychol* 1988;56:529–534.
50. Black DR, Gleser LJ, Kooyers KJ. A meta-analytic evaluation of couples weight-loss programs. *Health Psychol* 1990;9:330–347.
51. Wing RR, Marcus MD, Epstein LH, et al. A "family-based" approach to the treatment of obese type II diabetic patients. *J Consult Clin Psychol* 1991;59:156–162.
52. Wing RR, Jeffery RW. Benefits of recruiting participants with friends and increasing social support for weight loss maintenance. *J Consult Clin Psychol* 1999;67:132–138.
53. Wadden TA, Letizia KA. Predictors of attrition and weight loss in patients treated by moderate and severe caloric restriction. In: Wadden TA, Vanitallie TB, eds. *Treatment of the seriously obese patient.* New York: The Guilford Press, 1992:383–410.
54. French SA, Jeffery RW, Wing RR. Sex differences among participants in a weight-control program. *Addict Behav* 1994;19:147–158.
55. Hoie LH, Bruusgaard D. Predictors of long-term weight loss reduction in obese patients after initial very-low-calorie diet. *Adv Ther* 1999;16:285–289.
56. Pekkarinen T, Takala I, Mustajoki P. Two year maintenance of weight loss after VLCD and behavioral therapy for obesity: correlation to the scores of questionnaires measuring eating behavior. *Int J Obes Relat Metab Disord* 1996;20:332–337.
57. Carmichael HE, Swinburn BA, Wilson MR. Lower fat intake as a predictor in initial and sustained weight loss in obese subjects consuming an otherwise ad libitum diet. *J Am Diet Assoc* 1998;98:35–39.
58. Clark MN, Niaura RS, King TK, et al. Depression, smoking, activity level, and health status: pretreatment predictors of attrition in obesity treatment. *Addict Behav* 1996;21:509–513.
59. Neumark-Sztainer D, Kaufmann NA, Berry EM. Physical activity within a community-based weight control program: program evaluation and predictors of success. *Public Health Rev* 1995;23:237–251.
60. Kumanyika SK, Obarzanek E, Stevens VJ, et al. Weight-loss experience of black and white participants in NHLBI-sponsored clinical trials. *Am J Clin Nutr* 1991;53:1631–1638.
61. Yanovski SZ, Gormally JF, Leser MS, et al. Binge eating disorder affects outcome of comprehensive very-low-calorie diet treatment. *Obes Res* 1994;2:205–212.
62. Anglin K, Wing RR. Effectiveness of a behavioral weight control program for blacks and whites with NIDDM. *Diabetes Care* 1996;19:409–413.
63. Wadden TA, Foster GD, Wang J, et al. Clinical correlates of short and long-term weight loss. *Am J Clin Nutr* 1992;56:274S–277S.
64. Clark M, Guise BJ, Niaura RS. Obesity level and attrition: support of patient-treatment matching in obesity treatment. *Obes Res* 1995;3:63–64.
65. Ek A, Andersson I, Barkeling B, et al. Obesity treatment and attrition: no relationship to obesity level. *Obes Res* 1996;4:295–296.
66. Karlsson J, Hallgren P, Kral JG, et al. Predictors and effects of long-term dieting on mental well-being and weight loss in obese women. *Appetite* 1994;23:15–26.
67. Khan M, St. Peter J, Breen G, et al. Diabetes disease stage predicts weight loss outcomes with long term appetite suppressants. *Diabetes* 1999;48:A308.
68. Guare JC, Wing RR, Grant A. Comparison of obese NIDDM and nondiabetic women: short- and long-term weight loss. *Obes Res* 1995;3:329–335.
69. Marcus MD, Wing RR, Hopkins J. Obese binge eaters: affect, cognitions, and response to behavioral weight control. *J Consult Clin Psychol* 1988;56:433–439.
70. Poston WS 2nd, Eriksson H, Linder J, et al. Personality and the prediction of weight loss and relapse in the treatment of obesity. *Int J Eat Disord* 1999;25:301–309.

71. Berman WH, Berman ER, Heymsfield S, et al. The effect of psychiatric disorders on weight loss in obesity clinic patients. *Behav Med* 1993;18:167–172.
72. LaPorte DJ. A fatiguing effect in obese patients during partial fasting: increase in vulnerability to emotion-related events and anxiety. *Int J Eat Disord* 1990;9:345–355.
73. Wadden TA, Stunkard AJ, Brownell KD, et al. A comparison of two very-low-calorie diets: protein-sparing-modified fast versus protein-formula-liquid diet. *Am J Clin Nutr* 1985;41:533–539.
74. Yanovski SZ. Binge eating disorder: current knowledge and future directions. *Obes Res* 1993;1:306–324.
75. Sherwood NE, Jeffery RW, Wing RR. Binge status as a predictor of weight loss treatment outcome. *Int J Obes Relat Metab Disord* 1999;23:485–493.
76. Wadden TA, Bartlett S, Letizia KA, et al. Relationship of dieting history to resting metabolic rate, body composition, eating behavior and subsequent weight loss. *Am J Clin Nutr* 1992;56:2065–2115.
77. Drapkin RG, Wing RR, Shiffman S. Responses to hypothetical high risk situations: do they predict weight loss in a behavioral treatment program or the context of dietary lapses? *Health Psychol* 1995;14:427–434.
78. Kiernan M, King AC, Kraemer HC, et al. Characteristics of successful and unsuccessful dieters: an application of signal detection methodology. *Ann Behav Med* 1998;20:1–6.
79. Pasman WJ, Saris WH, Westerterp-Plantega MS. Predictors of weight maintenance. *Obes Res* 1999;7:43–50.
80. Yass-Reed EM, Barry NJ, Dacey CM. Examination of pretreatment predictors of attrition in a VLCD and behavior therapy weight loss program. *Addict Behav* 1993;18:431–435.
81. Foreyt JP, Goodrick KG. Factors common to successful therapy for the obese patient. *Med Sci Sports Exerc* 1991;23:292–297.
82. Fogelholm M, Kukkonen-Harjula K, Oja P. Eating control and physical activity as determinants of short-term weight maintenance after a very-low-calorie diet among obese women. *Int J Obes Relat Metab Disord* 1999;23:203–210.
83. Jeffery RW, Wing RR, Mayer RR. Are smaller weight losses or more achievable weight loss goals better in the long term for obese patients. *J Consult Clin Psychol* 1998;66:641–645.
84. Barnstuble JA, Klesges RC, Terbizan D. Predictors of weight loss in a behavioral treatment program. *Behav Ther* 1986;17:288–294.
85. Schoeller DA. Limitations in the assessment of dietary energy intake by self-report. *Metabolism* 1995;44:18–22.
86. Harris JK, French SA, Jeffery RW, et al. Dietary and physical activity correlates of long-term weight loss. *Obes Res* 1994;2:307–313.
87. Holden JH, Darga LL, Olson SM, et al. Long-term follow-up of patients attending a combination very-low calorie diet and behaviour therapy weight loss programme. *Int J Obes* 1992;16:605–613.
88. French SA, Jeffery RW, Forster JL, et al. Predictors of weight change over two years among a population of working adults: the Healthy Worker Project. *Int J Obes Relat Metab Disord* 1994;18:145–154.
89. Foster GD, Wadden TA, Swain RM, et al. The Eating Inventory in obese women: clinical correlates and relationship to weight loss. *Int J Obes Relat Metab Disord* 1998;22:778–785.
90. Bjorvell H, Aly A, Langius A, et al. Indicators of changes in weight and eating behaviour in severely obese patients treated in a nursing behavioural program. *Int J Obes Relat Metab Disord* 1994;18:521–525.
91. Clark M, Marcus BH, Pera V, et al. Changes in eating inventory scores following obesity treatment. *Int J Eat Disord* 1994;15:401–405.
92. Guare JC, Wing RR, Marcus MD, et al. Analysis of changes in eating behavior and weight loss in type II diabetic patients. *Diabetes Care* 1989;12:500–503.
93. Jeffery RW, Wing RR. Long-term effects of interventions for weight loss using food provision and monetary incentives. *J Consult Clin Psychol* 1995;63:793–796.
94. Wadden TA, Bell ST. Obesity. In: Kazdin A, ed. *International handbook of behavior modification and therapy.* Vol 2. New York: Plenum Publishing, 1990:449–472.
95. Spiegel TA, Wadden TA, Foster GD. Objective measurement of eating rate during behavioral treatment of obesity. *Behav Ther* 1991;22:61–67.
96. Smith CF, O'Neil PM, Rhodes SK. Cognitive appraisals of dietary transgressions by obese women: associations with self-reported eating behavior, depression, and actual weight loss. *Int J Obes Relat Metab Disord* 1999;23:231–237.

19

Nutrition and Obesity

Adam Drewnowski and Victoria A. Warren-Mears

One in two adults in the United States is overweight, and one in three is obese (1). Obesity has become the most common nutrition-linked disease in the United States, and it is rapidly becoming a global public health problem (2–4). Given the adverse health consequences of obesity and its economic cost to society, much effort has gone into clinical and public health strategies for obesity prevention and treatment (5–7). Whether such interventions ought to target genetic, metabolic, psychologic, environmental, or nutritional factors is not always clear. All of these factors affect the expression of obesity, although their relative contribution probably varies from one person to another (8–10).

In years past, definitions of obesity were framed solely within the biomedical paradigm (8,11). The focus was on genetic predisposition and on metabolic, physiologic, or behavioral abnormalities that might help one distinguish between obese individuals and persons of normal weight. However, the sharp rise in obesity rates suggests that environmental influences on energy balance are more directly responsible. The gene pool within the United States population has not changed much over the past decade, and neither has human physiology. In contrast, food choices, eating habits, and activity patterns continue to evolve. The combination of excess energy intakes and reduced physical activity drives the energy equation toward increased deposition of body fat. Innate mechanisms regulating appetite and satiety continue to be challenged by sedentary lifestyles and by an oversupply of energy-dense foods. Regulatory mechanisms that evolved to deal with scarcity and starvation may be ill adapted to the current conditions of nutrition excess.

As a result, obesity and dietary behaviors are directly linked (1). Obesity is sometimes defined as a disease of overnutrition or as a metabolic consequence of nutrition imbalance. The precise contribution of excess energy as opposed to that of excess macronutrient intakes to weight gain is still unclear. Researchers disagree whether a high proportion of a given macronutrient in the diet can lead to obesity, independent of energy intakes. At different times, obesity has been linked to the overconsumption of all three macronutrients—carbohydrate, protein, and fat—when expressed as percentage of dietary energy (1). Obesity has also been associated with overconsumption of specific foods and beverages, with more diversified diets, with a higher incidence of snacking, and with higher rates of eating away from home (12–14). Not surprisingly, some of these postulated links between obesity and dietary choices have proved controversial.

In most cases, the nutritional component of obesity had been defined in terms of abnormal nutrient selection or inappropriate dietary behaviors. Given a choice, obese persons were said to select sugar, starches, fats, or energy-dense foods in preference to more nutritious vegetables and fruit. Constant snacking and inappropriate food choices were said to be driven by metabolic events, heightened taste preferences, food compulsions, or food "cravings." Pharmaceutical treatment options were often designed to halt the consumption of starches or fats, whereas the goal of behavior-oriented therapy was to modify and to improve the pattern of food choices (15–17). The underlying premise, in both cases, was that better nutrition choices were freely available to the obese individual.

The current view in public health nutrition is that individual choices related to diet and physical activity are often limited, whether by virtue of education, income, or other socio-cultural characteristics. The available diet options are often dictated by the environment, and they have little to do with individual freedom to choose. Generally, socially advantaged people have more choices regarding diet and exercise options than do poor people. Any discussion of nutrition factors in obesity cannot stray too far from the basic premise that food choices and the quality of one's diet tend to follow a socioeconomic gradient. It is not a coincidence that obesity in the United States is to a large extent a disease of the minorities and the poor (18).

OBESITY AND DIET COMPOSITION

The current United States food supply produces 3,700 calories per person per day, far more than the estimated energy needs for a typical man, woman, or child. Although energy imbalance is the chief, and possibly the only, reason for body weight gain, studies have sought to link obesity rates with excess consumption of specific nutrients or foods. Studies on the contribution of diet and nutrition to obesity have tended to emphasize the macronutrient composition of the diet and the influence of macronutrients on brain chemistry among obese, as opposed to lean, persons (19–24). Table 19.1 outlines the proposed mechanisms linking dietary macronutrients and obesity. Unresolved issues exist, however, concerning the role that each macronutrient or a given food may potentially play in promoting excess weight gain (24–26).

TABLE 19.1. *Macronutrient composition and obesity*

Dietary component	Proposed relationship to obesity	Therapeutic diet
Carbohydrate	Excessive consumption of starches and simple sugars leads to obesity, regardless of total energy intake. Hyperinsulinemia caused by carbohydrates, primarily those low in fiber, causes excessive storage of fat in adipose tissue. Elevated sugar intake *per se* is also thought to cause weight gain.	Consume low-carbohydrate diet, focusing on simple sugars.
Protein	Obesity is due to excess protein consumption in early childhood, regardless of calories. Early high protein intakes may account for the increases in stature and muscle mass. This may involve hormonal changes, particularly insulin-like growth factor-1 and growth hormone.	Avoid excess protein, particularly at an early age.
Fat	Excessive consumption of fat energy leads to obesity, regardless of total energy intake. High energy density of fat (9 kcal/g) is responsible for "passive overeating."	Consume a low-fat diet to assist with caloric restriction.

Carbohydrates and Weight Gain

Excessive intake of carbohydrates has been suggested as a primary cause of obesity (27,28). Some researchers believe that excessive consumption of starches and simple sugars leads to obesity, regardless of total energy intake (29). The proponents of this theory suggest that hyperinsulinemia caused by carbohydrates, primarily those low in fiber, causes excessive storage of fat and resultant increases in adipose tissue. Elevated sugar intake *per se* is also thought to cause weight gain. One illustration of this approach comes from pediatric studies that have attributed excessive weight gain in children to an elevated intake of fruit juice (fructose) and juice-based drinks (fructose and sucrose) (27,28). Other studies have also attributed adolescent weight gain to an elevated consumption of sweetened soft drinks (30).

One potential mechanism may involve the glycemic index (GI) of foods (29). In a small clinical trial, 12 obese boys consumed isocaloric test meals at breakfast and lunch that had a low, medium, or high GI but that did not vary in palatability, macronutrient composition, or in fiber content. *Ad libitum* food intake in the 5 hours after lunch was 5.8 megajoule (MJ) after the meal with a high GI, compared to that after a meal with a medium GI (3.8 MJ), and it was 81% greater than it was after the meal with a low GI (3.2 MJ). The meal with a high GI resulted in higher serum insulin levels and lower plasma glucose and serum fatty acids levels, compared with the meal with a low GI. The researchers concluded that rapid glucose absorption induces a sequence of hormonal and metabolic changes that promote further food consumption among the obese (29). In this view, obesity is caused by a cycle of inappropriate food choices.

Recent epidemiologic studies have pointed to higher rates of cardiovascular disease and type II diabetes among persons deriving a greater percentage of energy from refined grains and simple sugars than from whole grains (31). Diets with lower GIs have been reported to lower postprandial glucose and insulin responses, to improve lipid profiles, and to increase insulin sensitivity (32). Moreover, diets with high GIs stimulate *de novo* lipogenesis and result in increased adipocyte size, whereas diets with low GIs have been reported to inhibit these responses (33). In this view, the GI of foods plays an important role in the metabolic fate of carbohydrates, thereby altering the risk of obesity, diabetes, and cardiovascular disease (34).

This view is not universally accepted, and no long-term studies have been done on this topic. Although short-term clinical studies suggest that the consumption of food with a high GI increases hunger and promotes food consumption, their relevance to the long-term regulation of body weight is not clear. Some investigators have called for an increased consumption of whole grains and complex carbohydrates as a way to reduce energy intakes through improved dietary choices (35).

Protein and Weight Gain

Other researchers believe that obesity is due to excess protein consumption in early childhood, regardless of calories (36–38). The only significant association between nutritional intake at the age of 2 years and the age at which adiposity rebound occurred is a high percentage of energy from protein (37). Early high-protein intakes may account for the increase in stature and muscle mass. The suggested mechanism involves hormonal changes, particularly those of insulin-like growth factor-1 and growth hormone.

Real-life diets that are high in protein also tend to be rich in fat. In the United States food supply, protein-rich foods (i.e., meat) are often among the major dietary sources of fat. McCarty (39), who focused on protein sources, as opposed to the nutrient itself, has proposed a role for animal protein in the development of obesity.

Dietary Fat and Weight Gain

Excessive fat consumption is also believed to be a key cause of human obesity. At 9 kcal per g, fat has the highest energy density of all the macronutrients. Diets that are high in energy are also likely to be rich in fat because consuming an energy-rich diet that is devoid of energy-rich foods is difficult. In a metaanalysis study, Hill et al. (24) found that numerous environmental factors promoted excess energy intake and discouraged energy expenditure. However, the authors noted that the consumption of a high-fat diet increased the likelihood of the development of obesity, whereas persons consuming low-fat diets displayed a reduced risk (24).

Many clinical and epidemiologic studies have likewise reported a relationship between the percent of dietary energy from fat and obesity, although the relationship appears to be highly variable (40). First, researchers have not decided whether the key intake variable is percent of energy from fat or the absolute amount of fat consumed in grams per day. To complicate matters, the consumption of dietary fat in the United States has declined recently, but only when expressed as percent of dietary energy. When expressed in terms of grams of fat per day, fat consumption has actually increased (1). As a result, the role of fat in the development of obesity continues to be questioned. Some researchers claim that, because dietary fat intake has dropped even as the obesity rates have increased, the two are most likely unrelated. Others have noted that rising obesity rates were indeed associated with increased energy consumption and higher absolute consumption of dietary fat (1,41).

Another argument turns on the role of low-fat diets in facilitating weight loss. The premise that overconsumption of a given nutrient leads to obesity has given rise to a corollary belief, namely that removing that nutrient from the diet is bound to lead to weight loss. If high-fat diets lead to weight gain, then equicaloric low-fat diets should lead to weight loss. Diets recommended by Ornish and Pritikin advocate this approach to weight reduction. However, little evidence indicates that the macronutrient composition of the diet has any direct metabolic effects that are separate from those of restricted calories. Rather, the monotony of low-fat diets and the limited food choices may be responsible for restricted energy intakes and weight loss (42).

One of the longest and most thoroughly documented intervention trials of weight loss was the Women's Health Trial, in which more than 300 women between the ages of 45 and 69 years participated. The intervention consisted of a comprehensive dietary and behavioral program to lower fat intake from a mean baseline of 39% to 20% of energy intake. According to food records, this goal was achieved, and fat intake was reduced to approximately 22% of calories. An associated 25% reduction in energy intake was also seen during the first 12 months. Although weight loss was neither encouraged nor discouraged, the authors noted that many women used the program as an opportunity to lose weight (an average of 1.9 kg was lost at the end of 2 years) (43,44). Several other studies have also shown that low-fat diets in the absence of conscious energy restriction can result in modest weight loss over a few months. Such data suggest that intentionally lowering the fat content of the diet can be an effective strategy for weight loss. However, the primary mechanism may not be a reduction in fat *per se*, but rather the resulting reduction in energy intakes.

A similar analysis of 28 clinical trials by Bray and Popkin (45) has been taken as evidence that dietary fat plays a role in both the development and the treatment of obesity. A 10% reduction in energy from dietary fat was associated with a weight loss of 16 g per day. Among the studies cited in the metaanalysis, two demonstrated a modest, sustained weight loss in individuals participating for more than 1 year (46,47). The authors concluded that reducing fat consumption helped to reduce the imbalance between energy intake and expenditure and that it was an effective strategy for obesity prevention and treatment.

Another metaanalysis of controlled trials lasting more than 2 months comparing *ad libitum* low-fat diets with control diets with either habitual or medium-fat intake showed that weight loss was related to pretreatment body weight and to the reduction of the percentage of energy as fat (48). Based on their analysis, the authors concluded that there was no evidence that a high intake of simple sugars contributed to excess energy intakes. Another suggestion was that increasing the protein content of the diet to 25% of total calories would also help reduce energy intakes. Their suggestion was that a low-fat, high-protein diet that was also high in complex carbohydrates from fiber-rich whole grains, vegetables, and fruit was the most appropriate dietary option for the treatment of obesity.

An additional metaanalysis of 37 dietary intervention studies showed that, when dietary fat was reduced by more than 10% of total calories (i.e., from >35% to <25%), a weight reduction was seen (49). For every 1% decrease in energy as total fat, a 0.28-kg decrease in body weight occurred. The effect of change in total fat explained 57% of the total variance in weight loss (49).

OBESITY AND ENERGY DENSITY

If people consume a given weight or volume of food per day, food choices high in energy density will lead to elevated energy intakes overall. In contrast, energy-dilute foods will promote satiety while delivering fewer calories per eating bout. *Energy density* refers to the energy (calories) in a given weight of food (29). For the same amount of energy, a greater weight of food can be consumed if the food or diet is low in energy density than if the food or diet is high in energy density. Energy density is affected by the macronutrient composition of foods—both carbohydrate and protein provide 4 kcal per g, whereas fat provides 9 kcal per g and alcohol, 7 kcal per g. Because fat has such a high energy density, fat and the energy density of foods are often correlated. Weight loss attributed to the consumption of low-fat foods could be due to the increased bulk and the lower energy density of the diet (19,23).

Water content of foods probably contributes more to energy density than fat does. The weight of foods is largely determined by their hydration and water content, so water content and energy density of foods or diets are highly correlated. Water contributes weight, but not energy, to foods. Generally, dry foods are higher in energy density than water-containing foods; for instance, a dry fat-free pretzel has the same energy density as high-fat cheddar cheese, a food that is higher in water content. Energy density of foods can also be reduced by fiber or even air. However, the influence of fiber is relatively modest, because only a limited amount of fiber can be added to foods (19,23).

No convincing evidence links the development of obesity to macronutrient selection or to specific food choices, independent of calories. Although obesity has been blamed on fat and sugar consumption, little evidence is available to suggest that obese persons have an innate and selective appetite for either sugar or fat. Indeed, the very nature of physiologic mechanisms regulating macronutrient selection has been called into question. Obesity may be associated with an appetite for palatable energy-dense foods, whatever their macronutrient content. Nonetheless, diet composition is widely viewed as the primary cause of obesity and the key to successful weight loss. Low-carbohydrate diets, high-protein diets, high-fiber diets, and low-fat diets have all been popular at different times over the last 50 years (50).

Energy-Restricted Diets

Energy restriction has been the cornerstone of obesity treatment. A deficit of 3,500 kcal roughly equals 1 lb of body weight. A reduction in intake of 500 kcal per day below the body's requirement should lead, in principle, to a loss of 1 lb per week. Whereas diets of 1,000 kcal per day or less are used in clinical settings, they carry certain risks when they are used without appropriate supervision (51,52). Very low calorie diets may cause side effects, including intolerance to cold, hair loss, gallstone formation, and menstrual irregularity. Supplementation with vitamins, minerals, and electrolytes can be an issue.

As with many dietary changes, both risks and benefits are associated with weight loss (51,53–55). Most health care professionals believe that the more calorie restrictive the diet, the greater the risk is of adverse events associated with weight loss. Moderate energy restriction has been shown to increase bone turnover in obese postmenopausal women, an effect that may be regulated in part by hormonal changes (54). Most diets manipulate macronutrient composition instead. Table 19.2 presents a summary of various popular diets. Options for weight reduction include reducing the percent of fat energy, increasing the carbohydrate content, or reducing the energy density of the diet to achieve a reduction in total energy intakes (24,25,48,56–65).

Low-Energy–Density Diets

The energy-density approach to dieting has been the topic of many articles and books. If people consume a constant weight of food each day, then choosing energy-dense foods will lead to higher energy intakes. Conversely, choosing foods with low energy densities should lead, in principle, to lower energy intakes and eventual weight loss (19–23,66). The idea that fat and protein differ in their effect of satiety have already been exploited by the weight loss industry. Some liquid formula diets are simply mixtures of protein, fiber, and water, with small amounts of carbohydrates. Although they represent a major commercial success, their availability has not reduced the growing rates of overweight and obesity (66).

Two main problems are associated with the energy-density approach to weight loss. First, the energy density of food is almost completely determined by the fat and water content (25,67). Energy-dense foods are generally dry and high in fat and sometimes sugar. In contrast, energy-dilute foods are generally high in water, fiber, and sometimes protein. In practice, the energy density of the diet can be reduced by increasing the consumption of low-energy–density items, mostly of vegetables and fruit.

However, the more-energy–dense foods are usually more palatable. Individuals frequently tend to list energy-dense foods on their list of favorite foods. Women with anorexia nervosa are an exception to this rule, since they often list energy-dilute vegetables and salads among their favorite foods (67).

TABLE 19.2. *Diet description*

Diet description	Macronutrient composition			Recommended caloric level	Potential nutrient deficits	Examples
	Fat (% kcal)	Carbohydrate (% kcal)	Protein (% kcal)			
High fat, low CHO (<100 g/day), high protein	55–65	less than 20 (less than 100 g)	25–30	*Ad libitum* intake	Vitamin E, A, thiamine, B6, folate, calcium, magnesium, iron, zinc, potassium, and dietary fiber	Dr. Atkins' new diet revolution, Protein power
Moderate fat reduction, high CHO, moderate protein	20–30	55–60	15–20	Variable, generally more than 1,500		USDA Food Guide Pyramid, DASH Diet, Weight Watchers
Low fat and very low fat, very high CHO, moderate protein	less than 10–19	more than 65	10–20	Variable, generally about 1,450	Vitamin B$_{12}$ (with low meat intake)	Dr. Dean Ornish's Program for Reversing Heart Disease; Eat More, Weigh Less; The New Pritikin Program

Abbreviations: CHO, carbohydrate; DASH, Dietary Approaches to Stop Hypertension; USDA, United States Department of Agriculture.

High-Carbohydrate, Low-Fat Diets

Medical professionals recommend the consumption of a moderate-fat diet, which is defined as a diet deriving less than 30% of the energy from fat (Table 19.3). Lower-fat diets, which derive as little as 10% energy from fat, have been recommended for specific populations, such as obese and dyslipidemic men. Both the American Heart Association and the United States Department of Agriculture have published guidelines for recommended macronutrient intakes (68). As an example, the stage II National Cholesterol Education Program diet derives only 25% of the energy from fat and 7% of its calories from saturated fat and includes less than 200 mg of cholesterol. Such a diet severely restricts the consumption of high-fat meats, dairy products, and condiments high in saturated fat. Likewise, the Therapeutic Lifestyle Change (TLC) diet, which was proposed in May 2001 by the National Heart, Lung, and Blood Institute, recommends that 25% to 35% of total calories come from fat, with less than 7% coming from saturated fats (1). The assumption behind the restriction of calories from fat is that the most energy dense calories come from high-fat foods, with fat representing 9 kcal/g. The restriction of fat, therefore, would lead to a restriction of the most dense calories, thus contributing to lowering calories from energy-dense fat.

Dietary fat restrictions result in a variable amount of weight loss, depending on the individual's genetic background. Shaefer et al. (69) showed that, when subjects in their study switched from a high-fat to an *ad libitum* low-fat diet, they experienced a wide range of weight changes, ranging from a gain of 1.5 kg to a loss of 13 kg, with an average loss of 3.3 kg. This may suggest the existence of "responders" and "nonresponders" to a low-fat diet.

The influence of dietary fiber on energy regulation remains controversial. Under conditions of fixed energy intake, most studies indicate that an increase in either soluble or insoluble fiber intake increases postprandial satiety (70). When energy intake is *ad libitum*, the mean values for published studies indicate that the consumption of an additional 14 g of fiber per day for more than 2 days is associated with a 10% drop in total energy intake and a weight loss of 1.9 kg over approximately 4 months (70). Additionally, obese individuals may exhibit a greater suppression of energy intake and weight loss (70).

Pereira and Ludwig (71) cite short-term studies that suggest that high-fiber foods induce greater satiety. Likewise, epidemiologic studies support a reduced incidence of

TABLE 19.3. *Fat grams for 30% of total dietary kilocalories*

Daily caloric intake	Recommended fat grams to equal 30% of total kilocalories
1,200	40
1,300	43
1,400	46
1,500	50
1,600	53
1,700	56
1,800	60
1,900	63
2,000	66
2,100	70
2,200	73
2,500	83
3,000	100

high body weight among free-living individuals consuming self-selected diets that are higher in fiber. Thus, further evidence supports the conclusion that fiber-rich diets containing nonstarchy vegetables, fruits, and whole grains may be effective in both the treatment and the prevention of obesity.

In a cross-sectional cohort study conducted in seven countries, the population averages for physical activity and dietary fiber intake were both strongly inversely related to population average skinfold thickness. A similar, but less strong, association was attained for population average body mass index (BMI) (56). Likewise, in the Coronary Artery Development in Young Adults (CARDIA) study (57) after adjustment for confounding factors, dietary fiber showed a linear association with body weight, waist to hip ratios, and the 2-hour post–glucose administration insulin level adjusted for BMI. The CARDIA study demonstrated that the relationship between fiber ingestion and body weight was negative—that is, the higher the fiber intake the lower the body weight. Authors, therefore, suggest that a high-fiber diet may protect against obesity and cardiovascular disease by lowering insulin levels.

In view of the fact that dietary fiber intake in the United States is approximately 15 g per day, or approximately one-half of the recommendation of the American Heart Association, the National Heart, Lung, and Blood Institute, and the American Dietetic Association, efforts to increase dietary fiber consumption in individuals consuming less than 25 g per day may be beneficial.

Low-Carbohydrate, High-Protein Diets

Several weight loss diets of the 1950s and 1960s were based on carbohydrate restriction, with unlimited intake of foods high in protein and fat. Some of these diets were based on the premise that carbohydrates, particularly sugar, had low satiety value. Others took the position that ketogenesis was a benefit, conferring a reduced sensation of hunger. Weight loss experienced by people after carbohydrate-free diets is often due to water loss. A recent revival has occurred in the use of low-carbohydrate, high-protein diets, which is documented by the success of popular diet books. Some of these diets are also high in fat and saturated fat.

Proteins are essential components of many body structures, including enzymes, hormones, and antibodies. They also function as important transport and structural components. Proteins are made up of amino acids, eight of which are termed *essential*; in other words, they must be obtained from the diet. The remaining 12 amino acids are nonessential, and these can be manufactured in the body. The nutritional value of proteins varies based on a food item's amino acid profile. Foods that have essential amino acids at levels appropriate to use in the human body are termed *complete proteins*. As such, they have a high biologic value. High–biologic-value proteins are well absorbed, retained, and used by the body. The highest biologic value is seen, in general, from animal protein sources, such as eggs, milk, meat, fish, and poultry. Most high-protein foods also contain fat (68).

A change in emphasis regarding the benefits of low-carbohydrate, high-protein diets has occurred. The current focus is on insulin resistance and hyperinsulinemia. Emphasis has also shifted from total carbohydrates to high-GI carbohydrates—that is, those carbohydrates that, when eaten individually, cause the highest rise in blood glucose and therefore in insulin levels.

High-protein diets carry some nutritional risks in the long term. First, by limiting carbohydrate-rich foods, trace micronutrients, phytochemicals, and plant sterols will be lacking in the diet. Second, the concept of GI poses some difficulty when used in actual situations. The GI of given foods is determined by testing individual foods. Generally, foods are consumed in mixed meals, thus changing the impact of the meal versus the individual foods. Third, high-protein diets can be ketogenic. The effects of ketosis include rapid loss of water due to the use of glycogen stores, suppression of the appetite, dizziness, fatigue, and nausea. High-protein diets also cause increased calcium turnover. This, in turn, may have negative implications for bone health. Individuals who choose to follow a high-protein, low-carbohydrate plan should be monitored for orthostatic hypotension, which can be caused by sodium depletion, excessive water loss, and depressed sympathetic nervous system activity (55). High-protein diets also put patients with preexisting kidney and liver disease at risk. Taal and Brenner (72) have long emphasized the role of high-protein diets in declining kidney function with age. To achieve maximal renal protection, clinicians advocate a low-protein diet (72). Thus, high-protein, low-carbohydrate diets would be contraindicated for preservation of renal function. Additionally, glycogen depletion, as a result of low carbohydrate intake, may result in decreased tolerance for exercise and physical activity.

When individuals embark on a high-protein diet, they may also consume much higher levels of fat. Recent evaluations of many popular diets have shown that those following these diets have consumed more than 50% of total calories as fat (73). Higher fat diets are higher in saturated fats and cholesterol than the levels advocated in the current dietary guidelines, and their long-term use increases serum cholesterol levels and the risk of coronary heart disease (CHD) (74). Diets restricted in sugar lower serum cholesterol levels and the long-term risk of CHD; however, diets that are higher in carbohydrate and fiber but lower in fat would have the greatest effect in decreasing the serum cholesterol concentrations and risk of CHD. For this reason, the American Heart Association recently issued a statement on dietary protein and weight reduction (68). The association concluded that high-protein diets are not recommended because they restrict healthful foods that provide the essential nutrients and they do not adequately provide the variety of foods necessary to meet nutritional needs. Although high-fat diets may promote short-term weight loss, the potential hazards for worsening the risk of progression of atherosclerosis override the short-term benefits. Individuals derive the greatest health benefits from diets low in saturated fat and high in carbohydrate and fiber; these increase sensitivity to insulin and lower the risk of CHD.

THE GREAT DIET DEBATE

A current controversy that has been extensively debated by scientists is the relative value of a high-protein diet (Atkins diet) versus a high-carbohydrate diet (Ornish diet) (75). The data from the Continuing Survey of Food Intake by Individuals (CSFII) from 1994 to 1996 were used to examine the relationship between prototype popular diets and diet quality as measured by the healthy eating index (HEI), consumption patterns, and BMI. The CSFII study of Kennedy et al. (76) was based on 10,014 adults above 19 years of age. The prototype diets included vegetarian (no meat, poultry, or fish on the day of the survey) and nonvegetarian. The nonvegetarian group was further subdivided into low carbohydrate (<30% of energy from carbohydrate), medium (30% to 55%), and high (>55% of energy). Groups were further subdivided into low fat (<15% of energy from fat) and moderate fat (15% to 30% of energy from fat). BMIs were lowest for women in the vegetarian group (24.6) and the high-carbohydrate and/or low-fat group (24.4); for men, the lowest BMIs were observed for vegetarians (25.2) and the high-carbohydrate group (25.2). The highest BMIs were noted in the low-carbohydrate groups.

CONCLUSION

Overweight and obesity represent a major challenge to medicine and public health nutrition. Whereas biomedical researchers address the metabolism of nutrients and the regulation of food intake at the individual level, public health nutritionists address the question of why individuals consume such foods and not others. Long thought to be a matter of choice, access to therapeutic diets may be limited for segments of society. The links between diet quality, nutritional status, and overweight are influenced by socioeconomic status. Education and income are likely to influence patient compliance with the prescribed therapeutic diets.

REFERENCES

1. National Heart, Lung, and Blood Institute, Obesity Initiative Task Force. Clinical guidelines on the identification, evaluation, and treatment of overweight and obesity in adults—the evidence report. *Obes Res* 1998;6: 1S–210S.
2. Flegal KM, Carroll MD, Kuczmarski RJ, et al. Overweight and obesity in the United States: prevalence and trends, 1960 to 1994. *Int J Obes* 1998;22:39–47.
3. Mokdad AH, Serdula MK, Dietz WH, et al. The spread of the obesity epidemic in the United States, 1991–1998. *JAMA* 1999;282:1519–1522.
4. Must A, Spadano J, Coakley EH, et al. The disease burden associated with overweight and obesity. *JAMA* 1999; 282:1523–1529.
5. Thompson D, Brown JB, Nichols GA, et al. Body mass index and future healthcare costs: a retrospective cohort study. *Obes Res* 2001;9:210–218.
6. Quesenberry CP Jr, Caan B, Jabobson A. Obesity, health services use, and health care costs among members of a health maintenance organization. *Arch Intern Med* 1998;158:466–472.
7. Black DR, Sciacca JP, Coster DC. Extremes in body mass index: probability of healthcare expenditures. *Prev Med* 1994;23:385–393.
8. Wood SC, Schwartz MW, Baskin DG, et al. Food intake and regulation of body weight. *Ann Rev Psychol* 2000; 51:255–277.
9. Weinsier RL, Hunter GR, Heini AF, et al. The etiology of obesity: relative contribution of metabolic factors, diet and physical activity. *Am J Med* 1998;105:145–150.
10. Perusse L, Bouchard C. Gene-diet interactions in obesity. *Am J Clin Nutr* 2000;72:1285S–1290S.
11. Perusse L, Bouchard C. Genotype-environment interaction in human obesity. *Nutr Rev* 1999;57:S31–S38.
12. Zizz C, Siega-Riz AM, Popkin BM. Significant increase in young adults' snacking between 1977–1978 and 1994–1996 represents a cause for concern. *Prev Med* 2001;32:303–310.
13. Binkley JK, Eales J, Jekanowski M. The relationship between dietary change and rising US obesity. *Int J Obes Relat Metab Disord* 2000;24:1032–1039.
14. McCrory MA, Fuss PJ, Hays NP, et al. Overeating in America: association between restaurant food consumption and body fatness in healthy adult mean and women ages 19 to 80. *Obes Res* 1999;7:564–571.
15. Campbell ML, Mathys ML. Pharmacologic options for the treatment of obesity. *Am J Health Syst Pharm* 2001; 58:1301–1308.
16. Hauner H. Current pharmacological approaches to the treatment of obesity. *Int J Obes Relat Metab Disord* 2001; 25:S102–S106.
17. Poston WS, Hyder ML, O'Byrne KK, et al. Where do diets, exercise and behavior modification fit in the treatment of obesity? *Endocrine* 2000;13:187–192.
18. Visscher TL, Seidell JC. The public health impact of obesity. *Annu Rev Public Health* 2001;22:355–375.
19. Bell EA, Rolls BJ. Energy density of foods affects energy intake across multiple levels of fat content in obese and lean women. *Am J Clin Nutr* 2001;73:1010–1018.
20. Levine AS. Energy density of foods: building a case for food intake management. *Am J Clin Nutr* 2001;73: 999–1000.
21. Westerp-Plantenga MS. Analysis of energy density of food in relation to energy intake regulation in human subjects. *Br J Nutr* 2001;85:351–361.
22. Stubbs J, Ferres S, Horgan G. Energy density of foods: effects on energy intake. *Crit Rev Food Sci Nutr* 2000; 40:481–515.
23. Rolls BJ. The role of energy density in the overconsumption of fat. *J Nutr* 2000;130:268S–271S.

24. Hill JO, Melanson EL, Wyatt HT. Dietary fat intake and regulation of energy balance: implications for obesity. *J Nutr* 2000;130:284S–288S.
25. Bray GA, Popkin BM. Dietary fat does affect obesity. *Am J Clin Nutr* 1998;68:1157–1173.
26. Willett WC. Dietary fat and obesity: an unconvincing relation. *Am J Clin Nutr* 1998;68:1149–1150.
27. Dennison BA, Rockwell HL, Baker SL. Excess fruit juice consumption by preschool-aged children is associated with short stature and obesity. *Pediatrics* 1997;99:15–22.
28. Ludwig DS, Peterson KE, Gortmaker SL. Relation between consumption of sugar-sweetened drinks and childhood obesity: a prospective, observational analysis. *Lancet* 2001;357:505–508.
29. Ludwig DS, Majzoub JA, Al-Zahrani A, et al. High glycemic index foods, overeating, and obesity. *Pediatrics* 1999;103:E26.
30. Troiano RP, Briefel RR, Carroll MD, et al. Energy and fat intakes of children and adolescents in the United States: data from the National Health and Nutrition Examination Surveys. *Am J Clin Nutr* 2000;72: 1343S–1353S.
31. Liu S, Manson JE. Dietary carbohydrates, physical inactivity, obesity, and the "metabolic syndrome" as predictors for coronary heart disease. *Curr Opin Lipidol* 2001;12:395–404.
32. Ebbeling CB, Ludwig DS. Treating obesity in youth: should dietary glycemic load be a consideration? *Adv Pediatr* 2001;48:179–212.
33. McCarty MF. Modulation of adipocyte lipoprotein lipase expression as a strategy for preventing or treating visceral obesity. *Med Hypotheses* 2001;57:192–200.
34. Morris KL, Zemel MB. Glycemic index, cardiovascular disease and obesity. *Nutr Rev* 1999;57:273–276.
35. Roberts SB. High-glycemic index foods, hunger, and obesity: is there a connection? *Nutr Rev* 2000;58:163–169.
36. Parizkova J, Rolland-Cachera MF. High proteins early in life as a predisposition for later obesity and further health risks. *Nutrition* 1997;13:818–819.
37. Rolland-Cachera MF, Deheeger M, Bellisle F. Increasing prevalence of obesity among 18-year-old males in Sweden: evidence for early determinants. *Acta Paediatr* 1999;88:365–367.
38. Rolland-Cachera MF, Deheeger M, Bellisle F. Nutrient balance and android body fat distribution: why not a role for protein? *Am J Clin Nutr* 1996;646:663–664.
39. McCarty MF. The origins of western obesity: a role for animal protein? *Med Hypotheses* 2000;54:488–494.
40. Larson DE, Hunter GR, Williams MJ, et al. Dietary fat in relation to body fat and intra-abdominal adipose tissue: a cross-sectional analysis. *Am J Clin Nutr* 1996;64:677–684.
41. Lissner L, Heitmann BL, Bengtsson C. Population studies of diet and obesity. *Br J Nutr* 2000;83:S21–S24.
42. Kumanyika SK. Minisymposium on obesity: overview and some strategic consideration. *Annu Rev Public Health* 2001;23:293–308.
43. White E, Shattuck AL, Kristal AR, et al. Maintenance of a low-fat diet: follow-up of the Women's Health Trial. *Cancer Epidemiol Biomarker Prev* 1992;1:315–323.
44. Urban N, White E, Anderson GL, et al. Correlates of maintenance of a low-fat diet among women in The Women's Health Trial. *Prev Med* 1992;21:279–291.
45. Bray GA, Popkin BM. Dietary fat affects obesity rate. *Am J Clin Nutr* 1999;70:572–573.
46. Sheppard L, Kristal AR, Kushi LH. Weight loss in women participating in a randomized trial of low-fat diets. *Am J Clin Nutr* 1991;54:821–828.
47. Siggard R, Raben A, Astrup A. Weight loss during 12 weeks' ad libitum carbohydrate-rich diet in overweight and normal weight subjects at a Danish work site. *Obes Res* 1996;4:347–356.
48. Astrup A, Ryan I, Grunwald GK, et al. The role of dietary fat in body fatness: evidence from a preliminary meta-analysis of ad libitum low-fat dietary intervention studies. *Br J Nutr* 2000;83:S25–S32.
49. Yu-Poth S, Zhao G, Etherton T, et al. Effect of the National Cholesterol Education Program's Step I and Step II dietary intervention programs on cardiovascular disease risk facts: a meta analysis. *Am J Clin Nutr* 1999;69: 632–646
50. Rolls BJ. Dietary approaches to the treatment of obesity. *Med Clin North Am* 2000;84:401–418.
51. Cheung ST. Possible dangers in a low fat diet: some evidence reviewed. *Nutr Health* 2000;14:271–280.
52. Kersetter JE. Change in bone turnover in young women consuming differing levels of dietary protein. *J Clin Endocrinol Metab* 1999;84:1052–1055.
53. Festi D, Colecchia A, Larocca A, et al. Review: low caloric intake and gall-bladder motor function. *Aliment Phamacol Ther* 2000;14:51–53.
54. Ricci TA, Heymsfield SB, Pierson RN Jr, et al. Moderate energy restriction increases bone resorption in obese post-menopausal women. *Am J Clin Nutr* 2001;73:347–352.
55. Ahmed W, Flynn MA, Alpert MA. Cardiovascular complications of weight reduction diets. *Am J Med Sci* 2001; 321:280–284.
56. Kromhout D, Bloemberg B, Seidell JC, et al. Physical activity and dietary fiber determine population body fat levels: the Seven Countries Study. *Int J Obes Relat Metab Disord* 2001;25:301–306.
57. Ludwig DS, Pereira MA, Kroenke CH, et al. Dietary fiber, weight gain, and cardiovascular disease risk factors in young adults. *JAMA* 1999;282:1539–1546.
58. Saltzman E, Roberts SB. Soluble fiber and energy regulation. Current knowledge and future directions. *Adv Exp Med Biol* 1997;66:1332–1339.
59. Pasman WJ, Saris WH, Wauters MA, et al. Effect of one week of fibre supplementation on hunger and satiety ratings and energy intake. *Appetite* 1997;29:77–87.

60. Shepherd TY, Weil KM, Sharp TA, et al. Occasional physical inactivity combined with a high-fat diet may be important in the development and maintenance of obesity in human subjects. *Am J Clin Nutr* 2001;73:703–708.
61. Hill JO, Melanson EL, Wyatt HT. Dietary fat intake and regulation of energy balance: implications for obesity. *J Nutr* 2000;130:284S–288S.
62. Green SM. Wales JK, Lawton CL, et al. Comparison of high-fat and high-carbohydrate foods in a meal or snack on short-term fat and energy intakes in obese women. *Br J Nutr* 2000;84:417–427.
63. Astrup A. Macronutrient balances and obesity: the role of diet and physical activity. *Public Health Nutr* 1999;2: 341–347.
64. Baba NH, Sawaya S, Torbay N, et al. High protein vs. high carbohydrate hypoenergetic diet for the treatment of obese hyperinsulinemic subjects. *Int J Obes Relat Metab Disord* 1999;23:1202–1206.
65. Purnell JQ, Knopp RH, Brunzell JD. Dietary fat and obesity. *Am J Clin Nutr* 1999;70:108–110.
66. Drewnowski A. Intense sweeteners and energy density of foods: implications for weight control. *Eur J Clin Nutr* 1999;53:757–763.
67. Drewnowski A. Energy density, palatability, and satiety: implications for weight control. *Nutr Rev* 1998;56: 347–353.
68. St. Jeor ST, Howard BV, Prewitt TE, et al. Dietary protein and weight reduction. *Circulation* 2001;104: 1869–1874.
69. Shaefer EJ, Lichtenstein AH, Lamon-Farva S, et al. Body weight and low-density lipoprotein cholesterol changes after consumption of a low-fat ad libitum diet. *JAMA* 1995;274:1450–1455.
70. Howarth NC, Saltzman E, Roberts SB. Dietary fiber and weight regulation. *Nutr Rev* 2001;59:129–139.
71. Pereira MA, Ludwig DS. Dietary fiber and body-weight regulation. Observations and mechanisms. *Pediatr Clin North Am* 2001;48:969–980.
72. Taal MW, Brenner BM. Achieving maximal renal protection in nondiabetic chronic renal disease. *Am J Kidney Dis* 2001;38:1365–1371.
73. Anderson JW, Konz EC, Jenkins DJ. Health advantages and disadvantages of weight-reducing diets: a computer analysis and critical review. *J Am Coll Nutr* 2000;19:578–590.
74. Fleming RM. The effect of high-protein diets on coronary blood flow. *Angiology* 2000;51:817–826.
75. Freedman MR, King J, Kennedy E. Popular diets: a scientific review. *Obes Res* 2001;9:1S–40S.
76. Kennedy ET, Bowman SA, Spence JT, et al. Popular diets: correlation to health, nutrition and obesity. *J Am Diet Assoc* 2001;101:411–420.

20

Treatment of Obesity with Drugs in the New Millennium

George A. Bray

Drug treatment for obesity has been tarnished by a number of unfortunate problems (1,2). Since the introduction of thyroid hormone to treat obesity in 1893, almost every drug that has been tried in obese patients has led to undesirable outcomes that has resulted in its termination. Thus, caution must be used in accepting any new drugs for treatment of obesity, unless the safety profile makes it acceptable for almost everyone.

An additional serious negative aspect to the use of drug treatment for obesity is the negative halo spread by the addictive properties of amphetamine (3). Amphetamine stands for *alpha-methyl—phenethylamine*. It is an addictive β-phenethylamine that reduces food intake. The addictiveness of amphetamine is probably related to its effects on dopaminergic neurotransmission. On the other hand, its anorectic effects appear to result from modulation of noradrenergic neurotransmission. Because amphetamine is addictive, other β-phenethylamine compounds have also been presumed to be addictive. Whether actually addictive or not, they have been considered guilty by association. This has led to restrictions on the use of this entire class of drugs by the United States Drug Enforcement Agency (DEA).

Drugs such as phentermine, diethylpropion, fenfluramine, sibutramine, and the antidepressant venlafaxine are all β-phenethylamines. Phentermine and diethylpropion are sympathomimetic amines, like amphetamine, but they differ from amphetamine because they have little or no effect on dopamine release or on its reuptake at the synapse. Abuse of either phentermine or diethylpropion is rare (1). Fenfluramine, on the other hand, has no effect on reuptake or release of either norepinephrine (NE) or dopamine in the brain. Rather, it increases serotonin release and partially inhibits serotonin reuptake. Sibutramine, likewise, has no evident abuse potential. Thus, derivatives of β-phenethylamine have a wide range of pharmacologic effects and a highly variable potential for abuse. However, if examined uncritically, they could all be lumped with amphetamine and could carry its negative halo. Thus, to use the term "amphetamine-like" in reference to appetite suppressant β-phenethylamine drugs is misleading, except in the cases of amphetamine and methamphetamine, because of the negative linguistic images and the inaccurate linguistic content.

A third issue surrounding drug treatment of obesity is the perception that, because patients regain weight when drugs are stopped, the drugs are ineffective (4). Quite the contrary is true. Overweight is a chronic disease that has many causes. A cure, however, is rare, and treatment is thus aimed at palliation. Clinicians do not expect to cure such diseases as hypertension or hypercholesterolemia with medications. Rather, they expect to palliate them. When the medications for any of these diseases are discontinued, the disease is expected to recur. This means that the medications work only when used. The same arguments apply for the medications used to treat overweight, which is a chronic, incurable disease for which drugs work only when used.

Reports of valvular heart disease associated with the use of fenfluramine, dexfenfluramine, and phentermine have provided the most recent problem for drug treatment of obesity (5). This is an example of the "law of unintended consequences." The report of valvulopathy in up to 35% of patients treated with the combination of fenfluramine and phentermine was totally unexpected. The finding, however, will add caution to any future drugs that are marketed to treat obesity and will provide support for those who believe drug treatment of obesity is inappropriate and risky.

The final issue is the plateau of weight that occurs with all treatments of obesity (6–12). Figure 20.1 shows the weight loss that can be achieved by various treatments in relation to the expectations of patients when they enter treatment. At the beginning of treatment, a weight loss of less than 15% is considered unsatisfactory by most patients (13). Yet the reality is that none of the treatments, except gastric bypass (12), reach this level of effectiveness. When weight loss plateaus, as it invariably does with all treatments, patients usually blame the treatment. The perceived loss of effectiveness often leads patients to terminate treatment with the inevitable slow regain of the weight that has been lost. This chapter reviews the currently available medications in the light of these limitations.

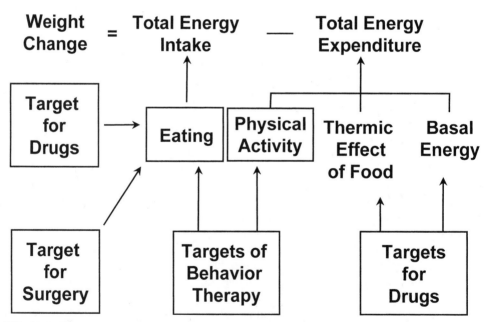

FIG. 20.1. Relation of plateaued weight during treatment of obesity and participant expectations in a weight loss program. The left hand ordinate shows the percent weight loss for each treatment. The right hand ordinate shows the cutpoints for weight loss expectations for each category. Only surgical treatment (11) produced a "dream" level of weight loss. The combination of fenfluramine and phentermine (9) produced acceptable weight loss, but the other treatments, including ephedrine combined with caffeine (10), phentermine (8), meal replacement (7), orlistat (6), and sibutramine (5), left patients disappointed.

MECHANISMS FOR DRUG TREATMENT OF OBESITY

Obesity results from an imbalance between energy intake and energy expenditure (EE). Drugs can shift this balance in a favorable way by reducing food intake, altering metabolism, and/or increasing EE. These three mechanisms are used to classify the drugs used for treating obesity (1,14).

Reducing Food Intake

Noradrenergic Receptors

A number of monoamines and neuropeptides are known to modulate food intake. Both noradrenergic receptors and serotonergic receptors have served as the site for clinically useful drugs to decrease food intake (Table 20.1) (1,14). Activation of the α_1-adrenoreceptors and β_2-adrenoceptors decreases food intake. On the other hand, stimulation of the α_2-adrenoceptor in experimental animals increases food intake. Direct agonists and drugs that release NE or block NE reuptake at the neuronal junction can activate one or more of these receptors, depending on where the NE is released. Phenylpropanolamine (PPA) is an α_1-agonist that decreases food intake by acting on α_1-adrenergic receptors in the paraventricular nucleus. The weight gain seen in patients treated with α_1-adrenergic antagonists for hypertension or prostatic hypertrophy indicates that the α_1-adrenoceptor is clinically important in regulation of body weight. Stimulation of the β_2-adrenoceptor by NE or by agonists such as terbutaline, clenbuterol, or salbutamol reduces food intake. The weight gain in patients treated with some β_2-adrenergic antagonists also indicates that this is a clinically important receptor for the regulation of body weight.

Serotonergic Receptors

The serotonin receptor system consists of seven families of receptors. Stimulation of receptors in the hydroxytryptamine (HT) 5-HT_1 and 5-HT_2 families produces the major effects on feeding. Activation of the 5-HT_{1A} receptor increases food intake, but this acute effect is rapidly downregulated, and it is not clinically significant in control of body weight. Activation of the 5-HT_{2C} and possibly the 5-HT_{1B} receptors decreases food intake. Direct agonists, such as quipazine, or drugs that block serotonin reuptake, such as fluoxetine, sertraline, or fenfluramine, will reduce food intake either by acting on these receptors or by providing the serotonin that modulates these receptors.

TABLE 20.1. *Mechanisms that reduce food intake*

System	Mechanism	Examples
Noradrenergic	α_1 Agonist	Phenylpropanolamine
	α_2 Antagonist	Yohimbine
	β_2 Agonist	Clenbuterol
	Stimulate NE release	Phentermine
	Block NE reuptake	Mazindol
Serotonergic	5-HT_{1B} or 5-HT_{1C} agonist	Metergoline
	Stimulate 5-HT release	Fenfluramine
	Block reuptake	Fluoxetine
Dopaminergic	D_2 agonist	Apomorphine
Histaminergic	H_1 antagonist	Chlorpheniramine

Abbreviations: 5-HT, 5-hydroxytryptamine; NE, norepeniphrine.

Altering Metabolism

Excess fat is the visible sign of obesity. Metabolic strategies have been directed at pre-absorptive and postabsorptive mechanisms for modifying fat or carbohydrate absorption or metabolism. Preabsorptive mechanisms that influence digestion and the absorption of macronutrients are the basis for orlistat, a drug that inhibits the intestinal digestion of fat and lowers body weight. The second strategy is to affect intermediary metabolism. Enhancing lipolysis, inhibiting lipogenesis, and affecting fat distribution between subcutaneous and visceral sites are strategies that can be developed (1,15).

Increasing Energy Expenditure

Increasing EE through exercise would be an ideal approach to treating obesity. Drugs that have the same physiologic thermogenic consequences as exercise could provide a useful pharmaceutical alternative for treating this intractable problem (1,15).

DRUGS THAT REDUCE FOOD INTAKE

Table 20.2 summarizes the effects of a number of drugs currently available in the United States to treat obesity (1,2,16). They are discussed in more detail in the following sections.

TABLE 20.2. *Drugs approved by the FDA for treatment of obesity*

Drug	Trade names	Dosage	DEA schedule	Cost per d
Pancreatic lipase inhibitor approved for long-term use				
Orlistat	Xenical	120 mg t.i.d. before meals	—	$3.56/d
Norepinephrine-serotonin reuptake inhibitor approved for long-term use				
Sibutramine	Meridia, Reductil	5–15 mg/d	IV	$2.98 to $3.68/d
Noradrenergic drugs approved for short-term use				
Diethylpropion	Tenuate, Tepanil	25 mg t.i.d.	IV	$1.27 to $1.52/d
	Tenuate Dospan	75 mg every morning		
Phentermine	Adipex, Fastin, Oby-Cap	15–37.5 mg/d	IV	$0.67 to $1.60/d
	Ionamin slow release	15–30 mg/d		$1.75 to $2.01/d
Benzphetamine	Didrex	25–50 mg t.i.d.	III	$1.19 to $2.38/d
Phendimetrazine	Bontril, Plegine, Prelu-2	17.5–70 mg t.i.d.	III	$1.20 to $5.25/d
	X-Trozine	105 mg q.d.		

Abbreviations: DEA, Drug Enforcement Agency; FDA, Food and Drug Administration; q.d., every day; t.i.d., three times a day.

Sympathomimetic Drugs Approved by the Food and Drug Administration to Treat Obesity

Pharmacology

The sympathomimetic drugs are grouped together because they can increase blood pressure (BP) and, in part, act like NE. Drugs in this group work by a variety of mechanisms, including the release of NE from synaptic granules (benzphetamine, phendimetrazine, phentermine, and diethylpropion), the blockade of NE reuptake (mazindol), the blockade of reuptake of both NE and 5-HT (sibutramine), or direct action on α_1-adrenoceptors (PPA).

All of these drugs are absorbed orally, and they reach peak blood concentrations within a short time. The half-life in blood is also short for each one, except the metabolites of sibutramine, which have a long half-life (1). The two metabolites of sibutramine are active, but this is not true for the metabolites of other drugs in this group. Liver metabolism inactivates a large fraction of these drugs before their excretion. Side effects include dry mouth, constipation, and insomnia. Food intake is suppressed either by delaying the onset of a meal or by producing early satiety. Sibutramine and mazindol have both been shown to increase thermogenesis as well.

Efficacy

The efficacy of an appetite-suppressing drug can be established through randomized, double-blind clinical trials that show a significantly greater weight loss than the placebo-treated group—more than 5% below that of the placebo-treated group (1). This is the basic criterion for approval by the United States Food and Drug Administration (FDA). A decrease in weight that is 10% below baseline and that is significantly greater than that occurring with a placebo is the major criterion for the European Committee on Proprietary Medicinal Products (CPMP). Clinical trials of sympathomimetic drugs conducted before 1975 were generally short term because the widespread belief was that short-term treatment would "cure obesity" (1,2,17). This was unfounded optimism, and, because the trials were of short duration and were often crossover in design, they provided few long-term data. In this review, the author focuses on more long-term trials lasting 24 weeks or more and uses only those trials in which an adequate control group was established. These data are displayed in Table 20.3.

Phentermine, Diethylpropion, Benzphetamine, and Phendimetrazine

Most of the data on these drugs come from short-term trials that were often crossover in design (1,14,18–23). The best and one of the longest of these clinical trials lasted 36 weeks and compared placebo treatment with continuous phentermine or intermittent phentermine (Fig. 20.2) (9). Both continuous and intermittent phentermine therapy produced more weight loss than did the placebo. In the drug-free periods, the weight loss of the patients treated intermittently slowed, only to lose weight more rapidly when the drug was reinstituted. Phentermine and diethylpropion are classified by the United States Drug Enforcement Agency (DEA) as schedule IV drugs, and benzphetamine and phendimetrazine, as schedule III drugs. This regulatory classification indicates the government's belief that these drugs have the potential for abuse, although this potential appears to be extremely low. Phentermine and diethylpropion are approved only for a "few weeks," which is usually interpreted as up to 12 weeks. Weight loss with phentermine and diethylpropion persists for the duration of treatment, suggesting that tolerance to these drugs does not develop. If tolerance were to develop, the drugs would be expected to lose their

TABLE 20.3. Long-term studies with noradrenergic drugs

Author	Year	No. of subjects Start Placebo/drug	No. of subjects Complete Placebo/drug	Dose (mg/d)	Duration of study (wk)	Initial weight (kg) Placebo	Initial weight (kg) Drug	Weight loss (kg) Placebo	Weight loss (kg) Drug	Weight loss (%) Placebo	Weight loss (%) Drug	Comments
Diethylpropion												
Silverstone and Solomon (18)	1965	16/16	6/5	75	52	78.8	80.7	-10.5	-8.9	-13.3%	-11.0%	Medication given on alternate months
McKay (19)	1973	10/10	6/10	75	24	84.5	92.3	-2.5	-11.7	-2.8%	-12.3%	—
Phentermine												
Munro et al. (9)	1968	36/36	25/17	30	36	92.3	94.1	-4.8	-12.2	-5.9%	-15%	Continuous drug group (top) lost as much as the intermittent therapy (bottom)
		36	22				97.3		-13.0		-16%	
Langlois et al. (20)	1974	35/35	29/30	30	14	87.0	85.1	-1.8	-7.3	-2.1%	-8.5%	1,000-kcal/d diet
Gershberg et al. (21)	1977	11/11		30	16	84.1	85.0	-2.9	-7.8	-3.4%	-9.2%	Obese diabetics
Campbell et al. (22)	1977	35/36	32/34	30	24	—	—	-1.5	-5.3	—	—	Obese diabetics; diet, biguanide or insulin
Williams and Foulsham (23)	1981	15/15	11/11	30	24	73.6	73.6	-4.5	-6.3	-9.2%	-12.6%	Elderly with osteoarthritis
Weintraub et al. (23a)	1984	20/20	10/14	30 (resin)	20	No baseline weights given	—	-4.4	-10.0	—	—	Four-arm trial: placebo, fenfluramine (F), phentermine (P), and F + P

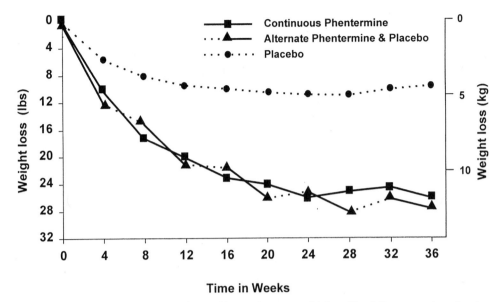

Time in Weeks

FIG. 20.2. Comparison of weight loss with continuous and intermittent therapy using phentermine (8). Overweight patients were randomized to receive either placebo or one of two dosing regimens with phentermine. One regimen provided 15 mg per day each morning for 9 months, and the other supplied 15 mg per day for 1 month and then a month of no treatment.

effectiveness, or increased amounts of drug would be required for patients to maintain weight loss. This does not occur.

Sibutramine

In contrast to the sympathomimetic drugs described in the previous section, sibutramine has been extensively evaluated in several multicenter trials lasting 6 to 18 months that are summarized in Table 20.4 (6,24–36).

In a clinical trial lasting 8 weeks, sibutramine produced a dose-dependent weight loss with doses of 5 and 20 mg per day (24). Several long-term, randomized, placebo-controlled, double-blind clinical trials have been conducted in men and women of all ethnic groups with ages ranging from 18 to 65 years and with a body mass index (BMI) between 27 kilograms per meter squared (kg/m^2) and 40 kg/m^2. In a 6-month dose-ranging study of 1,047 patients, 67% achieved a 5% weight loss, and 35% lost 10% or more. Data from this multicenter trial are shown in Fig. 20.3 (28).

A clear dose response is seen in this 24-week trial, and regain of weight occurred when the drug was stopped, indicating that the drug remained effective only when used. Nearly two-thirds of the patients treated with sibutramine lost more than 5% of their body weight from baseline, and nearly one-third lost more than 10%. In a 1-year trial that enrolled 456 patients who received either a placebo or sibutramine (10 or 15 mg per day), 56% of those who stayed in the trial for 12 months lost at least 5% of their initial weight, and 30% of the patients lost 10% of their initial body weight while taking the 10-mg dose (25). In a third trial of patients who initially lost weight eating a very low calorie diet before being randomized to sibutramine at 10 mg per day or a placebo, sibutramine produced additional weight loss, whereas the placebo-treated patients regained weight (29). The most recent clinical trial with sibutramine is the Sibutramine Trial of Obesity Reduc-

TABLE 20.4. Clinical trials with sibutramine

Author	Year	No. of subjects Start Placebo/ drug	Completers Placebo/ drug	Dose mg/d	Duration of study (wk)	Initial weight (kg) Placebo	Drug	Weight loss (kg) Placebo	Drug	Weight loss (%) Placebo	Drug	Comments
Weintraub et al. (24)	1991	20	19		8	97		-1.4		-1.3		Dose-ranging phase II
		20	18	5			97.9		-2.9		-3.0	
		20	18	20			102.4		-5.0		-5.1	
Jones et al. (25)	1995	163	76		52	87		-2.2		-2.5		Abstract
		161	80	10			87		-6.2		-7.1	
		161	93	15			87		-6.9		-7.9	
Bray et al. (26)	1996	24	23		24	92		-0.75		-0.77		Part of multicenter study. Data on completing women
		24	21	1			95.8		-2.96		-3.20	
		25	24	5			90.9		-2.87		-3.07	
		25	22	10			87.2		-6.19		-6.91	
		25	20	15			89.7		-6.89		-7.77	
		24	22	20			90.9		-7.30		-8.06	
		26	23	30			91.4		-8.24		-9.17	
Hannotin et al. (27)	1998	59	47		12	84		-1.4		-1.7		Multicenter trial
		56	47	5			83.3		-2.4		-2.9	
		59	49	10			85.0		-5.1		-6.0	
		62	52	15			88.3		-4.9		-5.5	

Study	Year	N randomized	N completed	Dose (mg)	Wk	Baseline wt (kg)	Change	Change	Change	Change	Comments
Bray et al. (28)	1999	148	87	0	24	95	−1.3	−2.4	−1.2	−2.7	Multicenter phase III trial
		149	95	1		94		−3.7		−3.9	
		151	107	5		94		−5.7		−6.1	
		150	99	10		91		−7.0		−7.4	
		152	98	15		93		−8.2		−8.8	
		146	96	20		93		−9.0		−9.4	
		151	101	30		95					
Apfelbaum et al. (29)	1999	181 / 82	48 / 60	10	52	97.7 / 95.7	+0.2	−6.1	+0.2	−6.4	Multicenter weight loss ≥6 kg after 4 wk VLCD were randomized
Finer et al. (34)	2000	44 / 47	40	15	12	82.5 / 84.6	−0.1	−2.4	–		Multicenter trial in diabetics
Fujioka et al. (33)	2000	86 / 89	43 / 61	5–20	24	98.2 / 99.3	−0.4	−3.7	−0.5	−4.5	Multicenter trial in diabetics
Fanghanel et al. (30)	2000	54 / 55	44 / 40	10	26	86.4 / 87.5	−4.6	−8.8	−4.8	−9.9	BMI >30 kg/m². Diet 30 kcal/kg of ideal body weight
McMahon et al. (6)	2000	74 / 150	69 / 142	5–20	52	95.5 / 97.0	−0.5	−4.4	−0.7	−4.7	Multicenter trial in hypertensives on calcium channel blockers
James et al. (31)	2000	115 / 232	57 / 204	10–20	78	102.1 / 102.3	−4.7	−10.2	−4.4	−10.0	Multicenter trial in subjects who lost ≥5% on 10 mg sibutramine in 6 months
Sramek et al. (33)	2001	32 / 29	(55)	5–20	12	95.9 / 94.2	−0.3	−4.2	−0.4	−4.5	Multicenter trial in hypertensives on β-blockers

Abbreviations: BMI, body mass index; VLCD, very low calorie.

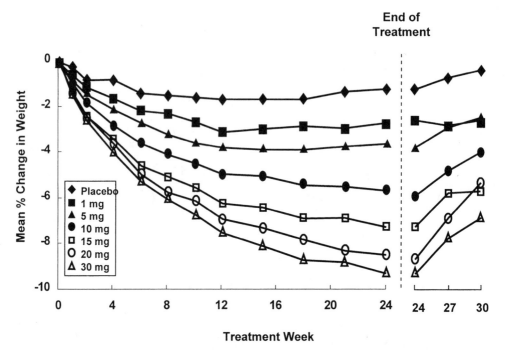

FIG. 20.3. Dose-related weight loss with sibutramine. A total of 1,047 patients were randomly assigned to receive placebo or one of six doses of sibutramine in a double-blind fashion for 6 months. By the end of the trial, weight loss had plateaued for most doses. When the drug was discontinued at 6 months, weight was regained, indicating that the drug remained effective during treatment (21).

tion and Maintenance (STORM trial) (31). Seven centers participated in this trial, in which patients were initially enrolled in an open-label fashion and were treated with 10 mg per day of sibutramine for 6 months. The patients who lost more than 5% of their initial body weight were then randomized as follows: two-thirds to sibutramine and one-third to a placebo. During the 18-month double-blind portion of this trial, the placebo-treated patients steadily regained weight, maintaining only 20% of their weight loss at the end of the trial. In contrast, the subjects treated with sibutramine maintained their weight for 12 months and then regained an average of only 2 kg, thus maintaining 80% of their initial weight loss after 2 years (31). In spite of the difference in weight at the end of the 18 months of controlled observation, the BP of the sibutramine-treated patients was still higher than that of the patients treated with the placebo, even though a weight difference of several kilograms existed.

Two trials using sibutramine to treat hypertensive patients have been reported (6,32,33). In a 3-month trial, all patients were receiving β-blockers with or without thiazides for their hypertension (33). The sibutramine-treated patients lost 4.2 kg (4.5%), compared with a loss of 0.3 kg (0.3%) in the placebo-treated group. Mean supine and standing diastolic and systolic BPs were not significantly different between the drug-treated and placebo-treated patients. Heart rate (HR), however, increased by 5.6 ± 8.25 (mean ± standard deviation) beats per minute in the sibutramine-treated patients, compared with an increase in HR of 2.2 ± 6.43 (mean ± standard deviation) beats per minute in the placebo-treated group (24). McMahon et al. (6) reported a 52-week trial of hypertensive patients whose BP was controlled with calcium channel blockers either with or without β-blockers or thiazides. Sibutramine doses were increased from 5 to 20 mg per day during the first 6 weeks. Weight loss was significantly greater in the sibutramine-treated patients, averaging 4.4 kg (4.7%), compared with 0.5 kg (0.7%) in the placebo-treated group. Diastolic BP decreased 1.3 mm Hg in the placebo-treated group and increased by 2.0 mm Hg in the sibutramine-treated group. The systolic BP increased by 1.5 mm Hg in the placebo-treated group and by 2.7 mm Hg in the sibutramine-treated group. HR was unchanged in the placebo-treated patients, but it increased 4.9 beats per minute in the sibutramine-treated patients (6).

In clinical trials, diabetics have been treated with sibutramine for 12 weeks or 24 weeks (34–36). In the 12-week trial, diabetic patients treated with sibutramine (15 mg per day) lost 2.4 kg (2.8%), compared with 0.1 kg (0.12%) in the placebo-treated group (27). In this study, the hemoglobin A_{1C} (HbA_{1C}) level fell by 0.3% in the drug-treated group and remained stable in the placebo-treated group. Corresponding fasting glucose values fell 0.3 mg per dL in the drug-treated group and rose 1.4 mg per dL in the placebo-treated group. In the 6-month trial (35), the dose of sibutramine was increased from 5 to 20 mg per day over 6 weeks. In those who completed the trial, the weight loss was 4.3 kg (4.3%) in the sibutramine-treated patients, compared with 0.3 kg (0.3%) in the placebo-treated patients (35). The HbA_{1C} level fell by 1.67% in the drug-treated group, compared with 0.53% in the placebo-treated group. These changes in glucose and HbA_{1C} levels were expected from the amount of weight loss associated with drug treatment.

Sibutramine has been studied as part of a behavioral weight loss program. With minimal behavioral intervention, the weight loss was about 5 kg over 12 months. When behavior modification was added, the weight loss increased to 10 kg; and, when a structured meal plan was added to the medication and behavior intervention, the weight loss increased further to 15 kg (37).

Sibutramine is available in 5-mg, 10-mg, and 15-mg pills; 10 mg per day as a single daily dose is the recommended starting level with titration up or down based on response. Doses of more than 15 mg per day are not recommended. Of the patients who lost 2 kg (4 lb) in the first 4 weeks of treatment, 60% achieved a weight loss of more than 5%, compared with less than 10% of those who did not lose 2 kg (4 lb) in 4 weeks (28). Combining data from the 11 studies on sibutramine showed a weight-related reduction in triglyceride (TG), total cholesterol, and low-density lipoprotein cholesterol (LDL-C) and a weight loss–related increase in high-density lipoprotein cholesterol (HDL-C) that was related to the magnitude of the weight loss (38).

Safety

The side-effect profiles for sympathomimetic drugs are similar (1,2). They produce insomnia, dry mouth, asthenia, and constipation. The safety of older sympathomimetic appetite-suppressant drugs has been the subject of considerable controversy because dextroamphetamine is addictive. The sympathomimetic drugs phentermine, diethylpropion, benzphetamine, and phendimetrazine have very little abuse potential as assessed by the low rate of reinforcement when the drugs are self-injected intravenously into test animals (1). In this same paradigm, neither PPA nor fenfluramine showed any reinforcing effects, and no clinical data show any abuse potential for either of these drugs. Sibutramine, likewise, has no abuse potential, but it is nonetheless a schedule IV drug.

Sympathomimetic drugs can increase BP. PPA is an α_1-agonist, and, at doses of 75 mg or more, it can increase BP. PPA has been associated with hemorrhagic stroke in women, and the FDA has proposed removing it from the market for both weight loss and as a decongestant (39). PPA has also been reported in association with cardiomyopathy. Sibutramine increases BP in normotensive and hypertensive patients or prevents the decrease that might have occurred with weight loss (28). The magnitude of the change may be dose related, thus suggesting that lower doses are preferred. In a 6-month trial with a fixed dose of 10 mg per day, Fanghanel et al. (30) found no significant changes in either systolic or diastolic BP. In placebo-controlled studies, systolic and diastolic BP increased by 1 to 3 mm Hg, and pulse increased by approximately 4 to 5 beats per minute (28). Caution should be exercised when combining sibutramine with other drugs that may increase BP. Sibutramine should not be used in patients with a history of coronary artery disease, congestive heart failure, cardiac arrhythmias, or stroke. A two-week interval should be allowed between the termination of monoamine oxidase inhibitors (MAOIs) and beginning sibutramine, and sibutramine should not be used with MAOIs or selective serotonin reuptake inhibitors (SSRIs). Because sibutramine is metabolized by the cytochrome P450 (CYP 450) enzyme system (isozyme CYP 3A4), it may interfere with the metabolism of erythromycin and ketoconazole.

Sympathomimetic Drugs Not Approved by the Food and Drug Administration to Treat Obesity

Several other sympathomimetic agents are also available that either carry warning labels (amphetamine and methamphetamine) or have never been approved by the FDA for the treatment of obesity (fenproporex, chlobenzorex). In December 2000, the FDA requested manufacturers of products such as cold remedies and weight loss drugs that contain PPA to remove the PPA from these products because of the alleged relation to the development of hemorrhagic strokes (39).

Serotonergic Drugs Not Approved by the Food and Drug Administration for Treating Obesity

No drugs working by this mechanism are currently approved by the FDA to treat obesity. Serotonergic drugs that act on specific serotonin receptors (i.e., 5-HT$_{1B}$ or 5-HT$_{2C}$) reduce food intake and, more specifically, reduce fat intake. Several drugs that influence serotonin release (fenfluramine and dexfenfluramine) or serotonin reuptake (fluoxetine and sertraline) have been used in obese patients. The clinical trial data are reviewed in detail elsewhere (1). At present, no drug that acts on the serotonin receptor system either directly or indirectly is approved for the treatment of obesity in the United States.

Combining Serotonergic and Noradrenergic Drugs

Efficacy

Drugs that act on either the noradrenergic or the serotonergic feeding system can reduce body weight. The possibility that combining a drug that acts on the serotonergic system with a drug that acts on the noradrenergic system was evaluated by Weintraub (40). Such a combination might produce more weight loss or may have fewer side effects if submaximal doses of one drug from each group are combined, than if full doses of a single agent are used (40). During the baseline run, patients received a program of behavior therapy, diet, and exercise that was demonstrably effective because they lost weight. When the patients were randomized, the drug-treated group lost 15.9% from baseline, compared with the placebo-treated group that lost only 4.9% from baseline during the first 34 weeks. When the placebo-treated patients began using the active drug in the open-label period, they too lost weight, indicating that the drug was active. Some patients received a long-term benefit by maintaining their weight at lower levels for up to 3.5 years during the time that the drug treatment was continued.

Safety

Following the report by Weintraub (40), the combination of phentermine and fenfluramine to treat obesity spread rapidly. More than 18 million prescriptions were written in 1996, and an estimated 3 to 4 million people were treated with this drug combination. In July 1997, 24 patients with a regurgitant type of valvular heart disease were reported to the medical profession (41). In the three patients in whom a histopathology of the heart valves was available, the valvular changes were similar to the changes seen in the carcinoid syndrome. Because early reports indicated that this valvulopathy might be present in more than 30% of the treated patients, fenfluramine and dexfenfluramine were withdrawn from the market on September 15, 1997. A series of 233 patients, including 91 with echocardiograms conducted before treatment, have been followed in the author's institution (5), and many reports have been published from other institutions (41). Figure 20.4 shows that 8% of the patients in the author's series had preexisting lesions and that

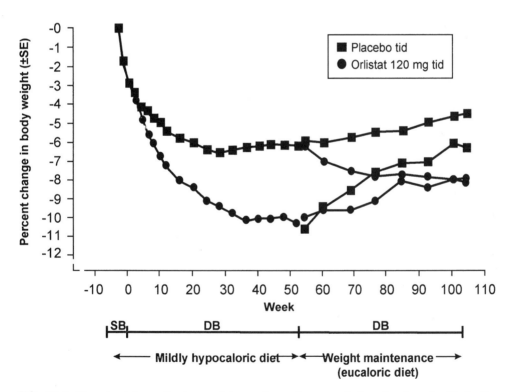

FIG. 20.4. Flowchart for patients receiving echocardiograms before treatment with fenfluramine and phentermine or mazindol (*upper lines*) or patients whose echocardiograms were obtained only after exposure to fenfluramine and phentermine or mazindol (*lower lines*). Longitudinal study includes 91 patients who had echocardiograms before initiation of treatment. In this group, 14 of 84 (16.5%) developed new lesions, and 3 have so far improved. The lower half includes patients in whom the first echocardiogram was done after beginning therapy, where just fewer than 25% had valvulopathy (4).

16.5% developed new lesions. With continued follow-up, some of the lesions have improved, and a few have completely regressed (5,42).

Current recommendations are that all symptomatic patients treated with fenfluramine or dexfenfluramine, either alone or in combination with phentermine, undergo an echocardiogram. Because careful clinical examination fails to detect a murmur in more than half of the patients with documented regurgitant lesions, conducting an echocardiogram on any patient who might need prophylactic antibiotics, as recommended by the American Heart Association, would be prudent.

Other Monoaminergic Drugs in Clinical Trial

Bupropion

Bupropion is a drug approved by the FDA for treatment of depression. In a short-term clinical trial, it was found to reduce body weight, prompting a 6-month multicenter trial. In this trial, a dose-related decrease in body weight was seen (43).

Topiramate

Topiramate is an antidepressant approved for monotherapy and for combination with other antiepileptic drugs. It is a carbonic anhydrase derivative that also has effects on the γ-aminobutyric acid (GABA$_a$) receptor. In clinical studies, the drug was noted to cause weight loss (44), and a controlled double-blind clinical trial is now underway.

Peptides That Reduce Food Intake and That Are in Early Stages of Drug Development—None Have Been Approved by the Food and Drug Administration to Treat Obesity

Leptin

Leptin is a peptide produced almost exclusively in adipose tissue. Absence of leptin produces massive obesity in mice (*ob/ob*) and in humans (45), and treatment with this peptide decreases food intake in the *ob/ob* mouse and the leptin-deficient human (46). The diabetes mouse (*db/db*) and the fatty rat, which have genetic defects in the leptin receptor, are also obese, but they do not respond to leptin. Leptin levels in the blood are highly correlated with body fat levels, yet obesity persists, suggesting that leptin resistance may be present. A dose-ranging clinical trial with leptin has been reported (47). In lean subjects treated for 4 weeks and in obese subjects treated for 24 weeks, a modest loss of weight was noted with doses ranging from 0.01 to 0.3 mg per kg. The side effects of local irritation at the site of injection limit the use of this preparation. A long-acting leptin preparation may provide an improved way to use this drug (48).

Ciliary Neurotrophic Factor

Ciliary neurotrophic factor is a cytokine-like peptide that will reduce food intake in animals that lack leptin or the leptin receptors (49). In a clinical trial for amyotrophic lateral sclerosis, the drug was noted to reduce weight, and a 3-month dose-ranging study demonstrated a significantly greater dose-related weight loss in the drug-treated patients (50).

Neuropeptide Y

Neuropeptide Y (NPY), which is one of the most potent stimulators of food intake, appears to act through NPY Y-5 and/or Y-1 receptors (1). Antagonists to these receptors might block NPY and may thus decrease feeding. Several pharmaceutical companies are attempting to identify antagonists to NPY receptors (15).

Cholecystokinin

Cholecystokinin (CCK) reduces food intake in humans and in experimental animals (1). This effect does not require an intact hypothalamic feeding control system, but it does appear to require an intact vagus nerve. Peptide analogs have been developed and tested experimentally, but clinical data have not yet been published. A second strategy to modify CCK activity is to reduce the degradation of CCK. This approach is likewise under evaluation.

Pancreatic Hormones

Glucagon and Glucagon-Like Peptide-1

Pancreatic glucagon produces a dose-related decrease in food intake (1). A fragment of glucagon (amino acids 6 through 29) called glucagon-like peptide-1 (GLP-1) reduced food intake when given either peripherally or into the brain (51). Exendin, an analog of GLP-1, has been used in humans because infusion of GLP-1 reduces food intake in humans (52).

Insulin

Circulating insulin levels are directly correlated with body fat, and the level of insulin in the cerebrospinal fluid has been proposed as a feedback signal to reduce food intake (53,54). Infusion of insulin into the brain's ventricular system lowers body weight. A drug that reduces insulin secretion has been found to reduce body weight. Somatostatin, a peptide that lowers insulin secretion, has been used to treat obesity with potentially promising results (55).

DRUGS THAT ALTER METABOLISM

Drugs Approved by the United States Food and Drug Administration

Orlistat (Xenical)

Pharmacology

Orlistat is a potent selective inhibitor of pancreatic lipase that reduces the intestinal digestion of fat. The drug has a dose-dependent effect on fecal fat loss, increasing it to about 30% for a diet in which 30% of energy intake comes as fat (56). Orlistat has little effect in subjects eating a low-fat diet, as might be anticipated from the mechanism by which this drug works (56).

Efficacy

A number of long-term clinical trials with orlistat that have lasted from 6 months to 2 years have been published (Table 20.5) (57–67). The results of one 2-year trial are shown in Fig. 20.5 (60). The trial consisted of two parts. In the first year, patients received a hypocaloric diet calculated to be 500 kcal per day below the patient's energy require-

TABLE 20.5. *Effect of orlistat in clinical trials of 1 and 2 years in duration*

Author	Year	No. of subjects (No. of participants beginning/no. completing) Placebo	Drug	Dose (mg/t.i.d.)	Duration of study (wks)	Run in (wks)	Diet	Initial weight (kg) Placebo	Drug	Weight loss Placebo	Drug	Comments
James et al. (58)	1997	23	23	120	52	4	600-kcal/d deficit	99	100	-2.6 kg	-8.4 kg	Weight loss at 12 mo
Van Gaal et al. (59)	1998	125	122 124 122 120	30 60 120 240	24	4	500-kcal/d deficit	35 BMI	35 34 35 34	-6.5%	-8.5% -8.8% -9.8% -9.3%	Multicenter dose ranging
Sjostrom et al. (60)	1998	340	343	120	104	4	600-kcal/d deficit (yr 1); maintenance (yr 2)	99.8	99.1	-6.1 kg -6.1%	-10.3 kg -10.2%	European multicenter crossover, 52-wk data
Hollander et al. (68)	1998	159	162	120	52	5	500-kcal/d deficit 30% fat	99.7	99.6	-4.3 kg -4.3%	-6.2 kg -6.2%	United States diabetic study
Davidson et al. (61)	1999	223	657	120	104	4	600-kcal/d deficit (yr 1); maintenance (yr 2) 30% fat	100.6	100.7	-5.8 kg -5.8%	-8.8 kg -8.7%	United States multicenter crossover, 52-wk data

Study	Year	N (enrolled/completed)	Dose (mg)	Wk		Diet	Baseline wt	Wt	Wt loss	Wt loss (dose)	Comments
Hill et al. (66)	1999	188/138		52	24	1,000-kcal/d deficit for 6 mo; Enrolled if weight loss >8%	90.8		−5.9 kg		Multicenter trial with initial dietary weight loss and test of maintenance of weight loss
		187/140	30					89.3		−5.15 kg	
		173/133	60					92.4		−6.16 kg	
		181/126	120					89.7		−7.24 kg	
Finer et al. (7)	2000	108		52	4	600-kcal/d deficit	98.4		−5.4%		British; 1 yr
		110	120					97.9		−8.5%	
Rossner et al. (63)	2000	243/136		104	4	600-kcal/d deficit (yr 1); maintenance (yr 2) 30% fat	97.7		−4.5%		Multicenter European trial
		242/140	60					99.1		−7.0%	
		244/159	120					96.7		−7.8% (2-yr data on completers)	
Hauptmann et al. (64)	2000	212/91		104	4	5020-kJ/d if weight <90 kg; or 6,275 kJ/d	101.8		−1.5 kg		Multicenter United States trial in family practice setting
		213/120	60					100.4		−4.6 kg	
		210/117	120					100.5		−5.2 kg	
Lindgarde (65)	2000	186		52	2	600-kcal/d deficit; 30% fat	95.9		−4.3 kg		Multicenter trial of individuals with high coronary heart disease risk
		190	120					96.1		−5.6 kg	

Abbreviation: BMI, body mass index; BMI units in kg/m².

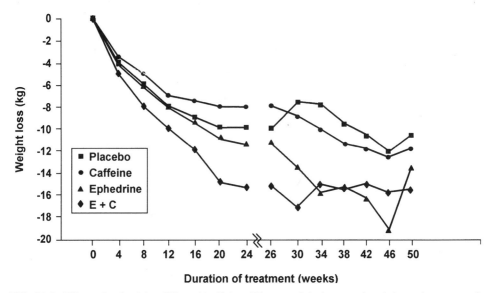

FIG. 20.5. Effect of ephedrine (E) and caffeine (C) on weight loss and weight maintenance for 1 year (10). A total of 180 patients were randomly assigned to four groups that were then treated in a double-blind fashion for 6 months and with an open-label protocol for another 6 months. The weight losses in the groups receiving placebo, ephedrine alone, and caffeine alone were not significantly different and were smaller than in the group receiving the combination of ephedrine and caffeine. During the 6-month open-label study with those who wished to receive ephedrine and caffeine, weight loss was maintained with no significant difference between groups.

ments. During the second year, the diet was adjusted to maintain weight. By the end of year 1, the placebo-treated patients had lost 6.1% of their initial body weight, and the drug-treated patients had lost 10.2%. The patients were rerandomized at the end of year 1. Those who had been switched from orlistat to the placebo gained weight from 10% below baseline to only 6.0% below baseline. Those switched from placebo to orlistat lost weight, dropping from 6% to 8.1% of their baseline weight, a result that was essentially identical to the 7.9% in the patients treated with orlistat for the full 2 years. In a second 2-year study, 892 patients were randomized (61). One group remained on the placebo throughout the 2 years (number of subjects [N] = 97 completers), and a second group remained on orlistat at a dosage of 120 mg, three times a day, for 2 years (N = 109 completers). At the end of 1 year, two-thirds of the orlistat-treated group were changed to orlistat at a dosage of 60 mg, three times a day (N = 102 completers), and the others to the placebo (N = 95 completers) (61). After 1 year, the weight loss was 8.67 kg in the orlistat-treated group and 5.81 kg in the placebo-treated group (p <0.001). During the second year, those switched to the placebo after 1 year regained to the same level of weight loss as those treated with placebo for 2 years (4.5% in those with placebo for 2 years and 4.2% in those switched to the placebo during year 2). In a third 2-year study, 783 patients enrolled in a trial in which they remained in the placebo-treated or the orlistat-treated groups at 60 or 120 mg, three times a day, for the entire 2 years (63). After 1 year on a weight loss diet, the completers in the placebo-treated group lost 7.0 kg, which was significantly less than the 9.6 kg lost by the completers treated with orlistat at 60 mg thrice daily or the 9.8 kg in the completers treated with orlistat at 120 mg thrice daily. During the second year, when the diet was liberalized to a "weight-maintenance" diet, all three groups regained some weight. At the end of 2 years, the completers in the placebo-treated group were 4.3 kg below baseline, the completers treated with orlistat at 60 mg thrice daily were 6.8 kg below baseline, and the completers treated with orlistat at 120 mg thrice daily were 7.6 kg below baseline. The final 2-year trial that has been published was carried out on 796 subjects in a general practice setting (64). After 1 year of treatment with orlistat at 120 mg per day, completers (N = 117) had lost 8.8 kg compared with 4.3 kg for the placebo completers (N = 91). During the second year, when the diet was liberalized to "maintain body weight," both groups regained some weight. At the end of 2 years, the orlistat group subjects receiving 120 mg thrice daily were 5.2 kg below their baseline weight, compared with 1.5 kg for the group treated with placebo.

Weight maintenance with orlistat was evaluated in a 1-year study (66). Patients who were enrolled had lost more than 8% of their body weight over 6 months by following a diet of 1,000 kcal per day (4,180 kJ per day). The 729 patients were randomized to receive a placebo or 30 mg, 60 mg, or 120 mg of orlistat thrice daily for 12 months. At the end of this time, the placebo-treated patients had regained 56% of their body weight, compared with 32.4% for the group treated with orlistat at a dosage of 120 mg thrice daily. The other two doses of orlistat showed no differences from the placebo in preventing the regain of weight.

Diabetics treated with orlistat at a dosage of 120 mg thrice daily for 1 year lost 6.5% of their baseline body weight, compared with 4.2% for the placebo-treated group (68). The diabetics also showed a significantly greater decrease in HbA_{1c}. In another look at the effect of orlistat and weight loss, Heymsfield et al. (69) pooled data on 675 subjects from three of the 2-year studies listed earlier in which glucose tolerance test (GTT) results were available. During treatment, 6.6% of the patients treated with orlistat converted from normal GTT results to impaired GTT results, compared with 10.8% of the patients in the placebo-treated group. None of the orlistat-treated patients who originally had normal GTT results became diabetic, compared with 1.2% of the patients in the placebo-treated group who became diabetic. Of those who initially had normal GTT results, 7.6% in the placebo-treated group, but only 3.0% in the orlistat-treated group, became diabetic. In a further analysis, Reaven et al. (70) divided patients who had participated in previously reported studies into those in the highest and lowest quintile for TG and HDL-C levels. Those with high TG and low HDL levels were labeled "syndrome X," and those with the lowest TG and highest HDL levels were the non–syndrome X controls. In this breakdown, almost no men were in the non–syndrome X group, compared with an equal gender breakdown in the syndrome X group. The other differences between these two groups included the slightly higher systolic and diastolic BP in the syndrome X group and the nearly twofold higher level of fasting insulin level. With weight loss, the only difference besides weight between placebo-treated and orlistat-treated patients was the drop in LDL-C levels. However, the syndrome X subgroups showed a significantly greater decrease in TG and insulin than did those patients without syndrome X. HDL-C levels rose more in the syndrome X subgroup, but LDL-C levels showed a smaller decrease than in the non–syndrome X group. A significant decrease in LDL-C level (i.e., usually more than can be accounted for by weight loss alone) has been observed in all of the clinical studies with orlistat (71). A recent abstract showed that orlistat reduced the absorption of cholesterol from the gastrointestinal (GI) tract, thus providing a mechanism for the clinical observations (72).

An analysis of quality of life in patients treated with orlistat showed improvements over the placebo-treated group in spite of concerns about GI symptoms. In addition, orlistat-treated patients showed a significant decrease in serum cholesterol and LDL-C levels that was greater than that which could be explained by weight loss alone.

Safety

Orlistat is not absorbed to any significant degree, and its side effects are thus related to the blockade of TG digestion in the intestine (56). Fecal fat loss and related GI symptoms are common initially, but they subside as patients learn to use the drug (63). During treatment, small, but significant, decreases in fat-soluble vitamin levels can occur, although these almost always remain within the normal range (67). However, a few patients may need supplementation with fat-soluble vitamins that can be lost in the stools. Because one cannot tell *a priori* which patients need vitamins, the author routinely provides a multivitamin with instructions to take it before bedtime. Absorption of other drugs does not seem to be significantly affected by orlistat.

Combining Orlistat and Sibutramine

Because orlistat works peripherally to reduce TG digestion in the GI tract and sibutramine works on noradrenergic and serotonergic reuptake mechanisms in the brain, their mechanisms do not overlap and thus combining them might result in additional weight loss. To test this possibility, Wadden et al. (73) randomly assigned patients to orlistat or a placebo after a year's worth of treatment with orlistat. During the additional 4 months of treatment, the patients achieved no further weight loss. This result was a disappointment, but additional studies are obviously needed.

Drugs Approved by the Food and Drug Administration for an Indication Other than Obesity

Androgens and Androgen Antagonists

Dehydroepiandrosterone

Dehydroepiandrosterone (DHEA) is a weak androgen that induces weight loss in several animal species. Clinical trials in humans have shown no effect (1).

Testosterone

In men, testosterone and the anabolic steroid, oxandrolone, have been reported to reduce visceral fat. A trial of an antiandrogen and nandrolone in women did not show any effects on visceral fat (1).

COMPARISON OF AVAILABLE DRUGS

Of the drugs discussed in this chapter, phentermine, orlistat, and sibutramine are the most widely used in the United States and other countries. The other drugs in the sympathomimetic category, benzphetamine, phendimetrazine, and diethylpropion, are less widely used, and less long-term information is available. Mazindol and PPA, which are also in this category, either are no longer manufactured, or they are under a request from the FDA to be removed from diet-drug and cold preparations.

Figure 20.6 provides a comparison of the three drugs available to the clinician, and it plots the weight loss of placebo-treated and drug-treated groups. All of the trials included in Fig. 20.6 lasted 6 months or more. The weight loss of the placebo-treated group is at the beginning of the arrow on the right, and the weight loss of the drug-treated group is at the tip of the arrowhead to the left. The length of the arrow is the magnitude of the difference between the drug and the placebo. In all of the studies plotted, the difference between the two groups was greater than 4 kg, except for one study with phentermine and one study with orlistat. Three trials with phentermine had weight losses exceeding 5 kg, whereas most of the others were around 5 kg.

The effect size, expressed as the difference between the drug-treated and the placebo-treated group in each study, is plotted in Fig. 20.7. The weight losses of the phentermine and orlistat groups were greater than that of the sibutramine group, but so was the weight loss of the placebo-treated group. When the difference is plotted (the right side of each of the three groups in Fig. 20.7), sibutramine and phentermine produced a similar amount of weight loss that was slightly greater than that seen with orlistat.

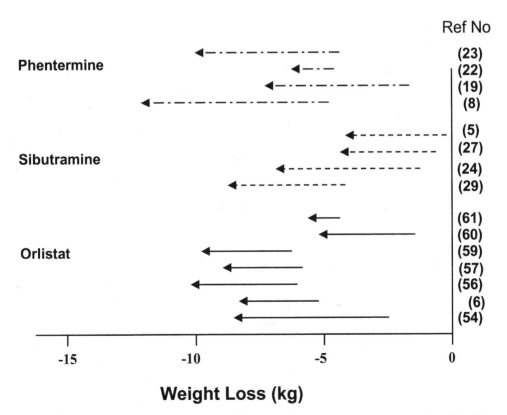

FIG. 20.6. Effect sizes for three weight loss drugs. Each line is a separate study with either phentermine, sibutramine, or orlistat. Reference to each study is in parenthesis. The right-hand end of the arrow is the weight loss of the placebo-treated group and the tip of the arrow is the weight loss of the drug-treated group. (Courtesy of George A. Bray, 2001.)

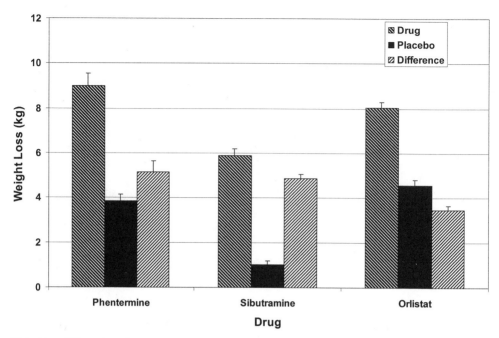

FIG. 20.7. Effect size of weight loss. The drug effect, the placebo effect, and the difference are plotted for the studies shown in Fig. 20.6. (Courtesy of George A. Bray, 2001.)

DRUGS THAT INCREASE ENERGY EXPENDITURE

Drugs Approved by the FDA for an Indication Other Than Obesity

Ephedrine and Caffeine

Pharmacology

Ephedrine is a derivative of PPA that is used to relax bronchial smooth muscles in patients with asthma. It also stimulates thermogenesis in humans (74). Caffeine is a xanthine that inhibits adenosine receptors and phosphodiesterase. In experimental animals, the combination of ephedrine and caffeine reduces body weight, probably through a stimulation of thermogenesis and a reduction in food intake.

Efficacy

One long-term, placebo-controlled clinical trial treated 180 patients with ephedrine, caffeine, or the combination of ephedrine and caffeine (11). Patients treated with the combination of ephedrine and caffeine lost more weight than the patients treated with ephedrine alone (Fig. 20.5). In a 6-month open-label extension, subjects who completed the initial trial were offered additional treatment with ephedrine and caffeine. Nearly two-thirds of the group opted for this treatment, and they were then able to maintain their initial weight loss for the next 6 months. No other long-term data are available using ephedrine and caffeine. During controlled metabolic studies, patients treated with ephedrine and caffeine lost less lean tissue than those in the placebo-treated group. Using the changes in body composition from these studies, Astrup et al. (75) have estimated the contribution of thermogenesis and food intake to the weight loss. They concluded that

60% to75% of the weight loss was due to a decrease in food intake and that 25% to 40% was due to the thermogenic effects of ephedrine and caffeine.

Safety

Although caffeine and ephedrine have a long record of clinical use separately, neither drug alone nor their combination is approved for treatment of obesity.

β₃-Adrenergic Receptor Agonists in Early Stages of Drug Development

The sympathetic nervous system has a tonic role in maintaining EE and BP. Blockade of the thermogenic part of this system reduces the thermic response to a meal. NE, the neurotransmitter of the sympathetic nervous system, may also decrease food intake by acting on β_2- or β_3-adrenergic receptors. Several synthetic β_3-agonists have been developed against rodent β_3-receptors, but the clinical responses have been disappointing (1). After cloning of the human β_3-receptor, a new round of compounds is being synthesized and will be tried in obese humans.

A clinical trial of the third-generation β_3-adrenergic drugs showed no significant effect on thermogenesis in humans when studied in a metabolic chamber after treatment for 28 days (76).

HERBAL PREPARATIONS FOR TREATMENT OF OBESITY

Several herbal preparations have been recommended for use in treating obesity. These include chromium picolinate, garcinia cambogia as a source of hydroxycitrate, chitosan as a fiber source that is claimed to reduce fat absorption, and ma huang as a source of ephedra alkaloids with or without guarana as a source of caffeine. Clinically controlled trials with these agents are few. These agents do not carry the approval of the FDA because the law allows them to be sold directly to the public through the over-the-counter route.

Chromium Picolinate

Because no clinical trials in humans with chromium picolinate as a single agent have been performed, this chapter does not include an evaluation of its effectiveness as a treatment for obesity (1).

Garcinia Cambogia

A single published randomized 3-month clinical trial with garcinia cambogia as a source of hydroxycitrate can be found in the literature (77). No difference was seen in the weight loss between the herbal-treated group and the placebo-treated group.

Chitosan

A recent study has evaluated the effect of this material on fecal fat loss. Using human subjects from whom fecal fat samples were collected, Guerciolini et al. (78) showed that chitosan did not increase fecal fat loss. In a 4-week dietary study, either chitosan or the placebo was given to subjects randomly with no dietary advice. At the end of this time, no difference in weight loss between the two groups was found, suggesting that chitosan has no effect independent of a lower calorie diet (79).

Ma Huang and Guarana

This combination is among the most widely used over-the-counter preparations for weight loss. No clinical trials with this combination have yet been published as full-length papers, but two abstracts of randomized, placebo-controlled clinical trials have been published. In an 8-week study with Metabolife 356 (80), the patients treated with the herbal preparation lost more weight and body fat, but the authors commented on the number of side effects and they urged caution until longer studies were available. A second trial was published recently (81). This was a 6-month trial comparing 90 mg of ephedra alkaloids from ma huang in three divided doses with 200 mg of guarana as a source of caffeine. The patients treated with the herbal medications again lost significantly more weight than the placebo-treated group. In this trial, Holter monitors were used to evaluate changes in cardiac rhythm at 1 week and 4 weeks of treatment. Compared with baseline, no significant changes were seen in any of the cardiac parameters that were measured. Pulse rate increased by 4 beats per minute from baseline in the groups treated with ephedra and guarana, but BP did not change significantly.

CONCLUSION

Only two drugs are currently approved for long-term treatment of obesity. Sibutramine inhibits the reuptake of serotonin and NE. In clinical trials, it produces a dose-dependent

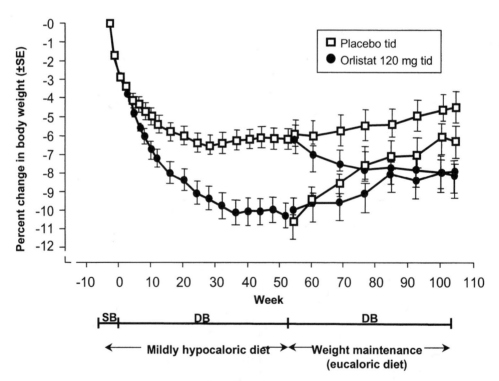

FIG. 20.8. Effect of orlistat on weight loss during year 1 and weight maintenance during year 2 (49). A total of 743 patients were randomized to receive either orlistat (120 mg three times daily) or a placebo for the first year and were then rerandomized to the same groups for a second year. After the 4-week single-blind (SB) run, the first double-blind (DB) period used a diet that was calculated to be 600 kcal per day below maintenance, and the second DB period used a diet that was intended to maintain body weight.

5% to 10% decrease in body weight. Its side effects include dry mouth, insomnia, asthenia, and constipation. In addition, sibutramine produces a small increase in BP and pulse, which is a contraindication to the use of this drug in some individuals with heart disease. Xenical is the other drug approved for long-term use in the treatment of obesity. It works by blocking lipase, thus increasing the fecal loss of TG. One valuable consequence of this mechanism of action is the reduction of serum cholesterol, which averages about 5% more than can be accounted for by weight loss alone. In clinical trials, it produces a 5% to 10% loss of weight. Its side effects are entirely due to undigested fat in the intestine, which can lead to increased frequency of and a change in the character of stools. It can also lower fat-soluble vitamins. The ingestion of a vitamin supplement before bedtime is a reasonable treatment strategy. The effect on weight loss during long-term trials with these two drugs is shown in Figs. 20.7 and 20.8. Also in these figures are data on phentermine, which was used in trials lasting 6 months or more. Although differences in mean weight losses with these drugs were seen, when the placebo effect was taken into account, they all had a surprisingly similar magnitude of weight loss.

REFERENCES

1. Bray GA, Greenway FL. Current and potential drugs for treatment of obesity [Review]. *Endocr Rev* 1999;20:805–875.
2. Yanovski SZ, Yanovski JA. Obesity. *N Engl J Med* 2002;346:591–602.
3. Weintraub M, Bray GA. Drug treatment of obesity [Review]. *Med Clin North Am* 1989;73:237–249.
4. Bray GA. Obesity—a time-bomb to be defused. *Lancet* 1998;352:160–161.
5. Ryan DH, Bray GA, Helmcke F, et al. Serial echocardiographic and clinical evaluation of valvular regurgitation before, during, and after treatment with fenfluramine or dexfenfluramine and mazindol or phentermine. *Obes Res* 1999;7:313–322.
6. McMahon FG, Fujioka K, Singh BN, et al. Efficacy and safety of sibutramine in obese white and African-American patients with hypertension. *Arch Intern Med* 2000;160:2185–2191.
7. Finer N, James WP, Kopelman PG, et al. One-year treatment of obesity: a randomized, double-blind, placebo-controlled, multicentre study of orlistat, a gastrointestinal lipase inhibitor. *Int J Obes Relat Metab Disord* 2000;24:306–313.
8. Flechtner-Mors M, Ditschuneit HH, Johnson TD, et al. Metabolic and weight loss effects of long-term dietary intervention in obese patients: four-year results. *Obes Res* 2000;8:399–402.
9. Munro JF, MacCuish AC, Wilson EM, et al. Comparison of continuous and intermittent anorectic therapy in obesity. *BMJ* 1968;1:352–354.
10. Greenway FL, Ryan DH, Bray GA, et al. Pharmaceutical cost savings of treating obesity with weight loss medications. *Obes Res* 1999;7:523–531.
11. Astrup A, Breum L, Tourbro S, et al. The effect and satiety of an ephedrine/caffeine compound compared to ephedrine, caffeine and placebo in obese subjects on an energy restricted diet. A double blind trial. *Int J Obes Relat Metab Disord* 1992;16:269–277.
12. Sjostrom CD, Lissner L, Wedel H, et al. Reduction in incidence of diabetes, hypertension and lipid disturbances after intentional weight loss induced by bariatric surgery: the SOS intervention study. *Obes Res* 1999;7:477–484.
13. Foster GD, Wadden TA, Vogt RA, et al. What is a reasonable weight loss? Patients expectations and evaluations of obesity treatment outcomes. *J Consult Clin Psychol* 1997;65:79–85.
14. Bray GA. Evaluation of drugs for treating obesity [Review]. *Obes Res* 1995;3:425S–434S.
15. Bray GA, Tartaglia LA. Medicinal strategies in the treatment of obesity [Review]. *Nature* 2000;404:672–677.
16. National on the Task Force Prevention and Treatment of Obesity. Long-term pharmacotherapy in the management of obesity [Review]. *JAMA* 1996;276:1907–1915.
17. Scoville B. Review of amphetamine-like drugs by the Food and Drug Administration: clinical data and value judgments. In: *Obesity in perspective*. Publication no. 75-708. Washington, D.C.: Department of Health, Education, and Welfare, 1975:441–443.
18. Silverstone JJ, Solomon T. The long-term management of obesity in general practice. *Br J Clin Pract* 1965;19:395–398.
19. McKay RHG. Long-term use of diethylpropion in obesity. *Curr Med Res Opin* 1973;1:489–493.
20. Langlois KJ, Forbes JA, Bell GW, et al. A double-blind clinical evaluation of the safety and efficacy of phentermine hydrochloride (Fastin) in the treatment of exogenous obesity. *Curr Ther Res* 1974;16:289–296.
21. Gershberg H, Kane R, Hulse M, et al. Effects of diet and an anorectic drug (phentermine resin) in obese diabetics. *Curr Ther Res* 1977;22:814–820.

22. Campbell CJ, Bhalla IP, Steel JM, et al. A controlled trial of phentermine in obese diabetic patients. *Practitioner* 1977;218:851–855.
23. Williams RA, Foulsham BM. Weight reduction in osteoarthritis using phentermine. *Practitioner* 1981;225: 231–232.
23a. Weintraub M, Hasday JD, Mushlin AI, Lockwood DH. A double-blind clinical trial in weight control. Use of fenfluramine and phentermine alone in combination. *Arch Intern Med* 1984;144:1143–1148.
24. Weintraub M, Rubio A, Golik A, et al. Sibutramine in weight control: a dose-ranging, efficacy study. *Clin Pharmacol Ther* 1991;50:330–337.
25. Jones SP, Smith IG, Kelly F, et al. Long-term weight loss with sibutramine. *Int J Obes* 1995;19:40.
26. Bray GA, Ryan DH, Gordon D, et al. A double-blind randomized placebo-controlled trial of sibutramine. *Obes Res* 1996;4:263–270.
27. Hanotin C, Thomas F, Jones SP, et al. Efficacy and tolerability of sibutramine in obese patients: a dose-ranging study. *Int J Obes Relat Metab Disord* 1998;22:32–58.
28. Bray GA, Blackburn GL, Ferguson JM, et al. Sibutramine produces dose-related weight loss. *Obes Res* 1999; 7:189–198.
29. Apfelbaum M, Vague P, Ziegler O, et al. Long-term maintenance of weight loss after a very-low-calorie diet: a randomized blinded trial of the efficacy and tolerability of sibutramine. *Am J Med* 1999;106:179–184.
30. Fanghanel G, Cortinas L, Sanchez-Reyes L, et al. A clinical trial of the use of sibutramine for the treatment of patients suffering essential obesity. *Int J Obes Relat Metab Disord* 2000;24:144–150.
31. James WPT, Astrup A, Finer N, et al, for the STORM study group. Effect of sibutramine on weight maintenance after weight loss: a randomized trial. *Lancet* 2000;356:2119–2125.
32. McMahon FG, Weinstein SP, Rowe E, et al. Sibutramine is safe and effective for weight loss in obese patients whose hypertension is well controlled with angiotensin-converting enzyme inhibitors. *J Hum Hypertens* 2002;16:5–11.
33. Sramek, JJ, Seiowitz MT, Weinstein SP, et al. Efficacy and safety of sibutramine for weight loss in obese patients with hypertension well controlled by β-adrenergic blocking agents: a placebo-controlled, double-blind, randomized trial. *Am J Hypertens* 2002;16:13–19.
34. Finer N, Bloom SR, Frost GS, et al. Sibutramine is effective for weight loss and diabetic control in obesity with type 2 diabetes: a randomised, double-blind placebo-controlled study. *Diabetes Obes Metab* 2000;2:105–112.
35. Fujioka K, Seaton TB, Rowe E, et al., and the Sibutramine/Diabetes Clinical Study Group. Weight loss with sibutramine improves glycemic control and other metabolic parameters in obese type 2 diabetes mellitus. *Diabetes Obes Metab* 2000;2:1–13.
36. Gockel A, Karakose H, Ertorer EM, et al. Effects of sibutramine in obese female subjects with type 2 diabetes and poor blood glucose control. *Diabetes Care* 2001;24:1957–1960.
37. Wadden RA, Berkowitz RI, Sarwer DB, et al. Benefits of lifestyle modification in the pharmacologic treatment of obesity: a randomized trial. *Arch Intern Med* 2001;161:218–227.
38. Wirth A, Krause J. Long-term weight loss with sibutramine: a randomized controlled trial. *JAMA* 2001;286:1331–1339.
39. Kernan WN, Viscoli CM, Brass LM, et al. Phenylpropanolamine and the risk of hemorrhagic stroke. *N Engl J Med* 2000;343:1826–1832.
40. Weintraub M. Long term weight control: the National Heart, Lung, and Blood Institute funded multimodal intervention study. *Clin Pharmacol Ther* 1992;51:581–585.
41. Connolly HM, Crary JL, McGoon MD, et al. Valvular heart disease associated with fenfluramine-phentermine. *N Engl J Med* 1997;337:581–588.
42. Mast ST, Jollis JG, Ryan T, et al. The progression of fenfluramine-associated valvular heart disease assessed by echocardiography. *Ann Intern Med* 2001;134:261–266.
43. Anderson JW, Greenway FL, Fujioka K, et al. Bupropion SR significantly enhances weight loss: a 24-week double-blind, placebo-controlled trial with placebo group randomized to bupropion SR during 24-week extension. *Obes Res* 2002;10:633–641.
44. Reife R, Pledger G, Wu S. Topiramate as add-on therapy: pooled analysis of randomized controlled trials in adults. *Epilepsia* 2000;41:S66–S71.
45. Montague CT Farooqi IS, Whitehead JP, et al. Congenital leptin deficiency is associated with severe early-onset obesity in humans. *Nature* 1997;387:903–908.
46. Farooqi IS, Jebb SA, Langmack G, et al. Effects of recombinant leptin therapy in a child with congenital leptin deficiency. *N Engl J Med* 1999;341:879–884.
47. Heymsfield SB, Greenberg AS, Fujioka K, et al. Recombinant leptin for weight loss in obese and lean adults: a randomized, controlled, dose-escalation trial. *JAMA* 1999;282:1568–1575.
48. Hukshorn CJ, Saris WH, Westerterp-Plantenga MS, et al. Weekly subcutaneous pegylated recombinant native human leptin (PEG-OB) administration in obese men. *J Clin Endocrinol Metab* 2000;85:4003–4009.
49. Lambert PD, Anderson KD, Sleeman MW, et al. Ciliary neurotrophic factor activates leptin-like pathways and reduces body fat, without cachexia or rebound weight gain, even in leptin-resistant obesity. *Proc Natl Acad Sci U S A* 2001;98:4652–4657.
50. Guler HP, Ettinger TW, Littlejohn SL, et al. Axokine causes significant weight loss in severely and morbidly obese subjects [Abstract]. *Int J Obes* 2001;25:S111.
51. Flint A, Raben A, Astrup A, Holst JJ. Glucagon-like peptide 1 promotes satiety and suppresses energy intake in humans. *J Clin Invest* 1998;101:515–520.

52. Al-Barazanji KA, Arch JR, Buckingham RE, et al. Central exendin-4 infusion reduces body weight without altering plasma leptin in (fa/fa) Zucker rats. *Obes Res* 2000;8:317–323.
53. Schwartz MW, Woods SC, Porte D, et al. Central nervous system control of food intake [Review]. *Nature* 2000;404:661–671.
54. Bruning JC, Gautam D, Burks DJ, et al. Role of brain insulin receptor in control of body weight and reproduction. *Science* 2000;289:2122–2125.
55. Lustig RH, Rose SR, Burghen GA, et al. Hypothalamic obesity caused by cranial insult in children: altered glucose and insulin dynamics and reversal by a somatostatin agonist. *J Pediatr* 1999;135:162–168.
56. Hauptmann JB, Jeunet FS, Hartmann D. Initial studies in humans with the novel gastrointestinal lipase inhibitor Ro18-0647 (tetrahydrolipstatin). *Am J Clin Nutr* 1992;5:309S–313S.
57. Drent ML, Larsson I, William-Olsson T, et al. Orlistat (Ro18-0647), a lipase inhibitor, in the treatment of human obesity: a multiple dose study. *Int J Obes Relat Metab Disord* 1995;19:221–226.
58. James WP, Avenell A, Broom J, et al. A one-year trial to assess the value of orlistat in the management of obesity. *Int J Obes Relat Metab Disord* 1997;21:S24–S30.
59. Van Gaal LF, Broom JI, Enzi G, et al. Efficacy and tolerability of orlistat in the treatment of obesity—a 6-month dose-ranging study. *Eur J Clin Pharmacol* 1998;54:125–132.
60. Sjostrom L, Rissanen A, Andersen T, et al. Randomised placebo-controlled trial of orlistat for weight loss and prevention of weight regain in obese patients. European Multicentre Orlistat Study Group. *Lancet* 1998;352:167–172.
61. Davidson MH, Hauptman J, DiGirolamo M, et al. Long-term weight control and risk factor reduction in obese subjects treated with orlistat, a lipase inhibitor. *JAMA* 1999;281:235–242.
62. Finer N, James WP, Kopelman PG, et al. One-year treatment of obesity: a randomized, double-blind, placebo-controlled, multicentre study of orlistat, a gastrointestinal lipase inhibitor. *Int J Obes Relat Metab Disord* 2000;24:306–313.
63. Rossner S, Sjostrom L, Noack R, et al., for the European Orlistat Obesity Study Group. Weight loss, weight maintenance, and improved cardiovascular risk factors after 2 years treatment with orlistat for obesity. *Obes Res* 2000;8:49–61.
64. Hauptmann J, Lucas C, Boldrin MN, et al., for the Orlistat Primary Care Study Group. Orlistat in the long-term treatment of obesity in primary care settings. *Arch Fam Med* 2000;9:160–167.
65. Lindgarde F, for the Orlistat Swedish Multimorbidity Study Group. The effect of orlistat on body weight and coronary heart disease risk profile in obese patients: the Swedish Multimorbidity Study. *J Intern Med* 2000;248:245–254.
66. Hill JO, Hauptmann J, Anderson JW, et al. Orlistat, a lipase inhibitor, for weight maintenance after conventional dieting: a 1-y study. *Am J Clin Nutr* 1999;69:1108–1116.
67. Drent ML, van der Veen EA. First clinical studies with orlistat: a short review. *Obes Res* 1995;3:S623–S625.
68. Hollander P, Elbein SC, Hirsch IB, et al. Role of orlistat in the treatment of obese patients with type 2 diabetes. *Diabetes Care* 1998;21:1288–1294.
69. Heymsfield SB, Segal KR, Hauptman J, et al. Effects of weight loss with orlistat on glucose tolerance and progression to type 2 diabetes in obese adults. *Arch Intern Med* 2000;160:1321–1326.
70. Reaven G, Segal K, Haputman J, et al. Effect of orlistat-assisted weight loss in decreasing coronary heart disease risk in patients with syndrome X. *Am J Cardiol* 2001;87:827–831.
71. Tonstad S, Pometta D, Erkelens DW, et al. The effects of gastrointestinal lipase inhibitor, orlistat, on serum lipids and lipoproteins in patients with primary hyperlipidaemia. *Eur J Clin Pharmacol* 1994;46:405–410.
72. Mittendorfer B, Ostlund R, Patterson BW, et al. Orlistat inhibits dietary cholesterol absorption. *Obes Res* 2000;8:43S.
73. Wadden TA, Berkowitz RI, Womble LG, et al. Effects of sibutramine plus orlistat in obese women following 1 year of treatment by sibutramine alone: a placebo-controlled trial. *Obes Res* 2000;8:431–437.
74. Astrup A, Bulow J, Madsen J, et al. Contribution of BAT and skeletal muscle to thermogenesis induced by ephedrine in man. *Am J Physiol* 1985;248:E507–E515.
75. Astrup A, Breum L, Toubro S. Pharmacological and clinical studies of ephedrine and other thermogenic agonists [Review]. *Obes Res* 1995;3:537S–540S.
76. Larsen TM, Toubro S, van Baak MA, et al. No thermogenic effect after 28 days treatment with L-796,568, a novel beta-3-adrenoceptor, in obese men. *Obes Res* 2000;8:44S.
77. Heymsfield SB, Allison DB, Vasselli JR, et al. Garcinia cambogia (hydroxycitric acid) as a potential antiobesity agent: a randomized controlled trial. *JAMA* 1998;280:1596–1600.
78. Guerciolini R, Radu-Radulescu L, Boldrin M, et al. Fecal fat excretion induced by treatment with orlistat or chitosan: a 3-week randomized crossover design study. *Obes Res* 2000;8:43S.
79. Pittler MH, Abbot NC, Harkness EF, et al. Randomized, double-blind trial of chitosan for body weight reduction. *Eur J Clin Nutr* 1999;53:379–381.
80. Boozer CN, Nasser JA, Heymsfield SB, et al. An herbal supplement containing ma huang-guarana for weight loss: a randomized, double-blind trial. *Int J Obes Relat Metab Disord* 2001;25:316–324.
81. Boozer CN, Daly PA, Blanchard D, et al. Herbal ephedra/caffeine for weight loss: a 6-month safety and efficacy trial. *Int J Obes Metab Disord* 2002;26:593–604.

21

Exercise

William J. Wilkinson and Steven N. Blair

Currently in the United States, an estimated 64% of adults are overweight or obese (defined as a body mass index [BMI] $\geq$ 25 kilograms per meter squared [kg/m^2]), and the prevalence rates are increasing (1,2). According to recent surveys, the prevalence of obesity (BMI $\geq$ 30 kg/m^2) in the United States increased by 61% between the years 1991 and 2000 (2,3). Overweight and obesity are directly related to an increased risk of several of the following medical conditions: insulin resistance, glucose intolerance, type II diabetes, hypertension, dyslipidemia, and impaired physical function (4,5). Some experts estimate that obesity is second only to cigarette smoking as a leading cause of death in the United States and that it is associated with approximately 300,000 deaths per year among adults (6). Physical inactivity and poor dietary habits appear to be the main lifestyle factors contributing to the excess deaths associated with obesity (7,8). Low cardiovascular fitness is also independently associated with premature mortality from all causes (9,10). The authors' studies of cardiorespiratory fitness, obesity, and mortality indicate that some, if not much, of the association between obesity and mortality may be due to low fitness (11,12).

Low levels of energy expenditure from physical activity appear to be a major contributing factor to the rapid increase in the prevalence of overweight and obesity (13–15). Although no direct data on the United States exist, a decline in energy expenditure has likely taken place because of obvious changes in occupational-related and household-related physical activity, as well as because of urban environments that are increasingly less conducive to leisure-time physical activity. In the United States, recent data indicate that 28.7% of adults report participating in no physical activity and that 45.9% participate in some leisure-time activity but at levels that are too low to confer significant health benefits. Only 25.4% of United States adults are physically active at recommended levels (16). Compared with normal-weight and overweight adults, obese individuals are more likely to report being inactive (24%, 26%, and 36%, respectively) (2). Cross-sectional and cohort studies suggest that differences in the amount of physical activity contribute to differences in body weight and body fatness and play an important role in whether obesity develops (15,17–20). Clinicians must have appropriate clinical and behavioral tools for increasing physical activity in overweight and obese patients.

This chapter examines evidence regarding the role of physical activity in the treatment of overweight and obesity. The review and discussion include (a) the role of physical activity in weight control and long-term maintenance of weight loss, (b) the influence of physical activity on health outcomes, and (c) physical activity intervention in clinical practice for overweight and obese patients.

PHYSICAL ACTIVITY IN WEIGHT MANAGEMENT

Because energy expenditure is an essential factor in the energy-balance equation, it plays a critical role in weight regulation. Total daily energy expenditure consists of resting energy expenditure, the thermic effect of food, and energy expenditure from physical activity. Energy expenditure from physical activity is the only component of total daily energy expenditure that is behaviorally modifiable. Because energy expenditure from daily activity accounts for up to 30% of total energy expenditure, it can have a significant impact on energy balance. Overweight and obesity result when dietary patterns create an average energy intake that is greater than the average energy expenditure. Increasing physical activity can help to establish the negative energy balance necessary for weight loss.

A large body of scientific evidence and consensus opinion indicates that physical activity is an essential element, along with dietary and behavioral modification, in the clinical strategy for weight management for patients who are overweight and obese (4,9,21,22). Recently, professional and government bodies have provided expert consensus recommendations on physical activity for the treatment of overweight and obesity and for health enhancement in the general population. The latest guidelines can be summarized as follows: all adults should increase their regular physical activity to a level appropriate to their capacities, needs, and interest. The long-term goal is to accumulate 30 minutes or more of moderate-intensity physical activity (e.g., brisk walking, leisurely cycling, swimming, recreational sports, home repair, and yard work) on most, and preferably all, days of the week. People who currently meet these recommended minimal standards may derive additional health and fitness benefits from becoming more physically active or including more vigorous activity (9,23,24).

The National Heart, Lung, and Blood Institute's (NHLBI) *Clinical guidelines on the identification, evaluation, and treatment of overweight and obesity in adults (Evidence report)* recommendation for physical activity as part of a comprehensive weight loss therapy and weight maintenance program is consistent with the previously mentioned summary statement (4). The *Evidence report's* recommendation is based on convincing scientific evidence that physical activity (a) modestly contributes to weight loss in overweight and obese adults, (b) may decrease abdominal fat, (c) increases cardiovascular fitness, and (d) may help with maintenance of weight loss. The *Evidence report* also states that, with time, larger volumes of physical activity can be performed to cause a greater weight loss as long as it is not compensated for by a higher caloric intake.

Based on the strength of evidence indicating the importance of physical inactivity to the increasing prevalence of overweight and obesity, the 2001 Surgeon General's *Call to action to prevent and decrease overweight and obesity* identified five national priority areas that require immediate action to assist Americans in increasing their physical activity levels (25). These priority areas include (a) ensuring daily quality physical education in all school grades, (b) assisting individuals in reducing time spent watching television and other similar sedentary behaviors, (c) ensuring that adults get at least 30 minutes of moderate physical activity on most days (children should get at least 60 minutes), (d) creating more opportunities for physical activity at work sites, and (e) making community facilities available and accessible for physical activity for all people.

Influence of Physical Activity on Weight Loss

Despite the importance of energy expenditure from physical activity in the energy-balance equation, available data suggest that physical activity, as a single treatment of overweight and obese adults, results in modest total weight losses on the order of 1 to 3 kg or an average of 0.06 to 0.1 kg per week (4,26–28). When physical activity is combined with dietary intervention, most studies have not found a statistically significant difference in weight loss, although the trend is usually in favor of increased weight loss compared with dietary intervention alone (27,29).

Despite the modest results suggested by cumulative data, several studies indicate that physical activity programs can result in large weight losses. Available evidence suggests that weight loss associated with physical activity occurs in a dose–response relationship; that is, weight loss increases as the number of kilocalories (kcal) expended in physical activity increases (30–32). Although higher intensity exercise may enhance weight loss through mechanisms such as appetite suppression, increased postexercise energy expenditure, or other metabolic factors, such as adrenergic or enzymatic stimulation of fat oxidation, most evidence supports the premise that the effect is related to the energy expenditure during physical activity participation (33,34). Unless the exercise intensity is sufficiently high, an increase in postexercise energy expenditure is unlikely to make a substantial contribution to weight loss (35). Physical activity does not consistently protect against the decrease in resting energy expenditure that is associated with diet-induced weight loss (36–39). Several studies suggest that, when combined with dietary change, exercise training increases total body fat loss and has favorable effects on the preservation of fat-free mass, compared with diet-induced weight loss alone (26,36,40,41). No consistent evidence suggests that exercise training in overweight and obese individuals results in significant changes in energy or macronutrient intake (42,43).

Studies that employed high volumes of physical training induced total weight losses up to 12.5 kg at rates between 0.6 and 1.8 kg per week (36,44,45). In one of the most recent studies, Ross et al. (36) conducted a 12-week randomized controlled trial to determine the effects of diet-induced or exercise-induced weight loss on subcutaneous fat, visceral fat, skeletal muscle mass, and insulin sensitivity in 52 obese men (mean BMI = 31.3 kg/m^2). Investigators matched both treatment groups for total energy deficit (a 700-kcal-per-day dietary deficit in the diet-only group and a 700-kcal-per-day exercise energy expenditure in the exercise-only group). The goal for both groups was to achieve a weekly weight loss of 0.6 kg. Participants in the exercise group performed daily exercise (brisk walking or light jogging) on a motorized treadmill. Exercising at an intensity of 77% of maximal heart rate, the exercise group was able to expend approximately 698 kcal in sessions lasting 60 minutes. Body weight decreased by 7.5 kg (8%) in both weight loss groups. Cardiovascular fitness (peak oxygen uptake) increased by 16% in the exercise group, compared with no change in the diet-only group. The average reduction in total fat was 1.3 kg greater in the exercise-induced weight loss group, and skeletal muscle was preserved compared to the diet-only group. Abdominal subcutaneous fat, visceral fat, and resting energy expenditure decreased and insulin sensitivity improved similarly in both weight loss groups.

The findings of Ross et al. (36) demonstrate that exercise-induced weight loss reduces total fat and improves cardiovascular fitness significantly more than an equivalent diet-induced weight loss. Also, exercise-induced weight loss without caloric restriction is an effective strategy for reducing obesity in moderately obese men. However, these obese men had a relatively high level of cardiovascular fitness at baseline and, consequently, a high energy expenditure during exercise (approximately 12 kcal per minute). In the authors' experience, this level of energy expenditure from physical activity exceeds the capacity of many sedentary and obese individuals.

Physical Activity and Weight Maintenance

One of the most significant roles of physical activity in the treatment of overweight and obesity is in the long-term maintenance of weight loss. Participation in regular exercise is frequently cited as one of the most important determinants of long-term weight main-tenance. Correlational data and prospective studies report that a higher percentage of weight maintainers than nonmaintainers engage in regular physical activity. Several prospective studies have found improved weight maintenance when exercise was included in a post–weight loss program (4,27). Wing (27) reviewed six randomized con-trolled studies that included follow-ups of 1 year or more. In all of the studies reviewed, weight loss at follow-up was greater in diet-plus-exercise groups than in diet-only groups. However, only two of the six studies reported a significantly greater weight loss at fol-low-up with diet plus exercise. Examination of the results from the review by Wing (27) suggests a 3.0-kg greater weight loss at follow-up when exercise is added to diet therapy. This finding is consistent with the conclusion of the NHLBI *Evidence report* that diet plus exercise is associated with a 1.5-kg to 3.0-kg greater weight loss at long-term fol-low-up, compared with diet alone (4).

Several correlational studies show a strong association between exercise at follow-up and maintenance of weight loss. In one of the most often cited studies, Kayman et al. (46) found that 90% of women who have lost weight and who have maintained their loss for more than 2 years reported exercising on a regular basis. Only 34% of women who regained their lost weight reported regular physical activity (46). Wadden et al. (47) reported that no significant differences were seen in weight loss between diet-plus-exer-cise groups and a diet-only group after 100 weeks of follow-up; however, subjects who reported regular exercise at follow-up maintained a weight loss of 12.1 kg compared with a loss of only 6.1 kg in those who reported no regular exercise. Weight loss maintenance was significantly enhanced in subjects who exercised regularly for 4.5 years after a very low calorie diet program, compared with those who avoided exercise (9.6 kg vs. 1.3 kg, respectively) (48).

In the National Weight Control Registry (NWCR), investigators surveyed nearly 800 men and women who had successfully lost 30 kg or more and who had maintained a min-imum 13.6-kg loss for an average of 5 years (49). Ninety percent of these successful maintainers reported participating in both dietary change and physical activity. This find-ing suggests that few individuals are able to maintain long-term weight loss successfully without participating in regular physical activity (10% of NWCR participants used dietary modification alone and 1% used modification of activity alone). Registry partic-ipants reported expending approximately 2,800 kcal per week in physical activity (equiv-alent to walking approximately 28 miles per week), with an average of 800 kcal per week coming from heavy activity. Seventy-two percent met or exceeded current public health consensus recommendations for at least 1,000 kcal in physical activity per week. The majority of energy expenditure came from walking (measured as blocks walked). Other commonly reported activities included stationary or road cycling, aerobics, treadmill walking, jogging, running, hiking, weight lifting, stair stepping, and step aerobics.

Schoeller et al. (50) conducted a prospective study to assess the effects of physical activity on weight maintenance and to determine how much physical activity was required to optimize maintenance. The investigators recruited 34 women who had recently lost an average of 23 kg. The average BMI at study entry was approximately 24 kg/m^2 (normal weight by current classifications). The researchers used measures of total energy expenditure, resting metabolic rate, and thermic effect of a meal to estimate energy expended in physical activity. Weight gain in the physically active group was sig-nificantly less than that in the sedentary group during the 1-year prospective observation. The data were analyzed retrospectively to determine the energy expenditure from physi-cal activity that provided the maximum differentiation between weight maintainers and gainers. Fewer than 20% of the women with an energy expenditure of more than 47 kJ per kg per day (11 kcal per kg per day) gained more than 4.5 kg, whereas nearly 71% of women who were less active gained more than 4.5 kg. The authors concluded that an energy expenditure from physical activity of 47 kJ per kg per day (11 kcal per kg per day) was the threshold for weight maintenance. Considering the difference in energy expenditure between the active and sedentary group, the investigators determined that the sedentary individuals would have to add 80 minutes per day of moderate activity, such as brisk walking, or 35 minutes of vigorous activity, such as fast cycling or aerobics, to maintain weight loss. This level of activity is comparable to that reported by the NWCR, and it is significantly higher than the current public health recommendations of at least 30 minutes of daily moderate-intensity physical activity (9). Whether individuals heavier than the women in this study need to perform more or less activity to achieve weight maintenance is not known.

Summary of Physical Activity in Weight Management

As reviewed herein, questions remain about the minimal and optimal doses of physical activity needed to achieve and to maintain significant weight loss. Evidence reviewed thus far suggests that public health recommendations for a minimum of 1,000 kcal per week in moderate-intensity physical activity, although associated with significant health benefits, may not be sufficient to produce significant weight loss or long-term weight maintenance (9,22). Overweight and obese individuals may need to accumulate 2,000 kcal or more of moderate-intensity and vigorous-intensity weekly physical activity to lose and maintain a significant weight loss (22,49,50). The authors caution, however, that this is a long-term goal and that individuals should be counseled to begin adding physical activity into their lifestyle no matter how low the initial level. In the authors' programs, sedentary individuals are encouraged to begin by cutting down on sitting time and adding moderate activities, such as brisk walking, in bouts as short as 2 minutes several times per day. In subsequent sections, evidence that low to moderate levels of physical activity are beneficial to long-term weight control and health enhancement is reviewed. The authors agree that more total activity and vigorous activity may offer additional benefits, but only to the degree that such participation is consistent with the goals, interests, and abilities of individual patients. The ultimate goal in behavioral interventions for physical activity is to promote long-term adherence to physical activity.

PHYSICAL ACTIVITY, OBESITY, AND HEALTH OUTCOMES

That physical activity and cardiorespiratory fitness have independent and beneficial effects on several of the adverse health outcomes of obesity, particularly those pertaining to cardiovascular disease (CVD), type II diabetes, and premature mortality, is well established (4,9,12,21). Physical activity plays an important role in weight management, not only because of its favorable effects on energy balance but also because it reduces the risk of obesity-related comorbidities and results in lower all-cause and CVD death rates (51). Following is a brief review of the effects of physical activity on the health outcomes of overweight and obesity.

Insulin Action and Glucose Tolerance

Epidemiologic and clinical trial data indicate that increased physical activity improves insulin action and thus reduces insulin resistance and improves glucose tolerance in obese individuals (12,21,52). The improvement in insulin action can occur independent of sig-

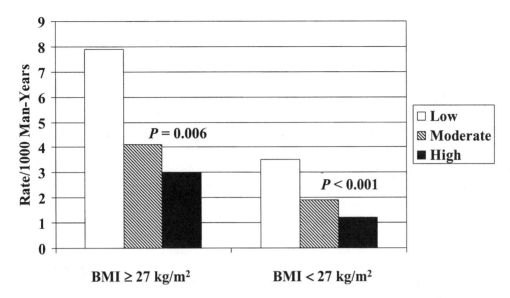

FIG. 21.1. Incidence of type II diabetes per 1,000 person-years by cardiorespiratory fitness levels, according to body mass index (BMI) (kilograms per meter squared [kg/m^2]). Included are low-fit men (least-fit 20%) (*white bars*), moderate-fit men (next 40%) (*diagonal lines*), and high-fit men (remaining 40%) (*black bars*). (Adapted from Wei M, Gibbons LW, Mitchell TL, et al. The association between cardiorespiratory fitness and impaired fasting glucose and type 2 diabetes mellitus in men. *Ann Intern Med* 1999;130:89–96, with permission.)

nificant changes in weight or body composition, but much of the benefit occurs in the presence of weight loss or of a change in body composition, particularly a reduction in abdominal or visceral fat (40,52–55). In 1999, Wei et al. (56) reported a greater than threefold risk for developing type II diabetes in men with low cardiorespiratory fitness, compared with the risk in high-fit men. These authors reported a steep inverse gradient of risk across fitness categories among individuals with a BMI of less than 27 kg/m^2 and of more than or equal to 27 kg/m^2 (Fig. 21.1). Fit men with a BMI of more than or equal to 27 kg/m^2 had a slightly lower incidence of type II diabetes than did unfit men with a BMI of less than 27 kg/m^2. With the publication of the Diabetes Prevention Project and the Finnish Diabetes Prevention Study, strong evidence from prospective randomized trials now indicates that physical activity combined with a weight-reducing diet can prevent the transition from impaired glucose tolerance to type II diabetes (57,58).

Blood Pressure and Hypertension

Observational studies suggest that physical activity reduces the risk of developing hypertension, independent of body habitus (12,21,59). Paffenbarger et al. (60,61) followed two cohorts of college alumni for up to 15 years for the development of incident physician-diagnosed hypertension. In general, active men in both studies had a lower risk of developing hypertension than did sedentary men, with the greatest protection occurring in men in the highest BMI categories. A review of 44 randomized controlled trials involving more than 2,600 participants revealed that aerobic exercise training reduces blood pressure by an average of 3.4/2.4 mm Hg, after controlling for weight loss and dietary change (59). The blood pressure reduction in response to exercise training is greater in hypertensive individuals (7.4/5.8 mm Hg) (59). Exercise training alone in overweight and obese individuals appears to be less effective for reducing blood pressure than does diet alone (59,62); however, a more recent study by Blumenthal et al. (63) found that the addition of a behavioral weight loss program enhanced the blood pressure–lowering effect of exercise (59,62). In a randomized clinical trial testing lifestyle interventions, including dietary change and physical activity, Stevens et al. (64) reported that individuals who maintained at least a 4.5-kg weight reduction also showed a persistent reduction in blood pressure over the 3 years of follow-up.

Dyslipoproteinemias

Physical activity does not appear to have a major independent effect on lipoprotein levels, apart from weight loss in overweight and obese individuals (55,65). Grundy et al. (21) concluded that physical activity of sufficient volume to result in at least a 4.5-kg weight loss is associated with an increase in high-density lipoprotein cholesterol (HDL-C) level and a decrease in triglycerides. The addition of physical activity to a caloric-deficit, low-fat diet may reverse the HDL-C–lowering effect associated with this eating pattern in overweight men and women. Physical activity significantly enhances the low-density lipoprotein cholesterol (LDL-C)–lowering effect of a weight-reducing, low-fat diet (21,65). Few available studies have examined the effects of physical activity in overweight or obese individuals with adverse lipoprotein profiles.

All-Cause and Cardiovascular Disease Mortality

Several prospective observational studies from the Aerobics Center Longitudinal Study (ACLS) cohort show an inverse relationship between cardiorespiratory fitness and all-cause and CVD mortality in normal-weight, overweight, and obese men and women. These data suggest that moderate to high levels of cardiorespiratory fitness protect against much, if not most, of the increased mortality associated with overweight and obesity. Following is a summary of the study methods and published data from the ACLS cohort.

The ACLS is an observational study of patients examined at least once at the Cooper Clinic from 1970 to 1993. All study participants came to the clinic for periodic health examinations and counseling about exercise, diet, and other lifestyle factors associated with increased risk of chronic disease. The participants were predominantly white, they were employed in executive and professional occupations, and they were college graduates from the mid to upper socioeconomic strata. All participants underwent a thorough evaluation, including a medical and family history, physical examination, anthropometry, clinical assessments, blood chemistry, and a determination of cardiorespiratory fitness by a maximal exercise test on a treadmill. Each participant's level of cardiorespiratory fitness was defined by criteria based on age, sex, and maximal time on the treadmill. The least-fit 20% were classified as unfit, the next 40% were classified as moderately fit, and the top 40% as high fit. Anthropometric measures included BMI (kg/m^2) calculated from directly measured height and weight, percent body fat determination by hydrostatic weight and/or the sum of seven skinfold measurements, and waist circumference measured at the umbilicus. Prevalence rates for normal-weight, overweight, and obesity were 41%, 46%, and 13%, respectively—a rate similar to a representative sample of United States men (66). Mailed follow-up surveys and the National Death Index were used to determine morbidity and mortality endpoints. For the studies reported herein, the average participant follow-up periods range from 5 to 10 years.

In 1989, Blair et al. (10) reported an inverse relationship between cardiorespiratory fitness and all-cause and CVD mortality. In this study, the authors calculated age-adjusted all-cause death rates across low, moderate, and high cardiorespiratory fitness categories in 10,224 men and 3,120 women who were apparently healthy at baseline. In all BMI strata (<20 kg/m^2, 20 to 25 kg/m^2, >25 kg/m^2), the least-fit men and women had higher death rates than did the participants in the moderate-fitness and high-fitness groups. In this report, high-fit men with a BMI of 25 kg/m^2 or more had an age-adjusted death rate from all causes of 20 per 10,000 man-years of observation, compared with a rate of 48 per 10,000 man-years in unfit men in this same BMI stratum. Although this study did not differentiate between overweight and obesity, it did provide evidence that being physically fit might reduce the risk of premature mortality in obesity.

To follow up on this line of evidence, Barlow et al. (67) specifically investigated the relation of cardiorespiratory fitness to mortality in overweight and obese men. In this report from the ACLS cohort, men who were overweight or obese (BMI ≥ 27 kg/m^2) and who had moderate to high levels of fitness did not have elevated mortality rates as compared with high-fit men who were normal weight (BMI < 27 kg/m^2). Specifically, obese men (BMI > 30 kg/m^2) who were at least moderately fit had an age-adjusted all-cause death rate of 18 per 10,000 man-years of observation, compared with a rate of 52 per 10,000 man-years in normal-weight men who were unfit. The highest death rate was observed in the unfit obese men (62.1 per 10,000 man-years of observation).

To determine whether changes in physical fitness significantly affect cardiovascular and all-cause mortality, the authors conducted a long-term follow-up study on a subset of ACLS men with at least two preventive medical examinations (68). Men who were unfit at baseline but who became more fit by follow-up had a reduction in mortality of 44%, compared with those men who remained unfit throughout the course of the study. This benefit was independent of age, health status, and other risk factors for premature mortality. In fact, improving fitness had a greater impact on mortality risk than losing weight, reducing blood pressure, reducing cholesterol, or quitting smoking.

Lee et al. (69) extended observations in 1999 with more detailed investigations of body habitus, cardiorespiratory fitness, and mortality in 21,925 men. Subjects were assigned to categories of lean, normal, or obese based on measures of percent body fat and waist circumference. In this study, the authors found a direct relationship between percent body fat and waist circumference measures and risk of all-cause mortality and CVD. Fit men had lower death rates than their unfit counterparts within each body fatness and waist circumference category. Obese men as classified by either body fatness ($\geq 25\%$) or waist circumference (≥ 99 cm) who were fit had a much lower risk of all-cause and CVD mortality than did unfit lean men (Fig. 21.2). All-cause mortality rates in the fit obese men were not significantly different from those of fit lean men; however, a tendency was observed, even in the fit men, for CVD death rates to be higher as the body habitus increased.

In the 1998 NHBLI *Evidence report,* physical inactivity is mentioned, along with high triglycerides, as "other risk factors" for which quantitative risk contribution is not available but that should heighten the need for weight reduction in obese persons (4). After the release of the *Evidence report,* Wei et al. (70) conducted a study of 25,714 men from the ACLS cohort (a) to provide a quantitative risk estimate of low cardiorespiratory fitness and (b) to compare low cardiorespiratory fitness with CVD and other established risk factors to assess its effect on mortality in normal-weight, overweight, and obese men. Obese men with baseline CVD, type II diabetes, elevated total cholesterol level (>240 mg per dL), hypertension, current smoking, and low cardiorespiratory fitness had a higher risk of all-cause and CVD mortality, compared with normal-weight men with none of these conditions. Low cardiorespiratory fitness was a strong predictor of mortality, with relative risks comparable to, if not greater than, the relative risks for type II diabetes, high cholesterol levels, hypertension, and current cigarette smoking (Fig. 21.3). Obese men

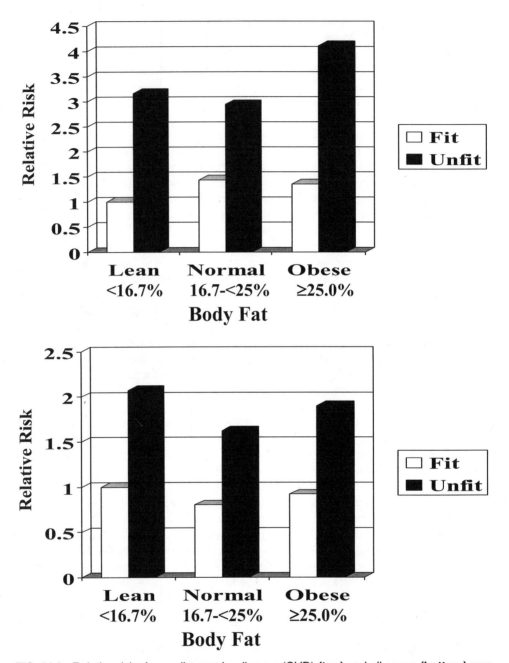

FIG. 21.2. Relative risks for cardiovascular disease (CVD) **(top)** and all-cause **(bottom)** mortality by percent body fat and cardiorespiratory fitness level in 21,925 men followed for 176,742 person-years of observation (428 deaths, 144 from CVD). Relative risks are adjusted for age (single year), examination year, smoking status, alcohol intake, and parental history of coronary heart disease. Unfit men (*black bars*) were the least fit (lowest 20% in each age-group), and all other men were classified as fit. (Data from Lee CD, Blair SN, Jackson AS. Cardiorespiratory fitness, body composition, and all-cause and cardiovascular disease mortality in men. *Am J Clin Nutr* 1999;69:373–380, with permission.)

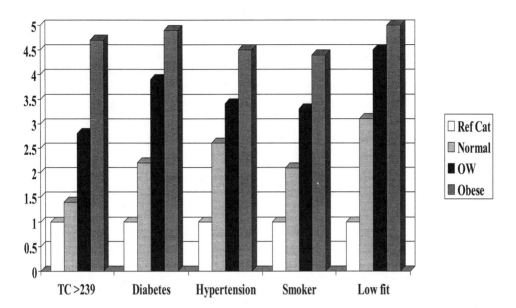

Co Morbidities of Obesity

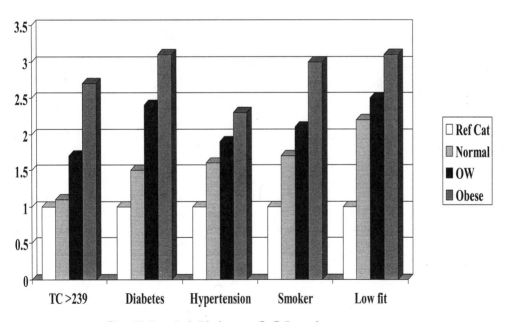

Co Morbidities of Obesity

FIG. 21.3. Relative risks for cardiovascular disease (CVD) **(top)** and all-cause **(bottom)** mortality in 25,714 men followed for 258,781 person-years of observation (1,025 deaths, 439 from CVD). Relative risks were adjusted for age and examination year. The reference category (Ref Cat) in each of the five analyses was normal-weight men (body mass index [BMI] = 18.5 to 24.9) who did not have the risk factor examined in the specific analysis. Overweight (OW) men were those with a BMI of 25.0 to 29.9 kilograms per meter squared (kg/m^2), and obese men were those with a BMI of 30.0 kg/m^2. Abbreviation: TC, total cholesterol. (Data from Wei M, Kampert JB, Barlow CE, et al. Relationship between low cardiorespiratory fitness and mortality in normal-weight, overweight, and obese men. *JAMA* 1999;282:1547–1553,with permission.)

with any of the risk factors had about a fivefold higher CVD death rate and a threefold higher all-cause death rate when compared with normal-weight men without the condition. In the 3,293 obese men, low fitness was the most common mortality predictor, with a prevalence rate about five times higher than that of type II diabetes, which was the least prevalent of the factors considered. About 50% of obese men in this study were unfit, whereas 16% had baseline CVD and 10% had type II diabetes. Because of its high prevalence and its strength as predictor of premature mortality, low cardiorespiratory fitness has the highest population attributable risk of the six mortality predictors evaluated in overweight and obese men in the ACLS cohort of men.

Summary of Obesity, Physical Activity, and Health Outcomes

Findings from the ACLS cohort suggest that higher levels of physical activity and cardiorespiratory fitness provide protection against many of the adverse health outcomes associated with overweight and obesity. These findings from the ACLS are supported by several other prospective observational studies (12,21). Available data indicate that overweight and obese individuals who are physically active and fit have a lower risk of morbidity and mortality than normal-weight individuals who are sedentary and unfit. Inactivity and low fitness may be as important as overweight and obesity, if not more so, in their adverse effects on health outcomes. All the findings reviewed herein suggest that the importance of clinician assessment of physical activity and fitness status in overweight and obese individuals is parallel to that of assessing for other obesity-related comorbidities. Evaluating physical activity and fitness allows for a more complete risk stratification in overweight and obese patients, and it can enhance clinical decision making and weight-management intervention. Clinicians should provide a physical activity prescription and counseling for physical activity, as they do for other comorbidities.

PHYSICAL ACTIVITY INTERVENTION IN CLINICAL PRACTICE: NEW APPROACHES TO EXERCISE PRESCRIPTION

Regular physical activity is clearly helpful for weight control, and it provides important health benefits, such as improved blood pressure and glucose tolerance, increased cardiorespiratory fitness, and reduced mortality risk, for overweight and obese individuals. Because of these benefits, professional and governmental groups have provided expert consensus documents and recommendations on physical activity, both for the treatment of overweight and obesity and for health enhancement in the general population (4,9,21–24,71). However, despite general consensus and expert guidelines, the barriers to physical activity counseling and participation present significant challenges for clinicians and patients, respectively. A recent survey of United States adults found that, of the 44% of the women and 29% of the men trying to lose weight at any given time, fewer than 40% report engaging in the recommended 150 minutes or more of leisure-time physical activity per week (72). Another survey found that more than 54% of overweight and obese patients are not receiving exercise counseling from their physicians (73). Research reveals that adherence to formal exercise programs is poor, particularly among obese individuals (74). Understanding the barriers to physical activity participation and applying sound behavioral interventions are important to improving these statistics. Alternative approaches to prescribing exercise, such as lifestyle physical activity and the accumulation of shorter bouts of exercise, may be better for promoting regular physical activity in overweight individuals than is the traditional structured exercise approach.

Current physical activity guidelines for public health emphasize moderate-intensity activity based on convincing evidence that significant health benefits, such as improved blood cholesterol levels, lower blood pressure, and reduced risk of mortality, occur when sedentary individuals move from low levels of physical activity and cardiorespiratory fitness to moderate levels (9,23,24,71). Data now indicate that health benefits associated with physical activity can be accrued at significantly lower intensities than those recommended by earlier consensus statements (9,71,75). The benefits of physical activity also apparently follow a dose–response curve across intensity levels and total duration, rather than appearing at specific thresholds (76). As the previous section reviewed, a similar pattern of benefit appears to occur in overweight and obese individuals. One novel feature of the latest consensus physical activity guidelines is the recommendation that allows for the accumulation of moderate-intensity physical activity over a 24-hour period.

Short Bouts of Physical Activity

Guidelines for accumulating physical activity are based on evidence indicating that comparable health and fitness benefits occur as long as the total amount of energy expenditure in moderate-intensity physical activity achieves the recommended levels (9,71). Several recent studies comparing longer (traditionally 30 minutes of continuous activity) versus shorter (5-minute to 15-minute) bouts of activity spread throughout the day reveal that comparable improvements in weight control, cardiorespiratory fitness, and cardiovascular risk occur when the total amount of physical activity is the same (31,77,78). In addition to comparable health and fitness benefits, multiple short bouts of physical activity may increase participation and adherence (79).

Jakicic et al. (79) randomly assigned 56 obese (33.9 kg/m^2) women to a standard 20-week behavioral intervention and one of two exercise treatments. Both groups were given a prescription of 40 minutes of exercise on 5 days per week. One group was instructed to perform 40 minutes of brisk walking that would be accomplished in one continuous bout (long-bout group). The other group was encouraged to divide their exercise into four 10-minute bouts (short-bout group). The main findings of the study after 20 weeks were that the short-bout group performed significantly more minutes of activity, exercised on more days of the week, and lost more weight than the long-bout group. These investigators extended this line of research by conducting an 18-month intervention comparing the effects of long-bout exercise with those of multiple short bouts both with and without home exercise equipment in 148 sedentary obese (BMI = 32.8 kg/m^2) women (31). At the end of the study, no significant differences were found between long-bout and short-bout groups with regard to weight loss, exercise participation, or cardiorespiratory fitness. One of the strongest predictors of weight loss in this study was the total minutes of activity performed per week. Weight loss was significantly greater in individuals who exercised 200 minutes or more per week, compared with the group that performed 150 minutes or more per week and the group that performed less than 150 minutes per week. Weight loss after 18 months was 13.1, 8.5, and 3.5 kg, respectively (Fig. 21.4). These results suggest a strong dose–response relationship between physical activity and weight loss. In this study, access to home exercise equipment facilitated compliance and long-term weight loss, compared with the use of short bouts alone. A long-term intervention conducted by Perri et al. (80) found that subjects randomized to home-based exercise adhered better and achieved greater weight loss than did those attending a supervised program. These studies indicate that nontraditional methods of exercise prescription, such as accumulating multiple short bouts of

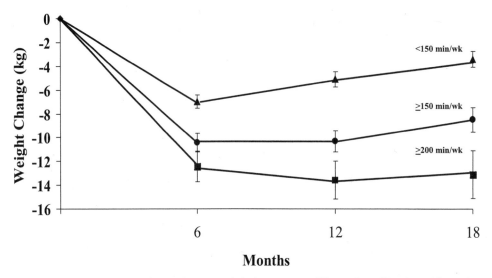

FIG. 21.4. Dose response of exercise on weight loss across 18 months of treatment based on self-reported exercise (mean [SEM]). Weight loss at 18 months was significantly greater in the exercise group that averaged 200 minutes per week, compared with the groups that averaged less than 150 minutes per week and 150 minutes per week ($p < 0.05$). Error bars indicate standard error of the mean *(SEM)*. (From Jakicic JM, Winters C, Lang W, et al. Effects of intermittent exercise and use of home exercise equipment on adherence, weight loss, and fitness in overweight women: a randomized trial. *JAMA* 1999;282:1554–1560, with permission.)

activity and home-based exercise, can be used as an option for incorporating physical activity and exercise into one's lifestyle.

A recent study by Levine et al. (81) demonstrated the potential impact of relatively low levels of physical activity on weight regulation. Sixteen nonobese men and women were fed 1,000 kcal per day in excess of weight-maintenance requirements for 8 weeks to determine which components of energy expenditure determine resistance to fat gain during overfeeding. Non–exercise-associated thermogenesis (NEAT) proved to be the principal mediator of resistance to fat gain with overfeeding. NEAT is the thermogenesis that accompanies physical activities other than volitional exercise, such as the activities of daily living, fidgeting, and spontaneous muscle contractions. Changes in NEAT directly predicted resistance to fat gain ($r = -0.77$, $p < 0.001$). Levine et al. (82) extended the previously mentioned investigation of NEAT by investigating the energy expenditure associated with fidgeting-like activities and strolling. Compared with sitting and standing motionless, fidgeting-like activities, such as hand and foot tapping, arm and leg swinging, and routine movements both in the sitting position and standing, significantly increased energy expenditure. The authors concluded that the energy expenditure associated with NEAT is sufficiently great to contribute substantively to energy balance. These results suggest that both clinical and population strategies to increase nonexercise physical activities, such as fidgeting and activities of daily living, may be helpful in an overall approach of prevention and treatment of overweight and obesity (83). The authors believe that behavioral counseling strategies aimed at increasing nonexercise physical activities, such as using fewer electronic devices that interfere with opportunities for household and occupational physical activity, may be an important adjunct to physical activity prescription for regulating energy balance.

Lifestyle Physical Activity

The authors have described a lifestyle approach to physical activity in which sedentary adults incorporate short bouts of moderate-intensity activity into their lifestyle, such as increasing the amount of walking in the daily routine, performing more yard work, and using the stairs when possible (84). A theoretical example of this approach is provided in Fig. 21.5. The advantage of this approach is that it provides various options for increasing physical activity, rather than limiting activity to the traditional structured exercise approach. A key feature of the lifestyle approach is the application of behavioral theory and counseling strategies to help individuals learn and apply the skills necessary to integrate beneficial levels of physical activity into their lives. Recent data suggest that this method of physical activity prescription is as effective as the traditional exercise prescription in increasing physical activity and fitness and in promoting weight loss and long-term maintenance (32,85).

The authors conducted Project Active, a 24-month randomized clinical trial, to compare the effects of a lifestyle physical activity intervention designed to help participants integrate moderate-intensity physical activity into their daily routine with those of a tra-

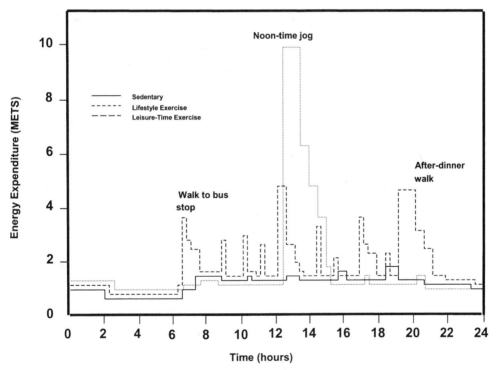

FIG. 21.5. Theoretical patterns of physical activity over 24 hours. Shown are the energy expenditure over the course of a day for a sedentary person (*solid line*); the energy expenditure of an individual who engages in planned vigorous exercise during leisure time but is otherwise sedentary (*dotted line*); and the energy expenditure for an individual with a sedentary job who seeks opportunities to integrate short bouts of physical activity into the daily routine (*dashed line*). Comparable health effects are expected for leisure-time exercise and lifestyle physical activity if the total daily energy expenditure is the same. (From Blair SN, Kohl HW III, Gordon NF. Physical activity and health: a lifestyle approach. *Med Exerc Nutr Health* 1992;1:54–57, with permission.)

ditional fitness center–based exercise program (85). Participants in both lifestyle (number of subjects [N] = 121) and structured (N = 114) groups received 6 months of intensive intervention, followed by 18 months of a minimal maintenance intervention. The lifestyle intervention used social cognitive theory (86) and the transtheoretical model (87) of behavior change in a group counseling format to encourage individuals to accumulate at least 30 minutes of moderate-intensity physical activity on most, and preferably all, days of the week. Individuals were encouraged to progress toward this goal in a manner best suited to their level of motivational readiness for change. Group facilitators worked with individuals weekly using a problem-solving approach that involved cognitive and behavioral strategies (e.g., developing skills to overcome barriers to physical activity) to help them initiate, adopt, and maintain a physical activity program. During the maintenance phase, lifestyle participants were encouraged to continue their physical activity. Participants in the structured exercise group received a traditional exercise prescription, with supervised exercise sessions 3 to 5 days per week for 6 months in a state-of-the-art fitness center in Dallas, Texas (88). During the maintenance phase, structured-exercise participants were encouraged to exercise on their own.

Both lifestyle and structured interventions produced significant and comparable benefits in physical activity, cardiorespiratory fitness, and cardiovascular risk profiles from baseline to 24 months with no significant differences between groups. The lifestyle group maintained cardiorespiratory fitness between months 6 and 24 better than did the structured group, which suggested that the structured group was not able to maintain its physical activity routines as effectively as the lifestyle group. In both groups, one of the strongest predictors of success was the percentage of weeks between months 6 and 24 that individuals reported regular moderate-intensity physical activity on at least 5 days of the week. For all outcomes, participants who reported that they were active 70% or more of the time had at least twice as much improvement in all measures as those who were less active. Weight decreased by nearly 1 kg for those who were active on 70% or more of the weeks compared with an increase of nearly 2.5 kg for those who were active on 30% or less. This study supports the hypothesis that a behavioral-based lifestyle physical activity intervention can significantly increase physical activity and fitness and can provide health benefits comparable to those of traditional fitness center–based exercise.

Andersen et al. (32) used a similar lifestyle physical activity approach in a 16-week randomized controlled trial with 1-year follow-up in 40 obese women (mean BMI = 32.9 kg/m^2). Women were randomized into a standard diet and behavioral intervention, which included a self-selected, low-fat, low-calorie diet of approximately 1,200 kcal per day, combined with either programmed aerobic exercise or lifestyle physical activity. Participants in the programmed aerobic exercise group attended three step-aerobics classes per week with an estimated 450 to 500 kcal energy expenditure per class. The participants in this group were assisted in developing a long-term individualized program of structured aerobic exercise after the 16 weeks of intervention. Participants in the lifestyle physical activity group were advised to increase their levels of moderate-intensity activity by 30 minutes per day on most days of the week. Lifestyle participants were taught to incorporate short bouts of activity into their daily schedules. For example, participants were encouraged to walk instead of drive short distances and to take the stairs instead of the elevator. Both groups attended four quarterly meetings during the 1-year follow-up.

Weight losses between the groups did not differ significantly at any time during the 68 weeks of treatment and follow-up. At week 16, weight loss in the lifestyle group was

7.9 kg, and, in the aerobic group, it was 8.3 kg. By the end of 16 weeks, the participants in the lifestyle group were performing an estimated 234-kcal-per-day energy expenditure from physical activity on 4.7 days of the week, for a weekly physical activity energy expenditure of approximately 1,100 kcal per week. This level of activity is consistent with current public health recommendations for physical activity (9). Although the trend was not statistically significant, the lifestyle group tended to regain less weight over the 1-year follow-up. Participants in the lifestyle group regained 0.08 kg from week 16 to the end of follow-up, whereas the aerobic group regained 1.6 kg (Fig. 21.6). Both groups significantly improved cardiovascular fitness and CVD risk profiles with no difference between groups. The principal finding of this study was that a program of diet plus lifestyle activity may be a suitable alternative to the traditional structured exercise approach in overweight and obese individuals. Interestingly, using combined group data, the researchers found a dose–response relationship between activity levels, as defined by the percentage of weeks that participants performed 30 minutes or more of moderate-intensity physical activity on at least 5 days of the week during the 12-month follow-up and long-term weight maintenance. At the end of 1-year follow-up, the least active one-third (moderately active for only 19% of the weeks) had regained significantly more of their lost weight than the middle and most active groups (Fig. 21.7). In summary, lifestyle physical activity and behavioral intervention techniques are appropriate options for exercise prescription for weight management and health enhancement.

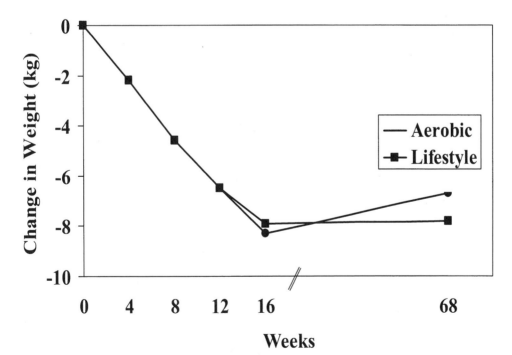

FIG. 21.6. Mean changes in body weight for the diet-plus-lifestyle group and diet-plus-aerobic group. Weight loss of the two groups did not differ significantly at any time. (From Andersen RE, Wadden TA, Bartlett SJ, et al. Effects of lifestyle activity vs structured aerobic exercise in obese women: a randomized trial. *JAMA* 1999;281:335–340, with permission.)

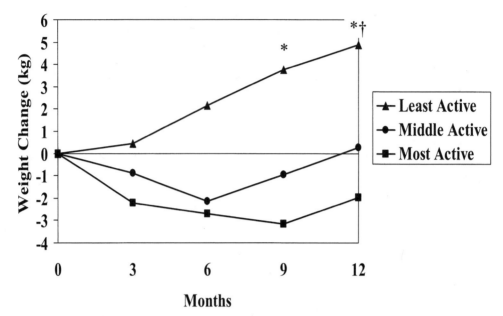

FIG. 21.7. Mean posttreatment changes in body weight according to the percentage of weeks that met or exceeded the Surgeon General's guidelines for physical activity in the year after completion of treatment. *, significantly different from most active group ($p < 0.05$); †, significantly different from middle active group ($p < 0.05$). (From Andersen RE, Wadden TA, Bartlett SJ, et al. Effects of lifestyle activity vs structured aerobic exercise in obese women: a randomized trial. *JAMA* 1999;281:335–340, with permission.)

Behavioral Approaches to Physical Activity

Physical activity is a behavior that is shaped and driven by multiple biologic, environmental, and psychosocial influences. Physical inactivity, as a behavior, may have been built up over many years under the influence of these same factors. The traditional prescriptive approach to exercise fails to consider fully the unique behavioral influences associated with physical activity. Simply giving a prescription to exercise at a specific intensity, frequency, and duration will work in only few individuals who are highly motivated to change. Many overweight and obese individuals experience barriers to physical activity that are in direct contrast with the traditional structured approach to exercise (Table 21.1). Because of the limitations of the traditional exercise prescription model, clinicians must develop new strategies to encourage meaningful levels of physical activity in overweight and obese patients. Current research is beginning to elucidate behavioral techniques for increasing physical activity participation and adherence (9,89). Applying validated behavior-modification techniques in clinical practice, in addition to

TABLE 21.1. *Common barriers to exercise participation*

Lack of time
Burden of excess weight
Lack of social support
Dislike of vigorous exercise
Inability to participate in vigorous exercise
Lack of access to exercise facilities
Embarrassment at taking part in activity
Unpleasant experiences with exercise

providing alternative physical activity options, such as lifestyle physical activity and accumulating several short bouts of moderate to vigorous activity each day, may improve patient participation in clinically beneficial levels of physical activity.

Transtheoretical Model Of Behavior Change

Traditionally, the practice of exercise counseling involves assessment, prescription, and expected action (e.g., increased physical activity). This approach assumes readiness for behavior changes. Studies reveal, however, that only about 20% of patients are ready to take action when advised to do so by a health care professional (90). Individuals must be psychologically and physically ready to commit themselves to a physical activity program. The transtheoretical model (Stages of Motivational Readiness) of behavior change, which was developed by Prochaska and DiClemente (87), is a comprehensive model of behavioral theory that provides intervention strategies based on an individual's motivational readiness to change. As presented earlier, the authors and others have successfully applied this model in the promotion of physical activity and weight management (32,85). The Stages of Motivational Readiness model integrates critical components of social cognitive theory, decisional balance, and relapse prevention; and it recognizes that behavior change is not a one-time event but that it takes place over time as individuals move back and forth between stages. As applied to physical activity, the five stages of change include the following:

1. Precontemplation: individuals who are not physically active and who do not intend to start soon, usually within 6 months. Individuals in this stage may be uninformed or unaware about the consequences of their behavior, or they may have tried to change and have been unsuccessful. These individuals usually perceive few personal benefits of physical activity, list many barriers to participation, and have a low self-confidence in their ability to change.
2. Contemplation: individuals who are not currently active but who intend to start soon, usually within the next 6 months. Individuals in this stage are usually aware of the benefits of becoming more physically active, but they are insufficiently motivated to overcome personal barriers to physical activity. Often, they are not aware of their options for physical activity and do not know how to get started.
3. Preparation: individuals who plan to start an activity program within the next month or who are currently participating in some activity, but not regularly. (The criterion measure for regular physical activity is usually defined as accumulating 30 minutes of moderate-intensity physical activity on 5 or more days of the week, or, using the more traditional exercise prescription, exercising on 3 or more days per week for at least 20 minutes or longer each time at a vigorous intensity.) Generally, these individuals have some plan of action and are gaining confidence in their ability to start and stick with a program of regular physical activity. This is the first stage in which individuals are ready for a specific physical activity prescription.
4. Action: individuals who are currently participating in regular physical activity (i.e., meeting the criterion measure for physical activity) but who have been doing so for less than 6 months. These individuals are motivated for activity, but they need to learn and develop behavioral skills to prevent relapse.
5. Maintenance: individuals who have participated in regular physical activity for 6 months or longer. These individuals have succeeded in long-term change and are becoming increasingly more confident that they can continue physical activity for a lifetime. These individuals need to develop behavioral skills to prevent relapse.

The transtheoretical model states that people vary in their readiness to change behavior, and counseling needs are different at each stage of change. To progress through the stages,

TABLE 21.2. *Cognitive and behavioral strategies for increasing physical activity*

Increasing knowledge—provide personalized messages on the benefits of and options for physical activity.
Decisional balance—help identify personal benefits and understand barriers to physical activity.
Problem solving—help identify barriers to physical activity; develop and practice potential solutions.
Relapse prevention—help identify high-risk situations for inactivity; develop plans to avoid or limit negative effects.
Cognitive restructuring—help identify and counter negative thoughts and rationalizations that facilitate physical inactivity and relapse.
Goal setting—help establish realistic and behaviorally specific short-term and long-term physical activity goals.
Self-monitoring—encourage keeping records of physical activity.
Stimulus control—help eliminate cues for inactivity and substitute alternatives for activity.
Social support—help identify and enlist the support of others; awareness of saboteurs.
Contingency management—help identify and provide appropriate rewards for success.

individuals use specific cognitive (e.g., evaluating personal benefits and barriers to physical activity participation) and behavioral (e.g., goal setting and self-monitoring) strategies in their efforts to change successfully. Table 21.2 lists several behavioral strategies that can be used to systematically help patients change thinking and behavior patterns that influence their participation in regular physical activity at each of these stages. Knowledge of where patients are in the process of change is critical for successful intervention. Prescribing activity and using counseling strategies that are not consistent with an individual's level of readiness or their needs, interests, and abilities will likely fail to produce desired results.

Programs to Help Clinicians Provide Behavioral Counseling

Several programs and tools are available to help clinicians provide behavioral counseling for physical activity in the clinical setting. A study by Wadden et al. (91) using the LEARN Program (American Health Publishing Co., Dallas, Texas) suggests that clinicians using behavioral strategies in brief individual counseling sessions are as effective as much more time-intensive group weight loss interventions. The Patient-Centered Assessment and Counseling for Exercise (PACE, San Diego State University Foundation and San Diego Center for Health Intervention, California) program was designed specifically for physicians to help them deliver effective guidance to patients about physical activity. This program can be used to promote physical activity within the limited time available for office visits. PACE includes an assessment form, a physician training manual, and behavior change protocols depending on a patient's stage of change and other personal characteristics. Program materials help clinicians and patients tailor the program based on individual needs, abilities, and interests.

PACE has been evaluated in 17 physician practices and 212 sedentary patients (92). Half of the practices were trained in using the program, and the other half provided standard medical care. A health educator supplemented provider counseling with a brief phone call 2 weeks later. Patients were assessed at baseline and 4 to 6 weeks after their first counseling session. Fifty-two percent of the PACE-counseled group moved into the action stage of change, compared with only 12% of the control group. The PACE group increased their overall physical activity level by 30%, whereas the control group changed very little (self-reported activity levels were confirmed with activity monitors). The PACE group increased from 37 minutes of walking per week to 75 minutes at follow-up. Controls increased from 34 minutes to 42 minutes. The investigators did not report on changes in weight or other health-related variables.

Figure 21.8 provides a brief lifestyle physical activity intervention that can be used in clinical practice to stage and counsel overweight and obese patients for physical activity.

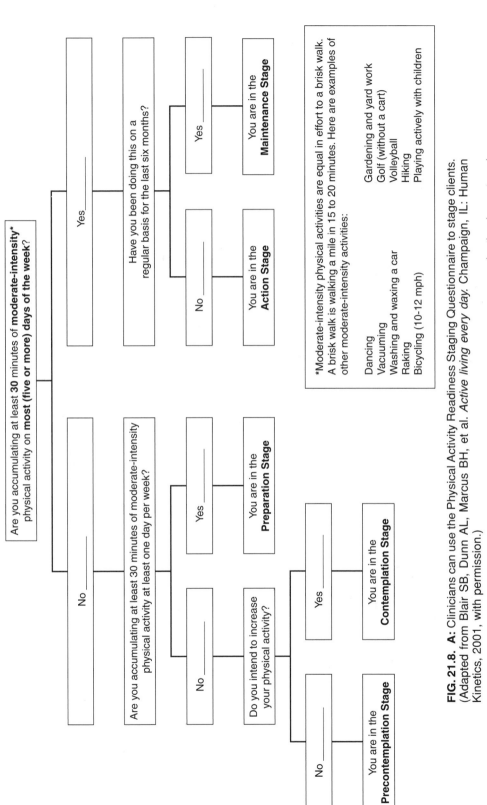

Are you accumulating at least **30** minutes of **moderate-intensity*** physical activity on **most (five or more) days of the week?**

No ___

Yes ___

Are you accumulating at least 30 minutes of moderate-intensity physical activity at least one day per week?

Have you been doing this on a regular basis for the last six months?

No ___

Yes ___

You are in the **Preparation Stage**

Do you intend to increase your physical activity?

No ___

Yes ___

You are in the **Precontemplation Stage**

You are in the **Contemplation Stage**

No ___

Yes ___

You are in the **Action Stage**

You are in the **Maintenance Stage**

*Moderate-intensity physical activities are equal in effort to a brisk walk. A brisk walk is walking a mile in 15 to 20 minutes. Here are examples of other moderate-intensity activities:

Dancing
Vacuuming
Washing and waxing a car
Raking
Bicycling (10-12 mph)

Gardening and yard work
Golf (without a cart)
Volleyball
Hiking
Playing actively with children

FIG. 21.8. A: Clinicians can use the Physical Activity Readiness Staging Questionnaire to stage clients. (Adapted from Blair SB, Dunn AL, Marcus BH, et al. *Active living every day.* Champaign, IL: Human Kinetics, 2001, with permission.)

(continued on next page)

A

PRECONTEMPLATION†

- **Goal:** Move to Contemplation
- **Strategies:**
  ✓ Increasing knowledge
  ✓ Decisional balance (barriers and benefits)
- **Clinician Messages:**
  ✓ Educate patient about benefits (i.e., weight control, personal health benefits, increased fitness) and options for physical activity (i.e., lifestyle activity, short-bouts, structured exercise)
  ✓ Help patient explore personal benefits of physical activity and ask about barriers (encourage them to develop a written list)
- **Possible Tools:**
  ✓ Physical activity handout
  ✓ Worksheet on barriers and benefits

CONTEMPLATION

- **Goal:** Move to Preparation
- **Strategies:**
  ✓ Increasing knowledge
  ✓ Decisional balance (barriers and benefits)
  ✓ Stimulus control
- **Clinician Messages:**
  ✓ Educate patient about benefits (i.e., weight control, personal health benefits, increased fitness) and options for physical activity (i.e., lifestyle activity, short-bouts, structured exercise)
  ✓ Review benefits and discuss patient's major barriers to physical activity (encourage them to develop a written list)
  ✓ Review amount of time patient spends in sedentary activity and encourage them to think about opportunities for becoming more active
  ✓ If patient is ready, encourage them to cut down on time spent sitting or to try 2-minute walks
- **Possible Tools:**
  ✓ Physical activity handout
  ✓ Worksheet on barriers and benefits

†Patients in precontemplation and contemplation are not ready for an action-oriented physical activity prescription.

PREPARATION

- **Goal:** Move to Action
- **Strategies:**
  - ✓ Increasing knowledge
  - ✓ Problem solving
  - ✓ Goal setting
  - ✓ Self-monitoring
  - ✓ Enlisting support
  - ✓ Stimulus control
- **Clinician Messages:**
  - ✓ Educate patient about benefits (i.e., weight control, personal health benefits, increased fitness) and options for physical activity (i.e., lifestyle activity, short-bouts, structured exercise)
  - ✓ Define the clinically desired activity goal (i.e., accumulate 30 minutes or more of moderate-intensity physical activity on most days of the week)
  - ✓ Help patient identify and plan a strategy to overcome one or two major barriers to physical activity (i.e., no time)
  - ✓ Help patient set realistic and behaviorally specific short-term goals (e.g., three 10-minute brisk walks per week for the next two weeks)
  - ✓ Encourage patient to schedule and keep track of physical activity (i.e., keep an activity log, step counter*)
  - ✓ Ask patient who can help them achieve their goals
- **Possible Tools:**
  - ✓ Physical activity handout
  - ✓ Written prescription or goal worksheet
  - ✓ Activity log, planning calendar, step counter

ACTION

- **Goal:** Move to Maintenance
- **Strategies:**
  - ✓ Self-monitoring
  - ✓ Enlisting support
  - ✓ Rewards
  - ✓ Relapse prevention
- **Clinician Messages:**
  - ✓ Praise patient for progress and explore personal rewards
  - ✓ Encourage patient to schedule and keep track of physical activity (i.e., keep an activity log, step counter*)
  - ✓ Ask patient who can help them achieve their goals
  - ✓ Help patient identify high-risk situations (i.e., travel, holidays) and to plan a strategy for potential lapses in physical activity
- **Possible Tools:**
  - ✓ Physical activity handout
  - ✓ Activity log, planning calendar, step calendar
  - ✓ Written prescription or goal worksheet

MAINTENANCE

- **Goal:** Stay in Maintenance, new behavior change goal
- **Counseling Strategies:**
  - ✓ As for action
- **Clinician Messages:**
  - ✓ As for action
  - ✓ Help patient set new goals as appropriate for weight management and risk reduction
- **Possible Tools:**
  - ✓ As for action

EVALUATION AND FOLLOW-UP

Follow-up is one of the keys to long-term success. Developing a system that facilitates patient follow-up is important. A brief office visit or a follow-up phone call or e-mail 2 to 6 weeks after each counseling session will help encourage compliance and provide an opportunity for addressing any problems. Focus on patient's positive steps and point out successes.

---

* The authors use an electronic pedometer (Yamax Digi-walker DW-500, Tokyo, Japan) as one tool to help individuals self-monitor physical activity. To meet current physical activity guidelines the authors recommend individuals accumulate 10,000 steps per day. For long-term weight management, individuals should aim for 15,000 to 20,000 steps (89). A realistic goal is to establish a baseline for number of steps accumulated during a typical day and then to set a goal to increase weekly physical activity by approximately 200 to 500 steps per day.

FIG. 21.8. *Continued.* **B:** The counseling algorithms should be used to deliver appropriate messages based on a client's stage of change. (Adapted from Insights to Multidimensional Strategies for Obesity Management Training Workshop. July 10, 1999, The Cooper Institute, Dallas, Texas, with permission.)

B

The authors have published specific guidelines and programs for using behavioral counseling to promote physical activity (85,93,94).

RECOMMENDATIONS

Conclusions

Clinicians must support and encourage individuals in developing the skills necessary to progress safely and effectively along the continuum of physical activity and exercise. The key is to match the physical activity prescription to the abilities, needs, and interests of the individual, with the ultimate clinical goal of achieving long-term weight management and health enhancement. The lifestyle approach helps the patient realize that physical activity can be integrated into daily life. Activity can gradually be increased as an individual becomes physically and psychologically ready. This moderate and gradual approach may help enhance confidence and long-term adherence and may facilitate the elimination of important barriers to physical activity, such as lack of time, low self-confidence, physical limitations, and lack of enjoyment of structured exercise. Helping individuals change their mindset about physical activity and exercise is important. Exercise does not have to be a structured or isolated activity, and it does not have to be hard to be beneficial.

For patients who are ready to change their physical activity, giving them specific advice on how to get started and what to expect is important. Significant health benefits can be achieved by accumulating at least 30 minutes of moderate-intensity physical activity on most, and preferably all, days of the week. This is an appropriate initial goal for all overweight and obese individuals. Brisk walking at 3 to 4 miles per hour (15 to 20 minutes per mile), or activities of an equivalent intensity, is a good way to accomplish this goal. Additionally, daily activities, such as taking stairs, doing more walking while working, participating in recreational sports, and performing more vigorous household chores and yard work, are likely to contribute to overall health and energy balance (9,32,71,81–83,85). Structured exercises, such as jogging, bicycling, aerobic dance, swimming, and other aerobic activities, are also appropriate. These exercises should be performed at moderate to vigorous intensities for at least 20 minutes on 3 days of the week. In addition, all individuals should be encouraged to include various activities such as strength training and flexibility exercises into their routines as they become physically and psychologically ready.

As this review indicates, improved long-term weight management and additional health benefits are likely to be realized when individuals perform more sustained and structured exercise than the minimum recommended levels (22). Accumulating 60 minutes or more of physical activity of at least moderate-intensity physical activity on 5 or more days of the week is an appropriate long-term goal. As an individual's fitness and activity tolerance improve, he or she may initiate more vigorous activity. The advantage of higher intensity activity is that higher levels of energy expenditure can be achieved in a shorter period. The clinician should encourage individuals to progress at a rate that minimizes the risk for orthopedic injury, metabolic complications, and adverse behavioral consequences (e.g., relapse). Non–weight-bearing and low-impact activities, such as water exercise, walking, cycle ergometry, and chair exercises, may be necessary. Individual preference and activities that are most likely to be sustained and enjoyed throughout life should determine the most appropriate type and intensity of exercise.

Although 60 minutes or more of physical activity on most days of the week may seem high, the individual must realize that this is a long-term goal for the purpose of weight maintenance. Also, the individual should work up to these levels of activity over a period of 1 to 2 years. The most important goal is to encourage long-term adherence to physical activity at any level. When prescribing physical activity for weight control, the clinician should help individuals avoid compensatory decreases in energy expenditure from nonexercise physical activities and increases in energy intake. Counseling directed at increasing nonexercise physical activity (e.g., moving more during occupational and leisure times) and on making appropriate food choices, such as reducing fat intake, will enhance the weight loss and health benefits of physical activity in the treatment of overweight and obesity (81,82,95).

Risk Assessment

Moderate-intensity physical activity is safe for most individuals; however, the authors recommend that sedentary overweight and obese individuals undergo an appropriate evaluation to identify underlying cardiovascular risk factors, functional and musculoskeletal limitations, and medications that may affect physical activity prescription and participation before initiating a physical activity program. Even with underlying risk factors, most individuals can safely begin a moderate-intensity program. If signs or symptoms of cardiovascular or metabolic disease are identified, further assessment, such as an exercise tolerance test, is indicated (96). Before beginning a vigorous exercise program, most at-risk patients should undergo exercise testing. The American College of Sports Medicine and the American Heart Association have released excellent guidelines on preexercise screening (97,98). Patients with underlying cardiovascular or severe metabolic disease, such as diabetes, may need to exercise under supervision initially. The clinician's familiarity with the patient and medical history should guide decisions on the extent of evaluation that is necessary before starting a physical activity program.

ACKNOWLEDGMENTS

The authors thank Melba Morrow, Stephanie Parker, and Thomas Olson for assistance with manuscript preparation and editorial review. They also thank Dr. Kenneth H. Cooper and the staff of the Cooper Aerobics Center for making this work possible. The work reported here is supported in part by grants AG06945 and HL48597 from the National Institutes of Health.

REFERENCES

1. National Center for Health Statistics. *Prevalence of overweight and obesity among adults: United States, 1999.* Hyattsville, MD: National Center for Health Statistics, 2001. Available at: http://www.cdc.gov/nchs/products/pubs/pubd/hestats/obese/obse99.htm. Accessed November 8, 2002.
2. Mokdad AH, Bowman BA, Ford ES, et al. The continuing epidemics of obesity and diabetes in the United States. *JAMA* 2001;286:1195–1200.
3. Mokdad AH, Serdula MK, Dietz WH, et al. The spread of the obesity epidemic in the United States, 1991–1998. *JAMA* 1999;282:1519–1522.
4. National Institutes of Health, National Heart, Lung, and Blood Institute. *Clinical guidelines on the identification, evaluation, and treatment of overweight and obesity in adults: the evidence report.* NIH Publication No. 98-4083. Bethesda, MD: National Institutes of Health, 1998:1–228.
5. Pi-Sunyer FX. Comorbidities of overweight and obesity: current evidence and research issues. *Med Sci Sports Exerc* 1999;31:S602–S608.
6. Allison DB, Fontaine KR, Manson JE, et al. Annual deaths attributable to obesity in the United States. *JAMA* 1999;282:1530–1538.
7. Hahn RA, Teutsch SM, Rothenberg RB, et al. Excess deaths from nine chronic diseases in the United States, 1986. *JAMA* 1990;264:2654–2659.

8. McGinnis JM, Foege WH. Actual causes of death in the United States. *JAMA* 1993;270:2207–2212.
9. Centers for Disease Control and Prevention. *Physical activity and health: a report of the Surgeon General.* Atlanta, GA: United States Department of Health and Human Services, Centers for Disease Control and Prevention, National Center for Chronic Disease Prevention and Health Promotion, 1996.
10. Blair SN, Kohl HW III, Paffenbarger RS Jr, et al. Physical fitness and all-cause mortality: a prospective study of healthy men and women. *JAMA* 1989;262:2395–2401.
11. Lee CD, Jackson AS, Blair SN. U.S. weight guidelines: is it also important to consider cardiorespiratory fitness? *Int J Obes Relat Metab Disord* 1998;22:S2–S7.
12. Blair SN, Brodney S. Effects of physical inactivity and obesity on morbidity and mortality: current evidence and research issues. *Med Sci Sports Exerc* 1999;31:S646–S662.
13. Weinsier RL, Hunter GR, Heini AF, et al. The etiology of obesity: relative contribution of metabolic factors, diet, and physical activity. *Am J Med* 1998;105:145–150.
14. Heini AF, Weinsier RL. Divergent trends in obesity and fat intake patterns: the American paradox. *Am J Med* 1997;102:259–264.
15. Hill JO, Melanson EL. Overview of the determinants of overweight and obesity: current evidence and research issues. *Med Sci Sports Exerc* 1999;31:S515–S521.
16. Centers for Disease Control and Prevention. Physical activity trends—United States, 1990–1998. *MMWR Morb Mortal Wkly Rep* 2001;50:166–169.
17. Williamson DF, Madans J, Anda RF, et al. Recreational physical activity and ten-year weight change in a US national cohort. *Int J Obes Relat Metab Disord* 1993;17:279–286.
18. DiPietro L, Kohl HW III, Barlow CE, et al. Improvements in cardiorespiratory fitness attenuate age-related weight gain in healthy men and women: the Aerobics Center Longitudinal Study. *Int J Obes Relat Metab Disord* 1998;22:55–62.
19. Ching PL, Willett WC, Rimm EB, et al. Activity level and risk of overweight in male health professionals. *Am J Public Health* 1996;86:25–30.
20. Coakley EH, Rimm EB, Colditz G, et al. Predictors of weight change in men: results from the Health Professionals Follow-up Study. *Int J Obes Relat Metab Disord* 1998;22:89–96.
21. Grundy SM, Blackburn G, Higgins M, et al. Physical activity in the prevention and treatment of obesity and its comorbidities. *Med Sci Sports Exerc* 1999;31:S502–S508.
22. Jakicic JM, Clark K, Coleman E, et al. American College of Sports Medicine position stand. Appropriate intervention strategies for weight loss and prevention of weight regain for adults. *Med Sci Sports Exerc* 2001;33:2145–156.
23. National Institutes of Health Consensus Development Panel on Physical Activity and Cardiovascular Health. NIH Consensus Conference: Physical activity and cardiovascular health. *JAMA* 1996;276:241–246.
24. Fletcher GF, Balady G, Blair SN, et al. Statement on exercise: benefits and recommendations for physical activity programs for all Americans: a statement for health professionals by the Committee on Exercise and Cardiac Rehabilitation of the Council on Clinical Cardiology, American Heart Association. *Circulation* 1996;94:857–862.
25. United States Department of Health and Human Services. *The Surgeon General's call to action to prevent and decrease overweight and obesity.* Rockville, MD: United States Department of Health and Human Services, Public Health Service, Office of the Surgeon General, 2001.
26. Garrow JS, Summerbell CD. Meta-analysis: effect of exercise, with or without dieting, on the body composition of overweight subjects. *Eur J Clin Nutr* 1995;49:1–10.
27. Wing RR. Physical activity in the treatment of the adulthood overweight and obesity: current evidence and research issues. *Med Sci Sports Exerc* 1999;31:S547–S552.
28. Ballor DL, Keesey RE. A meta-analysis of the factors affecting exercise-induced changes in body mass, fat mass and fat-free mass in males and females. *Int J Obes* 1991;15:717–726.
29. Miller WC, Koceja DM, Hamilton EJ. A meta-analysis of the past 25 years of weight loss research using diet, exercise or diet plus exercise intervention. *Int J Obes Relat Metab Disord* 1997;21:941–947.
30. Wing RR, Blair E, Marcus M, et al. Year-long weight loss treatment for obese patients with type II diabetes: does including an intermittent very-low-calorie diet improve outcome? *Am J Med* 1994;97:354–362.
31. Jakicic JM, Winters C, Lang W, et al. Effects of intermittent exercise and use of home exercise equipment on adherence, weight loss, and fitness in overweight women: a randomized trial. *JAMA* 1999;282:1554–1560.
32. Andersen RE, Wadden TA, Bartlett SJ, et al. Effects of lifestyle activity vs structured aerobic exercise in obese women: a randomized trial. *JAMA* 1999;281:335–340.
33. Tremblay A, Simoneau JA, Bouchard C. Impact of exercise intensity on body fatness and skeletal muscle metabolism. *Metabolism* 1994;43:814–818.
34. Arner P. Impact of exercise on adipose tissue metabolism in humans. *Int J Obes Relat Metab Disord* 1995;19:S18–S21.
35. Bahr R. Excess postexercise oxygen consumption—magnitude, mechanisms, and practical implications. *Acta Physiol Scand* 1992;605:1–70.
36. Ross R, Dagnone D, Jones PJ, et al. Reduction in obesity and related comorbid conditions after diet-induced weight loss or exercise-induced weight loss in men: a randomized, controlled trial. *Ann Intern Med* 2000;133:92–103.
37. Donnelly JE, Pronk NP, Jacobsen DJ, et al. Effects of a very-low-calorie diet and physical-training regimens on body composition and resting metabolic rate in obese females. *Am J Clin Nutr* 1991;54:56–61.

38. Whatley JE, Gillespie WJ, Honig J, et al. Does the amount of endurance exercise in combination with weight training and a very-low-energy diet affect resting metabolic rate and body composition? *Am J Clin Nutr* 1994;59:1088–1092.
39. Wadden TA, Vogt RA, Andersen RE, et al. Exercise in the treatment of obesity: Effects of four interventions on body composition, resting energy expenditure, appetite, and mood. *J Consult Clin Psychol* 1997;65:269–277.
40. Rice B, Janssen I, Hudson R, et al. Effects of aerobic or resistance exercise and/or diet on glucose tolerance and plasma insulin levels in obese men. *Diabetes Care* 1999;22:684–691.
41. Ballor DL, Poehlman ET. Exercise-training enhances fat-free mass preservation during diet-induced weight loss: a meta-analytical finding. *Int J Obes Relat Metab Disord* 1994;18:35–40.
42. Blundell JE, King NA. Physical activity and regulation of food intake: current evidence. *Med Sci Sports Exerc* 1999;31:S573–S583.
43. Tremblay A, Almeras N. Exercise, macronutrient preferences and food intake. *Int J Obes Relat Metab Disord* 1995;19:S97–S101.
44. Bouchard C, Tremblay A, Nadeau A, et al. Long-term exercise training with constant energy intake, I. Effect on body composition and selected metabolic variables. *Int J Obes* 1990;14:57–73.
45. Lee L, Kumar S, Leong LC. The impact of five-month basic military training on the body weight and body fat of 197 moderately to severely obese Singaporean males aged 17 to 19 years. *Int J Obes Relat Metab Disord* 1994;18:105–109.
46. Kayman S, Bruvold W, Stern JS. Maintenance and relapse after weight loss in women: behavioral aspects. *Am J Clin Nutr* 1990;52:800–807.
47. Wadden TA, Vogt RA, Foster GD, et al. Exercise and the maintenance of weight loss: 1-year follow-up of a controlled clinical trial. *J Consult Clin Psychol* 1998;66:429–433.
48. Walsh MF, Flynn TJ. A 54-month evaluation of a popular very low calorie diet program. *J Fam Pract* 1995;41:231–236.
49. Klem ML, Wing RR, McGuire MT, et al. A descriptive study of individuals successful at long-term maintenance of substantial weight loss. *Am J Clin Nutr* 1997;66:239–246.
50. Schoeller DA, Shay K, Kushner RF. How much physical activity is needed to minimize weight gain in previously obese women? *Am J Clin Nutr* 1997;66:551–556.
51. Bouchard C, Blair SN. Roundtable introduction: introductory comments for the consensus on physical activity and obesity. *Med Sci Sports Exerc* 1999;31:S498–S501.
52. Kelley DE, Goodpaster BH. Effects of physical activity on insulin action and glucose tolerance in obesity. *Med Sci Sports Exerc* 1999;31:S619–S623.
53. Segal KR, Edano A, Abalos A, et al. Effect of exercise training on insulin sensitivity and glucose metabolism in lean, obese, and diabetic men. *J Appl Physiol* 1991;71:2402–2411.
54. Dengel DR, Pratley RE, Hagberg JM, et al. Distinct effects of aerobic exercise training and weight loss on glucose homeostasis in obese sedentary men. *J Appl Physiol* 1996;81:318–325.
55. Katzel LI, Bleecker ER, Colman EG, et al. Effects of weight loss vs aerobic exercise training on risk factors for coronary disease in healthy, obese, middle-aged and older men. *JAMA* 1995;274:1915–1921.
56. Wei M, Gibbons LW, Mitchell TL, et al. The association between cardiorespiratory fitness and impaired fasting glucose and type 2 diabetes mellitus in men. *Ann Intern Med* 1999;130:89–96.
57. Knowler WC, Barrett-Connor E, Fowler SE, et al., for the Diabetes Prevention Program Research Group. Reduction in the incidence of type 2 diabetes with lifestyle intervention or metformin. *N Engl J Med* 2002;346:393–403.
58. Tuomilehto J, Lindstrom J, Eriksson JG, et al. Prevention of type 2 diabetes mellitus by changes in lifestyle among subjects with impaired glucose tolerance. *N Engl J Med* 2001;344:1343–1350.
59. Fagard RH. Physical activity in the prevention and treatment of hypertension in the obese. *Med Sci Sports Exerc* 1999;31:S624–S630.
60. Paffenbarger RSJ, Wing AL, Hyde RT, et al. Physical activity and incidence of hypertension in college alumni. *Am J Epidemiol* 1983;117:245–257.
61. Paffenbarger RS Jr, Jung DL, Leung RW, et al. Physical activity and hypertension: an epidemiological view. *Ann Med* 1991;23:319–327.
62. Gordon NF, Scott CB, Levine BD. Comparison of single versus multiple lifestyle interventions: are the antihypertensive effects of exercise training and diet-induced weight loss additive? *Am J Cardiol* 1997;79:763–767.
63. Blumenthal JA, Sherwood A, Gullette EC, et al. Exercise and weight loss reduce blood pressure in men and women with mild hypertension: effects on cardiovascular, metabolic, and hemodynamic functioning. *Arch Intern Med* 2000;160:1947–1958.
64. Stevens VJ, Obarzanek E, Cook NR, et al. Long-term weight loss and changes in blood pressure: results of the trials of hypertension prevention, phase II. *Ann Intern Med* 2001;134:1–11.
65. Stefanick ML. Physical activity for preventing and treating obesity-related dyslipoproteinemias. *Med Sci Sports Exerc* 1999;31:S609–S618.
66. Flegal KM, Carroll MD, Kuczmarski RJ, et al. Overweight and obesity in the United States: prevalence and trends, 1960–1994. *Int J Obes Relat Metab Disord* 1998;22:39–47.
67. Barlow CE, Kohl HW III, Gibbons LW, et al. Physical fitness, mortality and obesity. *Int J Obes Relat Metab Disord* 1995;19:S41–S44.
68. Blair SN, Kohl HW III, Barlow CE, et al. Changes in physical fitness and all-cause mortality: a prospective study of healthy and unhealthy men. *JAMA* 1995;273:1093–1098.

69. Lee CD, Blair SN, Jackson AS. Cardiorespiratory fitness, body composition, and all-cause and cardiovascular disease mortality in men. *Am J Clin Nutr* 1999;69:373–380.
70. Wei M, Kampert JB, Barlow CE, et al. Relationship between low cardiorespiratory fitness and mortality in normal-weight, overweight, and obese men. *JAMA* 1999;282:1547–1553.
71. Pate RR, Pratt M, Blair SN, et al. Physical activity and public health: a recommendation from the Centers for Disease Control and Prevention and the American College of Sports Medicine. *JAMA* 1995;273:402–407.
72. Serdula MK, Mokdad AH, Williamson DF, et al. Prevalence of attempting weight loss and strategies for controlling weight. *JAMA* 1999;282:1353–1358.
73. Wee CC, McCarthy EP, Davis RB, et al. Physician counseling about exercise. *JAMA* 1999;282:1583–1588.
74. Dishman RK, Sallis JF. Determinants and interventions for physical activity and exercise. In: Bouchard C, Shephard RJ, Stephens T, eds. *Physical activity, fitness, and health.* Champaign, IL: Human Kinetics, 1994:214–238.
75. Blair SN, Shaten J, Brownell K, et al. Body weight change, all-cause mortality, and cause-specific mortality in the Multiple Risk Factor Intervention Trial. *Ann Intern Med* 1993;119:749–757.
76. Blair SN, Connelly JC. How much physical activity should we do? The case for moderate amounts and intensities of physical activity. *Res Q Exerc Sport* 1996;67:193–205.
77. DeBusk RF, Stenestrand U, Sheehan M, et al. Training effects of long versus short bouts of exercise in healthy subjects. *Am J Cardiol* 1990;65:1010–1013.
78. Coleman KJ, Raynor HR, Mueller DM, et al. Providing sedentary adults with choices for meeting their walking goals. *Prev Med* 1999;28:510–519.
79. Jakicic JM, Wing RR, Butler BA, et al. Prescribing exercise in multiple short bouts versus one continuous bout: effects on adherence, cardiorespiratory fitness, and weight loss in overweight women. *Int J Obes Relat Metab Disord* 1995;19:893–901.
80. Perri MG, Martin AD, Leermakers EA, et al. Effects of group- versus home-based exercise in the treatment of obesity. *J Consult Clin Psychol* 1997;65:278–285.
81. Levine JA, Eberhardt NL, Jensen MD. Role of nonexercise activity thermogenesis in resistance to fat gain in humans. *Science* 1999;283:212–214.
82. Levine JA, Schleusner SJ, Jensen MD. Energy expenditure of nonexercise activity. *Am J Clin Nutr* 2000;72:1451–1454.
83. Yanovski JA, Yanovski SZ. Recent advances in obesity research. *JAMA* 1999;282:1504–1506.
84. Blair SN, Kohl HW III, Gordon NF. Physical activity and health: a lifestyle approach. *Med Exerc Nutr Health* 1992;1:54–57.
85. Dunn AL, Marcus BH, Kampert JB, et al. Comparison of lifestyle and structured interventions to increase physical activity and cardiorespiratory fitness: a randomized trial. *JAMA* 1999;281:327–334.
86. Bandura A. Self-efficacy: toward a unifying theory of behavior change. *Psychol Rev* 1977;84:192–215.
87. Prochaska JO, DiClemente CC. Transtheoretical therapy: toward a more integrative model of change. *Psychotherapy: Theory, Research, and Practice* 1982;20:161–173.
88. American College of Sports Medicine. The recommended quantity and quality of exercise for developing and maintaining cardiorespiratory and muscular fitness in healthy adults. *Med Sci Sports Exerc* 1990;22:265–274.
89. Marcus BH, Pinto BM, Clark MC, et al. Physician-delivered physical activity and nutrition interventions. *Med Exerc Nutr Health* 1995;4:325–334.
90. Velicer WF, Fava JL, Prochaska JO, et al. Distribution of smokers by stage in three representative samples. *Prev Med* 1995;24:401–411.
91. Wadden TA, Berkowitz RI, Vogt RA, et al. Lifestyle modification in the pharmacologic treatment of obesity: a pilot investigation of a potential primary care approach. *Obes Res* 1997;5:218–226.
92. Calfas KJ, Long BJ, Sallis JF, et al. A controlled trial of physician counseling to promote the adoption of physical activity. *Prev Med* 1996;25:225–233.
93. Blair SB, Dunn AL, Marcus BH, et al. *Active living every day.* Champaign, IL: Human Kinetics, 2001.
94. Leermakers EA, Dunn AL, Blair SN. Exercise management of obesity. *Med Clin North Am* 2000;84:419–440.
95. Tremblay A, Almeras N, Boer J, et al. Diet composition and postexercise energy balance. *Am J Clin Nutr* 1994;59:975–979.
96. Yamanouchi K, Shinozaki T, Chikada K, et al. Daily walking combined with diet therapy is a useful means for obese NIDDM patients not only to reduce body weight but also to improve insulin sensitivity. *Diabetes Care* 1995;18:775–778.
97. Franklin BA, Whaley MH, Howley ET, eds. *American College of Sports Medicine's guidelines for exercise testing and prescription,* 6th ed. Philadelphia, PA Lippincott Williams & Wilkins, 2000.
98. Fletcher GF, Balady G, Amsterdam EA, et al. Exercise standards for testing and training: a statement for healthcare professionals from the American Heart Association. Writing Group. *Circulation* 2001;104:1694–1740.

22

Surgical Treatment of Obesity

Rifat Latifi and Harvey J. Sugerman

THE PROBLEM

Approximately 97 million adults in the United States are overweight or obese; 32.6% are overweight, which is defined as a body mass index (BMI) of 25 to 29.9 kilograms per meter squared (kg/m^2), while 22.3% are obese with a BMI of more than or equal to 30 kg/m^2. Morbid obesity or clinically severe obesity is defined as 100 lb above ideal body weight, or as a BMI of 35 kg/m^2 or more. As the BMI increases, so does the mortality rate from all causes, particularly from cardiovascular disease, which is 50% to 100% higher than that of persons who have a BMI from 20 to 25 kg/m^2 (1). Severe obesity is a harbinger of multiple other diseases and disorders affecting every organ and system of the body, and it is associated with several significant clinical syndromes (Table 22.1), including the following: cardiovascular-related problems, such as coronary artery disease, heart failure, and increased complications after coronary artery bypass; respiratory insufficiency resulting from obesity-hypoventilation syndrome and obstructive sleep apnea syndrome (multiple nocturnal awakenings, loud snoring, falling asleep while driving, daytime somnolence); metabolic complications, such as diabetes mellitus, hypertension, elevated triglycerides, cholesterol, and gallstones; increased intraabdominal pressure that is manifested as stress overflow urinary incontinence, gastroesophageal reflux, nephrotic syndrome, increased intracranial pressure leading to pseudotumor cerebri, hernias, venous stasis, and probably hypertension and preeclampsia; hypercoagulopathy; sexual hormone dysfunction, such as amenorrhea, dysmenorrhea, infertility, hypermenorrhea, and Stein–Leventhal syndrome; an increased incidence of breast, uterine, colon, prostate, and other cancers; and debilitating joint disease involving the hips, knees, ankles, feet, and lower back.

The difficulties in diagnosing and treating surgical conditions in obese patients, such as peritonitis, necrotizing panniculitis, necrotizing fasciitis, diverticulitis, necrotizing pancreatitis, and other intraabdominal infectious catastrophes, are significant. Morbidly obese patients are clearly at higher risk of dying than other patients even from treatable infections.

Recent studies have demonstrated that obesity is associated with a low-grade systemic inflammatory state, as manifested by elevated proinflammatory cytokines, interleukin-6 (IL-6), and C-reactive protein, which are thought to contribute to cardiovascular morbidity (2). Furthermore, the elevated C-reactive protein levels have been associated with an increased risk of myocardial infarction, stroke, peripheral arterial disease, and coronary heart disease. The effect of surgically induced weight reduction on the serum levels of the cytokines has been reported (3).

Although the causes of severe obesity are multifactorial and the pathophysiology of morbid obesity syndrome is complex, the published success rate for all medical approaches, including pharmacotherapy and behavioral modification, for morbid obesity

503

TABLE 22.1. *Pathologic conditions associated with morbid obesity*

Cardiovascular dysfunction
 Coronary artery disease
 Increased complications after coronary bypass operation
 Cardiomyopathy
 Left ventricular concentric hypertrophy: hypertension
 Left ventricular eccentric hypertrophy: obesity
 Right ventricular hypertrophy pulmonary failure
 Prolonged QT interval with sudden death
 Heart failure
Respiratory insufficiency of obesity (pickwickian syndrome)
 Obesity–hypoventilation syndrome
 Obstructive sleep apnea syndrome
Metabolic complications
 Type II diabetes mellitus
 Hypertension
 Elevated triglycerides
 Elevated cholesterol
 Nonalcoholic hepatic steatosis (NASH) or nonalcoholic liver
  disease (NALD)
 Cholelithiasis
 Cholecystitis
Increased intraabdominal pressure
 Obesity-hypoventilation syndrome
 Gastroesophageal reflux
 Stress overflow urinary incontinence
 Thrombophlebitis
 Venous stasis ulcers
 Pulmonary embolism
 Pseudotumor cerebri
 Nephrotic syndrome
 Hernias (incisional, inguinal)
 Preeclampsia
Sexual hormone dysfunction
 Amenorrhea, hypermenorrhea
 Polycystic ovary syndrome (Stein–Leventhal syndrome)
 Infertility
Cancer
 Endometrial carcinoma
 Breast carcinoma
 Colon cancer
 Renal cell carcinoma
 Prostate cancer
Degenerative bone and joint disease
 Osteoarthritis of feet, ankles, knees, hips, back, shoulders
 Chronic lower back pain
Psychosocial impairment
 Decreased employability
 Work discrimination

is extremely poor. An estimated 95% of morbidly obese patients subjected to medical weight-reduction programs regain all of their lost weight, as well as additional excess weight, within 2 years of the onset of therapy (4).

INDICATIONS FOR SURGICAL TREATMENT OF MORBID OBESITY

Because of the extremely high failure rate of all nonsurgical attempts to correct morbid obesity, including diet, behavior modification, hypnosis, voluntary incarceration, jaw wiring, and intragastric balloons, the presence of morbid obesity itself is an indication for surgical correction. Based on medical evidence, the National Institutes of Health 1991 Consensus Conference concluded that the surgical treatment of patients with a BMI of more than 40 kg/m^2 or a BMI of more than 35 kg/m^2 with comorbid conditions has emerged as definitive therapy (5). The comorbidities that warrant surgical treatment in the authors' program include type II diabetes mellitus, severe degenerative joint disease pains that interfere with the patient's function, moderate to severe sleep apnea (respiratory disturbance index $\geq$ 20), pseudotumor cerebri, polycystic ovary syndrome not responsive to metformin, severe gastroesophageal reflux with esophagitis or Barrett esophagus, and nonalcoholic steatohepatitis. Patients with this BMI are unlikely to have severe venous stasis disease or obesity-hypoventilation syndrome, unless the latter is associated with chronic obstructive pulmonary disease or severe asthma. Bariatric surgery has gained acceptance among surgeons, physicians, and the public. No nonoperative program has had a long-term weight loss efficacy.

The presence of any endocrine disorder that may be responsible for obesity, albeit extremely rare, should be treated first. Most insurance companies require that patients have attempted but failed with nonsurgical attempts to reduce the weight. After surgery, the patient needs to make significant lifestyle changes, including increased exercise and dietary education.

HISTORICAL PERSPECTIVE

Surgical treatment of obesity has evolved over the last half a century, and it has been characterized by constant exploration, investigation, innovation, and revisions of surgical procedures. Although Henrikson (4) reported the first surgical treatment for morbid obesity in 1952, the work of Payne and De Wind (6) prompted other investigators to develop intestinal bypass surgery for morbid obesity. Payne and De Wind (6) reported the first series of patients who underwent jejunal anastomosis to the colon, which was abandoned shortly after its introduction because of the severe metabolic derangements it induced; this was then changed to the end-to-side jejunoileostomy. This approach created a long blind segment of small intestine. The end-to-side jejunoileostomy (7), or the so-called 14+4 operation (14 inches of jejunum anastomosed to the terminal 4 inches of the ileum), which was also known as the jejunoileal bypass (JIB), was the first popular surgical procedure for morbid obesity (8). It was widely adopted by general surgeons who were interested in bariatric surgery, but the blind intestinal segment produced by this procedure was prone to bacterial overgrowth and other metabolic complications. Although this operation produced weight loss by obligatory malabsorption via bypass of a major portion of the absorptive surface of the small intestine, it was associated with a number of serious early and late complications. The most serious postoperative complication was liver failure from cirrhosis. Other serious late sequelae were arthritis, gallstones, hypocalcemia, kidney stones, osteoporosis, intractable malodorous diarrhea with associated potassium and magnesium deficiencies, metabolic acidosis, vitamin B$_{12}$ deficiency, vitamin K deficiency, interstitial nephritis with renal failure, pneumatosis intestinalis and bypass enteritis associated with occult blood in the stools, and iron-deficiency anemia. Because of these significant complications, some have suggested that all JIB procedures should be reversed because cirrhosis can develop insidiously in the absence of abnormal liver function test results (9). However, others have found the liver dysfunction to be reversible with metronidazole therapy (10). In particular, if the patient has intractable diarrhea, gas-bloating syndrome or bypass enteritis, arthritis, nephrolithiasis or nephrocalcinosis, uncorrectable electrolyte problems (e.g., acidosis, hypokalemia, hypocalcemia, hypo-magnesemia), dermatitis, liver deterioration, anemia, malnutrition, hypoproteinemia, dif-ficulties with mental acuity, chronic weakness, and lethargy or fever of unknown origin, a reversal of the JIB should be conducted. In a study by Hocking et al. (11) of 43 patients with an intact JIB who were followed prospectively for 12.6 years, the adverse effects, such as hypokalemia, cholelithiasis, and vitamin B_{12} or folate deficiency, decreased over time. However, the incidence of diarrhea remained at 64%, hypomagnesemia increased to 67%, nephrolithiasis occurred in 33%, and progressive hepatic fibrosis occurred in 38% of the patients (11). Because of these and other significant complication rates, the JIB should no longer be performed. A randomized prospective study found that the gas-tric bypass (GBP) operation was associated with comparable weight loss and a signifi-cantly lower complication rate than JIB (12). Because complications from the JIB can develop at any time, careful follow-up should be conducted with these patients so that complications can be diagnosed and treated promptly. If a patient's cirrhosis is classified as Child's A, the patient should be converted from the JIB to a Roux-en-Y gastric bypass (RYGBP) because simple takedown of the JIB has been associated with the regain of all lost weight (13). A Child's B cirrhotic patient, especially one with esophageal varices, may carry an excessive risk with conversion to RYGPB, so a simple "takedown" of the JIB should be performed.

In 1969, Mason and Ito (14) introduced the concept of GBP, in which the stomach was compartmentalized into a small proximal segment and a much larger distal bypassed seg-ment with drainage of the proximal gastric pouch into the proximal jejunum. In 1982, Mason (15) introduced vertical banded gastroplasty (VBGP), in which the stomach is compartmentalized with the use of a vertical staple line parallel to the lesser curvature of the stomach. The outlet for drainage of the proximal gastric pouch into the distal gastric pouch was reinforced with a polypropylene mesh collar. This operation was superior to other pure gastric restrictive operations because it prevented stomal widening. Scopinaro et al. (16,17) reintroduced malabsorptive methods in a blended operation that they called *partial biliopancreatic diversion.* In this operation, the distal stomach was resected, and the proximal gastric pouch was drained into a Roux-en-Y limb in which the small intes-tine was divided 250 cm proximal to the ileocecal valve and the distal end was reanasto-mosed 50 cm from the ileocecal valve, while the proximal end was used for the gastroje-junostomy.

CURRENT OPERATIONS

Over the last decade, the safety and effectiveness of many surgical procedures has evolved. Currently, most bariatric surgical centers in North America and Europe perform RYGBP, VBGP, or adjusted gastric banding (AGB).

Gastroplasty

VBGP was introduced as an attempt to avoid the adverse long-term nutritional and ulcerogenic consequences of GBP (15). In gastroplasty, the upper stomach is stapled near the gastroesophageal junction, thus creating a small upper gastric pouch, which commu-nicates with the rest of the stomach and gastrointestinal tract through a small outlet. The concept and the technique of gastroplasty were suggested as a safer and relatively easier method for restricting food intake with virtually no reported metabolic complications, because the gastrointestinal tract remains in continuity. Gastroplasties are performed with either horizontal or vertical placement of the staples. Horizontal gastroplasty usually requires ligation and division of the short gastric vessels between the stomach and the spleen, it carries the risk of devascularization of the gastric pouch or splenic injury, and it has been associated with very high failure rates (42% to 70%). The VBGP, on the other hand, is a procedure in which a stapled opening 5 cm from the cardioesophageal junction is made in the stomach with an end to end anastomosis (EEA) stapling device (Fig. 22.1). The pouch is made between this opening and the angle of His that is constructed with a 90-mm stapling device, and a 1.5-cm × 5-cm strip of polypropylene mesh is wrapped around the stoma on the lesser curvature and is sutured to itself, but not to the stomach. VBGP can be associated with severe gastroesophageal reflux. VBGP is more effective than horizontal gastroplasty but it is significantly less effective than RYGBP, as randomized prospective trials in which several centers have demonstrated with reports of inferior weight reduction with this operation, as compared with the standard RYGBP (18–20).

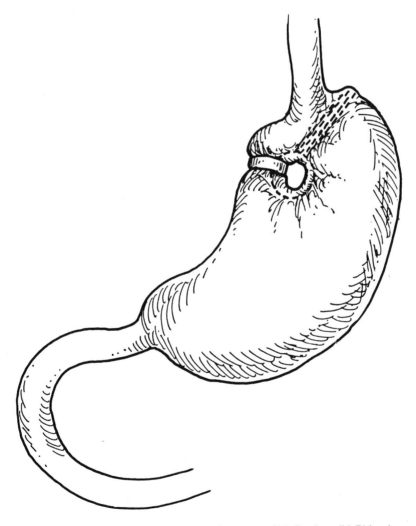

FIG. 22.1. Vertical banded gastroplasty. (From Sugerman HJ, Starkey JV, Birkenhauer RA. A randomized prospective trial of gastric bypass versus vertical banded gastroplasty for morbid obesity and their effects on sweets versus non sweets eaters. *Ann Surg* 1987;205:613–624, with permission.)

Gastric Banding

Gastric banding was introduced as a treatment for morbid obesity; in this approach, a Dacron tube or silicone band is used to compartmentalize the stomach into small proximal and large distal segments (21). This approach has the advantage of producing a pure restrictive operation using an extremely simple reversible technique, in which stapling with its inherent risk of staple-line disruption was avoided. More recent developments include the introduction of an adjustable silicone gastric banding device, which was originally described by Kuzmak (22), that can be placed laparoscopically. This band has a subcutaneous or subfascial reservoir. If weight loss is meager or if vomiting is excessive, the outlet diameter of the upper gastric segment can be adjusted.

Roux-En-Y Gastric Bypass

Recently, RYGBP has become the most common bariatric operation performed by bariatric surgeons in the United States (Fig. 22.2). The migration toward this operation

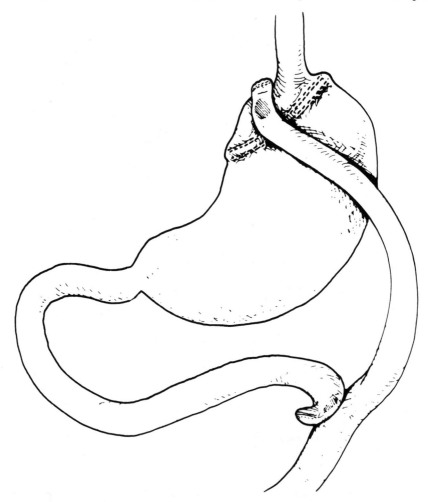

FIG. 22.2. Roux-en-Y gastric bypass. (From Sugerman HJ, Starkey JV, Birkenhauer RA. A randomized prospective trial of gastric bypass versus vertical banded gastroplasty for morbid obesity and their effects on sweets versus non sweets eaters. *Ann Surg* 1987;205:613–624, with permission.)

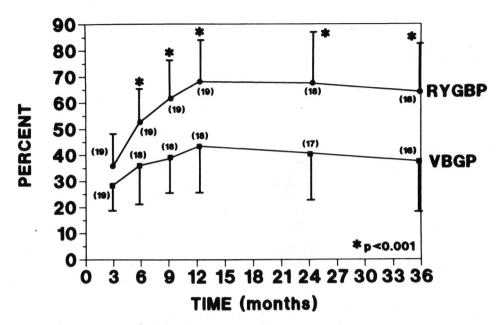

FIG. 22.3. The percentage of extra weight plus or minus standard deviation (n) over 3 years after Roux-en-Y gastric bypass (RYGBP), compared with vertical banded gastroplasty. (From Sugerman HJ, Starkey JV, Birkenhauer RA. A randomized prospective trial of gastric bypass versus vertical banded gastroplasty for morbid obesity and their effects on sweets versus non sweets eaters. *Ann Surg* 1987;205:613–624, with permission.)

has been based mainly on superior long-term weight loss effects of RYGBP, compared with those of VBGP (Fig. 22.3). In four randomized prospective trials and three retrospective studies, RYGBP was found to induce significantly greater weight loss than did VBGP. This was particularly true for patients addicted to sweets. "Sweet eaters" were found to lose less weight after VBGP than after RYGBP because most patients develop dumping syndrome symptoms after the ingestion of foods rich in sugar following RYGBP. When patients who were "non–sweet eaters" were assigned to VBGP and "sweets eaters" were designated to GBP, a significant improvement was seen in weight loss with VBGP, but these patients still lost significantly less weight than did the patients who underwent GBP (Fig. 22.4). Because of the high incidence of staple-line disruption and ulcer formation, some surgeons recommend transecting the stomach of patients who have undergone a GBP, particularly in those weighing more than 400 lb (23). Currently, the authors' group performs GBP by constructing a small gastric pouch (15 mL) with a 45-cm Roux-en-Y limb and stoma restricted to 1 cm. Superobese patients (BMI of 50 kg/m^2 or greater) achieve a significantly better weight loss with a 150-cm Roux limb (long-limb GBP) (24). The small gastric pouch has a limited volume of acid secretion, and it is associated with a low incidence of marginal ulcer. The GBP is associated with long-lasting weight loss in the vast majority of patients. The average weight loss is 66% of excess weight at 2 years, 60% at 5 years, and 50% at 10 years after surgery.

Operative Technique of Open Gastric Bypass

The abdomen is entered through a midline incision carried superiorly along the side of the xiphoid process and inferiorly to the umbilicus, or inferior enough to obtain adequate

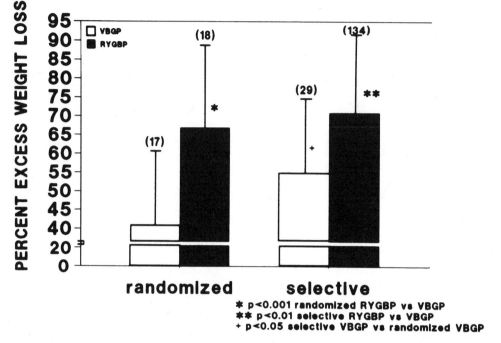

FIG. 22.4. Percentage excess weight loss at 2 years after selective assignment of sweet eaters to Roux-en-Y gastric bypass (RYGBP) and non–sweet eaters to vertical banded gastroplasty (VBGP), as compared with random assignment. (From Sugerman HJ, Felton WL, Sismanis A, et al. Effects of surgically induced weight loss on idiopathic intracranial hypertension in morbid obesity. *Neurology* 1995;45:1655–1659, with permission.)

access (25). Upon entering the peritoneal cavity, the surgeon performs a complete exploration to exclude unanticipated pathology before the GBP is begun. If gallstones, sludge, or polyps are present on palpation or are found on the intraoperative ultrasound, then a cholecystectomy is performed.

The distal esophagus is mobilized and is encircled with a soft rubber drain. The gastrohepatic omentum is entered where it overlies the caudate lobe. An aberrant left hepatic artery may be present, and it should be avoided. An opening that is large enough to admit a right-angled clamp is made in the mesentery along the stomach between the first and the second branch of the left gastric artery. After blunt dissection of the avascular space on the posterior stomach wall, a rubber tube that will serve as a guide for introduction of the stapling device is placed between the opening in the gastrohepatic omentum and the lateral angle of His. Before staplers are applied, all intraluminal tubes (the nasogastric tube, the esophageal stethoscope) must be removed by the anesthesiologist. The ligament of Treitz is identified, and the jejunum is divided with a gastrointestinal anastomosis (GIA) stapling device 45 cm distally and the Roux limb is created. A side-to-side jejunojejunostomy is created at 45 cm for the standard bypass or at 150 cm for superobese patients. With blunt dissection, an opening is created in the transverse colon mesentery and the Roux limb is brought through to the proximal stomach without tension. At this point, a 55-mm stapling device is placed across the stomach using the rubber tube as a guide. The stomach is then stapled three times with superimposed staple applications. A 1-cm gastrojejunal anastomosis is created between the proximal stomach and the Roux limb. This anastomosis is hand-sewn using a two-layer technique. Once the posterior layer of the anastomosis is sewn, a no. 30 French dilator is placed by anesthesia and is guided by the surgeon through the anastomosis. After completion of the anastomosis, methylene blue dye is injected through nasogastric tube to assess for a possible leak. All mesenteric defects are closed, including those at the jejunojejunostomy, at the mesocolon, and behind the Roux limb to prevent a Petersen hernia. The abdominal fascia is closed with a running stitch, while the skin is approximated with skin staples.

Laparoscopic Gastric Bypass

Laparoscopic bariatric surgery has developed rapidly in recent years (26–29). The weight loss at 1 to 3 years after this approach is equivalent to that of the open technique. The advantages include a decreased length of hospital stay, less pain, and a much lower risk of incisional hernia, which currently exceeds 20% following open obesity surgery or major wound infections. In addition, as with other laparoscopic surgeries, the hope is that this will cause fewer and less severe adhesions, with the potential for fewer subsequent small bowel obstructions. However, in several series, the risk of internal hernia with obstruction appears to be increased, possibly because of inadequate closure of these potential hernia defects with the laparoscopic approach.

Improved techniques appear to be resolving this problem, as well as that of the increased anastomotic leak rate that was reported in the early laparoscopic series. Wittgrove and Clark (26) reported 500 patients who have undergone laparoscopic RYGBP (LRYGBP) with follow-up from 3 to 60 months. In these, major complications were present in 11%, anastomotic leak in 5%, and no mortalities were reported. In a study by Schauer et al. (27), RYGBP was found to be safe and to have very low mortality and morbidity. Furthermore, the recovery time was short and the operative complications were comparable to those of the open technique. The conversion rate from LRYGBP to an open RYGBP was 1% in 275 consecutive patients, and the median hospital stay was 2 days, while the amount of days to return to work was 21 days. The frequency of early major and minor complications was 3.3% and 27%, respectively. Only one death, which was due to pulmonary embolus, was reported, and minor wound infections were observed in only 5%. The excess weight loss was comparable to that achieved by the open technique, with 83% and 77% of excess weight loss at 24 and 30 months, respectively. In addition, most of the comorbidities either improved or resolved, and 95% of patients reported significant improvements in quality of life. A randomized prospective trial comparing laparoscopic bypass to open GBP noted an equivalent weight loss, a shorter hospital stay, earlier improvement in quality-of-life assessment, and an improved early postoperative pulmonary function in the patients who underwent laparoscopic bypass (30–32).

Laparoscopic Adjustable Gastric Banding

The adjustable silicone gastric band has been developed to be placed laparoscopically. The device contains a balloon that is adjusted by injecting saline into a subcutaneously implanted port. Problems with band slippage leading to gastric obstruction and the need for reoperation, esophageal dilation, band erosion into the lumen of the stomach, and port infections, as well as inadequate weight loss, have been reported. The presence of hiatal hernia and esophageal dysmotility have been identified as independent risk factors for lap-band slippage (33). Other complications of gastric banding include food intolerance, reflux esophagitis, pouch dilation, and stoma occlusion. Thirty-five percent of patients who underwent adjustable silicone gastric banding in the authors' center have undergone removal of the gastric band and conversion to GBP (34). In some patients, removal of the gastric band and conversion to RYGBP can be performed laparoscopically; however, these operations are technically challenging, with an increased risks of complications. The Australians and Europeans have reported excellent results with laparoscopic gastric banding (35,36).

Partial Biliopancreatic Diversion and Duodenal Switch Operations

The partial biliopancreatic diversion has been developed as both a gastric restrictive and a malabsorptive procedure that does not have a blind intestinal limb in which bacterial overgrowth can occur (16,17). This operation involves a subtotal gastrectomy, leaving a 400-mL gastric pouch for the average obese patient and a 200-mL gastric pouch for the superobese patient. The distal small bowel is transected 250 cm proximal to the ileocecal valve, and the proximal bypassed bowel is anastomosed to the ileum 50 cm proximal to the ileocecal valve. This leaves a 200-cm "alimentary tract," a 300- to 400-cm "biliary tract" of bypassed intestine, and a 50-cm "common tract," where the ingested food mixes with bile and pancreatic juices for digestion and absorption. This operation has demonstrated excellent weight loss, and it does not appear to be associated with the high incidence of bacterial overgrowth and bacterial translocation problems of the JIB because the bile and pancreatic juices usually wash out the bypassed small intestine. However, the biliopancreatic diversion may be associated with severe protein-calorie malnutrition, necessitating hospitalization and total parenteral nutrition; frequent foul-smelling steatorrheic stools that float, leading to fat-soluble vitamin deficiencies and calcium loss secondary to chelation with fat; and subsequent severe osteoporosis. Because of frequent diarrhea and protein malnutrition, the common channel has been increased from 50 to 100 cm in some patients.

The authors have described a modification of biliopancreatic diversion in which the stomach is merely stapled, as in GBP, and the enteroenterostomy is placed 50 to 150 cm proximal to the ileocecal valve (37,38). This modification, which was termed distal GBP, was associated with superior weight loss in the "superobese," as compared with standard GBP. In a randomized prospective trial using a much smaller proximal stomach pouch (50 mL) without gastric resection and a longer common absorptive intestinal tract (150 cm) in superobese patients, the distal GBP was associated with much greater weight loss than was the standard GBP, but it had a 25% incidence of severe malnutrition (38). Of 14 patients, 4 required conversion to a standard GBP because of protein-calorie malnutrition. The authors therefore currently reserve this type of distal GBP for superobese patients who fail a standard GBP and who have persistent, severe obesity-related comorbidities (e.g., diabetes and pickwickian syndrome). These patients require fat-soluble vitamin supplementation, and they may develop severe malnutrition.

A modified surgical procedure, known as the biliopancreatic diversion with duodenal switch, that combines restriction and malabsorption has been developed with the hope that less protein and fat-soluble vitamin malabsorption will occur (39,40). This requires resection of the greater curvature of the stomach, combined with a "duodenal switch." This operation divides the duodenum at the distal bulb and the ileum 250 cm proximal to the ileocecal valve, with anastomosis of the proximal duodenum to the distal ileum segment; the distal end of the transected duodenum is closed as a duodenal stump. The proximal ileal segment, which carries the biliary and pancreatic secretions, is anastomosed end-to-side for an enteroenterostomy 100 cm proximal to the ileocecal valve. Whether this operation will prevent the protein malnutrition and calcium and fat-soluble vitamin deficiencies associated with the partial biliopancreatic bypass procedure is still unclear. This operation was performed in 440 patients as the initial bariatric procedure, and it was associated with weight loss of 70% at 8 years after surgery (39). Seventeen of these patients underwent second operations for excessive weight loss to correct severe protein malnutrition. This operation was associated with an improved quality of life, and no marginal ulcers or cases of dumping syndrome were found. The risks and benefits of the duodenal switch procedure have not been compared in a randomized prospective trial to those of the long-limb GBP.

COMPLICATIONS OF BARIATRIC SURGERY

Perioperative Complications

Although not common, perioperative complications of patients undergoing surgery for morbid obesity may be significant (Tables 22.2 and 22.3) (41). Operative mortality after GBP surgery is about 1% in most studies, but it increases significantly in patients with

TABLE 22.2. *Potential complications of bariatric surgery*

Perioperative
    Splenic or other organ injuries
    Dilation of excluded stomach
    Perforation of distal stomach (rare)
    Afferent limb obstruction
    Difficulties into recognizing abdominal catastrophe
    Deep venous thrombosis and pulmonary embolus
    Cardiac events
    Wound infections
    Wound dehiscence
    Anastomotic leak
    Abdominal sepsis
    Multiple system organ failure
    Gastrointestinal fistulas
    Prolonged ventilatory dependency
    Difficult tracheotomy
    Death
Nutritional
    Protein-calorie malnutrition
    Malabsorption of micronutrient
    Vitamin deficiencies (vitamin A, B_{12}, folate)
    Acute thiamine deficiency
    Severe anemia
    Mineral deficiencies (Ca, Mg)
    Dehydration
    Failure to lose weight
Gastrointestinal
    Food intolerance
    Dumping syndrome
    Nausea
    Vomiting
    Marginal ulcer
    Stomal stenosis
    Diarrhea
Long-term surgical
    Incisional hernia
    Gallstones
    Intraabdominal hernia
    Bowel obstruction

TABLE 22.3. *Pitfalls and pearls*

Preoperatively
  Select patients carefully.
  Have a frank conversations with the patient and his or her family.
Intraoperatively
  Have a good exposure.
  Explore entire abdomen.
  Remove all tubes from the esophagus before stapling the stomach.
  Close all intraabdominal spaces for potential hernias.
  Repair existing umbilical hernia.
  Convert to open technique, if needed, when the operation is attempted laparoscopically.
  Perform leak test at end of procedure.
Postoperatively
  Recognize subtle signs and symptoms of peritonitis, such as tachycardia or organ failure.
  Identify dilated bypassed gastric pouch and need for decompression.
  Beware of absent classic abdominal pain and tenderness.

---

respiratory insufficiency of obesity and in those with extremely high BMIs. Complications must be recognized and addressed promptly to minimize possible mortality and morbidity. Intraoperative injuries to the spleen or other organs are rare. After GBP for clinically severe obesity, the distal bypassed stomach occasionally will develop gaseous distention, secondary to afferent limb obstruction at the jejunojejunostomy, that may lead to gastric necrosis, gastric perforation, staple-line disruption, or disruption of the gastrojejunal anastomosis. This complication is usually heralded by frequent hiccups, and it can be diagnosed by noting a large gastric bubble on a plain abdominal roentgenogram. This requires urgent gastric decompression, which can be performed via percutaneous or open techniques. In patients who undergo reoperation, such as conversion from jejunoileal bypass to GBP, or in patients with extensive adhesions from previous abdominal surgery, a gastrostomy tube should be inserted prophylactically to prevent this complication. The gastrostomy tube also can be used for feeding until the patient's oral intake permits weight stabilization or for enteral nutritional support in patients who develop a leak from the proximal gastric pouch. The most feared early complication of GBP for morbid obesity is a postoperative leak from the gastrojejunostomy or peritonitis caused by the jejunojejunostomy.

The inability to recognize an abdominal catastrophe readily is one of the most significant aspects of the surgical care of morbidly obese patients. The classic signs and symptoms of peritonitis in these patients are often absent, and they may not become apparent for days. If a patient experiences worsening abdominal pain, back pain, left shoulder pain, urinary frequency, or rectal tenesmus, the clinician must suspect a leak. The presence of tachycardia, tachypnea, fever, leukocytosis, or metabolic acidosis also should raise the strong suspicion of an abdominal catastrophe. A leak may be confirmed with upper gastrointestinal (UGI) roentgenographic series using water-soluble contrast. If a leak is observed or even if the study results are negative but the index of suspicion is high, the patient's abdomen must be urgently explored. However, if the leak is in the bypassed stomach or at the jejunojejunostomy, a UGI may be normal. An attempt to repair the leak should be made, and a large sump drain should be placed nearby, because the repair frequently breaks down. This leads to a controlled fistula, which requires therapy with total parenteral nutrition, a feeding gastrostomy, or jejunostomy.

Additional complications include deep venous thrombosis, pulmonary embolus, and superficial or deep wound infections. Although these complications are not unique to gastric surgery for morbid obesity, they are more common in this patient population. The incidence of lower leg venous thrombosis and pulmonary embolism can be significantly reduced with the use of intermittent venous compression boots placed before the start of the operation and low-dose heparin or low-molecular-weight heparin (LMWH) given 30 minutes before surgery. Although no data currently support LMWH use in these patients, higher doses may be needed, based on heparin anti–factor XA levels, if LMWH is used (42). For patients with either obesity-hypoventilation syndrome, pulmonary hypertension, or severe venous stasis disease at the time of obesity surgery, a vena cava filter should be placed prophylactically. Early ambulation is also extremely important in all patients who undergo gastric surgery for morbid obesity.

A marginal ulcer develops in about 10% of patients who undergo GBP. This usually responds to acid-suppression therapy (H2-receptor or proton-pump blockers). In one report of 123 patients who underwent GBP, staple-line disruption occurred in 29%, while stomal ulcers occurred in 16% of patients (43,44). Stomal stenosis can develop in patients after RYGBP or VBGP. Outpatient endoscopic balloon stomal dilation should be attempted; it usually is successful in patients who have undergone GBP, but it is less effective in patients with stenosis after VBGP.

Late Complications

Rapid weight loss after either VBGP or GBP is associated with a high incidence (32% to 35%) of gallstone formation, with a need for subsequent cholecystectomy for acute biliary colic or cholecystitis within 3 to 5 years of the surgery for obesity in 10% of patients (45). Although some surgeons perform prophylactic cholecystectomy at the time of bariatric surgery, the authors' group and others perform cholecystectomy only with sonographic evidence of gallstones. In a randomized prospective trial, prophylactic ursodeoxycholic acid (300 mg orally, twice daily) has been shown to reduce the risk of gallstone formation from 32% to 2% when given for 6 months after GBP surgery; moreover, a very low risk of subsequent gallstone formation for the 6 months after discontinuation of the medication was seen (45).

After GBP, the patient is at risk of developing of an internal hernia with a closed-loop obstruction and strangulation. This may happen after open or laparoscopic GBP. These hernias usually occur in the following three locations: (a) through the mesenteric defect at the jejunojejunostomy site, (b) through the opening of transverse mesocolon through which the retrocolic Roux limb is brought, and (c) through the mesenteric defect located under the Roux limb, before it passes through the mesocolon, known as a Petersen hernia. These hernias may manifest principally with periumbilical abdominal pain, and their diagnosis may be difficult. A computed tomographic scan of the abdomen may be more helpful than upper gastrointestinal tract contrast studies in establishing the diagnosis. When the diagnosis is uncertain and the radiologic studies are not helpful, the safest course of action for the patient with recurrent crampy, periumbilical pain attacks is to reoperate because massive intestinal infarction has been seen with these internal hernias. Another significant complication of bariatric surgery is incisional hernia, which has an incidence of about 20% in open surgery.

Many patients desire abdominoplasty after weight loss; however, insurance coverage may be difficult to obtain for this procedure, which is viewed as cosmetic. Although abdominoplasty may be followed with complications in as many as 55% of patients, previous bariatric surgery does not influence the rate of complications after this operation (46). The most important factor influencing complications after abdominoplasty is the degree of obesity at the time of the surgery.

Nutritional Complications

After GBP for morbid obesity, significant micronutrient deficiencies can develop. A rare syndrome of polyneuropathy can occur after any bariatric procedure. This usually occurs in association with intractable vomiting and severe protein-calorie malnutrition, with subsequent acute thiamine deficiency (47). Although protein deficiency is the most serious problem after the malabsorption procedures, its true prevalence is unknown. The length of functional absorptive gut and the compromised role of pancreas and stomach in biliopancreatic bypass are the main factors causing this. Biliopancreatic bypass is associated with significant loss of endogenous nitrogen and decreased protein absorption, and, if these are persistent and resistant to medical treatment, revision is required.

Iron deficiency is a frequent complication of GBP in menstruating women, and vigilant monitoring and supplementation are required if severe consequences are to be avoided (48). Iron-deficiency anemia can be refractory to supplemental ferrous sulfate because iron absorption takes place primarily in the duodenum and upper jejunum or because patients avoid taking iron because it causes intestinal discomfort or severe constipation. Occasionally, iron–dextran injections may be necessary. Hysterectomy may be required in a woman with heavy menses and recurrent iron-deficiency anemia. All menstruating women should take two iron sulfate tablets (325 mg per day) by mouth after GBP as long as they continue to menstruate.

The risk of vitamin B_{12} deficiency mandates long-term follow-up with annual measurement of the vitamin B_{12} level (49,50). Vitamin B_{12} deficiency is probably due to decreased acid digestion of vitamin B_{12} from food, with the subsequent failure of coupling to intrinsic factor. Postoperatively, patients need to take 500 μg of oral vitamin B_{12}daily or 1 mg of vitamin B_{12} intramuscularly per month. Calcium deficiency is a potential serious consequence of surgery for morbid obesity because decreased calcium and vitamin D absorption will disturb normal calcium physiology and will affect the bone structure. To this end, supplementation is often necessary after any GBP procedure. Patients with either a long-limb gastric or a partial biliopancreatic bypass either with or without duodenal switch can develop calcium and fat-soluble vitamin deficiencies that need to be monitored and treated. Magnesium deficiency may also occur and may require supplementation.

OUTCOMES OF BARIATRIC SURGERY

Gastric procedures for morbid obesity can yield dramatic and long-term satisfactory weight reduction, with an average loss of two-thirds of excess weight within 1 to 2 years after GBP. Weight becomes stable at this level in most patients as the reduced caloric intake meets the caloric expenditure. The patients must be followed carefully to ensure adequate protein, vitamin, and other micronutrient levels.

Effect on Comorbidities

Weight loss corrects diabetes in 90% of morbidly obese patients who require insulin. No other therapy has produced more durable and complete control of diabetes mellitus (51). Hypertension is cured in two-thirds to three-fourths of the patients (52). The Swedish Obese Subjects (SOS) study, in which 2,000 patients have undergone surgical treatment of obesity as compared with matched control patients from a group of 8,000 who have not undergone surgery, also found correction of diabetes and hypertension 1 year after surgery, which contrasts with the increase in these medical problems in the control group. However, at 5 years after surgery, although the diabetes was still significantly improved in the surgical arm, the hypertension was not (53). In a subsequent publication, 94% of the patients were noted to have undergone gastric banding or gastroplasty, and 6% had had a GBP performed. As in other studies, the SOS patients who underwent GBP lost significantly more weight and continued to have significant decreases in both systolic and diastolic blood pressure at 5 years after surgery (54). Headaches and associated cerebrospinal fluid pressure elevation (Fig. 22.5) resolved in almost all patients with pseudotumor cerebri (55,56). The obstructive sleep apnea syndrome resolves with weight loss (Fig. 22.6) (57). The hypoxemia and hypercarbia seen in the obesity-hypoventilation syndrome return toward normal with weight loss (Fig. 22.7) (58). Elevated pulmonary artery and pulmonary capillary wedge pressures also improve significantly after weight loss with correction of abnormal arterial blood gases (59).

The loss of weight usually corrects female sexual hormone abnormalities, permits healing of chronic venous stasis ulcers associated with venous insufficiency, prevents reflux esophagitis, relieves stress overflow urinary incontinence, and improves low back pain and joint-related pain (Fig. 22.8) (60–63). Furthermore, weight loss can permit successful total artificial joint replacement. Patient self-image is often markedly improved after gastric surgery for obesity (64). Surgically induced weight reduction is associated with a significant improvement in left ventricular ejection fraction, chamber size, and ventricular thickness (65,66). Improvement in the lipid profile of morbidly obese patients has been documented (52,53,67).

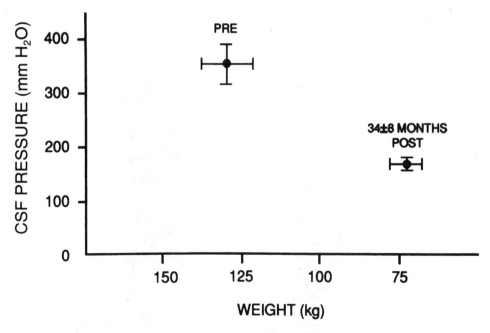

FIG. 22.5. Elevated cerebrospinal fluid (CSF) pressure before gastric bypass surgery and a significant ($p < 0.001$) decrease 34 months, plus or minus 8 months, after gastric surgery for severe obesity associated with pseudotumor cerebri. (From Sugerman HJ, Felton WL, Sismanis A, et al. Effects of surgically induced weight loss on pseudotumor cerebri in morbid obesity. *Neurology* 1995;45:1655–1659, with permission.)

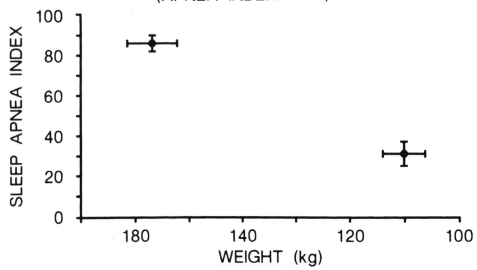

FIG. 22.6. Significant improvement in respiratory disturbance index (RDI) of sleep apnea in a group of patients with severe sleep apnea (RDI >40) 5 years after gastric bypass. (From Sugerman HJ, Fairman RP, Sood RK, et al. Long-term effects of gastric surgery for treating respiratory insufficiency of obesity. *Am J Clin Nutr* 1992;55:597S–601S, with permission.)

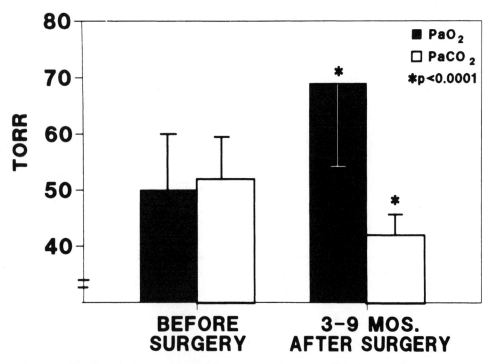

FIG. 22.7. Significantly improved partial pressure of oxygen (Pao_2) and of carbon dioxide ($Paco_2$) in 18 patients 3 to 9 months after gastric surgery induced loss of 42% of excess weight. (From Sugerman HJ, Baron PL, Fairman RP, et al. Hemodynamic dysfunction in obesity hypoventilation syndrome and the effects of treatment with surgically induced weight loss. *Ann Surg* 1988;207:604–613, with permission.)

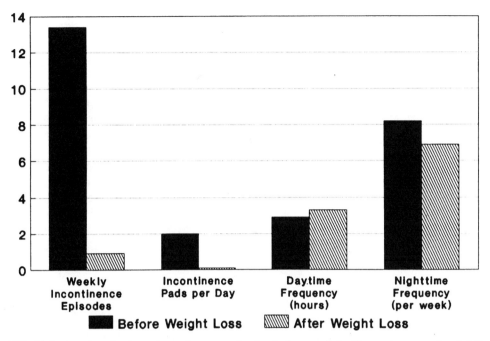

FIG. 22.8. Increased urinary incontinence episodes before and significant decrease (*p* <0.01) 1 year after gastric bypass for severe obesity in women with stress overflow urinary incontinence. (From Bump RC, Sugerman HJ, Fantl JA, et al. Obesity and lower urinary tract function in women: effect of surgically induced weight loss. *Am J Obstet Gynecol* 1992;167:392–399, with permission.)

FAILED GASTRIC BYPASS

Inability to lose more than 40% of the patient's excess weight at one year is considered a failure of obesity surgery. About 10% to 15% of patients regain their lost weight or fail to achieve an acceptable weight loss. The cause for this failure appears to be excessive constant nibbling on foods with a high caloric density or a failure to maintain regular exercise.

Reoperation

Reoperation for failed GBP can be extremely challenging, and it heralds significantly higher risk of morbidity and mortality. The operations to correct the failed GBP could be from restapling to revision of large upper gastric pouch. Rarely, the GBP has to be taken down. GBP revisions occur in 3% to 11% of patients. The risks of revision surgery are significantly higher than those of a primary procedure. A patient with a technically adequate GBP and weight loss failure needs further behavioral modifications, dietary counseling, and increased exercise. They may be candidates for conversion to a distal malabsorptive GBP; however, this can be associated with severe protein-calorie malnutrition steatorrhea, fat-soluble vitamin deficiencies, and osteoporosis, and thus it should be used only in a patient with a severe life-threatening (e.g., malignant hypertension) or debilitating comorbidity (38). Attempts to revise a failed gastroplasty are often unsuccessful. Reoperation in these patients may be extremely difficult because of extensive adhesions to the liver and spleen. Results appear to be significantly better when gastroplasty patients are converted to an RYGBP (68). Most patients who fail a GBP do so as a consequence of constant nibbling on high-fat junk foods or from drinking nondietetic liquids.

CONCLUSION

Surgery for severe obesity continues to be effective for long-term weight loss. The GBP has been more effective than gastroplasty procedures. The biliopancreatic bypass with duodenal switch may have a better long-term efficacy, but it may also be associated with greater nutritional problems than a GBP. No randomized studies comparing these procedures have been completed. Laparoscopic approaches are rapidly evolving. The laparoscopic adjustable silicone gastric band has been approved for use in patients in the United States. Concerns regarding complications and weight loss in the initial United States Food and Drug Administration trial have been voiced; however, the Australian and European data are quite favorable. Laparoscopic GBP has been developed into a safe procedure that is now being performed by larger numbers of bariatric surgeons. Surgically induced weight loss has been shown to treat most of the obesity-related comorbidity problems effectively.

REFERENCES

1. Allison DB, Fontaine KR, Manson JE, et al. Annual deaths attributable to obesity in the United States. *JAMA* 1999;282:1530–1538.
2. Wisser M, Bouter M, Mc Quillan GM, et al. Elevated C-reactive protein levels in overweight and obese adults. *JAMA* 1999;282:2131–2135.
3. Kyzer S, Binyamini J, Chaimoff C, et al. The effect of surgically induced weight reduction on the serum levels of the cytokines: interleukin-3 and tumor necrosis factor. *Obes Surg* 1999;9:229–234.
4. Henrikson V. Kan tunntarmresektion fosfars som terapi mot fettost. *Nord Med* 1952;47:744.
5. Gastrointestinal surgery for severe obesity: National Institutes of Health Consensus Development Conference Statement. *Am J Clin Nutr* 1992;55:615S–619S.
6. Payne JH, De Wind LT. Surgical treatment of obesity. *Am J Surg* 1969;118:141–147.
7. Scott HW Jr, Dean RH, Shull HJ, et al. Results of jejunoileal bypass in two hundred patients with morbid obesity. *Surg Gynecol Obstet* 1977;145:661–673.
8. Buchwald H, Campos CT. Reoperation following surgery for morbid obesity. In: McQuarrie DG, Humphrey EW, Lee TJ, eds. *Reoperative general surgery,* 2nd ed. St. Louis: Mosby, 1997:289–311.
9. Hocking MP, Duerson MC, O'Leary JP, et al. Jejunoileal bypass for morbid obesity. Late follow-up in 100 cases. *N Engl J Med* 1983;308:995–999.
10. Drenick EJ, Fisler J, Johnson D. Hepatic steatosis after intestinal bypass—prevention and reversal with metronidazole, irrespective of protein-calorie malnutrition. *Gastroenterology* 1982;82:535–549.
11. Hocking M, Davis GL, Franzini DA, et al. Long-term consequences after jejunoileal bypass for morbid obesity. *Dig Dis Sci* 1998;43:11:2493–2499.
12. Griffen WO, Young VL, Stevenson C. A prospective comparison of gastric and jejunoileal bypass for morbid obesity. *Ann Surg* 1977;186:500–505.
13. Halverson JD, Gentry K, Wise L, et al. Reanastomosis after jejunoileal bypass. *Surgery* 1978;84:241–249.
14. Mason EE, Ito CC. Gastric bypass. *Ann Surg* 1969;170:329–339.
15. Mason EE. Vertical banded gastroplasty for obesity. *Arch Surg* 1982;117:701–706.
16. Scopinaro N, Gianetta E, Civalleri D, et al. Two years of clinical experience with biliopancreatic bypass for obesity. *Am J Clin Nutr* 1980;33:506–514.
17. Scopinaro N, Gianetta E, Civalleri D, et al. Partial and total biliopancreatic bypass in the surgical treatment of obesity. *Int J Obes* 1981;5:521–429.
18. MacLean LD, Rhode BM, Sampalis J, et al. Results of the surgical treatment of obesity. *Am J Surg* 1993;165:155–162.
19. Sugerman HJ, Starkey JV, Birkenhauer RA. A randomized prospective trial of gastric bypass versus vertical banded gastroplasty for morbid obesity and their effects on sweets versus non sweets eaters. *Ann Surg* 1987;205:613–624.
20. Hall JC, Watts JM, O'Brien PE, et al. Gastric surgery for morbid obesity. The Adelaide study. *Ann Surg* 1990;211:419–427.
21. Bø Modalsli Ø. Gastric banding, a surgical method of treating morbid obesity: preliminary report. *Int J Obes* 1983;7:493–499.
22. Kuzmak LI. Stoma adjustable silicone gastric banding. *Probl Gen Surg* 1992;9:298–317.

23. Curry TK, Carter PL, Porter CL, et al. Resectional gastric bypass is a new alternative in morbid obesity. *Am J Surg* 1998;175:367–370.
24. Brolin RE, Kenler HA, Gorman JH, et al. Long-limb gastric bypass in the superobese. A prospective randomized study. *Ann Surg* 1992;215:387–395.
25. Sugerman HJ. Gastric surgery for morbid obesity. In: Zinner MJ, ed. *Maingot's abdominal operations.* Norwalk, CT: Appleton & Lange, 1997.
26. Wittgrove AC, Clark GW. Laparoscopic gastric bypass: a five year perspective study of 500 followed from 3 to 60 months. *Obes Surg* 1999;9:124.
27. Schauer PR, Ikramuddin S, Ramanathan R, et al. Outcomes after laparoscopic Roux-en-Y gastric bypass for morbid obesity. *Ann Surg* 2000;232:515–529.
28. Higa KD, Boone KB, Ho T. Complications of the laparoscopic Roux-en-Y gastric bypass: 1,040 patients—what have we learned? *Obes Surg* 2000;10:509–513.
29. DeMaria EJ, Sugerman HJ, Kellum JM, et al. Results of 281 consecutive total laparoscopic Roux-en-Y gastric bypasses to treat morbid obesity. *Ann Surg* 2002;235:640–645.
30. Nguyen NT, Goldman C, Rosenquist J, et al. Laparoscopic versus open gastric bypass: a randomized study of outcomes, quality of life, and costs. *Ann Surg* 2001;234:279–291.
31. Nguyen NY, Lee SL, Goldman C, et al. Comparison of pulmonary function and postoperative pain after laparoscopic versus open gastric bypass: a randomized trial. *J Am Coll Surg* 2001;192:469–472.
32. Nguyen NT, Ho HS, Palmer LS, et al. A comparison study of laparoscopic versus open gastric bypass for morbid obesity. *J Am Coll Surg* 2000;191:149–155.
33. Greenstein RJ, Nissan A, Jaffin B. Esophageal anatomy and function in laparoscopic gastric restrictive bariatric surgery: implications for patient selection. *Obes Surg* 1999;8:199–206.
34. DeMaria EJ, Sugerman HJ, Meador JG, et al. High failure rate following laparoscopic adjustable silicone gastric banding for treatment of morbid obesity. *Ann Surg* 2001;233:809–818.
35. O'Brien PE, Brown WA, Smith A, et al. Prospective study of a laparoscopically placed, adjustable gastric band in the treatment of morbid obesity. *Br J Surg* 1999;86:113–118.
36. Angrisani L, Alkilani M, Basso N, et al. Laparoscopic Italian experience with the Lap-Band. *Obes Surg* 2001; 11:307–310.
37. Liska TG, Sugerman HJ, Kellum J, et al. Risk/benefit considerations of distal gastric bypass [Abstract]. *Int J Obes Surg* 1988;12:604S.
38. Sugerman HJ, Kellum JM, DeMaria EJ. Conversion to distal gastric bypass for failed standard gastric bypass for morbid obesity. *J Gastrointest Surg* 1997;1:517–525.
39. Hess DS, Hess DW. Biliopancreatic diversion with a duodenal switch. *Obes Surg* 1998;8:267–282.
40. Marceau P, Hould FS, Simard S, et al. Biliopancreatic diversion with duodenal switch. *World J Surg* 1998;22:947–954.
41. Kellum JM, DeMaria EJ, Sugerman HJ. The surgical treatment of morbid obesity. *Curr Probl Surg* 1998;35: 791–858.
42. Martin LF, Finigan KM. Heparin antifactor XA levels in morbidly obese patients receiving Lovenox prophylaxis [Abstract]. *Obes Surg* 1999;9:128.
43. MacLean LD, Rhode BM, Nohr C, et al. Stomal ulcer after gastric bypass. *J Am Coll Surg* 1997;185:1–7.
44. Sanyal AJ, Sugerman HJ, Kellum JM, et al. Stomal complications of gastric bypass: incidence and outcome of therapy. *Am J Gastroenterol* 1992;87:1165–1169.
45. Sugerman HJ, Brewer WH, Shiffman ML, et al. A multicenter, placebo-controlled, randomized, double-blind, prospective trial of prophylactic ursodiol for the prevention of gallstone formation following gastric-bypass–induced rapid weight loss. *Am J Surg* 1995;169:91–97.
46. Vastine VL, Morgan RF, Williams GS, et al. Wound complications of abdominoplasty in obese patients. *Ann Plast Surg* 1999;42:34–39.
47. Oczkowski WJ, Kertesz A. Wernicke's encephalopathy after gastroplasty for morbid obesity. *Neurology* 1985;35: 99–101.
48. Halverson JD. Vitamin and mineral deficiencies following obesity surgery. *Gastroenterol Clin North Am* 1987; 15:307–315.
49. Boylan LM, Sugerman HJ, Driskell JA. Vitamin E, vitamin B_{12}, and folic acid status of gastric restriction surgery patients. *J Am Diet Assoc* 1988;88:579–582.
50. Rhode BM, Arsenau P, Cooper BA, et al. Vitamin B-12 deficiency after gastric surgery for obesity. *Am J Clin Nutr* 1996;63:103–109.
51. Pories WJ, Swanson MS, MacDonald KG, et al. Who would have thought it? An operation proves to be the most effective therapy for adult-onset diabetes mellitus. *Ann Surg* 1995;222:339–350.
52. Carson JL, Ruddy ME, Duff AE, et al. The effect of gastric bypass surgery on hypertension in morbidly obese patients. *Ann Intern Med* 1994;154:193–200.
53. Sjostrom CD, Lissner L, Wedel H, et al. Reduction in incidence of diabetes, hypertension, and lipid disturbances after intentional weight loss induced by bariatric surgery: the SOS intervention study. *Obes Res* 1999;7:477–484.
54. Sjostrom CD, Peltonen M, Sjostrom L. Blood pressure and pulse pressure during long-term weight loss in the obese; the Swedish Obese Subjects (SOS) intervention study. *Obes Res* 2001;9:188–195.
55. Sugerman HJ, Felton WL, Sismanis A, et al. Effects of surgically induced weight loss on pseudotumor cerebri in morbid obesity. *Neurology* 1995;45:1655–1659.

56. Sugerman HJ, Felton WL III, Sismanis A, et al. Gastric surgery for pseudotumor cerebri associated with severe obesity. *Ann Surg* 1999;229:634–642.
57. Sugerman HJ, Fairman RP, Sood RK, et al. Long-term effects of gastric surgery for treating respiratory insufficiency of obesity. *Am J Clin Nutr* 1992;55:597S–601S.
58. Charuzi I, Lavie P, Peiser J, et al. Bariatric surgery in morbidly obese sleep-apnea patients: short- and long-term follow-up. *Am J Clin Nutr* 1992;55:594S–596S.
59. Sugerman HJ, Baron PL, Fairman RP, et al. Hemodynamic dysfunction in obesity hypoventilation syndrome and the effects of treatment with surgically induced weight loss. *Ann Surg* 1988;207:604–613.
60. Deitel M, Toan BT, Stone EM, et al. Sex hormone changes accompanying loss of massive excess weight. *Gastroenterol Clin North Am* 1987;16:511–516.
61. Sugerman HJ, Sugerman EL, Wolfe L, et al. Risks/benefits of gastric bypass in morbidly obese patients with severe venous stasis disease. *Ann Surg* 2001;234:41–46.
62. Smith SC, Edwards CB, Goodman GN. Symptomatic and clinical improvement in morbidly obese patients with gastroesophageal reflux disease following Roux-en-Y gastric bypass. *Obes Surg* 1997;7:479–484.
63. Bump RC, Sugerman HJ, Fantl JA, et al. Obesity and lower urinary tract function in women: effect of surgically induced weight loss. *Am J Obstet Gynecol* 1992;167:392–399.
64. Stunkard AJ, Stinnet JL, Smoller JW. Psychological and social aspects of the surgical treatment of obesity. *Am J Psychiatry* 1986;143:417–429.
65. Sugerman HJ, Baron PL, Fairman RP, et al. Hemodynamic dysfunction in obesity hypoventilation syndrome and the effects of treatment with surgically induced weight loss. *Ann Surg* 1988;207:604–613.
66. Gleysteen JJ, Barboriak JJ, Sasse EA. Sustained coronary-risk-factor reduction after gastric bypass for morbid obesity. *Am J Clin Nutr* 1990;51:774–778.
67. Brolin RE, Kenler HA, Wilson AC, et al. Serum lipids after gastric bypass surgery for morbid obesity. *Int J Obes* 1990;14:939–950.
68. Sugerman HJ, Kellum JM Jr, DeMaria EJ, et al. Conversion of failed or complicated vertical banded gastroplasty to gastric bypass in morbid obesity. *Am J Surg* 1996;171:263–269.

23

The Economic Impact of Overweight, Obesity, and Weight Loss

Anne M. Wolf, JoAnn E. Manson, and Graham A. Colditz

HEALTH CARE ECONOMICS AND TERMINOLOGY

Overview

Health care economic studies evaluate the burden of disease (i.e., cost of illness) or the relative effectiveness of interventions designed to improve health in monetary terms. The following is a list of the definitions of more widely used methods. In the field of obesity, most of the published reports have been cost-of-illness studies.

Cost of illness: an analysis of the total costs incurred by a society due to a specific disease.
Cost-effectiveness analysis (CEA): an analytic tool in which costs and effects of a program and at least one alternative are calculated and presented in a ratio of incremental cost to incremental effect. Effects are health outcomes, such as cases of a disease prevented, years of life gained, or quality-adjusted life-years (QALYs).
Cost–benefit analysis (CBA): an analytic tool for estimating the net social benefit of an intervention as the incremental benefit of the program less the incremental costs, with all benefits and costs in dollars.

Cost-of-Illness Studies

Cost of illness is a tool used to estimate the cost impact of disease on the community (the "community" is broadly defined—it could be a nation, state, health insurance membership, or employer). The economic costs of a health condition, such as obesity, are categorized into the following:

Direct costs: the cost of preventive, diagnosis, and treatment services related to the disease (e.g., hospital care, physician services, and medications).
Indirect costs: the value of lost output resulting from cessation or reduction of productivity caused by morbidity and mortality. Morbidity costs are wages lost by people who are unable to work because of illness and disability. Mortality costs are the value of future earnings lost by people who die prematurely.

Cost-of-illness studies are useful in the development of public policy because they can identify how resources are being used, can assist health care decision makers in making comparisons between the relative economic burden of different diseases, and can highlight to both policymakers and health care decision makers the magnitude of the health problem in a language that they understand—money. Although cost-of-illness studies may suggest that a disease, such as obesity, has a high cost, they do not imply that this high-cost disease should be given preferential consideration for treatment because treatment may be ineffective or unacceptably expensive. Hence, priority setting for the treatment of disease should be based on the relative cost-effectiveness of interventions and not on the cost of the disease alone.

ECONOMIC IMPACT OF OVERWEIGHT AND OBESITY INTERNATIONALLY

The economic impact of overweight and obesity is observed internationally. Eight countries have assessed the economic burden of overweight or obesity in each of their countries (1–9). Seven of the studies used similar cost-of-illness methods to estimate costs. In cost-of-illness evaluations, the relationship of comorbidity to obesity is quantified using the population-attributable risk (PAR). The PAR has been used widely in economic evaluations, and it estimates the proportion of a disease attributable to obesity using relative risks from large epidemiologic studies. Hence, the spectrum of the disease is defined within the epidemiologic study versus the cost study; this could be a potential limitation. This "top-down" approach is limited by the availability of data relating obesity to various comorbid conditions, as well as to data on national cost. For instance, even though obesity is associated with a plethora of medical conditions, the cost-of-illness studies presented in Table 23.1 evaluate only 6 to 13 conditions because of a lack of incidence data to relate obesity to other diseases or of cost data for specific diseases.

TABLE 23.1. *The economic impact of overweight or obesity in different countries*

Author	Country, year of dollar equivalent	Definition of obesity (BMI, kg/m^2)	Conditions included	Total of national health care expenditure (%)
Segal et al. (1)	Australia, 1989	≥30	Type II DM; gallstones; hypertension; CHD; breast and colon cancer	2
Levy et al. (2)	France, 1992	≥27	Hypertension; MI; angina; stroke; venous thrombosis; type II DM; hyperlipidemia; gout; osteoarthritis; hip fracture; gallbladder dse; breast and genitourinary cancer	2
Birmingham et al. (4)	Canada, 1997	≥30	Postmenopausal breast, endometrial, and colorectal cancers; type II DM; CHD; hyperlipidemia; hypertension; gallbladder dse; pulmonary embolism; stroke	2.4
Swinburn et al. (5)	New Zealand, 1991	≥30	Type II DM; CHD; hypertension; gallstone dse; postmenopausal breast and colon cancer	2.5
Pereira et al. (6)	Portugal, 1996	≥30	Colon, breast, and endometrial cancer; type II DM; hyperlipidemia; hypertension; obesity; cardiovascular dse; gallbladder dse; arthropathies	3.5
Seidell (7)	Netherlands	≥25		4
Wolf and Colditz (9)	United States, 1995	≥29	Type II DM; hypertension; CHD; gallbladder dse; osteoarthritis; breast, endometrial, and colon cancer	5.7

Abbreviations: BMI, body mass index; CHD, coronary heart disease; DM, diabetes mellitus; dse, disease; MI, myocardial infarction.

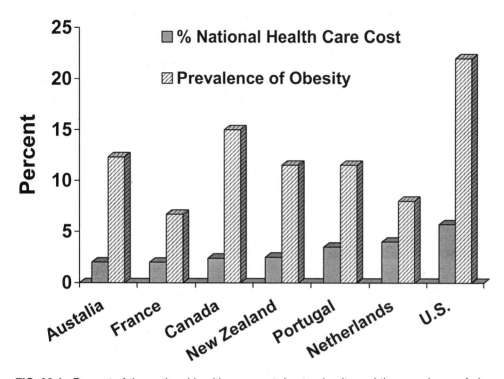

FIG. 23.1. Percent of the national health care cost due to obesity and the prevalence of obesity.

Cost-of-illness studies, therefore, estimate the proportion of several diseases that are attributable to obesity and then apply nation-specific cost and prevalence data to estimate the direct health care of obesity. However, when directly comparing the results (Table 23.1), one must be aware that the assumptions differ between studies. Additionally, the prevalence of obesity, which is a considerable determinant of the cost estimate, differs from country to country (Fig. 23.1). Despite the differences among studies, the variation in cost estimates is relatively narrow, ranging from 2% to 6% of total health care expenditure within that country.

Australia

The National Health and Medical Research Council (NHMRC) assessed the economic impact of obesity (body mass index [BMI] greater than or equal to 30 kilograms per meter squared [kg/m²]) by looking at six diseases associated with obesity (Table 23.1). The direct cost was estimated at AUD $464 million (1989 to 1990 dollar equivalent, or U.S. $250 million), and the indirect cost amounted to an additional AUD $272 million (U.S. $147 million) (1); this was 2% of the country's national health expenditure for that year. The population of Australia is more than 18 million people, and the potential years of life lost because of obesity was 29,855. Obesity was responsible for 50,931 hospital admissions, 433,165 hospital-stay days, 3.1 million medical consultations, 6.7 million pharmaceutical prescriptions, and 164,903 referrals to allied health professionals in Australia from 1989 to 1990. Coronary heart disease (CHD) and hypertension accounted for almost 60% of the total cost.

The NHMRC also estimated the cost of obesity treatment within the health care system in Australia, which accounted for 10% of the total cost of obesity. This approximation may be conservative, considering a 1992 survey by the Consumer Advocacy and Financial Counseling Association of Victoria (10) that estimated that 300,000 Australians purchased weight loss programs each year, a cost that was calculated to exceed AUD $500 million per year (U.S. $270 million). This highlights the fact that, in many developed countries, a substantial proportion of the cost of obesity lies outside the formal health care sector (11).

France

In France, Lévy et al. (2) estimated the cost of obesity (BMI greater than or equal to 27 kg/m^2) based on 13 diseases that have a well-established relationship with obesity (Table 23.1). The direct cost was estimated to be Fr 12 billion (U.S. $1.56 billion), which corresponds to approximately 2% of the total health care expenditure in France for 1992. Hypertension represented 53% of the total direct costs of obesity. The economic burden of obesity for France was recently reevaluated by Detourneay et al. (3), using a more direct analytical approach. The direct cost attributable to obesity (BMI greater than or equal to 30 kg/m^2) was slightly lower—Fr 4.2 to 8.7 billion (approximately U.S. $0.55 to $1.13 billion) or 0.7% to 1.5% of total health expenditures—but was within the range of the previous estimate.

Canada

The economic impact of obesity (BMI more than or equal to 27 kg/m^2) in Canada was estimated using various sources (4). The following ten comorbidities associated with obesity were considered: CHD, postmenopausal breast, colorectal and endometrial cancer, gallbladder disease, hyperlipidemia, hypertension, pulmonary embolism, stroke, and type II diabetes. The direct cost of obesity in 1997 was estimated to be more than Can $1.8 billion (U.S. $1.2 billion). This corresponds to 2.4% of the total health care expenditures for all diseases in Canada in 1997. The three largest contributors to the total cost of obesity were hypertension (36%), type II diabetes (23.5%), and coronary artery disease (19%).

New Zealand

The 1991 health care costs of six diseases—type II diabetes, CHD, hypertension, gallbladder disease, and postmenopausal breast and colorectal cancers—associated with obesity in New Zealand were estimated using various sources (5). The direct health care cost attributable to obesity in New Zealand was N.Z. $135 million (U.S. $55 million), which represents 2.5% of the nation's total health care costs.

Portugal

In Portugal, the cost of obesity (BMI of at least 30 kg/m^2) was estimated using various sources (National Health Survey, IMS-Portugal) (6). In 1996, the direct cost of obesity in Portugal was estimated to be PTE $46.2 billion (approximately U.S. $0.31 billion), which corresponds to 3.5% of the country's national health care expenditure for that year. The largest cost component was pharmaceutical use (43%), followed by hospitalization (29%) and ambulatory care (28%). Medication costs were attributable largely to circulatory system pathologies, in particular, hypertension. Annually, more than 35,000 inpatient episodes and 2 million physician visits were attributable to obesity, figures which are substantial in a population of 10 million people.

The Netherlands

In the Netherlands, Seidell and Deerenberg (7) assessed the excess use of medical care of overweight (BMI from 25 to 29.9 kg/m^2) and obesity (BMI greater than or equal to 30 kg/m^2) using data on 58,000 participants in the National Health Interview Surveys from 1981 to 1987. Overall, overweight and obese people in Holland were found to consult their doctor 20% and 40%, respectively, more than average-weight people did. They did not see medical specialists more frequently, and only obese *women* were admitted to the hospital more than nonobese women. Overweight persons were 1.4 to 2.4 times more likely to be on diuretics compared with nonoverweight persons, and obese persons were 4.6 to 4.8 times more likely to use these. Similarly, overweight persons were 1.5 to 2.5 times more likely to be on cardiovascular disease (CVD) medications than were nonoverweight persons. The authors estimated the direct cost associated with overweight and obesity to be 1 billion Dutch guilders per year (U.S. $390 million), or 4% of the total health care costs in the Netherlands.

Sweden

In the Swedish Obese Subjects (SOS) study, Narbro et al. (8) evaluated the economic consequences of sick leave and early retirement in obese Swedish women. Sick leave and disability pension rates were doubled in obese women compared with the Swedish population. In the Swedish population, the cost of the sick leave amounted to SEK $3.6 billion, which translates to approximately U.S. $300 million per 1 million women in the United States adult population. They also reported that medication use was 77% higher among the obese compared with a healthy body weight referent population and that the medication classes that were increased the most among the obese compared to the referent population were diabetes, cardiovascular, pain, and asthma medications (12). Finally, the authors evaluated the willingness to pay (WTP) for obesity treatment among the obese in Sweden and found that the average WTP for obesity treatment was twice the monthly income; a high WTP was associated with high income, high weight, and poor perceived health (13).

ECONOMIC IMPACT OF OBESITY IN THE UNITED STATES

Of all the countries that have completed cost-of-illness studies, the United States has the greatest prevalence of and economic burden from obesity (Fig. 23.1). Additionally, more economic analyses have been conducted in the United States to estimating the cost to the nation, the cost to managed care organizations (MCOs), and the cost to employers. The following sections review and focus on the direct health care costs, the lost productivity, and the functional impairment associated with obesity in the United States.

Direct Medical Costs of Obesity

Wolf and Colditz (9) estimated the proportion of several diseases that were attributable to obesity, as well as the direct health care cost of obesity (BMI greater than or equal to 29 kg/m^2) in the United States (Table 23.2). The diseases associated with obesity included in this estimate were type II diabetes, CHD, hypertension, osteoarthritis, gallbladder disease, postmenopausal breast cancer, and endometrial and colon cancers. The

TABLE 23.2. *Relative risk, percent of disease, and annual direct and indirect health care costs attributable to obesity[a] by disease in the United States (2001 dollars)*

Obesity comorbidity	Relative risk	Population-attributable risk (PAR %)	Direct cost ($ in billions)	Indirect cost ($ in billions)
Type II Diabetes	27.6	61	40.1	38.02
Coronary heart disease	3.5	17.3	8.8	–
Hypertension	3.9	17	4.08	–
Gallbladder disease	3.2	30	3.2	0.187
Breast cancer	1.3	11	1.05	1.83
Endometrial cancer	2.0	34	0.31	0.623
Colon cancer	1.5	11.3	1.26	2.20
Osteoarthritis	2.1	24	5.3	15.9
Total			**$64.1**	**$58.8**

[a]Obesity was defined as body mass index ≥ 29 kg/m^2.
The referent group's body mass index was ≤ 20 kg/m^2 for gallbladder disease, <21 kg/m^2 for coronary heart disease, <22 kg/m^2 for type II diabetes and colon cancer, and <23 kg/m^2 for hypertension.
Adapted from Wolf A, Colditz G. Current estimates of the economic costs of obesity in the United States. *Obes Res* 1998;6:97–106, with permission, and inflated to year 2000 United States dollars using the medical component of the Consumer Price Index.

PAR can be interpreted in the following way: the proportion of type II diabetes that is attributable to obesity was approximately 61%, whereas the proportion of CHD that was attributable to obesity was approximately 17%. In other words, if obesity were prevented or effectively treated, a *maximum* of 61% of type II diabetes and of 17% of CHD cases could potentially be prevented. The high attribution of type II diabetes to obesity should not be surprising, considering that 80% to 90% of people with type II diabetes are overweight and that 30% are obese (14).

The direct health care cost estimate attributable to obesity was approximately $51.6 billion in 1995, which was approximately 5.7% of the national health expenditure for that year in the United States. Inflating this estimate to current dollars, the direct health care cost of obesity in 2001 dollars would be $64.1 billion. Compared with other major chronic diseases, the direct cost of obesity is approximately the same as that of diabetes* (15–17) and is more expensive than those of CHD and hypertension (18). Most of the direct costs of obesity stemmed from type II diabetes (63%), CHD (14%), osteoarthritis (8%), and hypertension (6%). The direct health care costs of obesity increase as BMI increases (Fig. 23.2) (19).

Colditz (20) recently reestimated the cost of obesity using national prevalence rates for obesity based on the National Health and Nutrition Examination Survey III (NHANES-III) and updated the relative risk estimates for various disease states; he estimated the direct cost of obesity to be approximately $70 billion in 1995, or 7% of the national health care expenditure. The primary difference between the studies was a different prevalence rate of obesity and higher relative risk estimates. The difference in these cost estimates illustrates the great impact of the underlying assumptions on the variability of these national cost estimates. Therefore, the direct cost of obesity in the United States in 1995 dollars is estimated to be between $51.9 and $70 billion. However, these estimates are based on epidemiologic data, and therefore they are limited by data availability. Moreover, these estimates account only for eight diseases associated with obesity, whereas

---

*The direct cost estimates of diabetes in the United States vary considerably, ranging from $7.4 billion (1984 dollars) (13) to $85.7 billion (1992 dollars) (14). The cost estimate used was from the American Diabetes Association and was $44.1 billion (1997 dollars) (15).

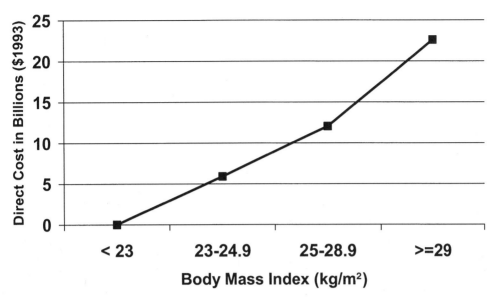

FIG. 23.2. Annual direct health care costs (1993 United States $) of obesity by body mass index (BMI) category. Costs based on the following four selected disease states: hypertension, coronary heart disease, type II diabetes, and gallbladder disease. (Adapted from Wolf AM, Colditz GA. Social and economic impact of body weight in the United States. *Am J Clin Nutr* 1996;63:466S–469S, with permission.)

obesity is associated with many more comorbid states (e.g., metabolic syndrome, sleep apnea, stroke, pregnancy complications, and low back pain). Other comorbid conditions were not included in these estimates because of a lack of national cost data or of incidence data linking obesity to other disease states.

The economic impact of obesity can also be evaluated more directly using large, nationally representative databases, such as the National Health Interview Survey (NHIS), or the NHANES or by linking the NHIS with the Medical Expenditure Panel Survey (MEPS). BMI can be calculated using self-reported weight and heights, and participants can be categorized by BMI into the World Health Organization (WHO)–established classification system for body weight (i.e., healthy body weight, BMI of 20 to 24.9 kg/m², overweight, BMI of 25 to 29.9 kg/m²; and obesity, BMI of at least 30 kg/m²) (11). The NHIS contains health-related information, such as the annual number of physician visits, disease state, workdays missed due to sickness, and activity-limitation variables. The NHANES database contains weight and height, dietary intake, and the presence of hypertension, diabetes, and hypercholesterolemia through self-reports and physical examinations. Wolf and Colditz (9) evaluated the number and the change in the number of physician visits associated with obesity (BMI of greater than or equal to 30 kg/m²) from 1988 to 1994 using the NHIS. In 1988, the annual number of physician visits because of obesity was 33.3 million; in 1994, the number of visits had increased by 88% to 62.6 million. The increase appeared secondary to an increase in the prevalence of obesity in the United States, as well as to an increase in the average number of annual visits among the obese. In 1994, obese women made 67% of office visits.

Thompson et al. (21) modeled the lifetime health and economic consequences of obesity for men and women from the ages of 35 to 64 years using NHANES-III, the Framingham Heart Study, and other secondary sources. Although they evaluated the disease

states that account for the major cost of obesity (i.e., type II diabetes, hypercholesterolemia, CHD, hypertension, and stroke), they were unable to evaluate many of the
other diseases associated with obesity because of lack of data; therefore, this study may
be considered an underestimate of the lifetime health and economic impact of obesity.
They reported that the disease risks and costs increased substantially with increased BMI
and age. The lifetime risks of developing hypertension were between 2.4 and 3.7 times
greater in the obese population, depending on age and gender, compared with the lean
population. The lifetime risks of developing type II diabetes were between 3.2 and 4.8
times greater in the obese, compared with the lean, population. Lastly, the lifetime risks
of developing hypercholesterolemia were lower than those of hypertension and type II
diabetes and were within the range of 1.3 to 1.4 times greater in the obese population as
compared with that of the lean population. The lifetime risk of developing CHD or stroke
was higher in the obese, than in the lean, population (approximately 1.35 and 1.2, respectively), but it was considerably less than that of hypertension and type II diabetes. Life
expectancy is reduced by approximately 1 year. The differences in disease risk translated
into differences in medical care costs. Mild obesity (BMI of 27.5 kg/m^2) increased the
expected lifetime medical care costs for the five disease states by approximately 20%,
whereas moderate obesity (BMI of 32.5 kg/m^2) increased them by about 50% and severe
obesity (BMI of 37.5 kg/m^2) almost doubled the costs. The estimated lifetime medical
care costs for persons with severe obesity compared with those of lean persons differed
by approximately $10,000. The age-specific and gender-specific costs of obesity were
comparable to those of smoking.

Gorsky et al. (22) estimated the excess health care costs associated with moderate
overweight (BMI of 25 to 28.9 kg/m^2) and severe overweight (BMI of at least 29 kg/m^2)
among a hypothetical cohort of 10,000 women from 40 to 65 years of age during a 25-
year interval by using the incidence of obesity and disease in women during this age
range. The diseases they specified in their model were CHD, hypertension, diabetes,
osteoarthritis, and gallstone disease. Compared to the nonoverweight group (BMI of 20
to 24.9 kg/m^2), the moderately overweight group incurred excess costs of $22 million and
had 212 excess deaths. The severely overweight group incurred excess costs of $53 mil-
lion and had 497 deaths over a 25-year period. The dominant sources of the costs were
type II diabetes, nonfatal heart disease, and hypertension. Extrapolating their findings to
the current United States population, the authors estimated that approximately $16.1 bil-
lion (in 1996 dollars) will be spent in the United States during the next 25 years for the
treatment of non–cancer-related illnesses in overweight women in the 40-year-old to 44-
year-old age-group. Therefore, using databases nationally representative of the United
States, obesity (BMI greater than or equal to 30 kg/m^2) has a substantial and growing
impact on the country's health care system.

Sturm (23) recently compared the economic impact of obesity with that of smoking
and problem drinking with regard to health care use and health status based on data from
Healthcare for Communities (HCC). The HCC was a national household telephone survey with approximately 10,000 respondents that was conducted in the United States in
1997 and 1998. Obesity was defined as a BMI of more than or equal to 30 kg/m^2, and
self-reported weights and heights were used—prevalence of obesity in this population
was 23%, which is similar to the 1999 NHANES. Smoking status was classified as "ever
smoking," "daily smoking," and "never smoking." Problem drinking was identified using
the Alcohol Use Disorders Identification Test. Age, gender, race, household income, and
education were included as explanatory variables. From this survey, the effects of obesity
on the number of chronic health conditions and declined health-related quality of life

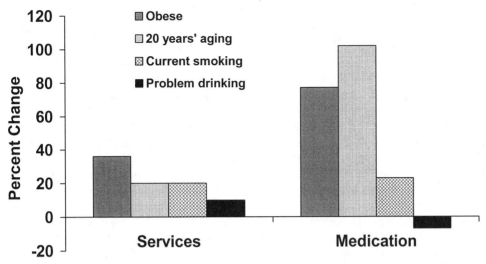

FIG. 23.3. Percent change in health care costs associated with obesity, aging, smoking, and drinking, as compared with a nonobese, nonaged, nonsmoking, and nondrinking population, 1998. (Adapted from Sturm R. The effects of obesity, smoking, and drinking on medical problems and costs. *Health Affairs* 2002;21:245–253, with permission.)

were shown to be significantly larger than the effects of current or past smoking or problem drinking (p <0.001) and are similar to those of 20 years of aging. In terms of economic consequences, obesity increased health care costs by 36% and medication costs by 77%, compared with people in the healthy weight range. Obesity's relative costs are much greater compared to 20 years' aging, current smoking, and problem drinking (Fig. 23.3). This is the first study that directly compares obesity with other behavioral risk factors, such as smoking and drinking, which also have an impact on chronic health conditions.

Models and Studies from the Managed Care Perspective

Although the body of literature on the health and economic impacts of obesity is growing, cost-of-illness studies may be too broad to be useful for administrators and health care policy decision makers in a MCO. Hence, models and studies that examine the health and economic impact from the managed care perspective are important. Currently, only one model estimates the health and economic burden of obesity in a managed care setting. Oster et al. (24) projected the impact of obesity on a MCO with 1 million members between of 35 and 84 years of age. They evaluated eight diseases associated with obesity—CHD, hypertension, hypercholesterolemia, gallbladder disease, stroke, type II diabetes, osteoarthritis of the knee, and endometrial cancer. Characteristics of a health plan membership (e.g., age, sex, and BMI) were obtained from a large MCO in the Pacific Northwest. The prevalence of obesity-related diseases was obtained from NHIS, NHANES-III, the Framingham Heart Study, the National Hospital Discharge Survey, and other published reports. The relative risks of diseases associated with obesity were obtained using published reports from major United States epidemiologic studies. Medical care costs were reported in 1996 dollars. In a health plan with 1 million members, 174,400 men (38%) and 132,900 women (25%) would be mildly obese (BMI of 25 to 28 kg/m^2), whereas 149,300 men (32%) and 168,800 women (32%) would be moderately to severely obese (BMI of at least 29 kg/m^2). This estimate, which utilizes BMI data from an MCO, is considerably higher than estimates within the general population (25). A total of 45% of all cases of hypertension were due to obesity, whereas 85% of cases of type II diabetes, 18% of cases of hypercholesterolemia, 35% of cases of CHD, 15% of cases of stroke, 45% of cases of gallbladder disease, 31% of cases of osteoarthritis of the knee, and 24% of cases of endometrial cancer were attributable to obesity. The estimated cost attributable to obesity of these eight diseases was $345.9 million per year, or 41% of the total cost for the eight diseases of interest (Table 23.3).

A few epidemiologic studies have been done in the managed care setting as well. Quesenberry et al. (26) evaluated the annual rate of health use and the direct costs of health services associated with BMI within the Northern California Kaiser Permanente Medical Care program. More specifically, the authors assessed the annual rate of inpatient hospital days and inpatient costs; outpatient visits and costs; and pharmacy, laboratory, surgery, and radiology services and costs (Table 23.4). The comorbidities associated with obesity that were evaluated were diabetes,* hypertension, high cholesterol, CHD, depression, and musculoskeletal pain. In persons with a BMI between 20 and 24.9 kg/m^2, 49.8% had at least one comorbid condition, compared with 70% of people with a BMI of 35 kg/m^2 or more who had at least one comorbid condition. Alternatively, only 6.3% of persons with a BMI between 20 and 24.9 kg/m^2 had three or more comorbid conditions, whereas 18.4% of persons with a BMI of more than or equal to 35 kg/m^2 had three or more comorbid conditions. A statistically significant association was found between BMI and the annual rate of inpatient hospital days (p <0.001), inpatient costs (p <0.001), outpatient visits (p <0.001), outpatient costs (p <0.001), pharmacy costs (p <0.001), laboratory costs (p <0.001), and total health care costs (p <0.001) (Table 23.5). A further analysis of pharmaceutical costs in this population reported significantly increased pharmaceutical costs with increased BMI for 10 of 16 drug categories. For those with a BMI of more than or equal to 35 kg/m^2, their total medication cost was twice that of their lean counterparts. The medications that were used the most among obese people were drugs for treating hypertension, diabetes, and CVDs; but increases were also seen for analgesics, antidepressants, and respiratory and ulcer medications (27). Relative to the group with BMIs between 20 and 25 kg/m^2, the mean annual costs were 25% greater among people with BMIs between 30 and 35 kg/m^2 and were 44% greater among people with BMIs of more than or equal to 35 kg/m^2. Most of these costs were largely explained by diabetes, hypertension, and CHD. The increased costs accounted for 6% of the total health care costs among the Northern California Kaiser population. The percent health care cost is comparable with the estimates for the United States population at large (9).

Future health care costs associated with obesity were also examined among 1,286 Kaiser Permanente Northwest members (28). Health plan members were nonsmoking, 35-year-olds to 64-year-olds with a BMI of more than or equal to 20 kg/m^2 in 1990. Members were excluded from the analysis if they had a history of CHD, stroke, human immunodeficiency virus, or cancer. Members were then stratified by baseline BMI (20 to 24.9 kg/m^2, 25 to 29.9 kg/m^2, and greater than or equal to 30 kg/m^2) and were evaluated for differences in their use and cost of health care services for the next 9 years (1990 to 1998). Cost ratios for prescription drugs and inpatient and outpatient services were assessed (Fig. 23.4). Although a trend of increased health care costs with increased BMI appeared to exist, only the prescription medications category was statistically significant; this may be due to a relatively small sample size for outcomes that have a great variability.

---

*A small proportion of type I diabetics were included because the type of diabetes was undifferentiated in the database.

TABLE 23.3. *Obesity[a] attributable cases and costs of selected diseases in a managed care organization with one million members*

Selected disease	Cases attributable to obesity	Annual medical care costs (1996 $ in millions)
Hypertension	132,900	72.3
Hypercholesterolemia	51,500	8.0
Type II diabetes	58,500	130.5
Coronary heart disease	16,500	83.5
Stroke	4,100	23.7
Gallbladder disease	1,701	10.2
Osteoarthritis of the knee	7,700	17.2
Endometrial cancer	53	0.5

[a]Obesity is defined as a body mass index (BMI) $\geq$29 kg/m^2.

Adapted from Oster G, Edelsborg J, O'Sullivan AK, Thompson D. The clinical and economic burden of obesity in a managed caresetting. *Am J Manag Care* 2000;6:681–689, with permission.

TABLE 23.4. *Relative rates (95% confidence interval) of health services costs associated with body mass index[a]*

Services	Body mass index (kg/m^2)			p
	25–29.9	30–34.9	$\geq$35	
Outpatient				
Visits	1.02 (0.96–1.07)	1.14 (1.06–1.23)	1.25 (1.14–1.38)	<0.001
Surgery	0.99 (0.84–1.17)	1.01 (0.79–1.29)	1.09 (0.78–1.54)	0.96
Radiology	0.68 (0.29–1.56)	1.40 (0.60–3.25)	1.73 (0.75–3.97)	0.24
Pharmacy	1.23 (1.15–1.32)	1.60 (1.48–1.74)	1.78 (1.60–1.99)	<0.001
Laboratory	0.97 (0.84–1.12)	1.24 (1.04–1.48)	1.85 (1.52–2.24)	<0.001
All outpatient	0.99 (0.88–1.13)	1.21 (1.03–1.42)	1.37 (1.11–1.68)	0.003
Inpatient services	0.83 (0.72–0.96)	1.33 (1.12–1.57)	1.70 (1.34–2.15)	<0.001
All	0.95 (0.85–1.05)	1.25 (1.10–1.41)	1.44 (1.22–1.71)	<0.001

[a]Referent group for rate ratios is body mass index 20 to 24.9 kg/m^2.

From Quesenberry CP, Caan B, Jacobson A. Obesity, health utilization and health care costs among members of a health maintenance organization. *Arch Intern Med* 1998;150:466–472, with permission.

TABLE 23.5. *Annual medical care costs (1996$) of specified health risks to the employer with 5,000 employees*

Health risk	Health risk (%)	Numbers of employees with health risk	Difference in cost (%)[a]	Annual medical care cost due to health risk ($)
Depression	2.2	110	70	129,690
High-risk body weight[b]	20	1000	21.4	337,000
Tobacco use	19.1	955	14.5	257,850
Hypertension	4	200	11.6	40,000

[a]Percentage difference in mean annual medical expenditure ($ in 1996) for high-risk versus low-risk employees.

[b]High-risk body weight defined as weight being either $\geq$30% above or $\geq$20% below the midpoint of a person's frame-adjusted desirable weight range for height.

From Goetzel RZ, Anderson DR, Whitmer RW, et al., for the HERO committee. The relationship between modifiable health risks and health care expenditures: an analysis of the multi-employer HERO health risk and cost database. *J Occup Environ Med* 1998;40:843–854, with permission.

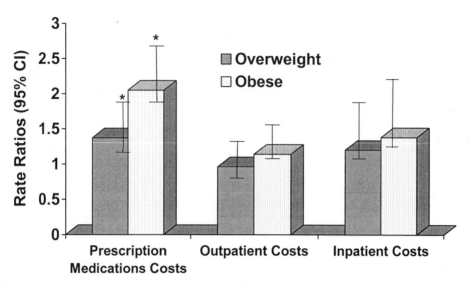

FIG. 23.4. Rate ratios (95% confidence interval [CI]) of prescription medication and outpatient and inpatient health care costs associated with overweight (body mass index [BMI] = 25 to 29.9 kg/m²) and obesity (BMI ≥ 30 kg/m²), as compared with lean managed care members (BMI = 20 to 24.9 kg/m²). *, statistically significant difference compared with lean persons. (Adapted from Thompson D, Brown JB, Nichols GA, et al. Body mass index and future health-care costs: a retrospective cohort study. *Obes Res* 2001;9:210–218, with permission.)

Pronk et al. (29) examined the impact of BMI, smoking, and physical activity on health care charges during an 18-month period among HealthPartners members who completed a 60-item questionnaire (number of subjects [n] = 5,689). They found a relatively modest increase in cost that was associated with BMI; this translated into an $11.26 increase in median charges for every 1-unit increase in BMI. This amount is lower than the costs associated with smoking ($107.81) or physical activity (−$27.99) and is much lower than other disease states, such as diabetes ($822.81) or heart disease ($901.60). This study, however, had one potential methodologic flaw in that it was statistically controlled for chronic disease (e.g., type II diabetes, CHD). Because obesity, with BMI used as a surrogate of obesity, is part of the causal pathway to the development of these diseases, inclusion of chronic disease in the model attenuates the impact of obesity. Hence, the full impact of obesity is underestimated. In a previous study among the same population, the authors noted that obesity was associated with an increase in costs of $135 per member per year (30). The homogeneous patient population (mostly white and middle to upper class) may limit the generalizability to the general population with indemnity insurance or Medicaid.

Not all studies have reported that BMI (as a surrogate for defining obesity) has an impact on health care costs. Researchers at Denver Health Medical Center measured height, waist circumference (WC), and the weight of 469 patients seen at their clinics. They reported a positive trend between BMI and annual health care costs, but it was statistically insignificant. However, they did see a significant association between health care costs and WC in this relatively small sample. People with a WC between 60 and 79 cm had average health care costs of $5,880 (±$820), whereas people with a WC between 80 and 99.9 cm and of more than 100 cm had average annual costs of $6,169 (±$668) and $7,958 (±$872), respectively (31).

In summary, from a managed care perspective, obesity (BMI of greater than or equal to 30 kg/m²) has an impact on health care use and cost, particularly pharmaceutical usage. The dominant sources of costs are type II diabetes, CHD, and hypertension. WC may be a more precise predictor of health care costs, as compared with BMI, but research in this area is only in the initial stages.

Studies from the Employer's Perspective

Employers are the major payers of health care in the United States, and hence they have a tremendous role in shaping the health care marketplace and in deciding which health care benefits to cover. Direct health care costs to the employer are in the form of premiums, which, in general, are influenced by the number and cost of claims that the employee base submits. In 1998, Burton et al. (32) evaluated the direct and indirect costs of obesity to one large employer, First Chicago National Bank (currently Bank One). A "high-risk" weight was defined as a BMI of more than or equal to 27.3 and 27.8 kg/m² for women and men, respectively. The First Chicago National Bank has an integrated health data management computer system that integrates sources of health information, including medical claims, health risk appraisal questionnaires, laboratory test results, short-term disability absences, illness days, demographic information, occupational nursing records, and more. Direct costs were evaluated among 843 employees with medical claim cost data. To reflect true medical costs, the amount charged in the claim was used and all dollars were adjusted to the 1996 value. The mean health care costs (3-year averages) for the BMI considered at risk was $6,822, compared with $4,496 for the population defined as not at risk. Hence, a 52% increase was seen in health care costs among the moderately overweight employees. The increased cost was primarily seen in women (difference in cost of $3,817), rather than men ($440). The greatest difference was seen in employees older than 45 years (Fig. 23.5). A BMI of more than 30 kg/m² represented

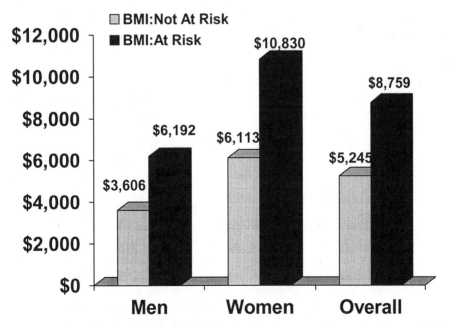

FIG. 23.5. Relation of body mass index (BMI) to health care costs for employees aged 45 and older. At-risk BMI is defined as 27.3 and 27.8 kg/m² for women and men, respectively. (Adapted from Burton WN, Chen CY, Schultz AB, et al. The economic costs associated with body mass index in a workplace. *J Occup Environ Med* 1998:786–792, with permission.)

18.7% of this population, but it had 28.9% of the total health care costs and 26.3% of the total number of health care claims. The elevated health care cost in this population was due to the increased number of claims, rather than the cost of claims, suggesting that people with higher BMIs are seeing their doctor more frequently for less expensive interventions than are those with lower BMIs. This association is more pronounced in women than men.

"Modifiable" health risks and health care expenditures were also examined among 46,026 employees from six large health care purchasers (33). Those people who reportedly had either a high or a low body weight[*] had 21% greater health care costs. Obesity compares with other conditions as follows: costs were increased by 70% for depression, by 35% for high blood glucose level, by 20% for current smokers, by 12% for hypertension, and by 10% for physical inactivity. Although body weight did not increase health care costs the most, it did affect a larger proportion of the employees (20%); hence, the health care costs associated with body weight in this population were higher than those for any other condition (Table 23.5). Overall, from the employer's perspective, obesity affects health care claims and the direct costs substantially.

Direct Medical Care Cost Savings of Weight Loss

The association between obesity and increased health care costs is robust. However, that association does not directly translate into a cost reduction or cost savings when obesity is treated. The following sections describe the models and studies that evaluate the health care cost changes associated with obesity treatment.

Models Projecting Cost Offset of Obesity Treatment

Models have been developed to estimate the cost offset associated with sustained weight loss. Models use short-term data from clinical and epidemiologic studies, and, by making specified assumptions, these models predict long-term costs and outcomes. Models are an accepted first-step method in health care economics before large-scale, long-term (longer than 5 years) clinical trials are used. Oster et al. (34) developed a two-stage model of the relationship between BMI and the risks and costs of the following five obesity-related diseases: hypertension, hypercholesterolemia, type II diabetes, CHD, and stroke. Lifetime health and economic benefits of a sustained 10% weight loss were estimated for men and women from the ages of 35 to 64 years with mild obesity (BMI of at least 27.5 kg/m²), moderate obesity (BMI of at least 32.5 kg/m²), and severe obesity (BMI of at least 37.5 kg/m²). Depending on age, gender, and initial BMI, a 10% weight loss would decrease the expected number of life-years with hypertension by 1.2 to 2.9, the expected number of years with type II diabetes by 0.5 to 1.7, and the expected number of years with hypercholesterolemia by 0.3 to 0.8 years. Lifetime risks of CHD would be decreased by 12 to 38 cases per 1,000, and stroke would be decreased by 1 to 13 cases per 1,000. The expected reduction in lifetime risk of CHD was similar among men and women, and it was greater among younger adults. Overall, a sustained 10% weight loss would increase life expectancy by 2 to 7 months for men and by 2 to 5 months for women. With regard to medical costs, a sustained 10% weight loss would decrease expected lifetime medical care costs of the five diseases by $2,300 to $5,300 per person for men and

---

[*]Most of the sample population had high body weights defined as more than 30% above the midpoint of their frame-adjusted desirable weight range for their height.

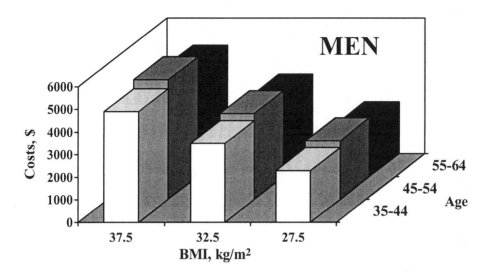

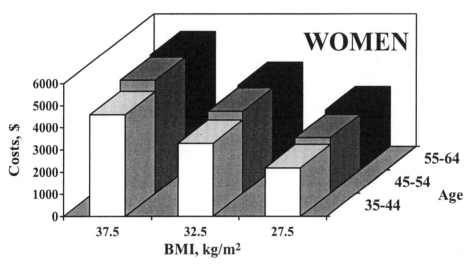

FIG. 23.6. Savings in expected lifetime medical care costs of specific obesity-related diseases (coronary heart disease, stroke, hypertension, type II diabetes, and hypercholesterolemia) with a sustained 10% weight loss by gender, age, and initial body mass index (BMI [kg/m²]) in 1996 United States dollars. (Adapted from Oster G, Thompson D, Edelsberg J, et al. Lifetime health and economic benefits of weight loss among obese persons. *Am J Public Health* 1999;89:1536–1542, with permission.)

by $2,200 to $5,200 per person for women (Fig. 23.6). Although this amount does not sound impressive, a cost savings for treating a chronic disease is rare. Most interventions cost money to save lives.

Studies Evaluating Cost Offset of Treating Obesity: Weight Loss

All of the studies that have been published have evaluated the cost offset associated with weight loss and have focused on pharmaceutical changes after weight loss. These studies are small but important to the growing body of literature; however, they are only a partial analysis of the cost offset associated with treating obesity. Collins and Anderson (35) evaluated the medication cost savings associated with a weight-management program among diabetic men and women. The study included 32 patients taking insulin (n = 8) or oral agents, and it estimated the medication costs for diabetes and hypertension medication only before the start of the study, after a 12-week weight-management program, and at the end of 1 year. At the end of the 12-week program, 75% of the people taking insulin were able to discontinue insulin use totally, and the remaining decreased their dosage by an average of 71%. At the end of the weight loss program, the average monthly cost for insulin therapy had dropped by 91%, and, after 1 year, only one patient had resumed insulin therapy. The average per patient medication cost savings was $443 per year.

Greenway et al. (36) determined the cost savings of pharmaceutical agents used to treat diabetes, hypertension, and hyperlipidemia, compared with that of pharmaceutical agents used to treat obesity. A modest weight loss (6% to 10%) produced a net cost savings of $122.64 per month for insulin-treated diabetics, of $42.92 per month for diabetics treated with sulfonylureas, of $61.07 per month for people treated for hyperlipidemia, and of $0.20 per month for people treated for hypertension.

Malone et al. (37) evaluated the changes in medication cost before and after gastric surgery. Before gastric surgery, an obese patient's medications cost was on average $391 per day. Cost for medications decreased to $230 per day by 3 months; medication costs were reduced by 60% from presurgical costs at 6, 9, and 12 months after gastric surgery.

In a large randomized clinical trial of orlistat in obese patients with type II diabetes who were taking sulfonylurea, Hollander et al. (38) secondarily evaluated the percentage of patients who reduced their dose or who discontinued sulfonylurea with a modest weight loss. People in the orlistat-treated group lost only 1.9% more body weight than the placebo group; however, 43.2% of them decreased their dose of sulfonylurea versus 28.9% in the placebo group, and 11.7% discontinued their use of sulfonylurea, compared with 0% in the placebo group. Although the authors did not translate this into costs, this provides further support for the idea that a modest weight loss decreases comorbid medication use.

The SOS study is the first large-scale study to provide economic information on the health care cost changes that occur after treating obesity, and its economic results are just beginning to be published. This study is an ongoing prospective study that compares the health and economic outcomes of 2,010 surgically treated patients with those of 2,038 matched conventionally treated obese patients. Because the treatment is surgery, which has substantial costs and health care use associated with it, the results may not be generalizable to behavioral or pharmaceutical treatment modalities.

Six years after intervention, the average weight loss was 15% in the surgically treated group and 1% in the conventionally treated group. The total medication cost increased in both groups over the 6-year period, and no significant difference was found in total pharmaceutical cost between groups. Average drug-specific costs were different between the groups, however. The surgically treated group had lower diabetes and CVD medication costs, but the costs for anemia and gastrointestinal disorder medications were higher than those of the conventionally treated group (39).

The SOS also compared changes in inpatient costs between the surgically treated group and the conventionally treated group. They reported that the aggregated cost of hospital care for 6 years of follow-up was U.S. $10,204 in the surgically treated group, compared with U.S. $2,827 in the conventionally treated group (40). The reduction in

TABLE 23.6. *The cost and effectiveness of obesity treatment in the United States*

Treatment modality	Mean weight loss (%)	Annual cost ($)	One time cost ($)
Lifestyle	6–8[a]		
Weight Watchers program		560	
Diet and Exercise with registered dietician		450–1,200	
Supervised program with doctor		2,000–3,500	
Very low calorie diet	8[a]	2,500	
Pharmacotherapy	7–10[b]		
		245–735[c]	
Phentermine			
Sibutramine		1,090–1,343[c]	
Orlistat		1,300[c]	
Gastric surgery	15–25[d]		20,000–25,000[e]

[a]Average weight loss provided in the National Heart, Lung, and Blood Institute Evidence Report on the Clinical Guidelines on the Identification, Evaluation and Treatment of Overweight and Obesity in Adults.
[b]Based on 1-year to 2-year randomized clinical trials by the manufacturer.
[c]Wholesale price of the medication. The cost does not include lifestyle counseling.
[d]Based on the Swedish Obesity Subjects (SOS) Study. Year 1 average weight loss was 21%, which decreased to 16% by year 4 (51).
[e]Based on price quoted for gastric bypass by gastric surgery centers in Kentucky and California for self-payers.
From Wolf A. Colditz G. Current estimates of the economic cost of obesity in the United States. *Obes Res* 1998,6:97–106, with permission.

inpatient care resulting from improved health with the 15% weight loss was not enough to offset the inpatient costs of gastric surgery and the complications that arose from gastric surgery. This study highlights the importance of accounting for the cost of treatment and the long-term cost reductions resulting from improvement in health (Table 23.6). Hence, initial reports from the SOS study do not support the idea that weight loss by gastric surgery will reduce future health care expenditures.

Long-term studies using various treatment modalities (e.g., behavioral therapy, pharmacotherapy, and surgery) that account for the cost of obesity treatment (Table 23.6) and that evaluate the impact of long-term weight loss on a fuller spectrum of economic outcomes are in progress, but the results will not be available for many years. In the meantime, models with solid assumptions can be developed that will help guide policy until these long-term studies are complete.

Cost-Effectiveness Models

CEAs evaluate the cost and the effects of an intervention and at least one alternative. For instance, the analysis might compare behavioral treatment to pharmacotherapy or to surgical intervention. The results are presented in a ratio of incremental costs (in dollars) to incremental effects ("incremental" meaning that one intervention is compared to the other, so the result represents the difference in costs and effects between interventions). The effects are long-term health outcomes, such as life-years gained (LYG), event-free LYG, or QALYs. For reference purposes, any cost to effectiveness ratio of less than or equal to $50,000 per QALY is considered a cost-effective therapeutic option.

To date, a few models have evaluated the cost-effectiveness of obesity treatments. The National Institutes of Clinical Excellence (NICE), which is part of the National Health System (NHS) in the United Kingdom, commissioned CEAs to determine the NHS policy on covering sibutramine and orlistat. The CEA for sibutramine came from the manufacturer, who estimated it to be U.S. $15,337 per QALY. The NICE evaluation panel considered some of the assumptions "optimistic" and adjusted the ratio to U.S. $22,000 to $44,000 per QALY. The terms of this ratio were that a patient had to lose at least 2 kg of absolute weight in the first 4 weeks and to achieve a weight reduction of 5% by 3 months (41). NICE also commissioned an independent (i.e., not from the manufacturer) CEA on the use of orlistat. The independent review estimated a cost per QALY gained of U.S. $68,000 if orlistat was used in all overweight people (defined as a BMI of at least 27 kg/m^2). If orlistat was used under the same conditions as sibutramine (initial weight loss in first 4 weeks and cumulative 5% weight loss by 3 months), the cost per QALY would be similar to that of sibutramine ($30,000 to $44,000) (42). The NHS in the United Kingdom provides both medications.

In Belgium, Lamotte et al. (43) estimated the cost-effectiveness of using orlistat in obese patients with type II diabetes and/or hypertension and hypercholesterolemia, as compared with diet and exercise alone (plus a placebo). The clinical effects of orlistat on hemoglobin A$_{Ic}$, blood pressure, and low-density lipoprotein cholesterol were taken from a 1-year randomized clinical trial (38). The data regarding the risk of microvascular and macrovascular complications were based on the United Kingdom Prospective Diabetes Study (UKPDS) substudy in obese patients treated with metformin (44). The cost per LYG was the best if the patient had type II diabetes, hypercholesterolemia, and hypertension (EUR $3,462 per LYG). The ratio remained favorable when a patient had two comorbid conditions (e.g., hypercholesterolemia and type II diabetes, EUR $7,407 per LYG; hypertension and type II diabetes, EUR $7,388 per LYG) and when they had type II diabetes without cardiovascular events (EUR $19,986 per LYG). This study suggests that the use of orlistat is cost-effective in the management of obese type II diabetic patients, particularly those with hypercholesterolemia and/or hypertension.

Another study that was based in the United States also estimates the cost-effectiveness of using orlistat, compared with dietary therapy, in obese patients with type II diabetes alone (45). Maetzel et al. (45) used clinical data from a metaanalysis of four randomized clinical trials (n = 1,749) of overweight and obese patients with type II diabetes taking diabetes medication. The data regarding risk of microvascular and macrovascular complications are based on the UKPDS (46). The model followed the patients' morbidity and mortality for 11 years. The authors report that, under the assumption of a 3-year persistence of the effect of orlistat (after 1 year of treatment), the cost per event-free LYG would be $7,594. If no persistence of the effect of orlistat was seen after treatment, the cost per event-free LYG would be $20,578. Hence, under the assumptions made, the cost-effectiveness of using orlistat supports its administration in overweight and obese type II diabetics.

Indirect Costs of Obesity

Morbidity Costs Lost Productivity, Functional Capability, and Health-Related Quality of Life

Illness affects one's abilities in profound ways; therefore, the "costs" associated with illness can be measured multidimensionally through productivity standards, short-term and long-term disability, functional capability, and health-related quality of life. Lost productivity and functional capability have a substantial impact at the individual and societal level because they have a tangible influence on the quality of life for individuals and affect the national workforce productivity. Approximately 27% of the United States labor force has a BMI of 29 kg/m^2 or more (35). Eight studies have evaluated the impact of obesity on indirect morbidity outcomes and costs (9,19,32,47–51).

Productivity and Functional Capability from a National Perspective

Published reports indicate that the indirect economic costs of obesity to business are substantial. Thompson et al. (47) estimated the cost of mild obesity (BMI of 25 to 28.9 kg/m^2) and moderate to severe obesity (BMI of greater than or equal to 29 kg/m^2) to United States businesses. Data were obtained from various secondary sources, including the NHIS, Bureau of Labor Statistics reports, and published reports on obesity from large United States epidemiologic studies. The diseases that were accounted for were CHD, hypertension, type II diabetes, hypercholesterolemia, stroke, gallbladder disease, osteoarthritis of the knee, and endometrial cancer. They found that, as body weight increases above a healthy body weight, greater amounts of lost productivity and disability are seen (Fig. 23.7). The cost of obesity to United States businesses in 1994 was estimated at $12.7 billion, 80% of which was due to moderate to severe obesity. By far, the greatest component of this expenditure was health insurance, which comprised $7.7 billion (61%) of the total. Paid sick leave, life insurance, and disability insurance amounted to $2.4 billion, $1.8 billion, and $800 million, respectively. The mean number of workdays lost and the level of disability increased as BMI and age increased.

Using the 1988 and 1994 NHIS, Wolf and Colditz (9) estimated the amount and costs associated with lost productivity, restricted activity, and bed days attributable to obesity over a 6-year period. Restricted activity and bed days are representative of a loss in functional capability. Restricted activity is defined as the number of days in which one's activity level is restricted because of illness or disability, whereas bed days are the number of days that a person is resigned to bed because of illness or disability. A substantial amount of lost productivity, restricted activity, and bed days was associated with being over-

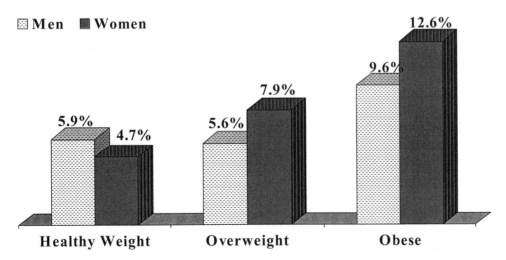

FIG. 23.7. Prevalence of disability (as measured by self-reported inability to work) by categories of body weight. Healthy body weight is defined as a body mass index (BMI) of less than 25 kg/m^2, overweight is defined as a BMI between 25 and 28.9 kg/m^2, and obese is defined as a BMI of 29 kg/m^2 or more. (Adapted from Thompson D, Edelsberg J, Kinsey KL, et al. Estimated economic costs of obesity to U.S. business. *Am J Health Promot* 1998;13:120–127, with permission.)

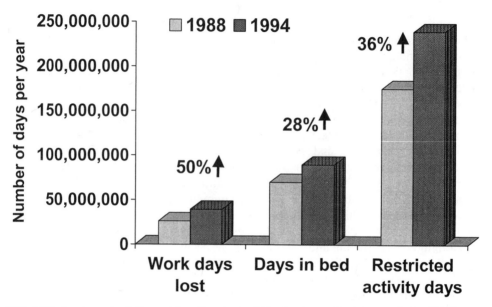

FIG. 23.8. Lost productivity and functional capability in obese (body mass index [BMI] ≥ 30 kg/m²) adults, compared with lean individuals (BMI < 25 kg/m²)—National Health Interview Survey, 1988 and 1994. (Adapted from Wolf A, Colditz G. Current estimates of the economic cost of obesity in the United States. *Obes Res* 1998;6:97–106, with permission.)

weight and obese in each given year; however, the striking finding was the increase in lost productivity and the loss in functional capability that occurred from 1988 to 1994 (Fig. 23.8). In 1994, among persons who were obese (BMI of greater than 30 kg/m²), 239 million excess restricted activity days, 89.5 million excess bed days, and 39.2 million excess workdays were lost compared with those of lean persons (BMI of less than 25 kg/m²). The cost of the lost productivity in 1995 dollars amounted to $3.93 billion. Comparing the 1988 and 1994 data for persons with a BMI of more than or equal to 30 kg/m², a 50% increase in lost productivity, a 36% increase in restricted activity, and a 28% increase in the number of bed days were observed during this 6-year period. Most of the increase appears to be a reflection of the increased prevalence of obesity among the United States population, with the only exception being for lost productivity, in which the increase was *also* due to an increase in the average number of workdays lost per obese person. In summary, the impact of obesity on the indirect morbidity cost and functional capability is measurable, and it is growing as the prevalence of obesity continues to rise.

Productivity from an Employer's Perspective

Four studies have evaluated the impact of body weight from an employer's perspective. Tucker and Friedman (48) evaluated the impact of obesity, as defined by the three-site skinfold technique, on the number of sick days among 10,825 employed adults. Obese employees were more than twice as likely to experience high-level absenteeism (defined as seven or more absences because of illness during the past 6 months) and were 1.49 times more likely to have moderate absenteeism (three to six absences because of illness during the past 6 months) than were lean employees. In day to day operations, this means that, if a company had 1,000 obese employees in an employee base of 3,500, the cost of high absenteeism among the obese would be $108,800 per year. Thus, based on an estimate of the difference in the cost of absenteeism between the obese and lean, an employer with an employee base of 3,500 pays an estimated $51,200 per year in lost productivity from obesity.

Shell Oil Company evaluated factors influencing illness among 2,287 employees at a manufacturing plant during a 9-year period (1986 to 1994) (49). Increased illness was associated with known health risk factors, such as smoking, elevated blood pressure, high cholesterol, and obesity (BMI greater than or equal to 27.2 kg/m^2 for men and greater than or equal to 26.9 kg/m^2 for women). Obese women had double the illness rate of nonobese women, an effect that was greater than that observed for smoking, hypertension, or hypercholesterolemia. Among male employees, the absence rate was 35% greater among the obese, which was comparable to the absence rate seen with hypertension and which was greater than that seen with hypercholesterolemia. Further analysis indicated that obesity had an impact on the risk of some common disease categories that in turn affected absenteeism. For instance, mental disorders were higher among obese women (1.1 versus 0.8 per 100), and musculoskeletal disorders and heart disease were higher among obese men (musculoskeletal disorders, 3.2 versus 2.0 per 100; and heart disease, 1.1 versus 0.7 per 100) than in their lean counterparts.

Burton et al. (32) also studied productivity in their analyses of the impact of obesity on the First Chicago National Bank (see "Direct Medical Costs of Obesity: Studies from the Employer's Perspective" above for methods). The study of indirect costs evaluated 3,066 employees who had 3 consecutive years of employment records and who did not experience pregnancy from 1989 to 1995. Employees at a "high risk" BMI had twice as many sick days (average of 8.45 days per year) as did employees with a healthy body weight (average of 3.73 days per year). The excess cost of sick leave to employers because of obesity was $863 per moderately overweight employee during a 3-year period (Fig. 23.9); this amount increases to $1,379 among older (i.e., over 45 years of age) over-

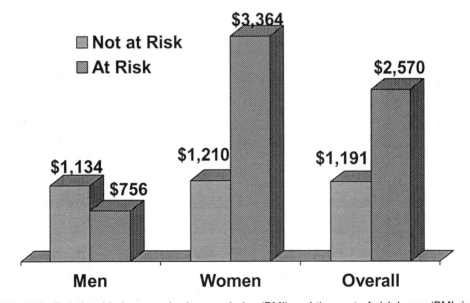

FIG. 23.9. Relationship between body mass index (BMI) and the cost of sick leave. (BMI risk is defined as ≥27.8 kg/m^2 for men and ≥27.3 kg/m^2 for women.) (Adapted from Burton WN, Chen CY, Schultz AB, et al. The economic costs associated with body mass index in a workplace. *J Occup Environ Med* 1998:786–792, with permission.)

Hours Lost per Week

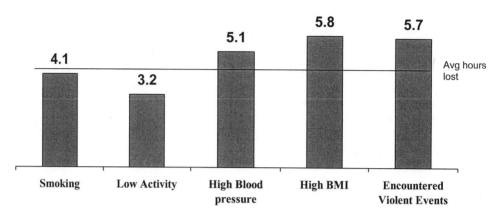

FIG. 23.10. Hours of productivity lost per week by selected health risk. (Adapted from Burton WN, Conti DJ, Chen CY, et al. The role of health risk factors and disease on worker productivity. *J Occup Environ Med* 1999;41:863–877, with permission.)

weight employees. Burton et al. (50) also observed that being moderately overweight affects a worker's productivity during the workday as measured by a productivity scale. Employees with "at-risk BMI" lost, on average, 5.79 hours per week, or 31% more time than the average employee (mean was 4.43 hours per week). Moderately overweight employees had productivity standards that were similar to those for other chronic disease risk factors (e.g., hypertension and hypercholesterolemia) and that were worse than many lifestyle risk factors (e.g., smoking and physical inactivity) (Fig. 23.10).

Thus, in general, absence rates among the obese are approximately double those among their lean counterparts. Why obese women tend to have greater amounts of workdays lost compared with obese men is not clear.

Weight Loss's Impact on Productivity

Only one published study, which was from the SOS study (51), has examined the impact of weight loss on productivity and disability. Before the intervention, the mean BMI of subjects was 41 kg/m². After 4 years of treatment, weight reduction in the surgically treated group was approximately 20%, whereas the controls maintained their weight. In the year before treatment, the average number of sick days and the amount of disability pension were similar in both groups. After treatment, the surgical group had 35% more days of sickness compared with the controls in the first year as a result of the recuperative process after the surgery, but it used 10% to 14% fewer days during years 2 and 3. During the fourth year, the days of sickness were lower (8%) in the surgical group, but this was not statistically significant (p =0.07).

Mortality Costs

Obesity has been associated with early mortality in many large epidemiologic studies (52–55). Thompson et al. (21) estimated that life expectancy would decrease by 0.2 to 1.8 years as compared with lean individuals, depending on gender, age, and current BMI. As BMI increased, the life expectancy decreased. No studies have evaluated the mortality costs of obesity. One study has estimated the indirect cost of obesity, including morbidity costs (lost productivity) and mortality costs. Using various secondary sources, Wolf and Colditz (9) estimated the indirect burden of obesity in 1995 dollars, accounting for six diseases associated with obesity as well—type II diabetes; gallbladder disease; osteoarthritis; and postmenopausal breast, endometrial, and colon cancers. The indirect cost associated with obesity was estimated to be $47.56 billion in 1995, which, in 2001 dollars, would be $58.8 billion. This figure may be a gross underestimate because it does not include major diseases, such as CHD and hypertension, which are felt to have large indirect costs. These were not included because the indirect cost data of these and many other disease states were unavailable.

Health-Related Quality of Life

Health-related quality of life is not typically a component of classic economic analyses. Although quality of life is a humanistic (versus economic) outcome measure, the authors briefly address this topic because quality of life affects cost to effectiveness ratios. Fontaine et al. (56) assessed the quality of life of 312 obese people and compared their scores with the United States normative values using the validated SF-36 (Medical Outcomes Study–Short Form-36 Health Survey). Obese individuals scored significantly lower on all of the scales—physical functioning, physical role, bodily pain, general health, vitality, social functioning, emotional role, and mental health. The impact of obesity was greatest on the vitality scale, bodily pain, and physical functioning. Moreover, when the obese population was stratified as mildly, moderately, and morbidly overweight, the moderately and morbidly overweight groups had significantly lower scores than the mildly overweight group for the following scales: physical functioning, physical role, bodily pain, general health, vitality, and social functioning (Table 23.7). This study indicates that obesity affects all aspects of quality of life but most predominantly the physical aspects. Additionally, the degree of obesity correlates with these variables, with the more obese enduring a poorer quality of life.

Recently, the Nurses Health Study evaluated the impact of a 4-year weight change (1992 to 1996) on health-related quality of life using the SF-36 among 37,429 registered nurses in the United States (57). In this group, 39% maintained their weight, 38% gained

TABLE 23.7. *Quality of life indicator (Short-form-36 scores): comparison of mildly, moderately, and morbidly obese people*

SF-36 item	Short-form (SF)-36 scores (mean, SD)			
	Mildly (n = 35)	Moderately (n = 163)	Morbidly (n = 80)	F-test
Physical functioning	85.6[a] (17.5)	79.4[b] (21.0)	51.9 (26.8)	45.6[c]
Role—physical	85.0[a] (26.1)	77.8[b] (33.1)	46.3 (37.6)	23.8[c]
Bodily pain	66.4[a] (27.7)	54.5[b] (27.5)	43.2 (22.1)	9.6[c]
General health	72.0[a] (20.5)	65.7[b] (20.3)	54.3 (18.0)	11.8[c]
Vitality	49.5[a] (18.6)	48.1[b] (21.3)	38.0 (19.1)	6.9[c]
Social functioning	84.9[a] (17.2)	79.3[b] (24.1)	67.9 (26.9)	7.3[c]
Role—emotional	85.4 (32.3)	75.3 (36.6)	69.3 (40.1)	2.4
Mental health	74.3 (11.8)	68.6 (18.7)	65.6 (19.6)	2.6

Higher scores indicate greater health-related quality of life. Total number of subjects was 278.
Abbreviations: n, number of subjects; sd, standard deviation.
[a]Mildly obese differed significantly (*p* <0.05) from morbidly obese.
[b]Moderately obese differed significantly (*p* <0.05) from morbidly obese.
[c]*p* <0.001, two-tailed probability.
From Fontaine KR, Chestin LJ, Barofsky L. Health-related quality of life in obese persons seeking treatment. *J Fam Pract* 1996;43:265–270, with permission.

between 5 and 20 lb, and 17% lost between 5 and 20 lb. Weight gain was associated with decreased physical function and vitality, as well as increased bodily pain, regardless of baseline weight. Even among the women who were lean at baseline, a weight gain of 20 lb or more was significantly associated with the development of role limitations because of physical problems (odds ratio, 2.05; 95% confidence interval, 1.69–2.49). Weight loss, both unintentional and intentional, in overweight women was associated with improved physical function and vitality, as well as decreased bodily pain. Weight change was more strongly associated with physical, rather than mental, health, a finding that has been consistent among all studies evaluating health-related quality of life and obesity. Because weight loss and the maintenance of the weight loss take an incredible amount of sustained effort (58), the difficultly in maintaining weight loss may diminish the improved mental health benefits of losing the weight.

Fontaine et al. (59) also examined the effect of weight loss on health-related quality of life. Thirty-eight moderately obese people (mean BMI of 31 kg/m^2) were treated for 13 weeks. Participants completed the SF-36 both before and after treatment,. Participants lost an average of 10% of their body weight during the 13 weeks. Modest weight loss was associated with significantly improved quality of life with respect to the following health domains of the SF-36: physical functioning, physical role, general health, vitality, and mental health. The largest improvements were observed in vitality, general health perceptions, and physical role. Hence, obesity decreases one's health-related quality of life, and weight loss improves quality of life.

CONCLUSION

From all published reports, the cost of obesity throughout the world is substantial. Across all countries that have estimated the economic impact of obesity, the cost is considerable, ranging from 2% to 6% of a country's national health expenditure. The countries that have the lowest prevalence of obesity tend to have a lower economic burden from this disease. Unfortunately, the prevalence and absolute number of persons who are overweight and obese in the United States now ranks among the highest in the world. In the United States, from all perspectives (e.g., government, MCO, and employers), health care use, health care costs, and indirect economic outcomes are associated with obesity. Published studies have reported that the dominant sources of the costs of obesity arise from type II diabetes, CHD, and hypertension, suggesting that targeting a segment of the population (those with these conditions) for treatment purposes may be the most cost-effective way of treating obesity. Cost-effectiveness models support this conclusion. Large long-term studies that will provide a cost to effectiveness ratio are underway so that the most cost-effective treatment modality may be determined.

To further the understanding of the health care economics of weight management, an evaluation of the direct and indirect cost offset of obesity prevention and treatment would be beneficial. As obesity continues to grow in epidemic proportions, the prevention of obesity in adults and children will become more pressing. Currently, in the United States, increased rates of type II diabetes are being observed in adults and children, mirroring the increased body weight and fatness among these groups (60,61). Furthermore, recent reports from the Diabetes Prevention Program and the Finnish Trial suggest that a modest weight loss (7%) can lower the development of type II diabetes by 58% in obese people who are at risk of developing diabetes (62,63). Moreover, modest weight gain (5 to 10 kg) in adults, independent of obesity, is associated with greater health care costs (19). Therefore, preventive efforts should focus on the cessation of adult weight gain, and the prevention of adulthood and childhood obesity may have major public health and potential health care cost ramifications.

More research is needed on both the costs and cost-effectiveness of obesity weight loss. Little information is available about the impact of weight loss on other dimensions of direct health care cost (e.g., physician visits, hospital care and length of stay, and laboratory costs) besides pharmaceutical use. Additionally, only one study (51) has evaluated the impact of weight loss on productivity and disability, and the only intervention evaluated was surgical. Because of the long recuperative process involved in gastric surgery, this study cannot be generalized to noninvasive obesity treatments; hence, no data is available on the indirect cost offset of noninvasive treatment for obesity. Finally, as treatments of obesity evolve, cost-effectiveness studies must be performed so that cost-effective methods will be used in the treatment of obesity.

REFERENCES

1. Segal L, Carter R, Zimmet P. The cost of obesity: the Australian perspective. *Pharmacoeconomics* 1994;5:45–52.
2. Levy E, Levy P, Le Pen C, et al. Economic cost of obesity: the French situation. *Int J Obes* 1995;19:788–792.
3. Detourneay B, Fagnani F, Phillippo M, et al. Obesity morbidity and health care costs in France: an analysis of the 1991–1992 Medical Care Household Survey. *Int J Obes Relat Metab Disord* 2000;24;151–155.
4. Birmingham CL, Muller JL, Palepu A, et al. The cost of obesity in Canada. *CMAJ* 1999;160:483–488.
5. Swinburn B, Ashton T, Gillespie J, et al. Healthcare costs of obesity in New Zealand. *Int J Obes Relat Metab Disord* 1997;21:891–896.
6. Pereira J, Mateus C, Amaral MJ. Direct costs of obesity in Portugal [Abstract]. *Value Health* 2000;3:64.
7. Seidell JC, Deerenberg I. Obesity in Europe: prevalence and consequences for use of medical care. *Pharmacoeconomics.* 1994;5:38–44.
8. Narbro K, Jonsson E, Larsson B, et al. Economic consequences of sick-leave and early retirement in obese Swedish women. *Int J Obes* 1996;20:895–903.
9. Wolf A, Colditz G. Current estimates of the economic cost of obesity in the United States. *Obes Res* 1998;6:97–106.
10. *Tipping the scales.* Melbourne: the Consumer Advocacy and Financial Counseling Association of Australia, 1992.
11. World Health Organization. The economic costs of overweight and obesity. *Obesity: preventing and managing the global epidemic.* Report of a WHO consultation on obesity, Geneva, June 3–5, 1997. Geneva: World Health Organization, 1998:83–103.
12. Narbro K, Ågren G, Jonsson E, et al. Pharmaceutical costs in the obese: a comparison with a randomly selected population sample, and long-term changes after conventional and surgical treatment. The SOS intervention study [Dissertation]. Sweden: Göteborg University, 2001.
13. Narbro K, Sjöström L. Willingness to pay for obesity treatment. *Int J Technol Assess Health Care* 2000;16:50–59.
14. National Institutes of Health. Consensus development conference on diet and exercise in non–insulin dependent type II diabetes mellitus. *Diabetes Care* 1987;10:639–644.
15. Entmacher PS, Sinnock P, Bostic E, et al. Economic impact of diabetes. In: Harris MI, Hamman RF, eds. *Diabetes in America.* NIH publication no. 85-1468. Bethesda, MD: National Diabetes Data Group, National Institutes of Health, 1985.
16. Rubin RJ, Altman WM, Medelson DN. Health care expenditures for people with diabetes mellitus, 1992. *J Clin Endocrinol Metab* 1994;78:809A–809F.
17. American Diabetes Association. Economic consequences of diabetes mellitus in the United States in 1997. *Diabetes Care* 1998;21:296–309.
18. Hodgson TA, Cohen AJ. Medical care expenditures for selected circulatory diseases: opportunities for reducing national health expenditures. *Medical Care* 1999;37:994–1012.
19. Wolf AM, Colditz GA. Social and economic impact of body weight in the United States. *Am J Clin Nutr* 1996;63:466S–469S.
20. Colditz GA. Economic costs of obesity and inactivity. *Med Sci Sports Exerc* 1999;31:S663–S667.
21. Thompson D, Edelberg J, Colditz GA, et al. Lifetime health and economic consequences of obesity. *Arch Intern Med* 1999;159:2177–2183.
22. Gorsky RD, Pamuk, E, Williamson DF, et al. The 25-year health care costs of women who remain overweight after 40 years of age. *Am J Prev Med* 1996;12:388–394.
23. Sturm R. The effects of obesity, smoking, and drinking on medical problems and costs. *Health Affairs* 2002;21:245–253.
24. Oster G, Edelsberg J, O'Sullivan AK, et al. The clinical and economic burden of obesity in a managed care setting. *Am J Manag Care* 2000;6:681–689.

25. Flegal KM, Carroll MD, Kuczmarski RJ, et al. Overweight and obesity in the United States: prevalence and trends, 1960–1994. *Int J Obes Relat Metab Disord* 1998;22:39–47.
26. Quesenberry CP, Caan B, Jacobson A. Obesity, health utilization and health care costs among members of a health maintenance organization. *Arch Intern Med* 1998;158:466–472.
27. Caan B, Quesenberry C, Stolcheck B, et al. Increases in pharmacy costs among obese members in an HMO. Presentation at NAASO annual meeting. November, 1999. Charleston, SC. *Obes Res* 1999;7:54S.
28. Thompson D, Brown JB, Nichols GA, et al. Body mass index and future health-care costs: a retrospective cohort study. *Obes Res* 2001;9:210–218.
29. Pronk NP, Goodman MJ, O'Connor PJ, et al. Relationship between modifiable health risks and short-term health care charges. *JAMA* 1999;282:2235–2239.
30. Pronk NP, Tan A, O'Connor P. Obesity, fitness, willingness to communicate and health care costs. *Med Sci Sports Exerc* 1999;31:1535–1543.
31. Tate CW, Bessesen DH. The relationship between body mass index, waist circumference and costs of medical care. Presentation at NAASO annual meeting. November, 1999. Charleston, SC. *Obes Res* 1999;7:54S.
32. Burton WN, Chen CY, Schultz AB, et al. The economic costs associated with body mass index in a workplace. *J Occup Environ Med* 1998;40:786–792.
33. Goetzel RZ, Anderson DR, Whitmer RW, et al.The relationship between modifiable health risks and health care expenditures: an analysis of the multi-employer HERO health risk and cost database. The Health Enhancement Research Organization (HERO) Research committee *J Occup Environ Med* 1998;40:843–854.
34. Oster G, Thompson D, Edelsberg J, et al. Lifetime health and economic benefits of weight loss among obese persons. *Am J Public Health* 1999;89:1536–1542.
35. Collins RW, Anderson JW. Medication cost savings associated with weight loss for obese non–insulin-dependent diabetic men and women. *Prev Med* 1995;24:369–374.
36. Greenway FL, Ryan DH, Bray GA, et al. Pharmaceutical cost savings of treating obesity with weight loss medications. *Obes Res* 1999;7:523–531.
37. Malone M, Alger S, Kispert P, et al. Changes in medication uses after gastric restrictive surgery. Presentation at NAASO annual meeting. November, 1999. Charleston, SC. *Obes Res* 1999;7:54S.
38. Hollander PA, Elbein SC, Hirsch IB, et al. Role of orlistat in the treatment of obese patients with type 2 diabetes. *Diabetes Care* 1998;21:1288–1294.
39. Narbro K, Ågren, G, Jonsson E, et al. Pharmaceutical costs in the obese: a comparison with a randomly selected population sample, and long-term changes after conventional and surgical treatment. In: Narbro K, ed. *Economic aspects on obesity. Results from the Swedish Obese Subjects Study* [Dissertation]. Göteburg, Sweden: Göteburg University, 2001.
40. Ågren G, Narbro K, Jonsson E, et al. Cost of in-patient care among the obese. A prospective study of surgically and conventionally treated patients in the Swedish Obese Subjects intervention study. In: Narbro K, ed. *Economic aspects on obesity. Results from the Swedish Obese Subjects Study* [Dissertation]. Göteburg, Sweden: Göteburg University, 2001.
41. National Institute for Clinical Excellence. *Guidance on the use of sibutramine for the treatment of obesity in adults.* Technology Appraisal Guidance, No. 31. London: National Institute for Clinical Excellence, 2001. Available at: http://www.nice.org.uk/Docref.asp?d=23004. Accessed September 30, 2002.
42. National Institute for Clinical Excellence. *Guidance on the use of orlistat for the treatment of obesity in adults.* Technology Appraisal Guidance, No. 22. London: National Institute for Clinical Excellence, 2001. Available at: http://www.nice.org.uk/cat.asp?c=15712. Accessed September 30, 2002.
43. Lamotte M, Annemans L, Lefever A, et al. A health economic model to assess the long-term effects and cost-effectiveness of orlistat in obese type 2 diabetic patients. *Diabetes Care* 2002;25:303–308.
44. United Kingdom Prospective Diabetes Study Group. Effect of intensive blood glucose control with metformin on complications in overweight patients with type 2 diabetes. *Lancet* 1998;352:854–865.
45. Maetzel A, Ruof J, Covington M, et al. Cost effectiveness of treatment of overweight and obese diabetic patients with orlistat [Abstract]. *Diabetes* 2002;51:A276.
46. Stratton IM, Adler AI, Neil HA, et al. Association of glycaemia with macrovascular and microvascular complications of type 2 diabetes (UKPDS 35): prospective observational study [see Comments]. *BMJ* 2000;321:405–412.
47. Thompson D, Edelsberg J, Kinsey KL, et al. Estimated economic costs of obesity to U.S. business. *Am J Health Promot* 1998;13:120–127.
48. Tucker LA, Friedman GM. Obesity and absenteeism: an epidemiologic study of 10,825 employed adults. *Am J Health Promot* 1998;12:202–207.
49. Tsai SP, Gilstrap EL, Colangelo TA, et al. Illness absence at an oil refinery and petrochemical plant. *J Occup Environ Med* 1997;39:455–460.
50. Burton WN, Conti DJ, Chen CY, et al. The role of health risk factors and disease on worker productivity. *J Occup Environ Med* 1999;41:863–877.
51. Nabro K, Agren G, Jonsson E, et al. Sick leave and disability pension before and after treatment for obesity: a report from the Swedish Obese Subjects (SOS) study. *Int J Obes Relat Metab Disord* 1999;23:619–624.
52. Manson JE, Willett WC, Stampfer MJ, et al. Body weight and mortality among women. *N Engl J Med* 1995;333:677–685.
53. Manson JE, Stampfer MJ, Hennekens CH, et al. Body weight and longevity: a reassessment. *JAMA* 1987;257:353–358.

54. Calle EE, Thun MJ, Petrelli JM, et al. Body mass index and mortality in a prospective cohort of U.S. adults. *N Engl J Med* 1999;341:1097–1105.
55. Allison DB, Fontaine KR, Manson JE, et al. Annual deaths attributable to obesity in the United States. *JAMA* 1999;282:1530–1538.
56. Fontaine KR, Cheskin LJ, Barofsky I. Health-related quality of life in obese persons seeking treatment. *J Fam Pract* 1996;43:265–270.
57. Fine JT, Colditz GA, Coakley EH, et al. A prospective study of weight change and health-related quality of life in women. *JAMA* 1999;282:2136–2142.
58. Klem ML, Wing RR, McGuire MT, et al. A descriptive study of individuals successful at long-term weight maintenance of substantial weight loss. *Am J Clin Nutr* 1997;66:239–246.
59. Fontaine KR, Barofsky I, Andersen RE, et al. Impact of weight loss on health-related quality of life. *Qual Life Res* 1999;8:275–277.
60. Mokdad AH, Ford ES, Bowman BA, et al. Diabetes trends in the U.S.: 1990–1998. *Diabetes Care* 2000;23: 1278–1283.
61. Type 2 diabetes in children and adolescents. American Diabetes Association. *Diabetes Care* 2000;22:381–389.
62. Knowler WC, Barrett-Connor E, Fowler SE, et al. Reduction in the incidence of type 2 diabetes with lifestyle intervention or metformin. *N Engl J Med* 2002;346:393–403.
63. Tuomilehto H, Lindstrom J, Eriksson JG, et al. Prevention of type 2 diabetes mellitus by changes in lifestyle among subjects with impaired glucose intolerance. *N Engl J Med* 2001;344:343–350.

24

Treatment of Childhood Obesity

Sarah E. Barlow

The prevalence of obesity in the United States has risen among both children and adults. Between 1980 and 1994, the percent of obese 6-year-old to 11-year-old children (body mass index [BMI] greater than or equal to the 95th percentile) increased from 7.5% to 10.8%. At the same time, the percent of obese 12-year-old to 17-year-old adolescents increased from 5.7% to 10.6% (1). Data from 1999 to 2000 show a continued increase to 15.3% and 15.5% in these two age-groups (2). This rapid increase has affected not only different age-groups but also diverse economic and racial and ethnic groups (3). Childhood obesity is a risk factor for adult obesity (4), and it increases the risk of many health conditions in adulthood, including cardiovascular disease risk factors (e.g., type II diabetes mellitus, hypertension, dyslipidemia), cardiovascular disease itself, type II diabetes mellitus, and mortality (5,6). Unfortunately, many overweight children experience obesity-related health problems before they reach adulthood. Hypertension or an abnormal lipid profile is present in most overweight children as young as 5 to 10 years of age (7). Central adiposity is associated with higher cardiovascular risk factor levels (8,9). Type II diabetes mellitus now accounts for as high as 45% of youths with newly diagnosed diabetes mellitus (10), and most of these cases arise in obese children. Life-threatening complications, such as obstructive sleep apnea, can affect severely obese children and adolescents (11). Effective interventions to treat childhood obesity and to prevent its development would have major health and economic benefits now and in the future.

Some argue against treatment of childhood obesity because those children destined to "outgrow" the obesity will receive unnecessary treatment and they may experience emotional harm from being labeled obese. Poor treatment efficacy is also a concern (12). However, the rising prevalence of obesity and obesity-associated medical conditions makes the lack of intervention increasingly difficult to justify. The risk of persistence of childhood obesity into adulthood is related to age and parental obesity (4). Obesity in older youths, particularly when both parents are obese, is unlikely to resolve spontaneously.

BMI is the recommended method for assessing obesity in children (13). BMI correlates with precise measures of body fat and the risk of obesity-associated medical conditions (14). Its use provides continuity in the assessment of obesity from childhood into adulthood. BMI is calculated by dividing weight by height squared (kilograms per meter squared [kg/m^2] or pounds by inches squared $\times$ 703 [$lb/in^2 \times 703$]). Because the normal range of BMI changes throughout childhood, the absolute BMI must be compared with normal percentiles for each child's age and sex. Current growth curves include BMI percentile curves for boys and girls from 2 to 20 years of age (15). An expert committee on childhood obesity recommended the use of 95th percentile BMI to define obesity. This cutoff minimizes the risk of misclassifying nonobese children because almost all children and adolescents with a BMI above this cutoff have excess fat. A BMI between the 85th and the 94th percentile defines a group "at risk of obesity" because many children with a BMI in this range will have excess fat, and therefore they require careful evaluation for obesity-related conditions and family risk factors (13).

Although the treatment of obesity in children is not simple or fast nor is it invariably successful, controlled studies of obese children have demonstrated good short-term and long-term outcomes (16). These outcomes were superior to the weight changes in parents who also participated in weight loss programs (17). Concerns remain about the stigma of obesity and the psychologic harm of being labeled obese (18–20). The impact of obesity on self-esteem and mood disorders seems to vary with age and ethnic background, but obesity in adolescence impairs quality of life in young adulthood, particularly for girls (21). Certainly, untreated obesity has demonstrable negative social consequences. Studies have not yet examined the impact of a diagnosis of obesity by a nurse, physician, or other health professional on self-esteem or occurrence of eating disorders. However, a prudent approach to therapy can balance the serious health risks associated with obesity and the potential psychologic harm to the child being labeled "obese" by using the safest methods that are available in a setting of empathy and encouragement. Such an approach would focus on the long-term goal of maintaining a healthy, well-functioning body, rather than on the short-term goals of rapid weight loss to achieve an esthetic ideal.

Programs that have achieved short-term and long-term successes used behavior-modification techniques to reduce caloric intake and to increase activity (22–27). The studies varied in detail, but most modified the diet to reduce total calories and calories from fat and to increase fruit and vegetable consumption. Approaches to improve caloric expenditure included reduced television viewing, increased programmed exercise, and increased daily activities. Commonly used strategies to change behavior included self-monitoring of eating and activity, modification of the environment to decrease the stimulus for eating or inactivity, and positive reinforcement for new behaviors. Rewards for diet and physical activity change, rather than for weight loss, were often recommended. Rewards generally were not food or expensive items but activities or special privileges instead. Figure 24.1 summarizes the kinds of interventions that have been studied and demonstrates the complexity of obesity treatment.

Work by Leonard H. Epstein represents the largest and longest studies in this field and serves as an example of a successful approach. Children from 6 to 12 years of age who were from 20% to 100% overweight participated in a series of studies. Treatment occurred weekly for 8 to 12 weeks and then monthly for 6 to 12 months from the start of the program. Families followed a balanced low-fat diet with moderate calorie restriction. Parent participation and type of physical activity were variables in the different studies. At the end of the active treatment period, children in the most successful groups of each study attained a 15% to 20% decline in weight (23,28–30). Ten years after the treatment programs, 30% of all children were nonobese, which was defined as less than 120% of the individual's ideal body weight.

These studies have demonstrated that behavior-based weight loss programs for children can succeed and that treatment nihilism is unwarranted. However, the success of some programs in some children does not necessarily define best practices. A recent review of studies of pediatric obesity treatment provides a useful summary of present knowledge, but this knowledge is incomplete for many reasons (31). The number of randomized controlled studies is small. Because successful interventions have approached the problem from many angles, they often did not establish the relative impact of different treatment components and they were not replicated to establish the effectiveness of the techniques in children of different ages, different economic or cultural backgrounds,

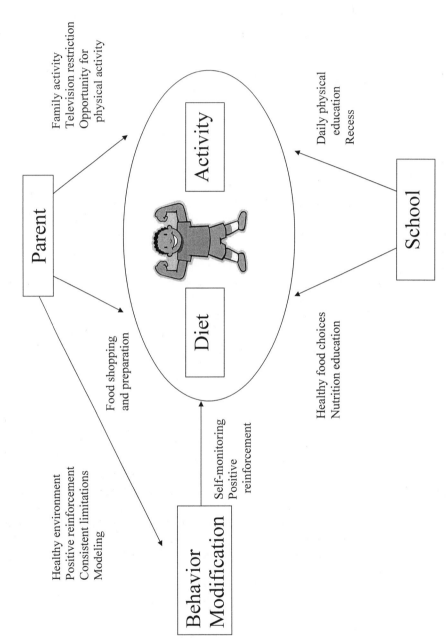

FIG. 24.1. Multifaceted approach to behavior-based treatment of childhood obesity. Published studies typically incorporate many aspects of this schema.

and different degrees of excess weight. Reproducing behavior-based interventions can be challenging because the interpersonal relationship between the professionals and the families they are educating and motivating may influence the outcome, particularly for individuals, in ways that are not quantifiable.

DIETARY INTERVENTIONS

Most studies of childhood obesity interventions have included diet changes, and many studies have demonstrated weight loss. Comparison across studies is limited by different caloric restrictions; different processes for educating, motivating, and reinforcing the diet changes; and different age-groups. In a small number of randomized trials of childhood obesity treatment, diets differed between the treatment and control groups. Among preadolescent children, one study demonstrated that 40 kcal per kg per day led to greater weight loss than 60 kcal/per kg per day did (32). Another study of this age-group found that the long-term outcome (12 months) was influenced more by the kind of activity intervention than by whether the children followed a structured diet (33). Among older youths, one study showed no statistical benefit for a reduced-calorie diet and behavior modification compared with a no-contact control (34). Another demonstrated that a structured diet was more effective than general nutrition education alone (35). A study of very low calorie diets demonstrated that the protein-modified fast (PMF) was more effective than a balanced hypocaloric diet in the intermediate follow-up but that the longer-term outcomes were equivalent (36). No one disputes the importance of dietary modification in weight-control programs, but, from published studies, one cannot identify a particular approach that is most effective.

A healthy permanent eating plan, the long-term goal of any weight loss program, is a diet that does not contain excess calories or high amounts of fat but that does contain adequate macronutrients and micronutrients to prevent nutritional deficiency. In the short-term, weight loss requires some calorie deficit. The National Academy of Science provides recommendations for daily caloric intake for different ages (Table 24.1). These recommendations are not precise, and therefore they cannot be considered prescriptive. The academy's guidelines group children by age and by body weight, without adjustment for different body composition. Because adipose tissue has little metabolic activity, obese patients have lower energy needs per kilogram of total body weight. However, they do have higher lean body mass (LBM) than do lean children of the same height, so they will have higher total resting energy expenditure (37). Physical activity also affects energy

TABLE 24.1. *Energy requirements*

	Age (yr)	Weight (kg)	Height (cm)	Estimated energy allowance	
				By weight (kcal/kg)	By height (kcal/cm)
Children	1–3	13	90	102	14.7
	4–6	20	112	90	16.1
	7–10	28	132	70	14.8
Males	11–14	45	157	55	15.8
	15–18	66	176	45	16.9
	19–24	72	177	40	16.3
Females	11–14	46	157	47	13.8
	15–18	55	163	40	13.5
	19–24	58	164	38	13.4

Adapted from *Recommended dietary allowances*, 10th ed. Washington, D.C.: National Academy Press, 1989, with permission.

needs. Despite the limitations of this table, it does provide standards with which to compare a child's reported intake. Assessed caloric intake that is markedly higher than expected, based on estimated LBM, provides some guidance for caloric reduction. The United States Department of Agriculture's (USDA) Food Guide Pyramid provides recommended quantities of grains, protein, vegetables, fruits, and milk products, and this is presently considered the guideline for a healthy diet in this country. The USDA also recommends that fat comprise less than 30% of the calories in the diet.

A more structured approach is the Traffic Light Diet (also known as the Stoplight Diet), which does not forbid any foods but which balances the amount of high-calorie and low-calorie foods (38). Leonard H. Epstein developed this diet for the studies of childhood obesity treatment, and other investigators have used it (23,28,30,35,39,40). This diet divides food into green-light, yellow-light, and red-light categories. Green-light foods contain at least 20 fewer kilocalories per average serving than the standard foods in its food group, yellow-light foods contain less than 20 kilocalories above the standard food in the food group, and red-light foods contain more than 20 kilocalories above the standard for food in that group. For example, in the fruit and vegetable group, red-light foods include French fried potatoes and creamed vegetables, yellow-light foods include baked potatoes, and green-light foods include carrots and lettuce. Patients are encouraged to consume no more than four servings per week of red-light foods and to have second servings at meals of green-light foods only.

Rarely, adolescents with marked obesity, usually with immediate serious complications such as obstructive sleep apnea or Blount disease (tibia vara), benefit from rapid weight loss. The PMF is a hypocaloric, ketogenic diet that is designed to provide enough protein to minimize the loss of LBM. The patient consumes 1.5 to 2.5 g of protein per kilogram of ideal body weight each day (37,41–43), which is the equivalent of 6 to 10 g of lean meat or fish per kilogram of ideal body weight. The protein intake can also occur as a protein drink. Intake of carbohydrate must be low enough to maintain ketosis. In the author's experience, patients can consume low-carbohydrate vegetables (e.g., lettuce, cruciferous vegetables) *ad libitum* and can maintain ketosis, as documented by ketonuria.

Benefits of this diet include relatively rapid weight loss (1 to 2 kg per week) and the anorexia induced by the ketosis. Complications include protein losses, hypokalemia, inadequate calcium intake, and orthostatic hypotension (37,42,44,45). Potassium and calcium supplementation and adequate calorie-free fluid intake can minimize these complications. Reports in the 1970s of sudden death among adults using protein drinks raised questions about the safety of these diets (46,47). Proposed but unproven explanations for the deaths included myocardial atrophy from low-quality protein (e.g., collagen) and arrhythmias from low total-body potassium (46,47). Use of lean meats and appropriate potassium supplementation may diminish the cardiac risks, but PMF is potentially harmful and thus it should be reserved for markedly obese adolescents who have serious comorbid conditions and who do not respond to more moderate interventions. Only physicians who are familiar with the diet and its potential complications should initiate and monitor this treatment.

ACTIVITY INTERVENTIONS

Increased physical activity will increase caloric expenditure. Most of the published weight loss programs for children included increased activity as part of the treatment, but, like diet changes, these activity changes often were not the focus of the study. Such studies cannot define the effect of activity independent of diet change or the effect of a particular kind of activity. The results of studies in which the activity differed between the treatment and control groups demonstrated mixed outcomes. Several studies showed a positive effect of activity programs when added to other diet and/or behavior changes (48,49). Other studies showed no additional benefit (34,50–52).

Approaches to activity modification vary widely. Epstein et al. (53) found that reinforcing decreased sedentary behavior was superior to reinforcing increased physical activity. They also showed that lifestyle exercise (e.g., walking to activities, using the stairs rather than elevators, and doing yard work), compared with programmed exercise (e.g., calisthenics), improved long-term outcomes (23,33). In a study of classes of third-grade and fourth-grade students that was not limited to overweight children, a classroom program to reduce television viewing led to significant relative decreases in BMI, compared with the control classes (54). Reduction of computer use might also improve weight, but this intervention has not been studied. Another study of overweight children demonstrated no benefit to gradually increasing activity frequency to a maintenance level, compared with more frequent activity initially that decreases to a maintenance level (55). These findings indicate that modest increases in activity, such as reduction of television viewing or lifestyle activity, may be superior in the long term to more intensive regimens, perhaps because these changes are easier to sustain. However, the process of increasing activity levels and sustaining them may be more important than a prescribed quantity of exercise.

BEHAVIOR MODIFICATION

Overview

More important than the specific dietary and activity recommendations is the process that children and families learn for modifying their eating and activity habits. Most weight loss studies use self-monitoring of behavior, modification of the environment to decrease stimulus for eating or inactivity, and positive reinforcement for new behaviors. Those studies in which the behavior component differed between the treatment and control groups demonstrated a benefit from behavior modification. Among prepubertal children, behavior modification techniques were superior to education alone (22,56). Although behavior modification techniques appeared no better than relaxation techniques in one study, they were significantly more effective in another (39,40). Among groups of older children, a combination of daily contact and monetary reinforcement for weight loss was better than weekly contact and money for calorie goals (57). Rewards for diet and behavior changes improved outcome (58). A perception of choice may be helpful (59). Group therapy for family-based behavior modification was less expensive than and as effective as a combination of group and individualized therapy (60).

Parental Participation

The usefulness of the parent's participation in obesity treatment was addressed in a number of studies, although results have been mixed. Among preadolescents, several studies suggested that participation of the child alone and the participation of the child with the mother were equivalent in the short term (28,61–63). However, long-term outcomes appeared better when parents were part of the interventions, although not all studies have confirmed this finding (25–27,62). In this preadolescent age-group, studies did not identify the best role a parent should take. Parents who participated by working on personal weight loss have appeared to be equivalent to parents who took a "helper" role

(26). Programs that emphasized a parent's control of the child's behavior have led to outcomes that were equivalent to those of programs that emphasized the child's control (63,64).

Among adolescents, only a few studies have examined the effect of parent participation in the child's weight loss program. One showed a benefit when the mothers participated in sessions separate from the adolescents, but others showed no benefit in this strategy when compared with no parent participation (57,65,66). The studies differed in baseline interventions common to both the control and the intervention groups, so the specific role a parent takes, the age of the child, and the kind of behavior changes that were promoted might have affected the parent's impact.

COMPREHENSIVE PROGRAMS: DIET, EXERCISE, AND BEHAVIOR MODIFICATION

Because of the paucity of studies and the diversity of age-groups and intervention components, the comparison of different strategies is difficult. Haddock et al. (67) performed a metaanalysis of 45 studies of childhood obesity treatment to identify components that predict successful weight loss. This analysis found that behavioral treatments that include behavior modification, a diet program, and an exercise program produced the best results and that programs that include behavior modification produced better outcomes than those that did not include behavior modification. Neither the intensity of parent participation nor the type of exercise program predicted better outcome. The small number of studies, the lack of inclusion of all variables in all studies, and the diversity of the studies (e.g., sample size, age, intervention, comparison groups) limit the reliability of the conclusions.

EXPERT COMMITTEE RECOMMENDATIONS

Faced with an epidemic of childhood obesity but incomplete data on the most efficacious treatment, the Maternal and Child Health Bureau, Health Resources and Services Administration convened a committee of experts in childhood obesity to provide those who care for children with practical directions on evaluation and treatment of overweight children (13). Health care providers can use these recommendations to address obesity in an office visit. The foundation of the treatment recommendations lies in the behavior-modification approaches of Epstein, which are supplemented by the clinical experience of many of the committee members. The recommendations emphasize the importance of

TABLE 24.2. *General approach to therapy*

Intervention should begin early.
The family must be ready for change.
Clinicians should educate families about medical complications of obesity.
Clinicians should involve the family and all caregivers in the treatment program.
Treatment programs should institute permanent changes, nor short-term diets or exercise programs aimed at rapid weight loss.
As part of the treatment program, a family should learn to monitor eating and activity.
The treatment program should help the family make small, gradual changes.
Clinicians should encourage and empathize, not criticize.

From Barlow SE, Dietz WH. Obesity evaluation and treatment: Expert committee recommendations. *Pediatrics* 1998;102:e29. Available at: http://www.pediatrics.org/cgi/content/full/102/3/e29, with permission. (Accessed October 2, 2002.)

TABLE 24.3. *Parenting skills for weight control*

Find reasons to praise the child's new behaviors.
Never use food as a reward.
Parents can ask for "rewards" for children in exchange for the changes in their own behavior.
Establish daily family meal and snack times.
Parents or caregivers should determine what food is offered and when, and the child should decide whether to eat.
Offer only healthy options.
Remove temptations.
Be a role model.
Be consistent.

From Barlow SE, Dietz WH. Obesity evaluation and treatment: Expert committee recommendations. *Pediatrics* 1998;102:e29. Available at: http://www.pediatrics.org/cgi/content/full/102/3/e29, with permission. (Accessed October 2, 2002.)

family readiness to change behavior. Published studies include only subjects who choose to participate, but clinicians in practice may identify obesity and may suggest intervention to families or children who have not sought help. Although families may welcome an opportunity to address the problem, some families may be unwilling or unable to make changes. Such families may not be concerned, they may feel that the excess weight is inevitable, or they may have personal circumstances, such as a move or family illness, that make eating and activity changes too difficult. Because lack of readiness generally leads to failure, frustration, and possibly reluctance to address the problem, the committee recommended that clinicians defer treatment or refer the family to a therapist who can address the family's readiness.

When clinicians begin treatment, the involvement of the entire family will create a healthy environment and will provide role models for children. The family should monitor eating and activity behaviors and should then make gradual but permanent changes to improve these behaviors. Table 24.2 presents the committee's general approach to treatment. To improve eating, families can reduce or eliminate specific high-calorie foods, rather than count calories, which is cumbersome and therefore is less likely to succeed. The Food Guide Pyramid is a helpful guide to healthy eating. Parents should take charge of meal times and food choices, but they should not force children to eat certain foods. To improve activity, parents should limit television viewing to 1 or 2 hours a day and should gradually add activity, such as walking to school or doing household chores, to the children's daily routines (68). Families must provide opportunities for enjoyable vigorous activity. Most children find periods of defined exercise (e.g., aerobic videos or treadmills) boring and unpleasant, so they may not continue the activity. Team sports; individualized sports, such as dance; family activity, such as bike riding; and unstructured outdoor play are all options that will appeal to different children. Because parents will institute the eating and activity changes, they need support and guidance in basic parenting skills, which are summarized in Table 24.3. Clinicians must consider each family's circumstances when they recommend changes; neighborhood safety, parent work schedules, and family finances will affect eating and activity options.

SCHOOL-BASED INTERVENTIONS

Treatment of obesity in a school setting is an attractive strategy because of the potential efficiency of addressing groups of overweight children in a place where they spend much of their time. A review by Story (69) summarized programs for weight loss among overweight children that included control groups and took place in schools. The sample size ranged from 10 to 119 children, and the age of the child varied from grade school to high school (70–74). Most employed weekly sessions for 2 to 3 months and included nutrition and exercise education and behavior modification (70–73,75). Weight change was reported using different metrics, but, with one exception (74), a study that used only an activity intervention with no diet education or behavior modification, the weight of the participants decreased by about 5% by the end the interventions (70–73,75). An intensive regimen of a protein-sparing modified fast for 2 months, followed by a balanced hypocaloric diet for a total of 6 months, led to a decrease of 24% of ideal body weight (76). Most studies did not include parents, and the one study in which parents were invited to participate in either five or two sessions through random assignment found no difference in weight loss in the two groups of children (73). The long-term effects of school-based studies were not reported. One study showed a sustained weight loss at 6 months, although the attrition was high during the treatment phase (70). School-based programs that target obese children deserve more study, particularly to establish their long-term effectiveness.

Rather than targeting overweight children, some school-based programs have made changes throughout a school or throughout a specific grade. Gortmaker et al. (77) developed Planet Health, a multidisciplinary curriculum for sixth-grade and seventh-grade students that encourages decreased television viewing, increased physical activity, and a lower fat diet with higher fruit and vegetable intake. This intervention improved obesity prevalence among girls, although not among boys. Many other schoolwide intervention trials have aimed primarily to improve cardiovascular disease risk factors, but these trials have assessed adiposity as a secondary outcome (78–84). Resnicow and Robinson (85) published a comprehensive review in 1997. These programs, like Planet Health, implemented curricula throughout the intervention schools to improve diet and physical activity. However, despite the similarity to Planet Health, these programs did not significantly improve the adiposity measures, with one exception (78). Most of the studies enrolled third-grade to fifth-grade classes. The students in the successful intervention and in Planet Health were older, but the impact of this difference on the outcomes of these generally similar programs is not known.

COMMERCIAL WEIGHT LOSS PROGRAMS

Many medical centers offer self-pay programs for weight control or weight loss in children. Examples include Shapedown and Way to Go Kids. Participants generally meet in groups weekly for about 3 months, and they receive guidance in eating, activity, and behavior modification. Often, parents participate through attendance either of sessions with their children or of parallel sessions for parents. Shapedown, a 3-month adolescent obesity program that uses behavioral techniques to change diet and exercise, showed a 5.9% change in relative weight at 3 months and a 9.9% decline at 15 months and reported a dropout rate of 16% (86). Committed to Kids also demonstrated significant weight loss in a 10-week program that included a very low calorie, high-protein diet (87). Neither of these reports included control groups. Other programs have not published their short-term and long-term outcomes. Some adolescents participate in adult commercial weight loss programs. Weight Watchers and Jenny Craig, for instance, accept adolescents of 15 years of age. However, studies of the effectiveness of these programs in teens have not been conducted.

MORE INTENSIVE TREATMENT

When children and adolescents must lose weight because of severe obesity-related complications like obstructive sleep apnea or tibia vara (Blount disease) and these children do not respond to comprehensive behavior-based programs, more intensive treatment may benefit these children if it is overseen by experienced clinicians (Table 24.4).

Protein-Sparing Modified Fast or Other Highly Restrictive Diet

The protein-sparing modified fast is discussed earlier in this chapter.

Pharmacologic Treatment

Studies of obese adults have demonstrated modest but significant benefits of pharmacologic interventions for weight loss. Randomized, controlled clinical trials of adults have shown the weight loss efficacy of orlistat, which blocks enteric lipase and therefore the absorption of about 30% of dietary fat, as well as sibutramine (88–91), which suppresses appetite by the inhibition of serotonin and noradrenaline reuptake. In these trials, subjects took the medication or a placebo while they participated in education and behavior modifications to increase physical activity and to decrease caloric intake. Trials of orlistat and sibutramine in children are forthcoming, but, at this time, the pharmacologic information that accompanies sibutramine indicates this its use is intended for patients 16 years and older. Other available appetite suppressants include phentermine and phendimetrazine. Fenfluramine, an agent that increases the release and blocks reuptake of serotonin, was used in combination with phentermine in adults, but it was withdrawn from the market in 1997 because of the occurrence of right-sided heart valve lesions. Small studies have demonstrated efficacy of phentermine and fenfluramine individually in adolescents (92–94). The use of metformin, an antihyperglycemic agent, has resulted in weight loss in obese adults with type II diabetes. In small studies, metformin, compared with a placebo, improved weight loss in obese adolescents with normal glucose tolerance test results who were on a restricted-calorie diet, and metformin resulted in significantly less weight gain compared with the placebo when given to obese adolescents with elevated fasting insulin levels on *ad libitum* diets (95,96). Lactic acidosis is a rare but serious complication of metformin, but this medication may eventually play a useful role in obesity therapy. Ephedra and its related compounds, such as ma huang, are active ingredients of many over-the-counter and herbal appetite suppressants. These agents have potential for abuse and dependence, and they may cause hypertension, palpitations, and coronary spasm (97). Because adolescents and families may assume that "natural" products are safe, clinicians should actively ask about their use of such products and should make the patients aware of their dangers. Use of Food and Drug Administration–approved prescription medications should await studies of safety and efficacy in children.

TABLE 24.4. *Additional treatment approaches when a comprehensive diet and exercise program is not effective for obese youth with severe medical complications*

- Medication, when Food and Drug Administration approved for the patient's age
- Protein-sparing modified fast
- Inpatient treatment
- Gastric bypass

Inpatient Programs

Inpatient programs have generally studied severely overweight children, particularly adolescents. In the published literature, the children participated in groups and generally received low-calorie diets that were in the range of 1,000 to 1,200 calories per day (98–102). In addition, the programs included 1 to 3 hours of exercise daily (37,98,100–103). Treatments were uniformly successful in the short term. However, few intermediate-term and long-term follow-up reports exist for these studies. The patients in one study maintained weight loss at 1 year, and another study demonstrated some weight regain at 4 months; however, patients on average remained below their pretreatment weight (42,102). These studies were not randomized trials.

Surgery

Bariatric surgery (e.g., gastric stapling, gastric bypass, and intestinal bypass operations) has been successful in morbidly obese adults. The adverse effects have included surgical complications, micronutrient deficiency, and the burden of consumption of small meals (104). In some cases, the patients did not lose weight or they regained weight because they consumed excessive quantities of high-fat, high-calorie fluids. Literature on obesity surgery in children is limited to case reports. Adolescents who underwent jejunoileal bypass in the 1970s had a high mortality and complication rate (105,106). Follow-up of 34 adolescents at 2 to 13 years after Roux-en-Y gastric bypass or vertical banded gastroplasty demonstrated substantial weight loss as a group, although at least one patient regained weight. No major postoperative complications were reported, and 85% said they were happy with the decision (107). A retrospective study of ten adolescents who underwent Roux-en-Y gastric bypass reported substantial weight loss (over 30 kg) in nine patients. One patient gained weight, and the complications included protein-calorie malnutrition, cholelithiasis, and small bowel obstruction (108). Gastric bypass should be reserved for superobese adolescents with life-threatening complications of obesity who do not respond to other treatment approaches. Such patients require counseling and education before the surgery and careful nutritional monitoring after the surgery.

TREATMENT GOALS

The most important goal is long-term good health—that is, an adulthood free of diabetes, early cardiovascular disease, sleep disorders, and the other conditions for which obesity increases risk. In an ideal situation, treatment improves a child's eating and activity behavior, and the child then loses weight, maintains that weight loss into adulthood, and avoids many medical problems. Such distant outcomes can be difficult to measure. Children with immediate medical problems benefit from weight loss to reduce fat rapidly. However, outcomes other than weight loss can indicate effective treatment. Weight maintenance with continued linear growth results in a gradual loss of body fat. Sustained weight maintenance is an appropriate initial weight goal for all children engaged in a weight-control program, and it is an appropriate long-term goal for certain children, depending on their degree of overweight and the presence of any obesity-related medical conditions (Fig. 24.2). The revised growth curves can demonstrate the an improvement in BMI percentile with weight maintenance. Resolution of any medical problems also signifies effective intervention. Improved eating and activity in the absence of significant weight loss or BMI percentile change may improve long-term health, and clinicians can

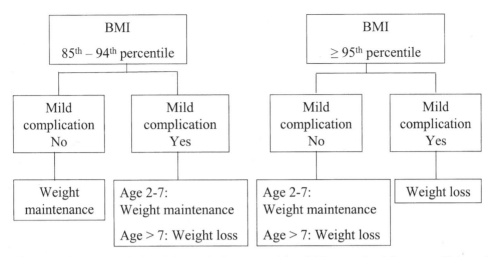

FIG. 24.2. Recommended weight goals for overweight children and adolescents. (Adapted from Barlow SE, Dietz WH. Obesity evaluation and treatment: Expert committee recommendations. Pediatrics 1998;102:e29. Available at: http://www.pediatrics.org/cgi/content/full/102/3/e29, with permission. [Accessed October 2, 2002.])

help families recognize the importance of such successful behavior changes. These behavior changes may also improve the individual's immediate quality of life and day-to-day functioning, although methods to measure this effect in children do not exist.

RISKS OF WEIGHT LOSS

Potential physiologic harm from weight loss includes the slowing or cessation of linear growth, a loss of LBM, inadequate nutrient intake, and gallstones. Height velocity decreased in a small group of children undergoing weight loss (109). However, most overweight children are tall, and long-term studies have indicated that weight loss has a minimal impact on the adult stature (110). In one short-term weight loss program, fat-free mass and bone mass did not change, and a similar maintenance of LBM was seen in a year-long program that led to approximately a 16% decline in body weight (111,112). However, PMFs do not completely "spare" protein losses, and they have led to a decline in LBM (37). In adults, very low calorie diets can lead to gallstone formation, and weight loss has been positively correlated with gallstone occurrence, although increased gallstones were not seen among moderately overweight adults on a low-calorie, but not very low calorie, diet (113,114). The Nurses Health Study also demonstrated a small risk of symptomatic gallstones associated with weight loss, and, in particular, it found an increased risk in women whose weight cycled (115,116). The risk of gallstones in children and adolescents with weight loss is not known.

Risk of inciting an eating disorder is a concern when engaging girls, in particular, in weight-control programs. Although dieting occurs more often in girls who later develop eating orders, whether dieting causes the eating disorders or is an early manifestation of the eating disorders is not known (117). Participation in an obesity program does not lead to a change in the symptoms of disordered eating, as measured by a standardized questionnaire (118).

CONCLUSION

All who observe the rapid rise in the number of obese children and the related health problems can find encouragement in the reports of sustained healthy weights achieved by some pediatric weight loss programs. However, these programs are complex and time consuming, and they require motivation and commitment from families. To consider enrolling all 15% of children who are obese into such programs is daunting. Even when families are motivated to participate, these programs, when not funded by research institutes, are expensive, and health insurance reimbursement for childhood obesity treatment is very low (119). Broad-based school and community programs and public awareness campaigns that promote more activity and better diets for all Americans may slow the rise in obesity prevalence. These kinds of programs will help children who are already obese by creating supportive environments, but many of these children need focused weight-loss programs to lose weight. Research supports the use of behavior-modification techniques to improve eating and activity. Future research should aim to define the most effective diets and activity programs, as well as the most efficient and low-cost process for implementing them. How best to use family group programs, group programs in a school setting, and individualized work with physicians, nurses, dietitians, and therapists; the ideal frequency of treatment sessions and maintenance sessions; and the influence of age, gender, degree of excess weight, and sociodemographic characteristics on the effectiveness of different treatment strategies are all important topics for research. If society does not address this problem now, it will pay the cost in 30 or 40 years when these obese children are obese adults with serious health problems.

REFERENCES

1. Troiano RP, Flegal KM, Kuczmarski RJ, et al. Overweight prevalence and trends for children and adolescents: the National Health and Nutrition Examination Surveys, 1963 to 1991. *Arch Pediatr Adolesc Med* 1995;149: 1085–1091.
2. Ogden CL, Flegal KM, Carroll MD, Johnson CL. Prevalence and trends in overweight among US children and adolescents, 1999–2000. *JAMA* 2002;288:1728–1732.
3. Troiano RP, Flegal KM. Overweight children and adolescents: description, epidemiology, and demographics. *Pediatrics* 1998;101:497–503.
4. Whitaker RC, Wright JA, Pepe MS, et al. Predicting obesity in young adulthood from childhood and parental obesity. *N Engl J Med* 1997;337:869–873.
5. Must A, Jacques PF, Dallal GE, et al. Long-term morbidity and mortality of overweight adolescents: a follow-up of the Harvard Growth Study of 1922 to 1935. *N Engl J Med* 1992;327:1350–1355.
6. Hoffmans MD, Kromhout D, de Lezenne Coulander C. The impact of body mass index or 78,612 18-year old Dutch men on mortality from all causes. *J Clin Epidemiol* 1988;41:749–756.
7. Freedman DS, Dietz WH, Srinivasan SR, et al. The relation of overweight to cardiovascular risk factors among children and adolescents: the Bogalusa heart study. *Pediatrics* 1999;103:1175–1182.
8. Morrison JA, Barton BA, Biro FM, et al. Overweight, fat patterning, and cardiovascular disease risk factors in black and white boys. *J Pediatr* 1999;135:451–457.
9. Morrison JA, Sprecher DL, Barton BA, et al. Overweight, fat patterning, and cardiovascular disease risk factors in black and white girls: the National Heart, Lung, and Blood Institute Growth and Health Study. *J Pediatr* 1999;135:458–464.
10. Types 2 diabetes in children and adolescents. American Diabetes Association. *Pediatrics* 2000;105:671–680.
11. Mallory GB, Fiser DH, Jackson R. Sleep-associated breathing disorders in obese children and adolescents. *J Pediatr* 1989;115:892–897.
12. Charney E. Childhood obesity: the measurable and the meaningful. *J Pediatr* 1998;132:193–195.
13. Barlow SE, Dietz WH. Obesity evaluation and treatment: Expert committee recommendations. *Pediatrics* 1998;102:e29. Available at: http://www.pediatrics.org/cgi/content/full/102/3/e29. Accessed October 2, 2002.
14. Dietz WH, Robinson TN. Use of body mass index as a measure of overweight in children and adolescents. *J Pediatr* 1998;132:191–193.
15. Kuczmarski RJ, Ogden CL, Grummer-Strawn LM, et al. *CDC growth charts: United States.* Hyattsville, MD: National Center for Health Statistics, 2000. Advance Data from Vital and Health Statistics, No. 314. Available at: http://www.cdc.gov/growthcharts. Accessed October 2, 2002.

16. Epstein LH, Valoski A, Wing RR, et al. Ten-year follow-up of behavioral, family-based treatment for obese children. *JAMA* 1990;264:2519–2523.
17. Epstein LH, Valoski AM, Kalarchian MA, et al. Do children lose and maintain weight easier than adults: a comparison of child and parent weight changes from six months to ten years. *Obes Res* 1995;3:411–417.
18. Erickson SJ, Robinson TN, Haydel KF, et al. Are overweight children unhappy? Body mass index, depressive symptoms, and overweight concerns in elementary school children. *Arch Pediatr Adolesc Med* 2000;154: 931–935.
19. French SA, Perry CL, Leon GR, et al. Self-esteem and change in body mass index over 3 years in a cohort of adolescents. *Obes Res* 1996;4:27–33.
20. Neumark-Stzainer D, Story M, Faibisch L. Perceived stigmatization among overweight African-American and Caucasian. *J Adolesc Health* 1998;23:264–270.
21. Gortmaker SL, Must A, Perrin JM, et al. Social and economic consequences of overweight in adolescence and young adulthood. *N Engl J Med* 1993;329:1008–1012.
22. Epstein LH, Wing RR, Steranchak L, et al. Comparison of family-based behavior modification and nutrition education for childhood obesity. *J Pediatr Psychol* 1980;5:25–36.
23. Epstein LH, Wing RR, Koeske R, et al. Effects of diet plus exercise on weight change in parents and children. *J Consult Clin Psychol* 1984;52:429–437.
24. Aragona J, Cassady J, Drabman RS. Treating overweight children through parental training and contingency contracting. *J Appl Behav Anal* 1975;8:269–278.
25. Epstein LH, Valoski A, Wing RR, et al. Ten-year outcomes of behavioral family-based treatment for childhood obesity. *Health Psychol* 1994;13:373–383.
26. Israel AC, Stolmaker L, Andrian CA. The effects of training parents in general child management skills on a behavioral weight loss program for children. *Behav Ther* 1985;16:169–180.
27. Israel AC, Stolmaker L, Sharp JP, et al. An evaluation of two methods of parental involvement in treating obese children. *Behav Ther* 1984;15:266–272.
28. Epstein LH, Wing RR, Koeske R, et al. Child and parent weight loss in family-based behavior modification programs. *J Consult Clin Psychol* 1981;49:674–685.
29. Epstein LH, Wing RR, Koeske R, et al. A comparison of lifestyle exercise, aerobic exercise, and calisthenics on weight loss in obese children. *Behav Ther* 1985;16:345–356.
30. Epstein LH, Wing RR, Koeske R, et al. Effects of parent weight on weight loss in obese children. *J Consult Clin Psychol* 1986;54:400–401.
31. Jelalian E, Saelens BE. Empirically supported treatments in pediatric psychology: pediatric obesity. *J Pediatr Psychol* 1999;24:223–248.
32. Amador M, Ramonth LT, Morono M, et al. Growth rate reduction during energy restriction in obese adolescents. *Exp Clin Endocrinol* 1990;96:73–82.
33. Epstein LH, Wing RR, Koeske R, et al. A comparison of life-style change and programmed aerobic exercise on weight and fitness changes in obese children. *Behav Ther* 1982;13:651–665.
34. Becque MD, Katch VL, Rocchini AP, et al. Coronary risk incidence of obese adolescents: reduction by exercise plus diet intervention. *Pediatrics* 1988;81:605–612.
35. Johnson WG, Hinkle LK, Carr RE, et al. Dietary and exercise interventions for juvenile obesity: long-term effect of behavioral and public health models. *Obes Res* 1997;5:257–261.
36. Figueroa-Colon R, von Almen TK, Franklin FA, et al. Comparison of two hypocaloric diets in obese children. *Am J Dis Child* 1993;147:160–166.
37. Brown MR, Klish WJ, Hollander J, et al. A high protein, low calorie liquid diet in the treatment of very obese adolescents: long-term effect on lean body mass. *Am J Clin Nutri* 1983;38:20–31.
38. Epstein LH, Squires S. *The Stoplight Diet for children.* Boston, MA Little, Brown and Company, 1988.
39. Duffy G, Spence SH. The effectiveness of cognitive self-management as an adjunct to a behavioral intervention for childhood obesity: a research note. *J Child Psychol Psychiatry* 1993;34:1043–1050.
40. Senediak S, Spence SH. Rapid versus gradual scheduling of therapeutic contact in a family-based behavioral weight control program for children. *Behav Psychother* 1985;13:265–287.
41. Merritt RJ, Blackburn GL, Bistrian BR, et al. Consequences of modified fasting in obese pediatric and adolescent patients: effect of a carbohydrate-free diet on serum proteins. *Am J Clin Nutr* 1981;34:2752–2755.
42. Stallings VA, Archibald EH, Pencharz PB, et al. One-year follow-up of weight, total body potassium, and total body nitrogen in obese adolescents treated with the protein-sparing modified fast. *Am J Clin Nutr* 1988;48:91–94.
43. Dietz WH, Schoeller DA. Optimal dietary therapy for obese adolescents: comparison of protein plus glucose and protein plus fat. *J Pediatr* 1982;100:638–644.
44. Dietz WH, Wolfe RR. Interrelationships of glucose and protein metabolism in obese adolescents during short-term hypocaloric dietary therapy. *Am J Clin Nutr* 1985;42:380–390.
45. Wadden TA, Stunkard AJ, Brownell KD. Very low calorie diets: their efficacy, safety, and future. *Ann Intern Med* 1983;99:675–684.
46. Sours HE, Frattali VP, Brand CD, et al. Sudden deaths associated with very low calorie weight reduction regimens. *Am J Clin Nutr* 1981;34:453–461.
47. Lantigua RA, Amatruda JA, Biddle TL, et al. Cardiac arrhythmias associated with a liquid protein diet for the treatment of obesity. *N Engl J Med* 1980;13:735–738.

48. Epstein LH, Wing RR, Penner BC, et al. The effect of diet and controlled exercise on weight loss in obese children. *J Pediatr* 1985;107:358–361.
49. Pena M, Bacallao J, Barta L, et al. Fiber and exercise in the treatment of obese adolescents. *J Adolesc Health Care* 1989;10:30–34.
50. Blomquist B, Borjeson M, Larsson Y, et al. The effect of physical activity on the body measurements and work capacity of overweight boys. *Acta Paediatr Scand* 1965;54:566–572.
51. Rocchini AP, Katch V, Anderson J, et al. Blood pressure in obese adolescents: effect of weight loss. *Pediatrics* 1988;82:16–23.
52. Hills AP, Parker AW. Obesity management via diet and exercise intervention. *Child Care Health Dev* 1988;14:409–416.
53. Epstein LH, Valoski A, Vara L, et al. Effects of decreasing sedentary behavior and increasing activity on weight change in obese children. *Health Psychol* 1995;14:109–115.
54. Robinson TN. Reducing children's television viewing to prevent obesity: a randomized controlled trial. *JAMA* 1999;282:1561–1567.
55. Emes C, Velde B, Moreau M, et al. An activity based weight control program. *Adapted Phys Activ Q* 1990;7:314–324.
56. Flodmark C, Ohlsson T, Ryden O, et al. Prevention of progression to severe obesity in a group of obese schoolchildren treated with family therapy. *Pediatrics* 1993;91:880–884.
57. Coates TJ, Jeffery RW, Slinkard LA, et al. Frequency of contact and monetary reward in weight loss, lipid change, and blood pressure reduction with adolescents. *Behav Ther* 1982;13:175–185.
58. Weiss AR. A behavioral approach to the treatment of adolescent obesity. *Behav Ther* 1977;8:720–726.
59. Mendonca PJ, Brehm SS. Effects of choice on behavioral treatment of overweight children. *J Soc Clin Psychol* 1983;1:343–358.
60. Goldfield GS, Epstein LH, Kilanowski CK, et al. Cost-effectiveness of group and mixed family-based treatment for childhood obesity. *Int J Obes Relat Metab Disord* 2001;25:1843–1849.
61. Kingsley RG, Shapiro J. A comparison of three behavioral programs for the control of obesity in children. *Behav Ther* 1977;8:30–36.
62. Kirschenbaum DS, Harris ES, Tomarken AJ. Effects of parental involvement in behavioral weight loss therapy for preadolescents. *Behav Ther* 1984;15:485–500.
63. Epstein LH, Wing RR, Valoski A, et al. Stability of food preferences during weight control: a study with 8- to 12-year-old children and their parents. *Behav Modif* 1987;11:87–101.
64. Israel AC, Guile CA, Baker JE, et al. An evaluation of enhanced self-regulation training in the treatment of childhood obesity. *J Pediatr Psychol* 1994;19:737–349.
65. Brownell KD, Kelman JH, Stunkard AJ. Treatment of obese children with and without their mothers: changes in weight and blood pressure. *Pediatrics* 1983;71:515–523.
66. Wadden TA, Stunkard AJ, Rich L, et al. Obesity in black adolescent girls: a controlled clinical trial of treatment by diet, behavior modification, and parental support. *Pediatrics* 1990;85:345–352.
67. Haddock CK, Shadish WR, Klesges RC, et al. Treatments for childhood and adolescent obesity. *Ann Behav Med* 1994;16:235–244.
68. Children, adolescents, and television. American Academy of Pediatrics, Committee on Communications. *Pediatrics* 1995;96:786–787.
69. Story M. School-based approaches for preventing and treating obesity. *Int J Obes Relat Metab Disord* 1999;23:S43–S51.
70. Zakus G, Chin ML, Cooper H, et al. Treating adolescent obesity: a pilot project in a school. *J School Health* 1981;51:663–666.
71. Lansky D, Brownell KD. Comparison of school-based treatments of adolescent obesity. *J School Health* 1982;52:384–387.
72. Lansky D, Vance MA. School-based intervention for adolescent obesity: analysis of treatment, randomly selected control and self-selected control subjects. *J Consul Clin Psychol* 1983;51:147–148.
73. Foster GD, Wadden TA, Brownell KD. Peer-led program for the treatment and prevention of obesity in the schools. *J Consult Clin Psychol* 1985;53:538–540.
74. Jette M, Varry W, Pearlman L. The effects of an extracurricular physical activity program on obese adolescents. *Can J Public Health* 1977;68:39–42.
75. Botvin GJ, Cantlon A, Carter BJ, et al. Reducing adolescent obesity through a school health program. *J Pediatr* 1979;95:1060–1062.
76. Figueroa-Colon R, Franklin FA, Lee JY, et al. Feasibility of a clinic-based hypocaloric dietary intervention implemented in a school setting for obese children. *Obes Res* 1996;4:419–429.
77. Gortmaker SL, Peterson K, Wiecha J, et al. Reducing obesity via a school-based interdisciplinary intervention among youth: Planet Health. *Arch Pediatr Adolesc Med* 1999;153:409–418.
78. Killen JD, Telch MJ, Robinson TN. Cardiovascular disease risk reduction for tenth graders: a multiple-factor school-based approach. *JAMA* 1988;260:1728–1733.
79. Walter HJ, Hoffman A, Vaughan R, et al. Modifications of risk factors for coronary heart disease. *N Engl J Med* 1988;318:1093–1100.
80. Bush PJ, Zuckerman AF, Theiss PK, et al. Cardiovascular risk factor prevention in black schoolchildren; two-year results of the Know Your Body program. *Am J Epidemiol* 1989;129:466–482.

81. Resnicow K, Cross D, Wynder E. The role of comprehensive school-based interventions. The results of four Know Your Body studies. *Ann N Y Acad Sci* 1991;623:285–298.
82. Donnelly JE, Jacobson DJ, Whatley JE, et al. Nutrition and physical activity program to attenuate obesity and promote physical and metabolic fitness in elementary school children. *Obes Res* 1996;4:229–243.
83. Harrell JS, McMurray RG, Bangdiwala SI, et al. Effects of a school-based intervention to reduce cardiovascular disease risk factors in elementary-school children: the Cardiovascular Health in Children (CHIC) Study. *J Pediatr* 1996;128:797–805.
84. Luepker RV, Perry CL, McKinlay SM, et al. Outcomes of a field trial to improve children's dietary patterns and physical activity: the Child and Adolescent Trial for Cardiovascular Health (CATCH). *JAMA* 1996;275: 768–776.
85. Resnicow K, Robinson TN. School-based cardiovascular disease prevention studies: review and synthesis. *Ann Epidemiol* 1997;7:S14–S31.
86. Mellin LM, Slinkard LA, Irwin CE. Adolescent obesity intervention: validation of the Shapedown program. *J Am Diet Assoc* 1987;87:333–338.
87. Sothern MS, von Almen TK, Schumacher HD, et al. A multidisciplinary approach to the treatment of childhood obesity. *Del Med J* 1999;71:255–261.
88. James WP, Avenell A, Broom J, et al. A one-year trial to assess the value of orlistat in the management of obesity. *Int J Obes Relat Metab Disord* 1997;21:S24–S30.
89. Sjostrom L, Rissanen A, Andersen T, et al. Randomised placebo-controlled trial of orlistat for weight loss and prevention of weight regain in obese patients. *Lancet* 1998;352:167–172.
90. Bray GA, Ryan DH, Gordon D, et al. A double-blind randomized placebo-controlled trial of sibutramine. *Obes Res* 1996;4:263–270.
91. Bray GA, Blackburn GL, Ferguson JM, et al. Sibutramine produces dose-related weight loss. *Obes Res* 1999; 7:189–198.
92. Rauh JL, Lipp R. Chlorphentermine as an anorexigenic agent in adolescent obesity. Report of its efficacy in a double-blind study of 20 teen-agers. *Clin Pediatr* 1968;7:138–140.
93. Pedrinola F, Cavaliere H, Lima N, et al. Is DL-fenfluramine a potentially helpful drug therapy in overweight adolescents subjects? *Obes Res* 1994;2:1–4.
94. Bacon GE, Lowrey GH. A clinical trial of fenfluramine in obese children. *Curr Ther Res Clin Exp* 1967;9: 626–630.
95. Kay JP, Alemzadeh R, Langly G, et al. Beneficial effects of metformin in normoglycemic morbidly obese adolescents. *Metabolism* 2001;50:1457–1461.
96. Freemark M, Bursey D. The effects of metformin on body mass index and glucose tolerance in obese adolescents with fasting hyperinsulinemia and a family history of type 2 diabetes. *Pediatrics* 2001;107:e55.
97. Adverse events associated with ephedrine-containing products—Texas, December 1993–September 1995. *MMWR Morb Mortal Wkly Rep* 1996;45:689–693.
98. Endo H, Takagi Y, Nozue T, et al. Beneficial effects of dietary intervention on serum lipid and apolipoprotein levels in obese children. *Am J Dis Child* 1992;146:303–305.
99. Fanari P, Somazzi R, Nasrawi F, et al. Haemorheological changes in obese adolescents after short-term diet. *Int J Obes* 1993;17:487–494.
100. Hoffman RP, Stumbo PJ, Janz FK, et al. Altered insulin resistance is associated with increased dietary weight loss in obese children. *Horm Res* 1995;44:17–22.
101. Wabitsch M, Braun U, Heinze E, et al. Body composition in 5–18 year-old obese children and adolescents before and after weight reduction as assessed by deuterium dilution and bioelectrical impedance analysis. *Am J Clin Nutr* 1996;64:1–6.
102. Rohrbacher R. Influence of a special camp program for obese boys on weight loss, self-concept, and body image. *Res Q* 1973;44:150–157.
103. Archibald EH, Harrison JE, Pencharz PB. Effect of a weight-reducing high-protein diet on the body composition of obese adolescents. *Am J Dis Child* 1983;137:658–662.
104. NIH Conference. Gastrointestinal surgery for severe obesity. Consensus Development Conference Panel. *Ann Intern Med* 1991;155:956–961.
105. Silber T, Randolph J, Robbins S. Long-term morbidity and mortality in morbidly obese adolescents after jejunoileal bypass. *J Pediatr* 1986;108:318–322.
106. Organ CH, Kessler E, Lane M. Long-term results of jejunoileal bypass in the young. *Am Surg* 1984;50:589–593.
107. Rand CS, MacGregor AM. Adolescents having obesity surgery: a 6-year follow-up. *South Med J* 1994;87: 1208–1213.
108. Strauss RS, Bradley LJ, Brolin RE. Gastric bypass surgery in adolescents with morbid obesity. *Arch Pediatr Adolesc Med* 1999;153:499–504.
109. Dietz WH Jr, Hartung R. Changes in height velocity of obese preadolescents during weight reduction. *Am J Dis Child* 1985;139:705–707.
110. Epstein LH, Valoski A, McCurley J. Effect of weight loss by obese children on long-term growth. *Am J Dis Child* 1993;147:1076–1080.
111. Figueroa-Colon R, Mayo MS, Aldridge RA, et al. Body composition changes in Caucasian and African American children and adolescents with obesity using dual-energy X-ray absorptiometry measurements after a 10-week weight loss program. *Obes Res* 1998;6:326–331.

112. Nuutinen O, Knip M. Weight loss, body composition and risk factors for cardiovascular disease in obese children: long-term effects of two treatment strategies. *J Am Coll Nutr* 1992;11:707–714.
113. Everhart JE. Contributions of obesity and weight loss to gallstone disease. *Ann Intern Med* 1993;119: 1029–1035.
114. Heshka S, Spitz A, Nunez C, et al. Obesity and risk of gallstone development on a 1200 kcal/d (5025 KJ/d) regular food diet. *Int J Obes Relat Metab Disord* 1996;20;450–454.
115. Stampfer MJ, Maclure KM, Colditz GA, et al. Risk of symptomatic gallstones in women with severe obesity. *Am J Clin Nutr* 1992;55:652–658.
116. Syngal S, Coakley E, Willett W, et al. Long-term weight patterns and risk for cholecystectomy in women. *Ann Intern Med* 1999;130:471–477.
117. Patton GC, Selzer R, Coffey C, et al. Onset of adolescent eating disorders: population based cohort study over 3 years. *BMJ* 1999;318:765–768.
118. Epstein LH, Paluch RA, Saelens BE, et al. Changes in eating disorder symptoms with pediatric obesity treatment. *J Pediatr* 2001;139:58–65.
119. Tershakovec AM, Watson MH, Wenner WJ, et al. Insurance reimbursement for the treatment of obesity in children. *J Pediatr* 1999;134:573–578.

Appendix A
Body Mass Index

Body Mass Index Table

Height (inches)	Normal						Overweight					Obese										Extreme Obesity														
BMI	19	20	21	22	23	24	25	26	27	28	29	30	31	32	33	34	35	36	37	38	39	40	41	42	43	44	45	46	47	48	49	50	51	52	53	54
	Body Weight (pounds)																																			
58	91	96	100	105	110	115	119	124	129	134	138	143	148	153	158	162	167	172	177	181	186	191	196	201	205	210	215	220	224	229	234	239	244	248	253	258
59	94	99	104	109	114	119	124	128	133	138	143	148	153	158	163	168	173	178	183	188	193	198	203	208	212	217	222	227	232	237	242	247	252	257	262	267
60	97	102	107	112	118	123	128	133	138	143	148	153	158	163	168	174	179	184	189	194	199	204	209	215	220	225	230	235	240	245	250	255	261	266	271	276
61	100	106	111	116	122	127	132	137	143	148	153	158	164	169	174	180	185	190	195	201	206	211	217	222	227	232	238	243	248	254	259	264	269	275	280	285
62	104	109	115	120	126	131	136	142	147	153	158	164	169	175	180	186	191	196	202	207	213	218	224	229	235	240	246	251	256	262	267	273	278	284	289	295
63	107	113	118	124	130	135	141	146	152	158	163	169	175	180	186	191	197	203	208	214	220	225	231	237	242	248	254	259	265	270	278	282	287	293	299	304
64	110	116	122	128	134	140	145	151	157	163	169	174	180	186	192	197	204	209	215	221	227	232	238	244	250	256	262	267	273	279	285	291	296	302	308	314
65	114	120	126	132	138	144	150	156	162	168	174	180	186	192	198	204	210	216	222	228	234	240	246	252	258	264	270	276	282	288	294	300	306	312	318	324
66	118	124	130	136	142	148	155	161	167	173	179	186	192	198	204	210	216	223	229	235	241	247	253	260	266	272	278	284	291	297	303	309	315	322	328	334
67	121	127	134	140	146	153	159	166	172	178	185	191	198	204	211	217	223	230	236	242	249	255	261	268	274	280	287	293	299	306	312	319	325	331	338	344
68	125	131	138	144	151	158	164	171	177	184	190	197	203	210	216	223	230	236	243	249	256	262	269	276	282	289	295	302	308	315	322	328	335	341	348	354
69	128	135	142	149	155	162	169	176	182	189	196	203	209	216	223	230	236	243	250	257	263	270	277	284	291	297	304	311	318	324	331	338	345	351	358	365
70	132	139	146	153	160	167	174	181	188	195	202	209	216	222	229	236	243	250	257	264	271	278	285	292	299	306	313	320	327	334	341	348	355	362	369	376
71	136	143	150	157	165	172	179	186	193	200	208	215	222	229	236	243	250	257	265	272	279	286	293	301	308	315	322	329	338	343	351	358	365	372	379	386
72	140	147	154	162	169	177	184	191	199	206	213	221	228	235	242	250	258	265	272	279	287	294	302	309	316	324	331	338	346	353	361	368	375	383	390	397
73	144	151	159	166	174	182	189	197	204	212	219	227	235	242	250	257	265	272	280	288	295	302	310	318	325	333	340	348	355	363	371	378	386	393	401	408
74	148	155	163	171	179	186	194	202	210	218	225	233	241	249	256	264	272	280	287	295	303	311	319	326	334	342	350	358	365	373	381	389	396	404	412	420
75	152	160	168	176	184	192	200	208	216	224	232	240	248	256	264	272	279	287	295	303	311	319	327	335	343	351	359	367	375	383	391	399	407	415	423	431
76	156	164	172	180	189	197	205	213	221	230	238	246	254	263	271	279	287	295	304	312	320	328	336	344	353	361	369	377	385	394	402	410	418	426	435	443

Body mass index. (Adapted from Clinical guidelines on the identification, evaluation, and treatment of overweight and obesity in adults: the evidence report. *Obes Res* 1998;6:51S–210S, with permission.)

Subject Index

Page numbers followed by *f* denote figures; those followed by *t* denote tables.

A

Acarbose, for management of diabetes mellitus, type II, 243*t*
    for management of diabetes mellitus, type II, 243*t*
Accidents, obesity-attributable mortality in adults, 5*t*
ACE. *See* Angiotensin-converting enzyme inhibitors.
Acetohexamide, for management of diabetes mellitus, type II, 251*t*
Acetylcholine, role in energy balance, 139
ACLS. *See* Aerobics Center Longitudinal Study.
Acylation-stimulating protein, 181
ADA. *See* American Diabetes Association.
Adenosine triphosphate (ATP), diabetes mellitus, type II, and, 240
Adipex. *See* Phentermine.
Adipocyte–arcuate–hypothalamic axis
    α-melanocyte–stimulating hormone, agouti-related protein, and melanocortin receptor system, 130–131
    leptin and
        discussion of, 131–135
        resistance, 135
    mutations in, as cause of obesity, 134*f*
    mutations causing obesity in humans, 134*f*
    other neuropeptides, 135–137
    in regulation of appetite, 130–137
Adipokines, insulin resistance and, 234–238
Adiponectin
    and adipose tissue as an endocrine organ, 181
    insulin resistance and, 236–237
Adipose tissue
    environmental influences, 9–10
    ethnic differences and admixture studies, 37–38
    functions, 8–9
    heart disease and
        adipose-tissue circulation, 181–182, 182*t*
        alterations in cardiac morphology, 184–185
        central hemodynamics, 182–184, 183*f*
        discussion of, 181–187
        effects on ventricular function, 185–187, 185*f*, 186*f*
        pathophysiology of obesity-related cardiomyopathy, 183*f*
        tissue blood flow during experimental hypovolemia, 182*t*
    leptin produced by, 462
    measurement, 124
    metabolic syndrome and, 379, 380, 386, 387
    renal compression in obesity and, 286, 287*f*
    roles of proteins secreted from, in humans, 8*t*
    type II diabetes and, 229, 233–238, 251–255, 256, 257–258, 260–261
    visceral, at the L4-L5 level, 108*f*
    waist-to-hip ratio, 260–261
Adiposis dolorosa. See Dercum disease.
Adipositas cordis (cardiomyopathy of obesity), 188–189
Adiposity
    measurement, 122–123, 123*t*
    pediatric, 95
Adolescents
    See also Pediatric obesity.
    adult consequences of obesity in, 96*t*
    criteria for identification of obesity in, 91
    energy expenditure, 96
    growth charts, 91–92, 92*t*
    nonalcoholic fatty liver disease and obesity, 321
    nonalcoholic steatohepatitis and obesity, 321
    obesity demographics, 3–4
    physical activity, 97
    prevalence of diabetes mellitus in, 98
    risk factors for adult obesity, 95
    weight goals, 560, 561*f*
    weight loss programs for, 554–556
Adoption studies, 33, 36–37
Adrenal axis, obesity and, 354–355
Aerobic exercise
    for blood pressure, 293
    for management of diabetes mellitus, type II, 247*f*
    for treatment of obesity, 293
Aerobics Center Longitudinal Study (ACLS), 482
Age
    prostate cancer and, 332–334
    as risk factor for gallbladder disease, 305*f*
    as risk factor for obstructive sleep apnea, 210
AHI. *See* Apnea-hypopnea index.
AICAR. *See* 5-Aminoimidazole-4-carboxamide ribonucleoside.
Air plethysmography (underwater weighing), for measurement of human body composition
    application of, 115–116
    history of, 114–115
Airway
    collapse, 205
    in obstructive sleep apnea, 202–203

Albright hereditary osteodystrophy, 52*t*, 53
Albuminuria, with coronary artery disease, 380
Alcohol, avoidance with sleep-disordered breathing,
    219
ALLHAT. *See* Antihypertensive and Lipid-Lowering
    treatment to prevent Heart Attack Trial.
α_1-adrenergic blocking agents, for management of
    obesity-related hypertension, 295
α-glucosidase inhibitors (Glyset; Precose)
    clinical profile, 255
    effects on adipose tissue and body weight, 256
    effects on insulin sensitivity, lipids, and
        cardiovascular risk factors, 255–256
    for management of diabetes mellitus, type II, 243*t*,
        255–256
α-melanocyte–stimulating hormone, 130–131
Alzheimer disease, obesity-attributable mortality in
    adults, 5*t*
American Academy of Pediatrics, in assessment of
    pediatric obesity, 91
American Cancer Society's Cancer Prevention Study
    II, 335
American Diabetes Association (ADA)
    recommendation on exercise, 250
    recommendation on nutrition, 244
American Heart Association, statement on obesity,
    192–193
American Medical Association, in assessment of
    pediatric obesity, 91
5-Aminoimidazole-4-carboxamide ribonucleoside
    (AICAR), 247
Amphetamines, in treatment of obesity, 449
Anabolism, insulin and, 19–20, 20*t*
Angelman syndrome, 52*t*, 53
AngII. *See* Angiotensin II receptor antagonists.
Angiotensin-converting enzyme (ACE) inhibitors, for
    management of obesity-related hypertension,
    294–295
Angiotensin II (AngII) receptor antagonists
    clinical trials, 295
    for management of obesity-related hypertension,
        295
Angiotensinogen, 181
Animal studies
    genetic influences on behavioral phenotypes,
        39–43, 40*t*–42*t*
    obesity-related traits that respond to selective
        breeding, 34*t*–35*t*
    quantitative trait locus mapping, 48–49
    of unusual obesity phenotypes, 54*t*
Anthropometry, for measurement of human body
    composition
    application of, 120–122, 120*t*, 121*t*, 122*t*
    history of, 119
Antidiabetic agents
    See also individual drug names.
    efficacy of oral agents as monotherapy, 243*t*
    metabolic effects of oral agents as monotherapy,
        244*t*
    oral agents as initial monotherapy, 243*t*
    side effects, 265, 265*f*
    sites of action of oral agents, 242*f*

Antihypertensive agents, for lowering blood pressure,
    293–294
Antihypertensive and Lipid-Lowering treatment to
    prevent Heart Attack Trial (ALLHAT), 295
Antiobesity agents, for management of diabetes
    mellitus, type II, 258–262
Antioxidants, for treatment of nonalcoholic
    steatohepatitis, 322
Antipsychotic drugs
    effect on body weight, 59, 59*t*
    endocrine complications of obesity and,
        352–353
Antiretroviral therapy, endocrine complications of
    obesity and, 352
Aortic aneurysm and/or dissection, obesity-
    attributable mortality in adults and, 5*t*
Apnea, definition of, 203*t*. *See also* Obstructive sleep
    apnea.
Apnea-hypopnea index (AHI)
    definition of, 203*t*
    obesity and, 210
Apomorphine, to reduce food intake, 451*t*
Appetite
    appetite-stimulating and appetite-suppressing
        molecules, 129*t*
    role of hypothalamus in regulation of, 128–141
Aquacultural studies
    obesity-related traits that respond to selective
        breeding, 34*t*–35*t*
    quantitative trait locus mapping, 48–49
Arrhythmias, with obesity, 191–192
Atherosclerosis, 192
ATP. *See* Adenosine triphosphate.
Australia
    economic impact of overweight or obesity, 524*t*,
        525
    percent of national health care cost due to obesity,
        525*f*
Axokine, effect on body weight, 59*t*

B
Back pain
    obesity and, 409–410
    and osteoarthritis, in obesity, 400
Bardet–Biedl syndrome
    association with obesity, 345–346
    and genetic causes of obesity, mental retardation
        in, 51, 52*t*
Bariatric surgery
    for children, 560
    for management of diabetes mellitus, type II,
        263–264
    for treatment of obesity
        complications of
            late, 515
            nutritional, 516
            perioperative, 513*t*, 513–515, 514*t*
        effect on comorbidities, 516–518, 517*f*, 518*f*,
            519*f*
        outcomes, 516–518
Behavior
    approaches to physical activity

cognitive and behavioral strategies for increasing physical activity, 494*t*

overview of, 492–494, 498

programs for behavioral counseling, 494, 495*f*–497*f*, 498

transtheoretical model, 493–494, 494*t*

behavioral measurement of food intake, 38–39

modification for childhood obesity, 555–556

patient and treatment predictors of outcome

discussion of, 426–432, 429*t*

patient characteristics, 427–429

treatment variables, 430–432

research on obesity-promoting, 60–61

support from spouses, 426

treatment of obesity

current programs, 416–417, 416*t*

history, 415–416

overview of, 415–435

strategies to improve outcome, 417–426, 418*t*, 419*t*, 420*t*, 422*f*, 424*f*

Beltsville One Year Dietary Intake Study, 75–76

Benzphetamine (Didrex)

efficacy, 453

to reduce food intake, 452*t*

Berardinelli–Seip syndrome, 50–51

β-adrenergic blockers, for management of obesity-related hypertension, 294

Betaine, for treatment of nonalcoholic steatohepatitis, 322

BIA. *See* Bioimpedance analysis.

Biguanide (metformin)

clinical profile, 253–254

effects on adipose tissue and body weight, 254–255

effects on insulin sensitivity, lipids, and cardiovascular risk factors, 254

for management of diabetes mellitus, type II, 243*t*, 253–255

Biguanides and the Prevention of the Risk of Obesity-1 trial, 254

Biliary colic, as a symptom of cholelithiasis, 310–311

Biliopancreatic diversion, for the treatment of obesity, 506, 512–513

Binge-eating disorder (BED)

diagnostic criteria, 366*t*

dieting and development of, 367–368

Diagnostic and statistical manual of mental disorders (DSM) classification, 366

introduction to, 365–366

psychosocial consequences of dieting and, 370

Bioimpedance analysis (BIA), for measurement of human body composition

application of, 118–119

history of, 118

Birth weight, as risk factor for childhood obesity, 94–95

Blood pressure

body mass index and, 273, 274*f*

in diagnosis of obesity, 5

hypertrophy with impaired systolic and diastolic function in obesity, 275–276, 276*f*

nonesterified fatty acids and, 281

physical activity and, 481–482

sodium and, 277

Blount disease

in children, 559

as an orthopedic complication of obesity, 99–100

BMI. *See* Body mass index.

Body image

dissatisfaction, 363–364

improvement, 370

psychosocial consequences of dieting and, 370

Body mass index (BMI)

annual direct health care costs of obesity by body mass index, 529*f*

blood pressure and, 273, 274*f*, 276*f*

changes in, 32–33, 32*f*

for children, 95*f*

definition of, 3

hyperplasia and, 4

hypertrophy and, 4

knockout mutants and transgenic models with effects on, 40*t*–42*t*

in pediatric obesity, 91

pediatric percentiles by age and gender, 92*t*

as a predictor of sleep-disordered breathing, 209, 209*f*

relation to health care costs, 535*f*

relationship between cost of sick leave and, 543*f*

relationship to incidence of cholecystectomy and symptomatic gallstones in women, 302*t*

relative rates of costs associated with body mass index, 533*t*

as risk factor for gallbladder disease, 305*f*

risk of diabetes mellitus, type II, and, 230*f*

table showing, 568*f*

uterine cancer and, 330–331

Body weight

as predictor of weight loss outcome, 428

regulation, 75–77, 76*f*

"set point," 76

settling point, 76–77

Bone minerals, measurement, 124

Bontril. *See* Phendimetrazine.

Börjeson–Forssman–Lehmann syndrome, 52, 52*t*

Breast, obesity and cancer, 329–330

Breathing

definitions in sleep-disordered, 202–205, 203*t*, 204*f*

periodic, 203*t*

Bright Futures: National Guidelines for Health Supervision of Infants, Children and Adolescents, 91

Bulimia nervosa

diagnostic criteria for, 367*t*

as an occurrence in obesity, 366

Bupropion, clinical trials of, 462

C

CAD. *See* Coronary artery disease.

Caffeine

effect of weight loss with ephedrine and, 466*f*

efficacy of, 470–471

pharmacology of, 470

safety of, 471

Calcium channel blockers, for management of
    obesity-related hypertension, 295–296
Calcium, supplementation recommendations, 340,
    340t
Calories
    expended per week in physical activity, 420t
    in management of diabetes mellitus, type II, 245
    as predictor of treatment outcome, 430
    values for 10 minutes of physical activity, 419t
Canada
    economic impact of overweight or obesity, 524t,
        526
    percent of national health care cost due to obesity,
        525f
Cancer
    breast, 329–330
    colon, 335–337
    comorbidity with obesity, 4–5
    esophageal, 337
    gallbladder, 312
    and interactions with endocrine, paracrine, and
        immune systems, 327–329, 328f
    obesity and, 327–344
    and obesity-attributable mortality in adults, 5t
    ovarian, 331–332
    pancreatic, 337–338
    and pediatric obesity, adult stature and relationship
        to, 338–340, 340t
    prostate, 332–334
    renal cell, 334–335
    uterine, 330–331
Carbohydrate-deficient glycoprotein syndrome, type
    IA (CDGSIA), 52t, 53
Carbohydrates
    dietary fat and, 82
    high-carbohydrate, low-fat diet, 443–444, 443t
    low-carbohydrate, high-protein diet, 444–445
    macronutrient composition and obesity, 437t
    metabolism, 150
    weight gain and, 438
CARDIA. See Coronary Artery Disease in Adults
    study.
Cardiac failure, as risk factor for obstructive sleep
    apnea, 211
Cardiac function, hemodynamics and obesity and
    cardiac hypertrophy with impaired systolic and
        diastolic function, 275–276, 276f
    increased heart rate and cardiac output, 275
Cardiac output
    exercise and, 184
    increased heart rate and, 275
Cardiomyopathy
    of obesity (adipositas cordis), 188–189
    pathophysiology of obesity-related, 183f
Cardiopulmonary system, complications of weight
    reduction therapy on, 195
Cardiovascular disease
    as chronic effect of obstructive sleep apnea,
        216–217
    physical activity and, 480–486
    risk in men, 484f
Cardiovascular system
    benefits of weight reduction on, 194–195, 195t
    obstructive sleep apnea and, 214–216, 214f–215f
Carpenter syndrome, 52, 52t
CBA. See Cost–benefit analysis.
CCK. See Cholecystokinin.
CDC. See Centers for Disease Control and
    Prevention.
CDGSIA. See Carbohydrate-deficient glycoprotein
    syndrome, type IA.
CEA. See Cost-effectiveness analysis.
Centers for Disease Control and Prevention (CDC), 91
Central apnea, 203, 205
Central event, definition, 203t
Central nervous system (CNS)
    effects of leptin in animal studies, 235f
    hyperinsulinemia and, 278, 280
    inputs that regulate appetite and energy
        homeostasis, 136f
Cerebrovascular diseases
    obesity-attributable mortality in adults, 5t
    as risk factor for obstructive sleep apnea, 211
CETP. See Cholesteryl ester transfer protein.
Cheyne–Stokes respiration, definition, 203t
CHF. See Congestive heart failure.
Childhood Obesity Working Group, 91
Children
    See also Pediatric obesity.
    energy expenditure in, 96
    growth charts for, 91–92, 92t
    growth hormone deficiency in, 349
    hypothyroidism and, 349
    nonalcoholic fatty liver disease and obesity, 321
    nonalcoholic steatohepatitis and obesity, 321
    obesity demographics in, 3
    physical activity of, 97
Chitosan, for treatment of obesity, 471
Chlorpheniramine, to reduce food intake, 451t
Chlorpropamide, for management of diabetes
    mellitus, type II, 251t
Cholecystectomy, incidence, 302t
Cholecystokinin (CCK)
    to reduce food intake, 463
    role in energy balance, 139
Cholelithiasis
    clinical manifestations and treatment, 310t
    epidemiology and risk factors
        age-adjusted and body mass index-adjusted risk
            of gallbladder disease related to ethnicity, 305f
        discussion of, 301–305
        incidence of cholecystectomy and symptomatic
            gallstones in women, 302t
        risk of gallbladder disease
            correlation to leptin concentration, 304f
            correlation to waist to hip ratio, 303f
    overview of, 301–312
    pathogenesis
        discussion of, 306–308, 306f
        gallbladder motility, 308, 308t
        nucleation factors, 307
        secretion of lithogenic bile by hepatocytes,
            306–307, 307t
    significance

asymptomatic cases, 309–310, 309f
gallbladder carcinoma, 312
gallbladder sludge, 311, 311f
spontaneous dissolution, 310
symptomatic cases, 310–311, 310t
types of gallstones, 305, 305f
Cholesterol
in diagnosis of obesity, 5
for management of diabetes mellitus, type II, 245
and reverse cholesterol transport, 386
Cholesteryl-ester transfer protein (CETP), 181, 384
Choroideremia, 52t, 53
Chromium picolinate, for treatment of obesity, 471
Chronic obstructive pulmonary disease (COPD), as
chronic effect of obstructive sleep apnea, 217
Chylomicronemia syndrome, as complication of
metabolic syndrome, 390
Ciliary neurotrophic factor, for reducing food intake,
462
Cirrhosis
nonalcoholic steatohepatitis as etiology of,
318–319
obesity-attributable mortality in adults, 5t
Clenbuterol, to reduce food intake, 451t
Clinical trials
for angiotensin II receptor antagonists, 295
Antihypertensive and Lipid-Lowering treatment to
prevent Heart Attack Trial (ALLHAT), 295
Biguanides and the Prevention of the Risk of
Obesity-1 trial, 254
for bupropion, 462
for diuretics, 294
Framingham Heart Study, 273
for garcinia cambogia, 471
for hormone replacement therapy, 352
of increasing physical activity as treatment for
obesity, 417–418, 418t
for ma huang and guarana, 472
of monoaminergic drugs, 462
on obesity, 273
for orlistat, 293, 463–468, 464t–465t
Prospective Cardiovascular Munster (PROCAM)
study, 290, 291f
for sibutramine, 456t–457t, 458–459
Sibutramine Trial of Obesity Reduction and
Maintenance (STORM), 260–261
for sympathomimetic drugs, 453
of third-generation β₃-adrenergic drugs, 471
for topiramate, 462
Treatment of Obese Patients with Hypertension
Study, 294
United Kingdom Prospective Diabetes Study
(UKPDS), 246, 254
weight loss to prevent and/or treat osteoarthritis,
407–408
Women's Health Trial, 439
Clonidine, for blockade of rise in blood pressure,
277–278
Clozapine, effect on body weight, 59, 59t
Cohen syndrome, 52, 52t
Colon, obesity and cancer, 335–337
Committed to Kids, 558

Computed tomography (CT), for measurement of
human body composition, 112–113
Congestive heart failure (CHF), risk with obesity,
187
Continuing Survey of Food Intake by Individuals
(CSFII), 445
Continuous positive airway pressure (CPAP), for
obstructive sleep apnea, 220–221
COPD. *See* Chronic obstructive pulmonary disease.
Coronary artery disease (CAD)
as complication of metabolic syndrome, 389
dietary fiber intake, increasing, as protection
against, 444
with obesity, 192–194
risk factors for, 192–193
Coronary Artery Disease in Adults (CARDIA) study,
85
Cor pulmonale
checking for, in the evaluation of the obese patient,
188
in obstructive sleep apnea, 203
Cost–benefit analysis (CBA), definition, 523
Cost–effectiveness analysis (CEA), definition, 523
Cost of illness
definition, 523
studies, 523–524
CPAP. *See* Continuous positive airway pressure.
CPMP. *See* European Committee on Proprietary
Medicinal Products.
CSFII. *See* Continuing Survey of Food Intake by
Individuals.
CT. *See* Computed tomography.
Cushing syndrome
See also Hypothalamic–pituitary–adrenal axis.
features, 347–348
metabolic syndrome and, 385
obesity and, 347–349
screening for, 348

D

DEA. *See* United States Drug Enforcement Agency.
"Deadly quartet," 273
Death
attributed to obesity, 4–5
homicide and, 5t
Dehydroepiandrosterone (DHEA), to induce weight
loss, 468
Demographics, as predictor of weight loss outcome,
427
De novo lipogenesis, 149
Dercum disease (*adiposis dolorosa*), 51
DEXA. *See* Dual-energy x-ray absorptiometry.
Dexfenfluramine
cardiac valve disorders and, 195
for decreased food intake and weight loss,
138–139
effect on body weight, 58
DHEA. *See* Dehydroepiandrosterone.
DHT. *See* Dihydrotestosterone.
Diabetes mellitus, type II
comorbidity with obesity, 4–5, 229–272
incidence of, 481f

Diabetes mellitus, type II (*contd.*)
  management of
    bariatric surgery, 263–264
    efficacy of oral antidiabetic agents as
      monotherapy, 243*t*
    exercise therapy, 246–250, 247*f*, 249*f*
    goals for glycemic control, 242*t*
    metabolic effects of oral antidiabetic agents as
      monotherapy, 244*t*
    nutrition therapy, 244–246, 244*f*
    oral antidiabetic agents as initial monotherapy,
      243*t*
    overview of, 241–264
    pharmacologic therapy in
      antidiabetic agents, 251–258
      antiobesity agents, 258–262
      role of, 250–262
    sites of action of oral antidiabetic agents, 242*f*
  metabolic syndrome and, 383
  and obesity-attributable mortality in adults, 5*t*
  obesity treatment with orlistat and, 467
  pathophysiology of
    hepatic glucose production, 239–241, 240*f*
    insulin resistance in
      adipocyte-secreted hormones and, 234–238,
        235*f*, 237*f*
      discussion of, 232–238
      free fatty acids and, 233–234, 233*f*
    insulin-secretory defects, 238–239
  prevalence in adolescent Native Americans, 98
  relationship between central abdominal fat and
    insulin sensitivity, 231*f*
  risk by body mass index, 230*f*
  sites of defects leading to hyperglycemia, 230*f*
  untreated, and metabolic syndrome, 384
Didrex (Benzphetamine)
  efficacy, 453
  to reduce food intake, 452*t*
Diet
  See also Nutrition.
  calorie goal choice, 421–422
  for childhood obesity, 556
  composition, 437–440
  debate regarding, 445–446
  eating control, 431
  high-carbohydrate, low-fat, 443–444, 443*t*
  and interventions for childhood obesity, 553–554,
    553*t*
  liquid, 424
  low-calorie versus very low calorie diets, 422–423,
    422*f*
  low-carbohydrate, high-protein, 444–445
  low-energy–density, 441
  low-fat, high-carbohydrate, 86–87
  macronutrient composition of, 245, 425, 437, 437*t*
  modifying intake in, 421–426
  and structured meal plans, 423–425, 424*f*
  support from spouses and, 426
  for treatment of nonalcoholic steatohepatitis, 322
  "Western," 327
Diet and Nutrition Survey of British Adults, 87
Dietary fat

breast cancer and, 329–330
cardiovascular, neurohumoral, and renal changes
  with high-fat diet, 275*t*
and dietary carbohydrate, 82
energy and, 80–82, 81*t*
energy density of, 80, 82
fat grams for 30% of total dietary kilocalories,
  443*t*
glucocorticoids and, 171
growth hormone storage and, 158
location of, and relationship to insulin sensitivity,
  231–232, 231*f*
in low-fat, high-carbohydrate diet, 86–87, 443–444,
  443*t*
macronutrient composition and obesity, 437*t*
measurement of, 120–121, 120*t*
in men, 484*f*
as predictor of treatment outcome, 430
storage and estrogens, 167–168
testosterone and, 163
and visceral fat in clinical assessment of pediatric
  obesity, 93–94
weight gain and, 439–440
Dietary fiber, role in weight loss, 245–246
Diethylpropion (Tenuate; Tepanil)
  efficacy, 453
  long-term studies, 454*t*
  to reduce food intake, 452*t*
  to treat obesity, 449
Dihydrotestosterone (DHT)
  fuel partitioning and, 161
  increase in, with age and benign prostate
    hyperplasia, 334
Direct costs, definition of, 523
Disability, productivity and functional capability in,
  541–542, 541*f*, 542*f*
Disease, definition of, 3
Diuretics
  clinical trials of, 294
  for management of obesity-related hypertension,
    294
Dopamine receptor D$_4$ (DRD4), as identified single-
  gene mutation for obesity, 50
Dopamine, role in energy balance, 138
Doppler imaging, for evaluation of heart disease, 186
Down syndrome, 52–53, 52*t*
DRD4. *See* Dopamine receptor D$_4$.
Drugs, for treatment of obesity
  See also individual drug names.
  for altering metabolism
    approved by the FDA, 463–468, 464*t*–465*t*, 466*f*
    drugs approved by the FDA for indications other
      than obesity, 468
    introduction to, 452
  and association with obesity, 351–353, 351*t*
  comparison of available drugs, 468–469, 469*f*,
    470*f*
  discussion of, 449–475
  for dyslipidemia, 391*t*
  effect on body weight, 58–59, 59*t*
  herbal preparations as, 471–472
  that increase energy expenditure, 452, 470–471

for management of diabetes mellitus, type II, 250–262
mechanisms of action for, 451–452
and obstructive sleep apnea, 222
to reduce food intake
combining serotonergic and noradrenergic drugs, 460–462, 461*f*
discussion of, 452–463
drugs approved by the FDA, 452*t*
mechanisms of, 451
monoaminergic drugs in clinical trials, 462
peptides not approved by the FDA to treat obesity, 462–463
serotonergic drugs not approved by the FDA to treat obesity, 460
sympathomimetic drugs
not approved by the FDA to treat obesity, 460
overview of, 453–460, 454*t*, 455*f*, 456*t*–457*t*, 458*f*
research on response to antiobesity medications, 62
Dual-energy x-ray absorptiometry (DEXA), for measurement of human body composition
application of, 116–118, 117*f*
history of, 116
Duodenal switch, for treatment of obesity, 512–513
Dyslipidemia
comorbidity with obesity, 4–5
coronary artery disease and, 192
diagnosis and assessment, 390
drug therapy for, 391*t*
and hepatic lipase promoter polymorphism, 384–385
lipoprotein physiology and, 385–386
mechanisms of, 385–389, 386*t*, 388*f*
of metabolic syndrome, 378–398
modifiers in central obesity, 384–385
and primary increase in hepatic triglyceride synthesis, 385, 385*f*
treatment of, 390–391, 391*t*
Dyslipoproteinemias, 482

E

Eating disorders, 365–367, 366*t*, 367*t*
ECG. *See* Electrocardiogram.
EEG. *See* Electroencephalogram.
Electrocardiogram (ECG)
changes with progressive obesity, 189*t*
detection of left ventricular hypertrophy by QRS in obesity, 190*t*
use of, in obesity, 189–191
Electroencephalogram (EEG), for evaluation of sleep-disordered breathing, 212
Electromyogram (EMG), for evaluation of sleep-disordered breathing, 212
Electrooculogram (EOG), for evaluation of sleep-disordered breathing, 212
EMG. *See* Electromyogram.
Employers
annual medical care costs to, 533*t*
health care costs to, 535–536, 535*f*

and perspective on employee productivity, 542–544, 543*f*, 544*f*
Endocrine disorders
as chronic effect of obstructive sleep apnea, 217–218
comorbidity with obesity, 4–5
that contribute to obesity
Cushing syndrome, 347—349
growth hormone deficiency, 349
hypothalmic obesity from tumors and/or damage to the hypothalamus, 346–347
hypothyroidism, 349
polycystic ovary syndrome, 350–351
prolactinomas, 351
pseudohypoparathyroidism, 349–350
and endocrine complications of obesity
adrenal axis, 354–355
effect on growth hormone, 354
effect on prolactin, 354
effects on female reproductive axis, 353–354
effects on male reproductive axis, 353
thyroid and, 354
vasopressin and, 354
genetic diseases associated with obesity and
Bardet–Biedl syndrome, 345–346
discussion of, 345–346
mutations in leptin and/or leptin receptor, 346
Prader–Willi syndrome, 345
and medications that contribute to obesity
antipsychotics, 352–353
antiretroviral therapy, 352
oral contraceptives, 351–352
overview of, 351–353, 351*t*
valproic acid, 352
obesity and, 345–357
obesity and cancer and, 327–329, 328*f*
synopsis of, 346–353
Endocrine system
control of fuel partitioning
effects of hormones on fuel balance, 148*f*
energy expenditure and metabolism, 150–151, 151*t*
processing of fuel, 149–150
synopsis of, 147–173
estrogens and
body composition, 167
physiology of, 164–168
regional fat storage, 167–168
replacement therapy and nutrient partitioning, 168–169
resting energy expenditure and thermic effect of food and exercise, 165–166
substrate availability, 166
substrate oxidation, 166–167
glucocorticoids and
cortisol and the hypothalamic–pituitary–adrenal axis, 170
hypothalamic–pituitary–adrenal axis and obesity, 172–173
managing glucocorticoid therapy in obese patients, 173
physiology of, 169–171, 171*f*

Endocrine system, glucocorticoids and (*contd.*)
  regional fat storage, 171
  resting energy expenditure and thermic effect of food and exercise, 170
  substrate availability and oxidation, 170–171
  growth hormone and
    administration in visceral obesity, 159–160
    insulin-like growth factors, 156–157
    physiology of, 156–158, 156*f*
    regional fat storage, 158
    resting energy expenditure and thermic effect of food and exercise, 157
    substrate availability and oxidation, 157–158
    visceral obesity in, 158–159
  insulin and
    intracellular effects on nutrient partitioning, 154
    nutrient partitioning in obesity, 155
    physiology of, 151–152, 152*f*
    resting energy expenditure and thermic effect of food and exercise, 153
    substrate availability and oxidation, 153–154
    tissue variability in insulin action, 154–155
  testosterone and
    administration in visceral obesity, 164
    physiology of, 161–163, 161*f*
    regional fat storage, 163
    resting energy expenditure and thermic effect of food and exercise, 161–162
    substrate availability and oxidation, 162
    visceral obesity in, 163–164
Endoscopic sphincterotomy, for cholelithiasis, 310*t*
Endotoxemia, steatohepatitis and, 321
Endstage renal disease (ESRD)
  and effect of food restriction on cumulative death rate, 288*f*
  glomerular hyperfiltration with renal injury in obesity and, 289
  obesity and, 288–291
  obesity as major cause of, 291, 292*f*
  risk factors for, obesity as, 273
  and structural and functional changes in glomeruli in early phases of obesity, 289–290, 290*f*, 291*f*
Energy
  See also Fuel.
  adipocyte–arcuate–hypothalamic axis, 130–137
  average daily consumption of, 79*t*
  average daily percentage of consumption, 81*t*
  changes that impact expenditure, 83–85, 83*f*
  changes that impact intake, 77–82
  comparisons of expenditure in children and adolescents, 96
  density and, 440–445
  dietary fat and, 80–82, 81*t*
  diets restricted in, 441, 442*t*
  drugs that increase expenditure, 452, 470–471
  expenditure and metabolism, 150–151, 151*t*
  glycemic index and, 82
  imbalance, 85
  low-energy–density diet, 441
  monoamine neurotransmitters and, 137–139
  peptidergic systems and, 129–130, 129*t*, 130*t*

physical activity and, 476
requirements in children, 553*t*
resting
  expenditure and thermic effect of food and exercise on, 153
  thermic effect of food and exercise on, 165–166
and role of the hypothalamus in appetite regulation, 128–141
total daily expenditure of, 83*f*
Environment
  alternatives to obesity and
    discussion of, 86–87
    low-fat, high-carbohydrate diets, 86–87
    physical activity and weight gain, 87
    self-monitoring and weight gain, 87
  changes in
    that impact energy expenditure, 83–85, 83*f*
    that impact energy intake
      average daily consumption of energy, 79*t*
      dietary fat, 80–82, 81*t*
      glycemic index, 82
      overview of, 77–82
      for prevention of obesity, 87–88
  effect on genetics, 43–45, 44*f*
  impact on physiologic regulatory system, 77
  implications for prevention and treatment of obesity, 87
  increased prevalence of pediatric obesity and, 94
  influences on adipose tissue mass, 9–10
  influences on obesity, 75–88
  metabolic consequences, 85–86
  research on obesity and, 61
EOG. *See* Electrooculogram.
Ephedrine
  effect of weight loss with caffeine and, 466*f*
  efficacy of, 470–471
  pharmacology of, 470
  safety of, 471
Epinephrine, role in energy balance, 137–138
Esophagus, obesity and cancer, 337
ESRD. *See* Endstage renal disease.
Estrogens
  and adipose tissue as an endocrine organ, 181
  body composition and, 167
  breast cancer and, 329–330
  effect on endocrine system, 164–169
  physiology of, 164–168
  regional fat storage and, 167–168
  replacement therapy and nutrient partitioning, 168–169
  resting energy expenditure and thermic effect of food and exercise, 165–166
  substrates and
    availability, 166
    oxidation, 166–167
Ethics, in genetic research, 62
Ethnicity
  breast cancer and, 329–330
  endocrine complications of obesity and, 353–354
  and epidemiology and risk factors of cholelithiasis, 301
  ethnic differences and admixture studies, 37–38

obesity and
    endstage renal disease, 291, 292*f*
    environmental influences associated with,
      9–10
    in various populations, 3
    ovarian cancer and, 332
    as predictor of weight loss outcome, 427
    prevalence of diabetes mellitus in pediatric obesity
      and, 98
    psychosocial complications of obesity and,
      360–361
    and research with diverse samples, 61
    as risk factor for gallbladder disease, 305*f*
European Committee on Proprietary Medicinal
    Products (CPMP), 453
Exercise
    amount of activity, 419–420
    caloric values for 10 minutes of physical activity,
      419*t*
    for childhood obesity, 556
    choice of, 419
    effect on weight loss and maintenance, 418*t*
    glucocorticoids and, 170
    heart disease and, 184
    lifestyle and structured exercise, 418
    for management of diabetes mellitus, type II,
      246–250, 247*f*, 249*f*
    physical activity intervention in clinical practice
      behavioral approaches to physical activity
        cognitive and behavioral strategies for
          increasing physical activity, 494*t*
        programs for behavioral counseling, 494,
          495*f*–497*f*, 498
        summary of, 492–494, 498
        transtheoretical model, 493–494, 494*t*
      common barriers to exercise, 492*t*
      lifestyle physical activity, 489–491, 489*f*, 491*f*,
        492*f*
      short bouts of physical activity, 487–488, 488*f*
      synopsis of, 486–494, 498
    physical activity, obesity, and health outcomes
      all-cause and cardiovascular disease mortality,
        482–486, 484*f*, 485*f*
      blood pressure and hypertension, 481–482
      discussion of, 480–486
      dyslipoproteinemias and, 482
      insulin action and glucose tolerance, 480–481,
        481*f*
    physical activity in weight management
      discussion of, 476–480
      influence of physical activity on weight loss,
        477–478
      physical activity and weight maintenance,
        478–480
    as predictor of treatment outcome, 430–431
    for prevention and treatment of hypertension,
      292–293
    for prevention and treatment of osteoarthritis, 408
    recommendations for, 498–499
    risk assessment for, 499
    self-monitoring versus supervised physical activity,
      420
    strategies to increase adherence, 420–421
    as a therapeutic approach to obesity, 476–502
    thermic effect
      of food and, 165–166
      of insulin on, 153
      of testosterone and, 161–162
    for treatment of nonalcoholic steatohepatitis, 322
Expert Committee on Clinical Guidelines for
    Overweight in Adolescent Preventive Services,
    91

F

Familial combined hyperlipidemia (FCHL), metabolic
    syndrome and, 381–383, 382*f*
Family studies, 33, 36–37
Fastin. *See* Phentermine.
Fasting plasma glucose (FPG), in management of
    diabetes mellitus, type II, 246
Fat
    See also Dietary fat.
    definition, 104
Fat and fat-free mass (FFM), 104
"The fatty streak," 192
FCHL. *See* Familial combined hyperlipidemia.
FDA. *See* United States Food and Drug
    Administration.
Fenfluramine
    cardiac valve disorders and, 195
    for decreased food intake and weight loss,
      138–139
    to reduce food intake, 451*t*
    safety, 461–462, 461*f*
    for treatment of obesity, 293, 449
FFAs. *See* Free fatty acids.
FFM. *See* Fat and fat-free mass.
Fiber. *See* Dietary fiber.
Fluoxetine
    for decreased food intake and weight loss, 138
    to reduce food intake, 451*t*
Food Guide Pyramid, 554
Food intake, drugs that reduce, 451, 452–463
FPG. *See* Fasting plasma glucose.
Framingham Heart Study, 273
France
    economic impact of overweight or obesity, 524*t*,
      526
    percent of national health care cost due to obesity,
      525*f*
Free fatty acids (FFAs)
    diabetes mellitus, type II, and, 232–233
    fat metabolism and, 149
    hepatic glucose and, 241
    insulin resistance and, 233–234, 233*f*
Fuel
    See also Energy.
    control of
      and effects of hormones on fuel balance,
        148*f*
      energy expenditure and metabolism and,
        150–151, 151*t*
      and processing of, 149–150
      overview of, 147–173

G

Gallbladder
  age-adjusted and body mass index-adjusted risk of
      disease related to ethnicity, 305*f*
  cancer, 312
  motility
      during diet-induced weight loss, 308*t*
      in obesity and weight loss, effects of, 308
  and risk of disease
      correlation to leptin concentration, 304*f*
      correlation to waist to hip ratio, 303*f*
  sludge, 311, 311*f*
Gallstones
  cholesterol and, 305*f*
  incidence of cholecystectomy and symptomatic
      gallstones, 302*t*
  types of, 305, 305*f*
  ultrasonogram for
      depiction of, 309*f*
      of sludge, 311*f*
GAPS. *See* Guidelines for Adolescent Preventive
      Services.
Garcinia cambogia, for treatment of obesity, 471
Gastric banding, laparoscopic adjustable, for
      treatment of obesity, 511–512
Gastric binding, for treatment of obesity, 508
Gastric bypass, for treatment of obesity
  failed, 519–520
  laparoscopic, 511
  open operative technique, 509–511
  roux-en-y, 508–509, 508*f*, 509*f*, 510*f*
Gastrin-releasing peptide (GRP), role in energy
      balance, 139
Gastroplasty, for treatment of obesity, 506–507, 507*f*
Gender, as risk factor for obstructive sleep apnea,
      210. *See also* Men; Women.
Genes
  effects of targeted ablation or transgenic
      overexpression on energy homeostasis, 130*t*
  and obesity from single gene defects, 4
  obesity-resistant, 43, 44*f*
  research on response to antiobesity medications
      and, 62
Genetics
  diseases associated with obesity and, 345–346
  environment and, 43–45, 44*f*
  and ethnic differences and admixture studies,
      37–38
  influence on obesity, 31–62
  influences on behavioral phenotypes
      animal studies, 39–43, 40*t*–42*t*
      human studies, 38–39
      overview of, 38–43
  knockout mutants and transgenic models with
      effects on body composition, 40*t*–42*t*
  lipodystrophies, 50–51
  microarray gene-expression studies and
      data analysis, 56–57
      definition, 56
      examples, 57
      uses, 57–58
  models of obesity with leptin abnormalities, 284*t*

mutation detection, 40*t*–42*t*, 53–55, 54*t*
pharmacogenomics
  definition of, 58
  drugs and/or classes of drugs with effects on
      body weight, 59*t*
  methodologic issues in, 60
quantitative trait locus mapping studies
  in agricultural and aquacultural species, 48–49
  in humans, 49
  introduction to, 45–49
  in mice
      backcrosses, 47
      congenic strains, 48
      intercrosses, 47
      model, for mapping, 45, 46*f*
      outbred populations, 47
      recombinant inbred strains, 47
      selected lines, 47
      trait loci identification, 46*f*, 47
research
  combining databases, 61
  environmental interactions and obesity, 61
  ethical issues, 62
  obesity genes and response to antiobesity
      medications, 62
  on obesity-promoting behaviors, 60–61
  single-gene syndromes versus gene phenotypes
      of obesities, 61–62
  suggestions for future, 60–62
  use of ethnically diverse samples, 61
response to phenotypically or genotypically
      unusual obese persons in the clinic, 55–56
as risk factor for obstructive sleep apnea, 210
selection studies, 32–33, 32*f*, 34*t*–35*t*
single-gene mutations, 49–50
syndromes associated with mental retardation,
      51–53, 52*t*
and twin, family, and adoption studies, 33, 36–37
Genotype
  biologic considerations of pleiotropic, 19–24,
      20*f*–22*f*, 20*t*, 23*t*
  obesity and, 18–19, 19*f*
  response to unusual obese persons in the clinic,
      55–56
  "thrifty," 18–19, 19*f*
GHIH. *See* Growth hormone–inhibiting hormone.
Ghrelin, role in energy balance, 140–141
GHRH. *See* Growth hormone–releasing hormone.
GI. *See* Glycemic index.
Gilbenclamide, for management of diabetes mellitus,
      type II, 251*t*
Gliclazide, for management of diabetes mellitus, type
      II, 251*t*
Glimepiride, for management of diabetes mellitus,
      type II, 251*t*
Glipizide, for management of diabetes mellitus, type
      II, 251*t*
Glipizide XL, for management of diabetes mellitus,
      type II, 251*t*
Glomerular filtration rate (GFR), renal medullary
      compression in obesity and, 286–287, 287*f*
GLP-1. *See* Glucagon-like peptide 1.

Glucagon, to reduce food intake, 463
Glucagon-like peptide 1 (GLP-1)
  to reduce food intake, 463
  role in energy balance, 140
Glucocorticoids
  endocrine system and, 169–173
  hypothalamic–pituitary–adrenal axis
    cortisol and, 169*f*, 170
    obesity and, 172–173
  managing therapy with, in obese patients, 173
  physiology of, 169–171, 171*f*
  regional fat storage and, 171
  and resting energy expenditure and thermic effect
    of food and exercise, 170
  substrate availability and oxidation and, 170–171
Glucose
  normal tolerance, 241
  physical activity and, 480–481, 481*f*
  production and diabetes mellitus, type II, 239–241,
    240*f*
Glucose transporter-4 (GLUT-4), insulin resistance
    and, 234
Glyburide, for the management of diabetes mellitus,
    type II, 251*t*
Glycemic index (GI)
  carbohydrates and, 438
  energy and, 82
  for management of diabetes mellitus, type II,
    242*t*
Glyset. *See* α-glucosidase inhibitors.
Green tea, supplementation recommendations, 340,
    340*t*
Growth hormone–inhibiting hormone (GHIH)
  See also Prader–Willi syndrome.
  deficiency and obesity, 349
  endocrine complications of obesity and, 354
  fuel partitioning and, 156
Growth hormone–releasing hormone (GHRH), fuel
    partitioning and, 156, 156*f*
Growth hormones
  See also Hormones.
  administration in visceral obesity, 159–160
  and impaired secretion in obesity, 217
  insulin-like growth factors, influence on,
    156–157
  physiology of, 156–158, 156*f*
  regional fat storage and, 158
  and substrate availability and oxidation,
    157–158
  visceral obesity and, 158–159
GRP. *See* Gastrin-releasing peptide.
Guarana, for treatment of obesity, 472
Guidelines for Adolescent Preventive Services
    (GAPS), 91
Gut peptides, role in energy balance, 139–140

H
HCC. *See* Healthcare for Communities.
HDL. *See* High-density lipoprotein.
Health care
  annual direct health care costs of obesity by body
    mass index, 529*f*

annual medical care costs to employers, 533*t*
budget for obesity, 6–7
cost and effectiveness of obesity treatment, 539*t*
economics
  cost-of-illness studies, 523–524
  international perspective, 524–527
  overview of, 523
obesity cases and costs in managed care
  organizations, 533*t*
percent change in health care costs associated with
  obesity, 531*f*
percent of national health care cost due to obesity,
  525*f*
relation of body mass index to costs, 535*f*
relative rates of costs associated with body mass
  index, 533*t*
relative risk, percent of disease, and annual direct
  and indirect health care costs attributable to
  obesity, 528*t*
Healthcare for Communities (HCC), 530
Healthy eating index (HEI), 445
Healthy People 2010, 6
Heart disease
  adipose tissue as an endocrine organ, 181
  and benefits of weight reduction on the
    cardiovascular system, 194–195, 195*t*
  cardiac morphology, 184–185
  cardiopulmonary complications of weight
    reduction therapy and, 195
  cardiovascular impact of increased adipose tissue
    mass
    adipose-tissue circulation, 181–182, 182*t*
    alterations in cardiac morphology, 184–185
    central hemodynamics in, 182–184, 183*f*
    effects on ventricular function, 185–187, 185*f*,
      186*f*
    pathophysiology of obesity-related
      cardiomyopathy, 183*f*
    tissue blood flow during experimental
      hypovolemia and, 182*t*
  in children
    cardiovascular comorbidities, 99
    cardiovascular risk factors, 98–99
  clinical and laboratory assessment of obese
    individuals
    cardiomyopathy of obesity (*adipositas cordis*),
      188–189
    electrocardiogram
      changes with progressive obesity, 189*t*
      detection of left ventricular hypertrophy by
        QRS in obesity, 190*t*
      discussion of, 189–191
    history and physical examination, 187–188
  as a comorbidity with obesity, 4–5
  coronary artery disease, 192–194
  energy imbalance and, 85
  malignant arrhythmias, 191–192
  obesity and, 181–196
  and obesity-attributable mortality in adults, 5*t*
  with use of drugs to treat obesity, 450
HEI. *See* Healthy eating index.
Hepatic fibrosis, 319–321, 319*t*

Hepatic glucose (HGP)
  increase in production with diabetic compared to
    nondiabetic controls, 240*f*
  production and diabetes mellitus, type II, 239–241,
    240*f*
Hepatobiliary disease
  cholelithiasis, 301–312
  as comorbidity with obesity, 4–5
  discussion of, 301–326
  nonalcoholic fatty liver steatohepatitis, 312–323
Heritability, definition of, 33
HGP. *See* Hepatic glucose.
High-density lipoprotein (HDL)
  in diagnosis of obesity, 5
  fuel partitioning and, 160
  for management of diabetes mellitus, type II, 245
  pediatric, 93–94
Hip
  obesity and outcome of total hip replacement,
    408–409
  obesity and prevalence of bilateral and unilateral
    osteoarthritis, 402*t*
  osteoarthritis, 402–403, 402*t*, 403*t*
  studies of weight and prevalent clinical hip
    osteoarthritis, 403*t*
HIV-1. *See* Human immunodeficiency virus, type 1.
Homicide, obesity-attributable mortality in adults, 5*t*
Hormone replacement therapy
  after menopause, 352
  clinical trials of, 352
Hormones
  See also Growth hormones.
  adipocyte-secreted, and insulin resistance, 234–238
  effects on fuel balance, 148*f*
  and obesity and cancer, 328–329, 328*f*
  to reduce food intake, 463
Hormone-sensitive lipase (HSL), fat metabolism and,
    149
Human body composition
  body components, 103–109, 103*f*, 104*f*, 105*f*, 106*f*,
    107*f*, 108*f*
  at the cellular level, 105, 105*f*
  component measurement
    adipose-tissue distribution, 124
    adiposity, 122–123, 123*t*
    bone mineral, 124
    skeletal muscle, 124
    visceral organs, 124
  levels, 103, 103*f*
  measurement methods for
    anthropometry
      application of, 120–122, 120*t*, 121*t*, 122*t*
      history of, 119
    bioimpedance analysis
      application of, 118–119
      history of, 118
    dual-energy x-ray absorptiometry
      application of, 116–118, 117*f*
      history of, 116
    hydrometry
      application of, 113–114
      history of, 113

imaging
  application of, 112–113
  history of, 112
for optimizing precision, 122*t*
potassium-40 counting
  application of, 109–110
  history of, 109
qualitative characteristics of body composition
  methods, 123*t*
underwater weighing or air plethysmography
  application of, 115–116
  history of, 114–115
in vivo neutron-activation analysis
  application, 110–112
  history, 110
models of, 104
at the molecular level, 104, 104*f*
overview of, 103–124
at the tissue-organ level, 105–106, 105*f*
Human immunodeficiency virus, type 1 (HIV-1), 51
Human studies
  genetic influences on behavioral phenotypes,
    38–39
  as models for livestock genetics, 48
  and quantitative trait locus mapping, 49
Hydrometry, for measurement of human body
    composition
  application of, 113–114
  history of, 113
Hyperglycemia
  coronary artery disease and, 192
  sites of defects leading to, 230*f*
Hyperinsulinemia
  central nervous system and, 278, 280
  obesity-related hypertension and, 278, 280, 280*f*
  in pediatric obesity, 98–99
Hyperleptinemia, hypertension and, 281–282, 282*f*,
    283*f*, 284*t*
Hyperlipidemia, metabolic syndrome and, 381–383,
    382*f*
Hyperplasia, body mass index and, 4
Hypertension
  association with obesity, 273–275, 274*f*, 275*t*
  as chronic effect of obstructive sleep apnea, 216
  comorbidity with obesity, 4–5
  hyperleptinemia and, 281–282, 282*f*, 283*f*, 284*t*
  impaired renal pressure natriuresis and
    hyperinsulinemia and, 278, 280, 280*f*
  hyperleptinemia and, 281–282, 282*f*, 283*f*, 284*t*
  and increased blood pressure caused by renal
    compression, 286–287, 287*f*
  leptin resistance and, 284–285, 284*f*
  mechanisms of sympathetic activation,
    278–285
  nonesterified fatty acids and, 281
  overview of, 277–287
  pharmacologic blockade of adrenergic activity
    and, 277–278
  and renal denervation, attenuated sodium
    retention and, 278, 279*f*
  renal sensory nerves and, 281
  renal sympathetic activity and, 277

and renin-angiotensin system activation in
    obesity
    discussion of, 285–286
    hypertension and, 285
    renal injury and, 286
    and sodium retention and blood pressure,
        277–278
lifestyle changes for prevention and treatment of,
    292–293
obesity-attributable mortality in adults and, 5*t*
physical activity and, 481–482
and treatment of obesity-related and renal disease
    lifestyle modification, 292–293
    pharmacotherapy of hypertension in obese
        patients, 293–296. *See also individual drug
        names.*
    synopsis of, 292–296
Hypertriglyceridemia, associated with visceral
    obesity, 387
Hypertrophy
    body mass index and, 4
    impaired systolic and diastolic function in obesity,
        275–276, 276*f*
Hypopnea, definition, 203*t*
Hypothalamic–pituitary–adrenal axis
    See also Cushing syndrome.
    cortisol and, 170
    glucocorticoids and, 170, 172–173
    obesity and, 172–173, 346–347
Hypothalamus
    feeding behavior and, 128*f*
    role in appetite regulation, 128–141
Hypothyroidism
    in infants, 349
    juvenile, 349
    obesity and, 349
    as risk factor for obstructive sleep apnea, 211
Hypoventilation
    definition of, 203*t*
    obstructive sleep apnea and, 202–228
Hypovolemia, tissue blood flow during experimental,
    182*t*

I
ICAM. *See* Intracellular adhesion molecule gene.
IGF-binding proteins (IGFBPs), fuel partitioning and,
    159
IGFs. *See* Insulin-like growth factors.
IL-6. *See* Interleukin-6.
Imaging, for measurement of human body
    composition
    application of, 112–113
    history of, 112
Immune system, obesity and cancer and, 327–329,
    328*f*
Indirect costs, definition of, 523
Infants, hypothyroidism and, 349
Influenza, obesity-attributable mortality in adults and,
    5*t*
Insulin
    action in insulin-sensitive tissues, 20*t*
    anabolism and, 19–20, 20*t*

in endocrine control of fuel partitioning, 151–155
exercise therapy and, 246–250, 247*f*, 249*f*
intracellular effects on nutrient partitioning, 154
and nutrient partitioning in obesity, 155
physical activity and, 480–481, 481*f*
physiology of, 151–152, 152*f*
and progression of sensitivity in leanness, 20*f*–22*f*
to reduce food intake, 463
relationship between central abdominal fat and,
    231*f*
resistance in diabetes mellitus, type II
    adipocyte-secreted hormones and, 234–238,
        235*f*, 237*f*
    free fatty acids and, 233–234, 233*f*
    introduction to, 232–238
resistance syndrome
    and coronary artery disease, treatment of, 194
    with nonalcoholic steatohepatitis, 322
    and resting energy expenditure and thermic effect
        of food and exercise, 153
    role in energy balance, 140
    secretory defects, 238–239
    substrate availability and oxidation and, 152*f*,
        153–154
    tissue variability in action of, 154–155
    weight reduction and, 11
Insulin-like growth factor–binding protein-3, 181
Insulin-like growth factors (IGFs), 156–157, 181
Insulin receptor substrate-1 (IRS-1), 247
Insulin resistance syndrome
    metabolic syndrome and, 381–384, 381*t*
    renal disease as part of, 273
"Insulin sensitizers." *See* Thiazolidinediones.
Interleukin-6 (IL-6)
    and adipose tissue as an endocrine organ, 181
    insulin resistance and, 236
International Obesity Task Force (IOTF), 91
Intracellular adhesion molecule (ICAM) gene, 53–54
IOTF. *See* International Obesity Task Force.
Iron, role in nonalcoholic steatohepatitis, 320
IRS-1. *See* Insulin receptor substrate-1.

J
Jejunoileal bypass (JIB)
    nonalcoholic steatohepatitis and, 318–319
    and perspective on use of surgery for obesity
        treatment, 505
Jenny Craig, 558
JIB. *See* Jejunoileal bypass.

K
Knee
    obesity and outcome of total knee replacement,
        408–409
    osteoarthritis, 401–402

L
Laparoscopic surgery, for treatment of obesity
    gastric banding, 511–512
    gastric bypass, 511
Launois–Bensaude syndrome (Madelung disease,
    multiple symmetric lipomatosis), 51

LCAC. *See* Long-chain acyl-coenzyme A.
LDL. *See* Low-density lipoprotein.
LEARN Program, 494
Left ventricular hypertrophy in obesity, detection by
    QRS, 190*t*
Legislation, on obesity, 6
Leptin (LEP)
    adipocyte–arcuate–hypothalamic axis, role in,
        131–135
    and adipose tissue as an endocrine organ, 181
    central nervous system and, 235*f*
    effect on body weight, 59*t*
    genetic models of obesity with leptin
        abnormalities, 284*t*
    and genetic mutations associated with obesity, 346
    hyperleptinemia and hypertension, 281–282, 282*f*,
        283*f*, 284*t*
    as an identified single-gene mutation for obesity,
        50
    insulin resistance and, 234–235, 235*f*
    in insulin-sensitive tissues, 22
    and monogenic (mendelian) causes of obesity in
        humans and mice, 133*t*
    mutations causing obesity in humans and, 134*f*
    obstructive sleep apnea and, 218
    to reduce food intake, 462
    resistance to
        discussion of, 135
        and obesity, 284–285, 284*f*
    risk of gallbladder disease, correlation to leptin
        concentration, 304*f*
Life expectancy
    relationship of obesity to, 14–16
    relationship to specific metabolic rate, 16, 17*f*
Lifestyle
    decreased sodium intake for prevention and
        treatment of hypertension, 292–293
    decreasing sedentary behavior, 421
    effect on obesity, 9–10
    exercise for prevention and treatment of
        hypertension, 292–293
    intervention with diabetes mellitus, type II,
        249–250
    management of diabetes mellitus, type II and, 244
    physical activity and, 489–491, 489*f*, 491*f*, 492*f*
    psychologic status of obese individuals and, 365
    structured exercise, 418
    and weight loss
        maintenance of, 418
        for prevention and treatment of hypertension,
            292–293
Lipid, definition of, 104
Lipodystrophies
    congenital, 50–51
    definition of, 50
Lipogenesis, *de novo*, 149
Lipolysis, regulation of, 149–150
Lipoprotein lipase (LPL)
    and adipose tissue as an endocrine organ, 181
    fat metabolism and, 149
    reduced obese state and, 12, 12*f*
Liquid diet, 424

Lithium, effect on body weight, 59*t*
Liver disease
    hepatic effects of pediatric obesity, 99
    and obesity-attributable mortality in adults, 5*t*
    transplantation with, 322–323
Long-chain acyl-coenzyme A (LCAC), insulin
    resistance and, 234
Look AHEAD (Action for Health in Diabetes) study,
    248–249
Low-density lipoprotein (LDL), pediatric, 93–94
LPL. *See* Lipoprotein lipase.
Lung disease, as chronic effect of obstructive sleep
    apnea, 217

M
Macronutrients, composition of, 245, 425, 437, 437*t*
Madelung disease (Launois–Bensaude syndrome,
    multiple symmetric lipomatosis), 51
MADs. *See* Mandibular advancement devices.
Magnetic resonance imaging (MRI)
    for identification of glucose transport site, 232–233
    for measurement of human body composition,
        112–113
Ma huang, for treatment of obesity, 472
Malignant arrhythmias, with obesity, 191–192
Managed care
    obesity cases and costs in managed care
        organization, 533*t*
    perspective of, with regard to costs of obesity,
        531–535, 533*t*, 534*f*
Mandibular advancement devices (MADs), for
    obstructive sleep apnea, 221
Mapping studies
    through admixture linkage disequilibrium, 38
    quantitative trait locus, 39, 43
    review of, 45–49
Maternal and Child Health Bureau (MCHB), 91
Maxillofacial surgery
    for obstructive sleep apnea, 222
    as risk factor for obstructive sleep apnea, 210
Maximum lifespan potential (MLP), relationship to
    specific metabolic rate, 16, 17*f*
Mazindol, to reduce food intake, 451*t*
MCH. *See* Melanin-concentrating hormone (MCH).
MCHB. *See* Maternal and Child Health Bureau.
MC4R. *See* Melanocortin-4 receptor.
Meals, structured, 423–425, 424*f*
Medical Expenditure Panel Survey (MEPS), 529
Meglitinides, for management of diabetes mellitus,
    type II, 243*t*
MEHMO (mental retardation, epileptic seizures,
    hypogonadism, microcephaly, and obesity)
    syndrome, 52*t*, 53
Melanin-concentrating hormone (MCH), role in
    energy balance, 136–137
Melanocortin-4 receptor (MC4R)
    as cause of obesity, 4
    as identified single-gene mutation for obesity,
        49–50
    leptin and, 22–23
Melanocortin receptor system, 130–131
Men

adult consequences of obesity in adolescence, 96*t*
degree of worry about typical concerns of male
  high-school students, 359*t*
and dietary fat, 484*f*
effects of endocrine complications of obesity on
  male reproductive axis, 353
multiple symmetric lipomatosis in, 51
prostate cancer, 332–334
risk of cardiovascular disease in, 484*f*
risk of gallbladder disease
  correlation to leptin concentration, 304*f*
  correlation to waist to hip ratio, 303*f*
semistarvation in, 13–14, 14*t*
Menopause
  metabolic syndrome and, 384
  and obesity and risk of osteoarthritis, 406
  weight gain and, 352
Mental retardation, syndromes associated with,
  51–53, 52*t*
MEPS. *See* Medical Expenditure Panel Survey.
Meridia. *See* Sibutramine.
Metabolic syndrome
  complications of
    chylomicronemia syndrome, 390
    nonalcoholic fatty liver disease, 389–390
    premature coronary artery disease, 389
  components of, 379–381, 380*t*
  Cushing syndrome and, 385
  and diagnosis and assessment of dyslipidemia, 390
  dyslipidemia in, 378–398
  history of, 378
  mechanism of dyslipidemia of
    discussion of, 385–389, 386*t*, 388*f*
    and lipoprotein physiology, 385–386
  modifiers of dyslipidemia in central obesity and
    hepatic lipase promoter polymorphism,
    384–385
    primary increase in hepatic triglyceride
    synthesis, 385, 385*f*
    untreated diabetes mellitus, type II, 384
  in oligogenic disorders
    associated with visceral obesity and insulin
    resistance, 381–384, 381*t*
    diabetes mellitus, type II, 383
    essential hypertension, 383
    familial combined hyperlipidemia, 381–383,
    382*f*
    menopause, 384
    polycystic ovary syndrome as oligogenic
    disorder, 383–384
  renal disease as part of, 273
  treatment of dyslipidemia, 390–391, 391*t*
  visceral obesity and insulin resistance as precursors
    of, 379, 379*f*
Metabolism
  of carbohydrates, 150
  in children, 96
  differences between lean and obese individuals
    during starvation, 16, 17*t*
  drugs that alter, 452, 463–468
  energy expenditure and, 150–151, 151*t*
  environmental consequences and, 85–86

of proteins, 150
and relationship to maximum lifespan potential, 16,
  17*f*
Metergoline, to reduce food intake, 451*t*
Metformin (Biguanide)
  clinical profile of, 253–254
  effects on adipose tissue and body weight,
    254–255
  effects on insulin sensitivity, lipids, and
    cardiovascular risk factors, 254
  efficacy as monotherapy for management of
    diabetes mellitus, type II, 243*t*
  for management of diabetes mellitus, type II, 243*t*,
    253–255
Methylphenidate, effect on body weight, 59*t*
Microarray gene-expression studies
  data analysis, 56–57
  definition of, 56
  examples of, 57
  uses for, 57–58
Miglitol, for management of diabetes mellitus, type
  II, 243*t*
Minnesota Experiment, 13, 14
MLP. *See* Maximum lifespan potential.
Models
  cost-effectiveness models of obesity, 539–540
  of direct medical care cost savings of obesity
    treatment, 536–537, 537*f*
  of human body composition, 104
  of human studies for livestock genetics, 48
  knockout mutants and transgenic models with
    effects on body composition, 40*t*–42*t*
  leptin genetic models of obesity with leptin
    abnormalities, 284*t*
  mice, quantitative trait locus mapping studies, 45,
    46*f*
  of obesity with leptin abnormalities, 284*t*
  of Stages of Motivational Readiness, 493
  "stealth model," 36
  transtheoretical behavioral, 493–494, 494*t*
Molecules, appetite-stimulating and appetite-
  suppressing, 129*t*
MOMO (macrosomia, obesity, macrocephaly, and
  ocular abnormalities) syndrome, 52*t*, 53
Monoamine neurotransmitters, in energy balance,
  137–139
Monoamine oxidase inhibitors, effect on body weight,
  59*t*
Monoaminergic drugs, in clinical trials, 462
Monobutyrin, 181
Monounsaturated fatty acids (MUFAs), for
  management of diabetes mellitus, type II,
  245
Mood, psychosocial consequences of dieting and,
  368–369, 369*t*
Mortality, attributed to obesity, 5*t*
MRI. *See* Magnetic resonance imaging.
MUFAs. *See* Monounsaturated fatty acids.
Multicomponent models, of human body
  composition, 104
Multiple symmetric lipomatosis (Launois–Bensaude
  syndrome, Madelung disease), 51

Musculoskeletal complications of obesity
  excess weight and risk of osteoarthritis
    hip osteoarthritis, 402–403, 402t, 403t
    knee osteoarthritis, 401–402
    mechanical effects of excess weight, 404–405, 405f
    metabolic concomitants of adiposity, 406–407
    obesity as cause of osteoarthritis, 403–407
  obesity and back pain, 409–410
  obesity and outcomes of total knee and hip replacement, 408–409
  overview of, 399–412
  pain and osteoarthritis, 399–401, 400f
  weight loss to prevent and/or treat osteoarthritis, 407–408
Mutations
  detection of, 40t–42t, 53–55
  knockout mutants and transgenic models with effects on body composition, 40t–42t
  single-gene, 49–50

N

NAFL. See Nonalcoholic fatty liver disease.
Nasal dilator strips, for obstructive sleep apnea, 219–220
Nasal ventilation, for obstructive sleep apnea, 223, 224f
NASH. See Nonalcoholic steatohepatitis.
Nateglinide
  clinical profile of, 253
  effects on adipose tissue and weight gain, 253
  effects on insulin sensitivity, lipids, and cardiovascular risk factors, 253
  efficacy as monotherapy for management of diabetes mellitus, type II, 243t
  for management of diabetes mellitus, type II, 252–253
National Association to Advance Fat Acceptance, 362
National Cancer Institute, 335
National Cholesterol Education Program (NCEP)
  Adult Treatment Panel III, 380–381
  metabolic syndrome and, 378
National Health and Medical Research Council (NHMRC), 525–526
National Health and Nutrition Examination Survey-II (NHANES-II), 93, 292f, 483
National Health and Nutrition Examination Survey-III (NHANES-III), 78, 79t, 301, 380–381, 528
National Health Interview Survey (NHIS), 529
National Heart, Lung, and Blood Institute (NHLBI), guidelines on obesity, 477
National Institutes of Health (NIH)
  clinical guidelines for prevention and treatment of obesity, 293
  lifestyle interventions, 248–249
National Weight Control Registry (NWCR), 86, 88, 425, 479
NCEP. See National Cholesterol Education Program.
NEAT. See Non–exercise-associated thermogenesis.
NEFAs. See Free fatty acids (FFAs); Nonesterified fatty acids.

Nephritis, and obesity-attributable mortality in adults, 5t
Nephrosis, and obesity-attributable mortality in adults, 5t
Nephrotic syndrome, and obesity-attributable mortality in adults, 5t
Netherlands
  economic impact of overweight or obesity, 524t, 527
  percent of national health care cost due to obesity, 525f
Neuropeptides, role in energy balance, 135–137
Neuropeptide Y (NPY),
  to reduce food intake, 462
  role in energy balance, 135–137, 136f
Neutron-activation analysis, in vivo, for measurement of human body composition
  application of, 110–112
  history of, 110
New Zealand
  economic impact of overweight or obesity, 524t, 526
  percent of national health care cost due to obesity, 525f
NGT. See Normal glucose tolerance.
NHANES-II. See National Health and Nutrition Examination Survey-II.
NHANES-III. See National Health and Nutrition Examination Survey-III.
NHIS. See National Health Interview Survey.
NHLBI. See National Heart, Lung, and Blood Institute.
NHMRC. See National Health and Medical Research Council.
Niacin, for dyslipidemia, 391t
Nicotine, effect on body weight, 59t
Night eating syndrome, 366–367
NIH. See National Institutes of Health.
Nonalcoholic fatty liver disease (NAFL)
  childhood and adolescent obesity and, 321
  as complication of metabolic syndrome, 389–390
  definition of, 315–316, 315t, 316t
  natural history of, 316–317
  pathogenesis of, 319–321
  prevalence of, 316
Nonalcoholic steatohepatitis (NASH)
  case presentation, 312, 313f–314f
  childhood and adolescent obesity and, 321
  clinical characteristics of, 319
  clinical predictors of advanced fibrosis, 317t
  definition of, 315
  as etiology of cryptogenic cirrhosis, 318–319
  fibrosis staging in, 316t
  histology features of, 315t
  and implications for liver transplantation, 322–323
  insulin resistance with, 322
  after jejunoileal bypass for morbid obesity, 318–319
  natural history of, 317–318, 317t
  pathogenesis of, 319–321, 319t
  prevalence of, 316
  role of iron in, 320
  treatment for, 322

Nonesterified fatty acids (NEFAs), blood pressure and, 281 *See also* Free fatty acids (FFAs).
Non–exercise-associated thermogenesis (NEAT)
  increase in overfeeding, 10
  physical activity and, 488
Nonrapid eye movement (NREM) sleep, 202. *See also* Obstructive sleep apnea.
Nonshared environment, definition of, 33
Noradrenergic drugs
  combining with serotonergic drugs, 460–462, 461*f*
  long-term studies of, 454*t*
  to reduce food intake, 451, 451*t*
Norepinephrine, role in energy balance, 137–138
Normal glucose tolerance (NGT), 241
NPY. *See* Neuropeptide Y.
NREM. *See* Nonrapid eye movement sleep.
Nurses Health Study, 246–247, 249, 561
Nutrient partitioning
  and intracellular effects of insulin, 154
  in obesity, 155
Nutrition, obesity and
  See also Diet.
  colon cancer and, 337
  complications in bariatric surgery, 516
  diet composition
    carbohydrates and weight gain, 438
    dietary fat and weight gain, 439–440
    discussion of, 437–440
    macronutrient composition, 437, 437*t*
    protein and weight gain, 438–439
  diet debate, 445–446
  energy density and
    energy-restricted diets, 441, 442*t*
    high-carbohydrate, low-fat diets, 443–444, 443*t*
    low-carbohydrate, high-protein diets, 444–445
    low-energy–density diets, 441
    overview of, 440–445
  for management of diabetes mellitus, type II, 244–246, 244*f*
  overfeeding and, 10
  and portion size, 79–80
  synopsis of, 436–448
NWCR. *See* National Weight Control Registry.

O

OA. *See* Osteoarthritis.
Obesity
  adipose tissue functions and, 8–9
  administration of growth hormones in, 159–160
  and adult consequences of obesity in adolescence, 96*t*
  alternatives to, 86–87
  behavioral treatment of, 415–435
  and biologic considerations of pleiotropic genotype, 19–24, 20*f*–22*f*, 20*t*, 23*t*
  cancer and, 327–344
  chronic renal disease and, 288–291
  comorbidities and, 4–5. *See also individual diseases.*
  costs of
    cost-effectiveness models, 539–540
    indirect, 540–546
  deaths attributed to, 4–5
  definitions of, 3, 5–7
  diagnosis of, 5
  as a disease, 3–7
  and dyslipidemia of the metabolic syndrome, 378–398
  economic consequences of, 88
  economic impact of
    assessment of, 523–549
    cost-of-illness studies, 523–524
    international perspective, 524–527
    overview of, 523
    in the United States, 527–546
  effect of starvation on, 7*f*
  endocrine disorders and, 345–357
  environmental implications for prevention and treatment of, 87
  environmental influences
    on adipose tissue mass, 9–10
    discussion of, 75–88
  ethnicity and, 3
  evidence that obesity promotes survival, 12–17, 13*f*, 14*f*, 15*f*, 16*f*, 17*f*, 17*t*, 18*f*
  exercise and, 476–502
  genetics and, 31–62
  genotype and, 18–19, 19*f*
  health care budget and, 6–7
  heart disease and, 181–196
  hepatobiliary complications of, 301–326
  human body composition and, 103–124
  and hypertension and renal disease, 273–300
  in *International Classification of Diseases*, 6
  and legislation for health care coverage, 6
  lifestyle and, 9–10
  monogenic (mendelian) causes in humans and mice, 133*t*
  mortality attributed to, 5*t*
  musculoskeletal complications of, 399–412
  and neuroendocrine control of energy balance, 128–141
  nutrition and, 436–448
  and obstructive sleep apnea and central hypoventilation, 202–228
  overfeeding and, 10
  pediatric, 91–100, 550–566
  pregnancy and, 9–10
  psychosocial complications of, and dieting, 358–377
  and reduced obesity as predictor of resumption of obese state, 11–12, 11*t*, 12*f*
  and related traits that respond to selective breeding, 34*t*–35*t*
  and roles of proteins from human adipose tissue, 8*t*
  from single gene defects, 4
  social consequences of, 361–363, 362*t*
  stigmatization because of, 372
  surgical treatment of, 293, 503–522
  as survival advantage, 7–24
  and treatment with drugs, 449–475
  type II diabetes mellitus and, 229–272
Obesity-hypoventilation syndrome (OHS), 206–208, 207*f*

Obstructive event, definition of, 203*t*
Obstructive sleep apnea (OSA)
   central hypoventilation and, 202–228
   in children, 559
   clinical aspects
      cardiovascular effects, 214–216, 214*f*–215*f*
      chronic effects, 216–218
      diagnosis of, 212–214, 213*f*, 213*t*
      psychosocial effects, 214
      signs and symptoms, 211–212, 211*t*
   comorbidity with obesity, 4–5
   effects of weight change on severity of, 219*t*
   epidemiology of
      in the general community, 208, 208*t*
      in the obese population, 209–210, 209*f*
   and improvement in respiratory disturbance index,
      517, 518*f*
   one-hour recording during sleep for, 213*f*
   pathogenesis of
      definitions in sleep-disordered breathing,
         202–205, 203*t*, 204*f*
      obesity-hypoventilation syndrome, 206–208,
         207*f*
      and physiology of sleep, 202
      role of obesity and, 205–206
   risk factors for
      age, 210
      comorbid conditions, 211
      familial, genetic, and maxillofacial factors, 210
      gender, 210
   tracing of patient with typical severe, 204*f*
   treatment for
      continuous positive airway pressure, 220–221
      with daytime respiratory failure, management of,
         222–223, 224*f*
      discussion of, 218–223
      mandibular advancement devices, 221
      pharmacologic, 222
      surgery
         tracheostomy, 221
         uvulopalatopharyngoplasty, 221–222
      weight loss, 218–219, 219*t*
Oby-Cap. *See* Phentermine.
OHS. *See* Obesity-hypoventilation syndrome.
Oligogenic disorders, metabolic syndrome and,
   381–385
Oral contraceptives
   effect on body weight, 59*t*
   endocrine complications of obesity and, 351–352
Organs, visceral, measurement of, 124
Organ transplantation, liver, 322–323
Orlistat (Xenical)
   clinical trials of, 293, 463–468, 464*t*–465*t*
   combining with sibutramine, 468
   effects of, on
      body weight, 59*t*
      diabetes prevention, 262, 263*f*
      glycemic control, 261
      insulin sensitivity, 261–262
      lipids, 262
      weight loss and weight maintenance, 471*f*
   effect sizes, comparison of, 469*f*

   efficacy of, 463–468
   for management of diabetes mellitus, type II,
      261–262, 263*f*
   pharmacology of, 463
   quality of life with, 467–468
   to reduce food intake, 452*t*
   safety of, 468
   for treatment of obesity, 293
   weight maintenance with, 467
Orthopedic complications
   comorbidity with obesity, 4–5
   with pediatric obesity, 99–100
OSA. *See* Obstructive sleep apnea.
Osteoarthritis (OA)
   course of, 400
   discussion of, with obesity, 399–412
   effect of counterbalancing forces of body weight
      and joint shock absorption, 405*f*
   etiology of, 400
   excess weight and risk of
      hip osteoarthritis, 402–403, 402*t*, 403*t*
      knee osteoarthritis, 401–402
      and mechanical effects of excess weight,
         404–405, 405*f*
      metabolic concomitants of adiposity and,
         406–407
      obesity as cause of, 403–407
   pain and, 399–401, 400*f*
   treatment of, 400
   weight loss to prevent and/or treat, 407–408
Ovaries, obesity and cancer of, 331–332
Overfeeding
   for determination of genetic predisposition to
      obesity, 10
   experiments in animals, 10
   experiments in humans, 10–11
"Overlap syndrome," 217
Overweight, definitions of, 93
Oxandrolone, to reduce visceral fat, 468

P

PACE. *See* Patient-Centered Assessment and
   Counseling for Exercise.
PAI-1. *See* Plasminogen activator inhibitor-1.
Pain
   musculoskeletal, 399–401
   from osteoarthritis, 399–401, 400*f*
Pancreas
   and hormones to reduce food intake, 463
   obesity and cancer of, 331–332
PAR. *See* Population-attributable risk.
Paracrine system, obesity and cancer of, 327–329, 328*f*
Parents
   participation in treatment of childhood obesity,
      555–556
   skills for weight control, 557*t*
Patient
   demographics, 427
   dieting history, 429
   ethnicity, 427
   initial body weight, 428
   medical status, 428

predictors of weight loss outcome, 426–432, 429*t*
  psychologic variables, 428–429
  social factors, 429
  stress and coping, 429
Patient-Centered Assessment and Counseling for
    Exercise (PACE), 494, 498
PCR. *See* Transcriptase polymerase chain reaction.
Pediatric obesity
  adolescent demographics, 3–4
  aggressive therapy for, 99–100
  assessment of, 91–94, 92*t*
  body mass index percentiles by age and gender, 92*t*
  cancer and
    clinical considerations with, 339–341, 340*t*
    implications of, on risk for, 338
  cardiovascular risk factors, 98–99
  and child abuse and neglect, 98
  childhood demographics, 3
  complications of, 97–99
  criteria for identification of, 91
  definitions of, 93
  factors associated with increased prevalence of,
      94
  hepatic effects of, 99
  orthopedic complications of, 99–100
  pathophysiology of, 96–97
  periods of risk for, 94–96, 95*f*, 96*t*
  physical effects of, 98
  psychologic effects of, 98
  social effects of, 97
  treatment of
    activity interventions, 554–555
    additional treatment approaches to, with failure
        of diet and exercise programs, 559*t*
    behavior modification, 555–556
    commercial weight loss programs, 558
    dietary interventions in, 553–554, 553*t*
    diet, exercise, and behavior modification, 556
    expert committee recommendations for,
        556–557, 556*t*, 557*t*
    goals of, 560–561, 561*f*
    inpatient programs for, 560
    multifaceted approach to behavior-based
        treatment of childhood obesity, 551, 552*f*
    overview for, 550–566
    parental participation in, 555–556
    pharmacologic, 559
    and risks of weight loss, 561
    school-based interventions for, 557–558
    surgery for, 560
  visceral fat in clinical assessment of, 93–94
  weight loss goals, 560, 561*f*
Peptidergic systems
  appetite-stimulating and appetite-suppressing
      molecules, 129, 129*t*
  effects of targeted gene ablation or transgenic
      overexpression on energy homeostasis
      phenotype of mice, 130*t*
  role in energy balance, 129–130, 129*t*, 130*t*
Peptides
  appetite-stimulating and appetite-suppressing
      molecules, 129*t*

not approved by the FDA to treat obesity,
    462–463
  role in energy balance, 139–140
  starvation and, 132
Peroxisome proliferator-activated receptor γ (PPARγ)
  activation of, 23–24, 23*t*
  as identified single-gene mutation for obesity, 50
  insulin resistance and, 237–238, 237*f*
Pharmacogenetics. *See* Pharmacogenomics.
Pharmacogenomics
  definition of, 58–59
  drugs and/or classes of drugs with effects on body
      weight, 59*t*
  methodologic issues, 60
Phendimetrazine (Bontril; Plegine; Prelu-2; X-
    Trozine)
  efficacy of, 453
  to reduce food intake, 452*t*
Phenotypes
  genetic influences on behavior
    animal studies of, 39–43, 40*t*–42*t*
    human studies of, 38–39
    overview of, 38–43
  research on single-syndromes versus gene
      phenotypes of obesities, 61–62
  and response to unusual obese persons in the
      clinic, 55–56
Phentermine (Adipex; Fastin; Oby-Cap)
  comparison of weight loss with, 455*f*
  and effect on body weight, 59*t*
  effect sizes, comparison of, 469*f*
  efficacy of, 453
  long-term studies with, 454*t*
  to reduce food intake, 451*t*, 452*t*
  for treatment of obesity, 293, 449
Phenylpropanolamine (PPA), to reduce food intake,
    451, 451*t*
Phosphatidylinositol-3 kinase (PI-3K), 247
PHT. *See* Pulmonary hypertension.
Physical activity
  in children and adolescents, 97
  effect on obesity, 9
  environmental influence on, 83–84
  with pediatric obesity, 94
  weight gain and, 87
Physical examination, of heart disease in obese
    individuals, 187–188
Physicians' Health Study, 246–247
Physiologic regulatory system, environmental impact
    on, 77
Phytonutrients, recommendations during weight loss
    and maintenance, 340*t*
Pickwickian syndrome, 206–207. *See also* Obesity-
    hypoventilation syndrome.
Pierre Robin syndrome, as risk factor for obstructive
    sleep apnea, 210
PI-3K. *See* Phosphatidylinositol-3 kinase.
Pioglitazone, for management of diabetes mellitus,
    type II, 243*t*
Plasminogen activator inhibitor-1 (PAI-1), 181
Plegine. *See* Phendimetrazine.
Pleiotropic gene, "thrifty," 18–19, 19*f*

Plethysmography, air (underwater weighing), for
    measurement of human body composition
    application of, 115–116
    history of, 114–115
PMF. See Protein-modified fast.
Pneumonia, obesity-attributable mortality in adults,
    5t
Polycystic ovary syndrome (PCOS)
    metabolic syndrome and, 383–384
    with metformin, 255
    obesity and, 350–351
    pathophysiology of, 350
    treatment of, 351
Polysomnography, for evaluation of sleep-disordered
    breathing, 212
POMC. See Proopiomelanocortin gene.
Population-attributable risk (PAR), 524
Portugal
    economic impact of overweight or obesity, 524t,
        526–527
    percent of national health care cost due to obesity,
        525f
Positional therapy, for obstructive sleep apnea, 219
Potassium-40 counting, for measurement of human
    body composition
    application of, 109–110
    history of, 109
PPA. See Phenylpropanolamine.
PPARγ. See Peroxisome proliferator-activated
    receptor γ.
Prader–Willi syndrome (PWS)
    See also Growth hormone–inhibiting hormone.
    association with obesity, 51, 52t, 345
Precose. See α-glucosidase inhibitors.
Pregnancy
    See also Women.
    food deprivation and obesity, 9–10
Prelu-2. See Phendimetrazine.
PROCAM. See Prospective Cardiovascular Munster
    study.
Productivity
    from employer's perspective, 542–544, 543f, 544f
    functional capability and, 541–542, 541f, 542f
    hours lost per week by selected health risk, 544f
    weight loss impact and, 544
Prolactin, endocrine complications of obesity and,
    354
Prolactinomas, obesity and, 351
Proopiomelanocortin (POMC) gene
    as identified single-gene mutation for obesity, 50
    role in energy balance, 130–134
Prospective Cardiovascular Munster (PROCAM)
    study, 290, 291f
Prostate, obesity and cancer, 332–334
Prostate-specific antigen (PSA) test, 332
Protease inhibitors, effect on body weight, 59t
Protein-modified fast (PMF), 553
Proteins
    agouti-related, 130–131
    low-carbohydrate, high-protein diet, 444–445
    macronutrient composition and obesity, 437t
    metabolism of, 150

    secreted by human adipose tissue, roles of, 8t
    weight gain and, 438–439
PSA. See Prostate-specific antigen test.
Pseudohypoparathyroidism, obesity and, 349–350
Psychologic problems, with pediatric obesity, 98
Psychosocial disturbances
    comorbidity with obesity, 4–5
    complications of obesity and dieting, 358–377
    instruments to assess psychosocial factors of
        obesity, 373t
    with obstructive sleep apnea, 214
    psychologic status of obese individuals in general
        population
        behavioral complications, 367–368
        eating disorders and, 365–367, 366t, 367t
        overview of, 363
        and quality of life, 365
    psychosocial consequences of weight loss and
        dieting
        binge eating, 370
        body image, 370
        mood, 368–369, 369t
        quality of life, 370
        sexuality, 369–370
        social relationships, 369
        with weight cycling, 371–372
        weight loss and psychosocial improvement,
            370–371
        with weight regain, 371
    psychosocial status of obese individuals who seek
        treatment
        body image dissatisfaction, 363–364
        discussion of, 363–365
        level of obesity, 364
        social factors and psychologic distress, 365
        trauma, sexual abuse and other forms of,
            364
    social consequences of obesity, 361–363, 362t
    social pressures to be thin, 358–361, 359t, 360f,
        361f
    stigmatization of obesity, 372
Pulmonary hypertension (PHT)
    as chronic effect of obstructive sleep apnea, 217
    in obstructive sleep apnea, 203
PWS. See Prader–Willi syndrome.

Q
QTL. See Quantitative trait locus.
Quality of life
    health-related, 545–546, 545t
    indicator, 545t
    with orlistat, 467–468
    psychologic status of obese individuals, 365
    psychosocial consequences of dieting and, 370
Quantitative trait locus (QTL)
    in animal studies, 39–43, 40t–42t
    identification for body weight measures, 46t,
        47
    mapping studies, 45–49
Quipazine
    for decreased food intake and weight loss, 138
    to reduce food intake, 451

R

Randle glucose fatty acid (FA) cycle, 233
Rapid eye movement (REM) sleep, 202, 207*f. See also* Obstructive sleep apnea.
Reductil. *See* Sibutramine.
REE. *See* Resting energy expenditure.
Reference man, definition of, 104
Renal cell cancer, obesity and, 334–335
Renal disease
    hypertension and obesity with, 273–300
    and obesity-attributable mortality in adults, 5*t*
    treatment of obesity-related hypertension and
        lifestyle modification, 292–293
        overview of, 292–296
        pharmacotherapy of hypertension in obese
            patients, 293–296. *See also individual drug
            names.*
Renin–angiotensin system, activation in obesity
    hypertension and, 285
    introduction to, 285–286
    renal injury and, 286
Repaglinide
    clinical profile, 253
    effects
        on adipose tissue and weight gain, 253
        on insulin sensitivity, lipids, and cardiovascular
            risk factors, 253
    efficacy as monotherapy for management of
        diabetes mellitus, type II, 243*t*
    for management of diabetes mellitus, type II,
        252–253
Resistin
    and adipose tissue as an endocrine organ, 181
    insulin resistance and, 236
Respiratory diseases, obesity-attributable mortality in
    adults, 5*t*
Respiratory disturbance index (RDI), 517, 518*f*
Resting energy expenditure (REE)
    environmental influence on, 85–86
    and thermic effect of food and exercise, 153
Resting metabolic rate (RMR)
    See also Metabolism.
    in children, 96
    energy expenditure and, 150–151
Retinal-binding protein, 181
RMR. *See* Resting metabolic rate.
Rosiglitazone, for management of diabetes mellitus,
    type II, 243*t*
Roux-en-y gastric bypass, for treatment of obesity,
    508–509, 508*f*, 509*f*, 510*f*

S

S-adenosylmethionine (SAMe), for treatment of
    nonalcoholic steatohepatitis, 322
SAECG. *See* Signal-averaged electrocardiogram.
School-based interventions, for childhood obesity,
    557–558
Secretagogues, as monotherapy for management of
    diabetes mellitus, type II, 243*t*
Sedatives, avoidance with sleep-disordered breathing,
    219
Selection studies, 32–33, 32*f*, 34*t*–35*t*

Selective serotonin reuptake inhibitors, effect on body
    weight, 59*t*
Selenium, supplementation recommendations, 340,
    340*t*
Self-monitoring
    as predictor of treatment outcome, 431–432
    versus supervised physical activity, 420
    for treatment of obesity, 417
Septicemia, and obesity-attributable mortality in
    adults, 5*t*
Serotonergic drugs
    combining with noradrenergic drugs, 460–462,
        461*f*
    not approved by the FDA to treat obesity, 460
    to reduce food intake, 451, 451*t*
Serotonin, role in energy balance, 138–139
Serum glucose concentration, in diagnosis of obesity,
    5
Sexuality, psychosocial consequences of dieting and,
    369–370
Shapedown, 558
Shared environment, definition of, 33
Sibutramine (Meridia; Reductil)
    clinical trials of, 456*t*–457*t*, 458–459
    for decreased food intake and weight loss, 138
    dose-related weight loss, 458*f*
    effect on,
        adipose tissue, 260–261
        body weight, 59, 59*t*
        glycemia, 259–260
        insulin sensitivity, 260
        lipids, 260
    effect sizes, comparison of, 469*f*
    efficacy, 455–459
    for management of diabetes mellitus, type II,
        259–261
    to reduce food intake, 452*t*
    for treatment of obesity, 293, 449
    for weight reduction, 195
Sibutramine Trial of Obesity Reduction and
    Maintenance (STORM), 260–261
Sick leave
    hours lost per week by selected health risk, 544*f*
    relationship between body mass index and, 543*f*
Signal-averaged electrocardiogram (SAECG),
    191–192
Skeletal muscle, measurement of, 124
Skin, measurement of, 121, 121*t*
Sleep
    See also Obstructive sleep apnea.
    definitions of normal and abnormal, 212
    obesity and, 205–206
    physiology of, 202
    reasons for false-negative sleep study results, 213*f*
    sleepiness in the obese patient, 208*f*
Sleep-disordered breathing
    body mass index as predictor of, 209, 209*f*
    pathogenesis of, 202–205, 203*t*, 204*f*
    symptoms of, 210–211, 211*f*
    terminology with, 203*t*
Sludge, gallbladder, 311, 311*f*
Smoking, 192

SMR. *See* Specific metabolic rate.
Snoring, 202. *See also* Obstructive sleep apnea;
    Sleep-disordered breathing.
Social problems
    with pediatric obesity, 97
    as predictor of weight loss outcome, 429
    social pressures to be thin, 358–361, 360*f*, 361*f*
Social relationships, psychosocial consequences of
    dieting and, 369
Sodium
    blood pressure and, 277
    decreased intake for prevention and treatment of
        hypertension, 292–293
    restriction for prevention and treatment of
        hypertension, 293
SOS. *See* Swedish Obesity Study.
Specific metabolic rate (SMR), relationship to
    maximum lifespan potential, 16, 17*f*
Stages of Motivational Readiness model, 493
Starvation
    death from, 12–17
    effect of famine, 13–14, 15*f*
    effect on obesity, 7*f*
    effect on plasma molar ratio, 17, 18*f*
    metabolic differences between lean and obese
        individuals during, 16, 17*t*
    recovery from, 14, 16*f*
    in regulation of peptides, 132
Statin, for dyslipidemia, 391*t*
Stoplight Diet (Traffic Light Diet), 554
STORM. *See* Sibutramine Trial of Obesity Reduction
    and Maintenance.
Stress, as predictor of weight loss outcome, 429
Stroke
    comorbidity with obesity, 4–5
    and obesity-attributable mortality in adults, 5*t*
Substrates
    estrogens and, 166–167
    glucocorticoids and, 170–171
    growth hormone and, 157–158
    insulin and, 153–154
    testosterone and, 162
Suicide, and obesity-attributable mortality in adults,
    5*t*
Sulfonylureas (SUs)
    clinical profile, 251, 251*t*
    effects on adipose tissue and body weight, 252
    effects on insulin sensitivity, lipids, and other
        cardiovascular risk factors, 251–252
    efficacy as monotherapy for management of
        diabetes mellitus, type II, 243*t*
    for management of diabetes mellitus, type II, 243*t*,
        251–252
Surgeon General, physical activity and, 477
Surgery
    for childhood obesity, 560
    for cholelithiasis, 310*t*
    for obstructive sleep apnea, 221–222
    for treatment of obesity
        complications of bariatric
            late, 515
            nutritional, 516

        perioperative, 513–515, 513*t*, 514*t*
        failed gastric bypass, 519–520
        gastric banding, 508
        gastroplasty, 506–507, 507*f*
        history of, 505–506
        indications for, 504–505
        laparoscopic
            adjustable gastric banding, 511–512
            gastric bypass, 511
        operative technique of open gastric bypass,
            509–511
        outcomes of bariatric
            discussion of, 516–518
            effect on comorbidities, 516–518, 517*f*, 518*f*,
                519*f*
        overview of, 503–522
        partial biliopancreatic diversion and duodenal
            switch operations, 512–513
        pathologic conditions associated with morbid
            obesity, 504*t*
        and renal disease, 293
        reoperation, 519–520
        roux-en-y gastric bypass, 508–509, 508*f*, 509*f*,
            510*f*
SUs. *See* Sulfonylureas.
Swedish Obese Subjects (SOS) Study, 264, 527
Sympathomimetic drugs
    clinical trials of, 453
    efficacy of, 453–459
    not approved by the FDA to treat obesity, 460
    pharmacology of, 453
    safety of, 459–460
    side effects of, 459–460
    to treat obesity, 453–460, 454*t*, 455*f*, 456*t*–457*t*, 458*f*
Syndrome X, 273, 378. *See also* Metabolic syndrome.
Systemic hormones, role in energy balance, 139–141

T
Technetium-99m, for evaluation of coronary artery
    disease with obesity, 193–194
TEF. *See* Thermic effect of food.
Tenuate. *See* Diethylpropion.
Tepanil. *See* Diethylpropion.
Testosterone
    administration in visceral obesity, 164
    fuel partitioning and, 161, 161*f*
    physiology of, 161–163, 161*f*
    to reduce visceral fat, 468
    regional fat storage and, 163
    and resting energy expenditure and thermic effect
        of food and exercise, 161–162
    substrate availability and oxidation and, 162
    visceral obesity in, 163–164
Thallium-201, for evaluation of coronary artery
    disease with obesity, 193–194
Thermic effect of food (TEF), energy expenditure
    and, 150–151
Thiazolidinediones
    clinical profile, 256
    for dyslipidemia, 391*t*
    effects on adipose tissue and body weight,
        257–258

effects on insulin sensitivity, lipids, and cardiovascular effects, 257
for management of diabetes mellitus, type II, 243*t*, 256–258, 258*f*
"Thrifty Genotype," 18–19, 19*f*
Thyroid, endocrine complications of obesity and, 354
Tibia vara, 559
Tissue, variability in insulin action of, 154–155
TKR. *See* Total knee replacement.
TNF-α. *See* Tumor necrosis factor α.
Tolazamide, for management of diabetes mellitus, type II, 251*t*
Tolbutamide, for management of diabetes mellitus, type II, 251*t*
Topiramate
    clinical trials of, 462
    and effect on body weight, 59*t*
Total joint arthroplasty, for treatment of osteoarthritis, 408–409
Total joint replacement, for treatment of osteoarthritis, 408–409
Total knee replacement (TKR), for treatment of osteoarthritis, 408–409
Tracheostomy, for obstructive sleep apnea, 221
Traffic Light Diet (Stoplight Diet), 554
Transcriptase polymerase chain reaction (PCR), 252
Transplantation. *See* Organ transplantation.
Trauma, psychosocial status of obese individuals and, 364
Treatment of Obese Patients with Hypertension Study, 294
Tricyclic antidepressants, effect on body weight, 59*t*
Triglycerides
    in diabetes mellitus, type II, 233, 240, 245, 254, 255, 257, 260
    definition of, 104
    in metabolic syndrome, 378, 385. *See also* Hypertriglyceridemia.
Trisomy 21, 52–53, 52*f*
Tumor necrosis factor α (TNF-α)
    and adipose tissue as an endocrine organ, 181
    insulin resistance and, 235
Twin studies
    overview of, 33, 36–37
    "stealth model," 36
    "virtual twins," 36

U
UDCA. *See* Ursodeoxycholic acid.
UKPDS. *See* United Kingdom Prospective Diabetes Study.
Ultrasonogram
    of gallstones, 309*f*
    of gallstone sludge, 311*f*
Underwater weighing (air plethysmography), for measurement of human body composition
    application of, 115–116
    history of, 114–115
United Kingdom Prospective Diabetes Study (UKPDS), 246, 254
United States
    annual direct health care costs of obesity by body

mass index, 529*f*
cost and effectiveness of obesity treatment, 539*t*
economic impact of overweight or obesity, 524*t*
percent change in health care costs associated with obesity, 531*f*
percent of national health care cost due to obesity, 525*f*
relative risk, percent of disease, and annual direct and indirect health care costs attributable to obesity, 528*t*
United States Drug Enforcement Agency (DEA), 449, 453
United States Food and Drug Administration (FDA)
    approval for metformin as monotherapy for diabetes mellitus, type II, 254
    drugs approved for treatment of obesity, 452*t*
    guidelines for sibutramine for treatment of obesity, 293
    serotonergic drugs not approved to treat obesity, 460
    sympathomimetic drugs not approved to treat obesity, 460
UPPP. *See* Uvulopalatopharyngoplasty.
Ursodeoxycholic acid (UDCA), for treatment of nonalcoholic steatohepatitis, 322
Uterus, obesity and cancer of, 330–331
Uvulopalatopharyngoplasty (UPPP), for obstructive sleep apnea, 221–222

V
Valproate (valproic acid)
    effect on body weight, 59*t*
    endocrine complications of obesity and, 352
Valproic acid. *See* Valproate.
Vasopressin, endocrine complications of obesity and, 354
Venlafaxine, to treat obesity, 449
Ventricular function, heart disease and, 185–187, 185*f*, 186*f*
Very low calorie diet (VLCD)
    binge-eating disorder and, 368
    insulin resistance and, 236
    versus low-calorie diet, 422–423, 422*f*
    for management of diabetes mellitus, type II, 245
    and risk of forming gallstones, 302–303
Very low density lipoprotein (VLDL), fat metabolism and, 149
Visible Man, and body composition, 106–107, 106*f*, 107*f*
Vitamin C, supplementation recommendations, 340, 340*t*
Vitamin E, supplementation recommendations, 340, 340*t*
Vitamins, supplementation recommendations, 340*t*
VLCD. *See* Very low calorie diet.
VLDL. *See* Very low density lipoprotein.

W
Waist to hip (WHR) ratio
    and risk of gallbladder disease, 303*f*
    sibutramine treatment, visceral obesity, and, 260–261

Way to Go Kids, 558
Weight cycling, psychosocial consequences of dieting
  and, 371–372
Weight gain
  carbohydrates and, 438
  dietary fat and, 439–440
  and increased heart rate and cardiac output, 275
  mechanical effects of excess weight, 404–405, 405*f*
  after menopause, 352
  physical activity and, 87
  proteins and, 438–439
  psychosocial consequences of dieting and weight
    regain, 371
  risk of osteoarthritis and, 401–407
  self-monitoring, 87
Weight loss
  See also Behavior.
  behavioral therapy for, 422, 422*f*
  calories expended per week in physical activity for
    successful weight loss maintainers, 420*t*
  commercial programs, 558
  comparison with phentermine, 455*f*
  direct medical care cost savings with
    models of obesity treatment, 536–537, 537*f*
    overview of, 536–539
    studies evaluating cost offset of treating obesity
      and, 537–539, 539*f*
  with dose-related sibutramine, 458*f*
  economic impact of, 523–549
  effect of exercise on weight loss and maintenance,
    418*t*
  effect of weight change on severity of obstructive
    sleep apnea, 219*t*
  gallbladder motility during diet-induced weight
    loss, 308*t*
  goals of, 560, 561*f*
  influence of physical activity on, 477–478
  and lithogenic index during diet-induced weight
    loss, 307*t*
  macronutrient composition in, 245
  phytonutrient recommendations during, as well as
    for maintenance, 340*t*
  plateaued weight during treatment, 450, 450*f*
  as predictor of treatment outcome, 430
  for prevention and treatment of hypertension,
    292–293
  for prevention and treatment of osteoarthritis,
    407–408
  problem-solving in, 417
  psychosocial consequences of dieting and, 368–372
  relapse prevention following, 417
  risks of, in childhood obesity, 561
  short-term, 244, 244*f*
  for treatment of nonalcoholic steatohepatitis, 322
  for treatment of obstructive sleep apnea, 218–219,
    219*t*
  vitamin supplementation recommendations with,
    340*t*

Weight maintenance
  orlistat and, 467, 472*f*
  physical activity and, 478–480
Weight reduction
  benefits on the cardiovascular system, 194–195,
    195*t*
  cardiopulmonary complications of therapy for,
    195
  with low-fat, high-carbohydrate diet, 86–87
  resumption of obesity, prognosis for, with, 11–12,
    11*t*, 12*f*
Weight Watchers, 558
WHR. *See* Waist to hip ratio.
Wilson–Turner syndrome, 52*t*, 53
Wisconsin Sleep Cohort Study, 208
Women
  See also Pregnancy.
  adult consequences of obesity in adolescence,
    96*t*
  breast cancer, 329–330
  Cushing syndrome in, 348–349
  degree of worry about typical concerns of female
    high-school students, 359*t*
  effect of endocrine complications of obesity on
    female reproductive axis, 353–354
  effect of food restriction on cumulative death rate
    with endstage renal disease, 288*f*
  epidemiology and risk factors of gallbladder
    disease in, 301–302, 302*t*
  estrogen-replacement therapy and nutrient
    partitioning for, 168–169
  after m enopause, 352
  and metabolic syndrome after menopause, 384
  obesity and risk of osteoarthritis after menopause,
    406
  ovarian cancer, 331–332
  and risk of gallbladder disease
    correlation to leptin concentration, 304*f*
    correlation to waist to hip ratio, 303*f*
  semistarvation in, 13–14, 14*t*
  and use of metformin with polycystic ovary
    syndrome, 255
  uterine cancer, 330–331
Women's Health Trial, 439

X

Xenical. *See* Orlistat.
X-ray absorptiometry, dual-energy, for measurement
    of human body composition
  application of, 116–118, 117*f*
  history of, 116
X-Trozine. *See* Phendimetrazine.

Y

Yohimbine, to reduce food intake, 451*t*

Z

Ziprasidone, effect on body weight, 59, 59*t*